D0998646

SECOND EDITION

Color Atlas of Medical Bacteriology

SECOND EDITION

Color Atlas of Medical Bacteriology

Luis M. de la Maza
Professor, Department of Pathology and Laboratory Medicine
Director, Division of Medical Microbiology
University of California, Irvine, School of Medicine
Orange, California

Marie T. Pezzlo
Clinical Associate, Department of Pathology and Laboratory Medicine
University of California, Irvine, School of Medicine
Orange, California

Janet T. Shigei
Administrative Director, Department of Pathology and Laboratory Medicine
University of California, Irvine, Medical Center
Orange, California

Grace L. Tan
Senior Supervisor, Division of Medical Microbiology
Department of Pathology and Laboratory Medicine
University of California, Irvine, Medical Center
Orange, California

Ellena M. Peterson
Professor, Department of Pathology and Laboratory Medicine
Associate Director, Division of Medical Microbiology
University of California, Irvine, School of Medicine
Orange, California

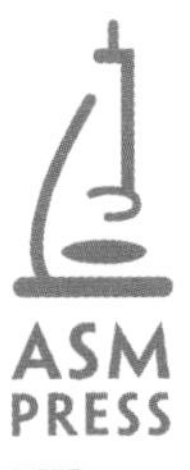

ASM
PRESS
WASHINGTON, DC 20036

Disclaimer: To the best of the publisher's knowledge, this publication provides information concerning the subject matter covered that is accurate as of the date of publication. The publisher is not providing legal, medical, or other professional services. Any reference herein to any specific commercial products, procedures, or services by trade name, trademark, manufacturer, or otherwise does not constitute or imply endorsement, recommendation, or favored status by the American Society for Microbiology (ASM). The views and opinions of the author(s) expressed in this publication do not necessarily state or reflect those of ASM, and they shall not be used to advertise or endorse any product.

Library of Congress Cataloging-in-Publication Data

Color atlas of medical bacteriology / by Luis M. de la Maza ... [et al.]. — 2nd ed.
p. cm.
Includes index.
ISBN 978-1-55581-475-5
1. Medical bacteriology—Atlases. I. De la Maza, Luis M.
[DNLM: 1. Bacteria. 2. Atlases. QW 17]
QR46.C773 2013
616.9'2010222—dc23
2013006836

Printed in the United States of America

10 9 8 7 6 5 4 3 2 1

Address editorial correspondence to: ASM Press, 1752 N St., N.W., Washington, DC 20036-2904, USA.
Send orders to: ASM Press, P.O. Box 605, Herndon, VA 20172, USA.
Phone: 800-546-2416; 703-661-1593. Fax: 703-661-1501.
E-mail: books@asmusa.org
Online: http://estore.asm.org

This book is dedicated to all past and present members of the Division of Medical Microbiology, Department of Pathology and Laboratory Medicine, at the University of California, Irvine, Medical Center who made this book possible.

Contents

Preface

At the dawn of the third millennium, when the names of Watson and Crick are more familiar to students than Koch and Pasteur, when the jargon terms NAAT, RFLP, and MALDI-TOF are part of everyday conversation, and when many hands-on identification methods are part of history, who needs an atlas of bacteriology?

Traditionally, microbiology—especially medical bacteriology—has been dependent on the subjective interpretation of a Gram stain or growth on an agar plate. While there are several excellent textbooks on the subject, they usually are composed of written descriptions of microorganisms with few images. In part, we were motivated to publish the first edition of this atlas by the challenge to find illustrations for our own lectures and laboratory presentations. But since medical bacteriology is dynamic, with changes occurring frequently, especially in classification, nomenclature, and methodology, we accepted the challenge of an update. Following uncountable hours of planning and several missed deadlines, this second edition went to press. We extend a special thanks to ASM Press for their patience and understanding.

With this second edition we have attempted to provide updated illustrations of typical Gram stains, colony morphologies, and biochemical reactions of bacteria most frequently encountered in the clinical laboratory. Furthermore, since the time of our first edition, the continuous and alarming emergence of antibiotic resistance has resulted in the need for more antimicrobial susceptibility testing. As well, the rapid development of molecular techniques has brought these principles into wide use in medical bacteriology. Accordingly, we have written two additional chapters to incorporate these concepts.

Each chapter has a brief introduction to provide some context for the illustrations; for in-depth background on individual organisms, the reader should consult one of the many excellent textbooks and manuals available. This second edition was structured with reference to a number of sources, listed below, and particularly to the *Manual of Clinical Microbiology*, 10th edition (MCM10). However, we are responsible for any errors that appear. The number of photos of a particular organism does not necessarily correlate with the frequency of its isolation or its clinical relevance. Certain bacteria have variable, distinctive, or unique pictorial characteristics, and we have tried to provide a representative sampling of these. We hope you will find this atlas a useful reference tool.

With the increasing use of nucleic acid techniques, the remarkable forms, shapes, and colors of bacteria in the laboratory are rapidly being replaced by signals only measurable by instruments. The time is very near when we will be showing our grandchildren many of the images in this atlas that have become a distant memory. In the meantime, let us enjoy the beauty of the colorful bacterial world.

References

Allen, S. D., W. M. Janda, E. W. Koneman, P. C. Schreckenberger, and W. C. Winn. 2005. *Koneman's Color Atlas and Textbook of Diagnostic Microbiology*, 6th ed. Lippincott Williams & Wilkins, Philadelphia, PA.

Forbes, B. A., D. F. Sahm, and A. S. Weissfeld. 2007. *Bailey and Scott's Diagnostic Microbiology*, 12th ed. Mosby, St. Louis, MO.

Jousimies-Somer, H. R., P. Summanen, D. M. Citron, E. J. Baron, H. M. Wexler, and S. M. Finegold. 2002. *Wadsworth-KTL*

Anaerobic Bacteriology Manual, 6th ed. Star Publishing Co., Inc., Redwood City, CA.

Mahon, C. R., D. C. Lehman, and G. Manuselis, Jr. 2010. *Textbook of Diagnostic Microbiology*, 4th ed. W. B. Saunders Co., Philadelphia, PA.

Murray, P. R., K. S. Rosenthal, and M. A. Pfaller. 2013. *Medical Microbiology*, 7th ed. Saunders, Elsevier, Philadelphia, PA.

Versalovic, J., K. C. Carroll, G. Funke, J. H. Jorgensen, M. L. Landry, and D. W. Warnock (ed.). 2011. *Manual of Clinical Microbiology*, 10th ed. ASM Press, Washington, DC.

Acknowledgments

We would like to thank many individuals who have made this book possible. First and foremost, we want to thank all the staff in the Division of Medical Microbiology at the University of California, Irvine Medical Center. In the laboratory, "The Book" became an obsession that for some was almost the equivalent of finding the Holy Grail. Now that it is complete, we can all relax! We also want to thank our colleagues at the Orange County Health Department and in particular Douglas Moore, Paul Hannah, Douglas Schan, and Tamra Townsen. Over the years we have worked with them on a daily basis on public health-related issues. Their help with the first edition of this atlas covering highly pathogenic organisms was invaluable. We also would like to acknowledge the contributions of Alan G. Barbour, Philippe Brouqui, J. Stephen Dumler, Ted Hackstadt, Barbara McKee, James Miller, and Christopher D. Paddock, who provided key images and specimens and made our work much easier. Additionally, we would like to thank AdvanDX, Inc., Anaerobe Systems, BD Diagnostic Systems, bio-Mérieux, Inc., Dade Behring Inc., EY Laboratories, Hardy Diagnostics, Thermo Scientific Remel Products, Inc., and Roche Diagnostics Systems for contributing various organisms, media, and reagents.

Technical Note

The microscopic pictures were taken with a Zeiss Universal microscope (Carl Zeiss, Inc., West Germany) equipped with Zeiss and Olympus (Olympus Optical Corp., Ltd., Japan) lenses. The macroscopic images were captured with a Contax RTS camera with a Carl Zeiss S-Planar 60 mm f/2.8 lens and a Nikon EL camera with a Micro-Nikkor 55 mm f/3.5 lens. Provia 100F and 400F Professional Fujichrome film (Fuji Photo Film Co., Ltd., Tokyo, Japan) and Kodachrome 25 Professional film (Eastman Kodak Co., Rochester, N.Y.) were used for most of the images. The final magnification of the Gram and acid-fast stains is ×1,200.

Staphylococcus and *Micrococcus* 1

Members of the genera *Staphylococcus* and *Micrococcus* are characterized as being catalase-positive, gram-positive cocci in pairs and clusters. These organisms commonly colonize the surface of skin and mucosal membranes of mammals and birds. *Micrococcus* is generally considered to be a saprophyte, while *Staphylococcus*, particularly *Staphylococcus aureus*, is an important and frequently encountered human pathogen. The genus *Staphylococcus* includes organisms with a low G+C content. In contrast, *Micrococcus* and the genera *Alliococcus*, *Rothia*, and *Kocuria*, all members of the family *Micrococcineae*, are of less human importance and have a high G+C content.

The species of *Staphylococcus* most frequently associated with human infections are *S. aureus*, *Staphylococcus epidermidis*, *Staphylococcus saprophyticus*, *Staphylococcus haemolyticus*, *Staphylococcus lugdunensis*, and *Staphylococcus schleiferi*. Of these, *S. aureus* is the most virulent, being a major cause of morbidity and mortality. It can produce disease mediated by toxins or by direct invasion and destruction of tissues. *S. aureus* infections range from superficial skin infections to fatal systemic infections that can occur when the integrity of the skin is damaged, thus giving this pathogen access to sterile sites. Among the more common *S. aureus* infections are boils, folliculitis, cellulitis, and impetigo. Immunocompromised hosts are at particular risk of infection. Systemic infections include septicemia, which can result in the seeding of distant sites, producing osteomyelitis, pneumonia, endocarditis, scalded-skin syndrome, and toxic shock syndrome. The last two are caused by toxigenic strains. *S. aureus* is also capable of producing food poisoning due to the elaboration of enterotoxins in foods such as potato salad, ice cream, and custards. Intense vomiting and diarrhea usually occurs within 2 to 8 h after ingestion of food containing the toxin.

An increasing problem with *S. aureus* is its resistance to antimicrobial agents, in particular methicillin. In the majority of methicillin-resistant *S. aureus* (MRSA) strains, this is due to an alteration in penicillin binding protein PBP2a, which is encoded by the *mecA* gene. Overproduction of β-lactamase accounts for a smaller percentage of MRSA strains. In recent years, *S. aureus* strains with decreased susceptibility to vancomycin have been identified. These strains are referred to as VISA (vancomycin-intermediate *S. aureus*) or, when addressing their susceptibility to the glycopeptide class of antimicrobials as a whole, GISA (glycopeptide-intermediate *S. aureus*). Although only a few of these strains have been isolated, they pose a potential threat to effective treatment of serious *S. aureus* infections.

Testing for MRSA can be difficult due to heteroresistance, in which the resistance is expressed to a different extent among subpopulations. A molecular test to directly detect the *mecA* gene and rapid assay formats employing monoclonal antibodies to the altered PBP2a protein have been used to circumvent the problems of in vitro susceptibility testing for MRSA. In addition, screening agar plates incorporating 6 μg of either oxacillin or vancomycin are commercially available to screen for MRSA and VISA strains, respectively. Selective chromogenic agars have facilitiated the detection of MRSA from nares specimens. Due to the importance of rapidly identifying blood cultures positive for *S. aureus*, peptide nucleic acid fluorescent in situ hybridization (PNA FISH) and nucleic acid amplification protocols have also been developed. These tests can be performed directly from blood cultures positive for gram-positive cocci in pairs and clusters.

Coagulase-negative staphylococci (CNS), in particular *S. epidermidis*, are recognized as the leading cause of nosocomial infections, with immunocompromised hosts at increased risk. Because CNS are members of the normal skin and mucosal membrane flora, they are frequently considered a contaminant when isolated from clinical specimens and therefore may be overlooked as a cause of infection. This is compounded by the fact that their clinical presentation is subacute, unlike that of *S. aureus*. An important virulence property of CNS is their ability to form a biofilm on the surface of indwelling or implanted foreign bodies, making them frequent agents of intravascular infections. *S. epidermidis* has also been implicated as a cause of endocarditis and is associated with right-side endocarditis in intravenous drug users. *S. saprophyticus* is a leading cause of noncomplicated urinary tract infections in young, sexually active females, second only to *Escherichia coli* in this patient population. Of the more recently described CNS human pathogens, *S. lugdunensis* and *S. schleiferi* have been implicated in serious infections including endocarditis, septicemia, arthritis, and joint infections. *S. lugdunensis*, which at times can behave more like *S. aureus* than CNS, has been associated with aggressive infections that have a high mortality rate; therefore, rapid recognition of this species is important for initiation of appropriate antimicrobial therapy. While other species of CNS have been implicated in a variety of infections, they occur with less frequency.

Micrococcus spp. are common inhabitants of the skin and have a fairly low pathogenic potential. However, infections with these organisms have occurred in immunocompromised hosts. *Micrococcus luteus* and related organisms have been implicated in a variety of infections, including meningitis, central nervous system shunt infections, endocarditis, and septic arthritis.

Upon incubation in air at 35°C for 24 to 48 h, staphylococci grow rapidly on a variety of media, with colonies that range from 1 to 3 mm in diameter. On blood agar, staphylococci produce white to cream opaque colonies. *S. aureus* colonies typically are cream in color but occasionally have a yellow or golden pigment, a phenotypic characteristic that led to the species name. *S. aureus* can be beta-hemolytic, and it is not uncommon to see both large and small colonies in the same culture, a phenotypic characteristic shared by several MRSA strains. CNS, in particular *S. epidermidis*, produce white colonies; however, other CNS strains and species can have colonies with a slight cream pigment. In general, CNS strains are nonhemolytic; however, some produce a small zone of beta-hemolysis on blood agar.

Since *S. aureus* is frequently isolated in mixed cultures, selective and differential media are used to facilitate the detection of these organisms in clinical material, particularly in nasal swabs, which are used to screen for carriage of this bacterium. Mannitol salt agar is an example of this, and here the high concentration of salt (7.5%) inhibits many other organisms. Mannitol, along with the phenol red indicator in the medium, facilitates the discrimination of *S. aureus*, which can ferment mannitol, from most CNS. However, since other organisms can grow on this medium and strains of CNS can also ferment mannitol, additional testing is required. Chromogenic media selective and differential for MRSA are more commonly used when screening nasal cultures.

In addition to their distinctive Gram stain morphology (gram-positive cocci in pairs and clusters), a common characteristic of these organisms is that they are catalase positive. The coagulase test, which measures the ability to clot plasma by converting fibrinogen to fibrin, is useful in distinguishing *S. aureus* from other bacteria that appear similar. A suspension of the organism to be identified is made in rabbit plasma containing EDTA and incubated at 35°C for 4 h. The tube is tilted gently, and the presence or absence of clot formation is noted. If the test is negative at 4 h, the suspension is incubated for up to 24 h. The 4-h reading is important because some strains produce fibrinolysin, which can dissolve a clot upon prolonged incubation, causing a false-negative result. Some strains of MRSA produce a very weak coagulase reaction, resulting in a negative reading. Bound coagulase (clumping factor) can be detected by a slide agglutination test, in which a suspension of the organism is emulsified on a slide with a drop of plasma. If bound coagulase is present, the organisms agglutinate. For correct interpretation of this test, a control in which saline is used instead of plasma is needed to check for autoagglutination. Of the CNS, *S. lugdunensis* and *S. schleiferi* can also test positive for bound coagulase but can be differentiated from *S. aureus* by a negative tube coagulation test. Alternatively, commercially available tests can be used that are based on a latex particle that has been coated with plasma, immunoglobulin, and in some versions of this test antibodies to the more common polysaccharide antigens. The plasma detects bound clumping factor, while the immunoglobulin binds protein A and the antibody to the polysaccharide antigens binds serotype antigens present on the surface of *S. aureus*. Some strains of MRSA, however, may be negative by this method because of low levels of bound coagulase and protein A, and false-positive reactions can occur due to the presence of the polysaccharide antigens present on some CNS isolates.

Strains of *S. aureus* that produce a weak coagulase reaction can be further tested by the DNase or a thermostable-endonuclease test. *S. aureus* and *S. schleiferi* possess enzymes that can degrade DNA, a DNase and a thermostable endonuclease. Both tests use the same basic medium containing agar that incorporates DNA and the metachromatic dye toluidine blue O. A heavy suspension of organisms is spotted onto the plate; after 24 h of incubation at 35°C, a pink haze appears around the colony, in contrast to the azure blue of the medium. When testing for the thermostable endonuclease, a suspension of the organism is boiled before being placed on the DNA plate.

CNS can be identified to the species level on the basis of their susceptibility profiles in response to selected agents, most notably novobiocin, as well as key biochemicals. A variety of commercial systems combine several biochemical tests to allow differentiation among the CNS. While most of the CNS of clinical importance are novobiocin susceptible, *S. saprophyticus* is novobiocin resistant. Other tests that can be used to differentiate among the species are phosphatase, production of acetoin, polymyxin susceptibility, pyrrolidonyl arylamidase activity (PYR test), and acid production from carbohydrates.

Micrococcus and related species, in addition to forming pairs and clusters, can appear as tetrads. Like the staphylococci, they can be easily grown in the laboratory and can be recovered from a variety of media. However, in comparison to staphylococci, they are slower growing with smaller colonies present after 24 h of incubation at 35°C. In addition, depending on the species, the colony color can range from cream to yellow (*M. luteus*) or rose red. As with CNS, a variety of commercial systems that incorporate several tests, including urease, acid production from carbohydrates, esculin, and gelatin, have been employed to aid in the differentiation of this group. Bacitracin, lysostaphin, and furazolidone have been used to aid in differentiating *Staphylococcus* from *Micrococcus*. In general, *Staphylococcus* is resistant to bacitracin (0.04-U disk), in contrast to *Micrococcus*, which is susceptible, while the opposite is found with furazolidone (100-μg disk) and lysostaphin (200-μg/disk), where *Micrococcus* is resistant.

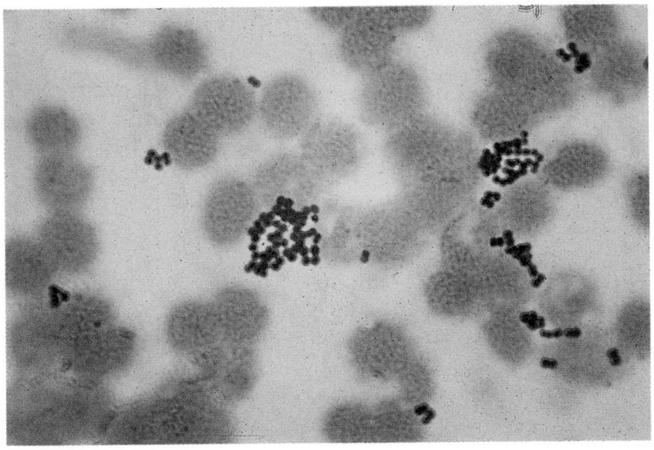

Figure 1-1 Gram stain of *Staphylococcus aureus*. A Gram stain of a positive blood culture shows gram-positive cocci in grape-like clusters. On subculture to solid media, *S. aureus* was isolated.

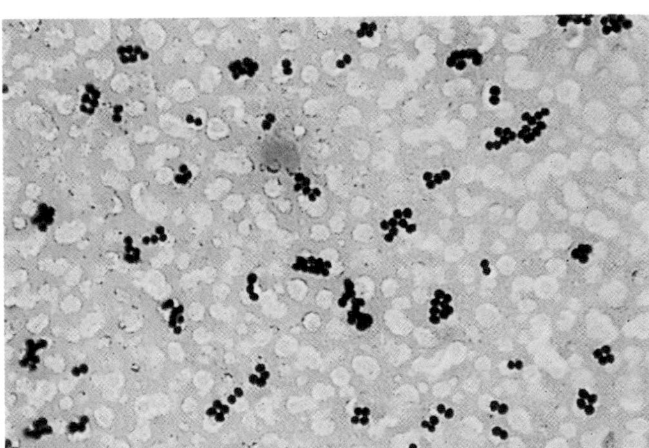

Figure 1-2 Gram stain of *Micrococcus luteus*. *M. luteus* organisms are gram-positive cocci that, like *S. aureus*, can appear in pairs and clusters. However, they also tend to form tetrads, as depicted in this Gram stain.

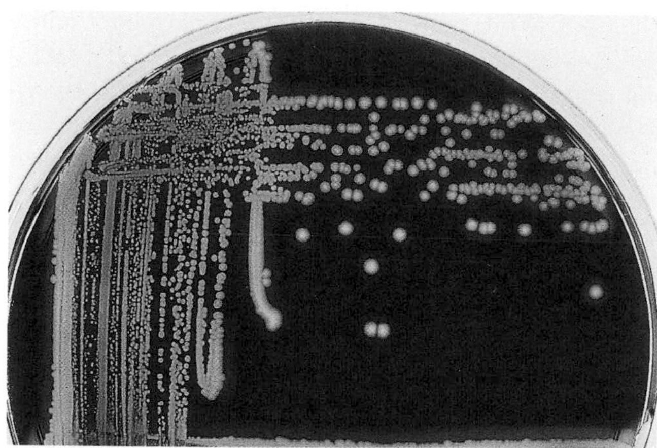

Figure 1-3 ***Staphylococcus aureus*** **on blood agar.** In the culture shown, *S. aureus* was grown overnight at 35°C on blood agar. The colonies are cream colored and opaque and have a smooth entire edge. A zone of beta-hemolysis surrounds the colony.

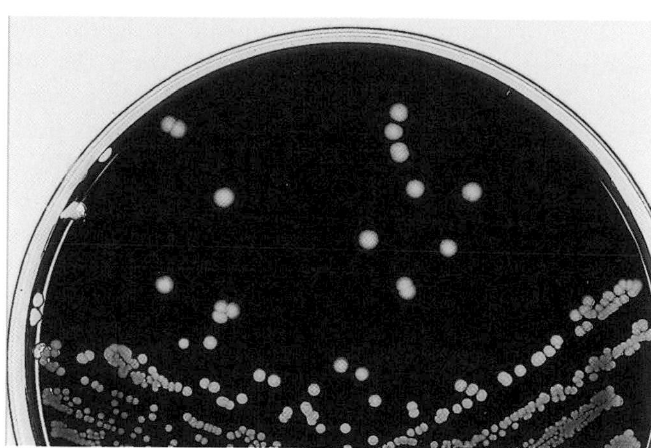

Figure 1-4 Golden pigment of ***Staphylococcus aureus.*** *S. aureus* is capable of producing the golden pigment that led to its species name. In practice, strains with this degree of pigment are not frequently isolated from clinical specimens. The isolate shown was incubated for 24 h on blood agar at 35°C and then left at room temperature for an additional day. When left at room temperature or refrigerated following incubation, isolates tend to develop more intense pigment.

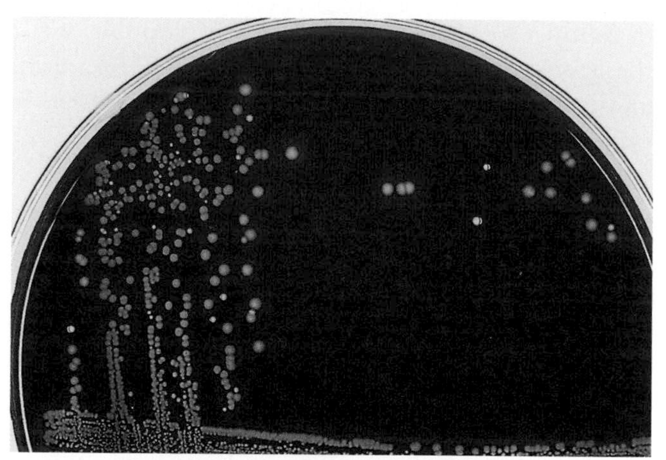

Figure 1-5 Size variation of ***Staphylococcus aureus*** **colonies.** It is not uncommon for strains of *S. aureus*, in particular MRSA strains, to produce colonies that are heterogeneous in size and the degree of hemolysis. Colonies shown were grown on blood agar for 24 h at 35°C.

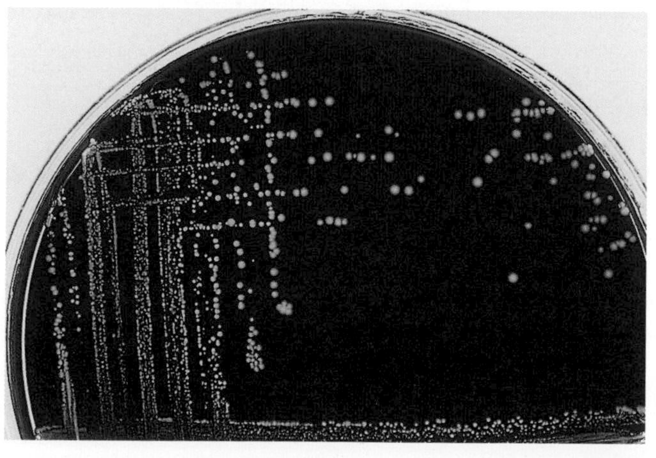

Figure 1-6 ***Staphylococcus epidermidis*** **on blood agar.** *S. epidermidis*, in contrast to both *S. aureus* and other CNS, produces a white colony with little or no pigment. The isolate shown here was grown on blood agar for 24 h at 35°C. This strain of *S. epidermidis* exhibits some variation in colony size.

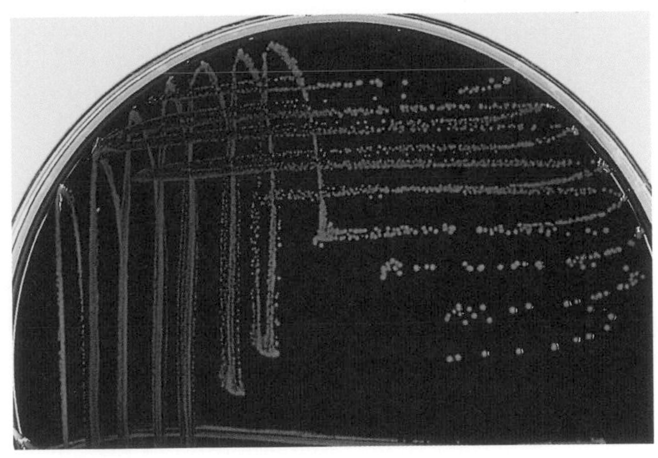

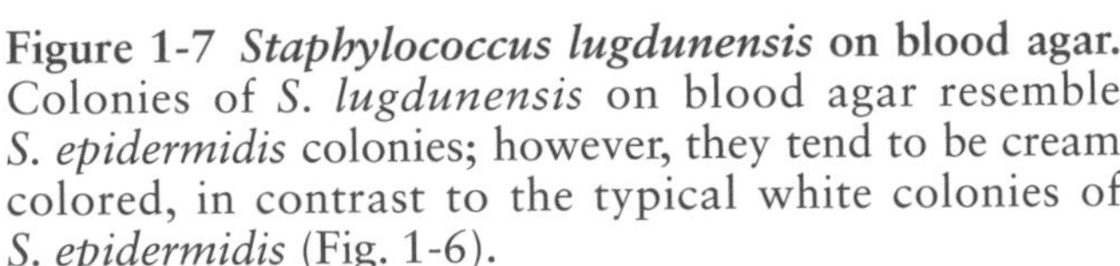

Figure 1-7 ***Staphylococcus lugdunensis*** **on blood agar.** Colonies of *S. lugdunensis* on blood agar resemble *S. epidermidis* colonies; however, they tend to be cream colored, in contrast to the typical white colonies of *S. epidermidis* (Fig. 1-6).

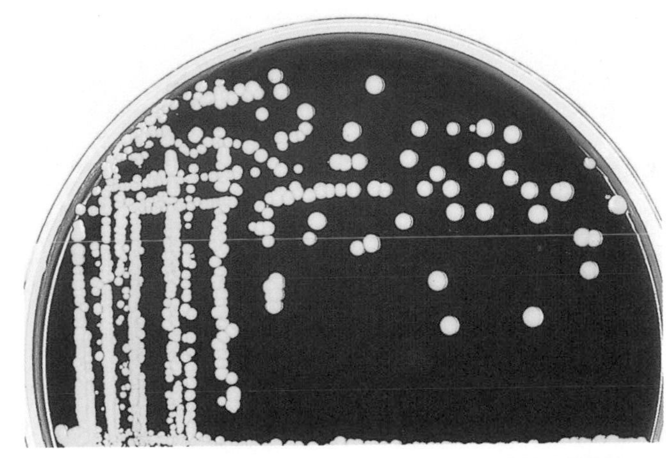

Figure 1-8 ***Micrococcus luteus*** **on blood agar.** A distinguishing feature of *M. luteus* is the vivid yellow colonies it produces. The isolate shown here was grown on blood agar for 72 h at 35°C. In general, *Micrococcus* is slower growing than *Staphylococcus*.

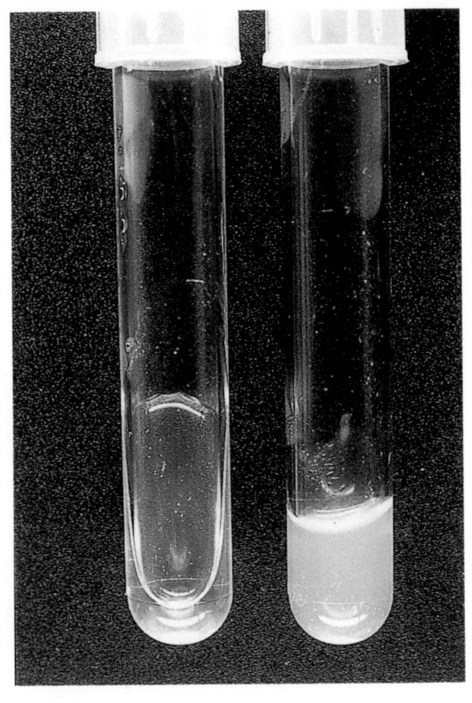

Figure 1-9 Coagulase test. A common method used to distinguish *S. aureus* from other *Staphylococcus* spp. is the tube coagulase test shown here. *S. aureus* is positive, and CNS are negative. Colonies of the isolate to be identified were emulsified in 0.5 ml of rabbit plasma. The tube was incubated at 35°C for 4 h and tipped gently to look for clot formation. The tube on the left is negative, with the plasma remaining liquid, while the tube on the right is positive, as evidenced by the clot formation. Tubes giving negative results at 4 h should be incubated for up to 24 h.

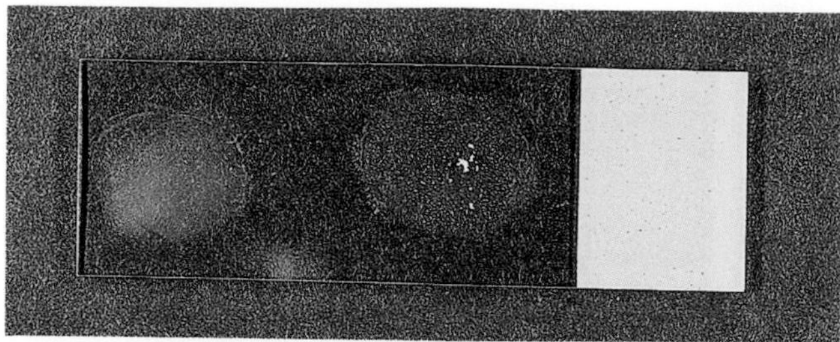

Figure 1-10 Slide coagulase test. The slide coagulase test is a rapid assay that tests for clumping factor on the surface of the organism. The test is performed by emulsifying the organism to be identified in both saline, which serves as a control for autoagglutination (left), and rabbit plasma (right). Agglutination of the organisms only in plasma is a positive test. *S. aureus*, as shown in this figure, and strains of *S. lugdunensis* and *S. schleiferi*, are positive by this test.

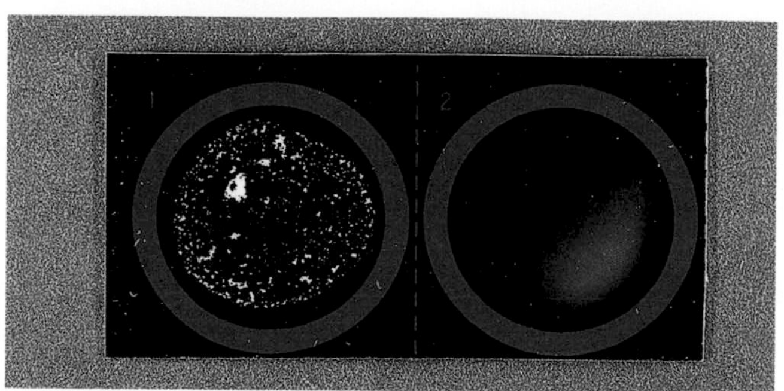

Figure 1-11 Latex test for the identification of *Staphylococcus aureus*. In the test depicted here, latex particles have been coated with antibody that can recognize bound coagulase as well as immunoglobulin that will bind to protein A present on the surface of most strains of *S. aureus*. The isolate to be identified (left) and *S. epidermidis* (right), which serves as a negative control, were emulsified with coated latex beads. The isolate shown here was identified as *S. aureus*. As with the slide coagulase test, some strains of MRSA may be negative and some strains of CNS, namely, *S. lugdunensis* and *S. schleiferi* strains, may be positive.

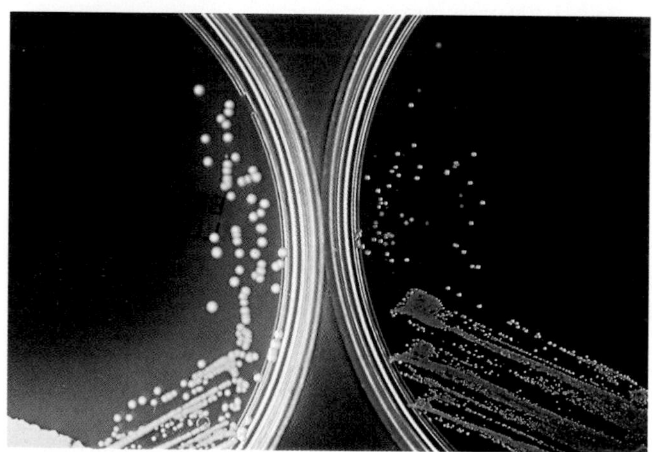

Figure 1-12 Mannitol salt agar. Mannitol salt agar is a selective and differential medium used for the isolation and presumptive identification of *S. aureus*. The high salt concentration inhibits the growth of many organisms that inhabit skin and mucosal membranes. The phenol red indicator incorporated into the medium detects acid production (yellow) resulting from the fermentation of mannitol by *S. aureus*. As shown here, CNS (right) and *S. aureus* (left) were inoculated on the agar and then were incubated overnight.

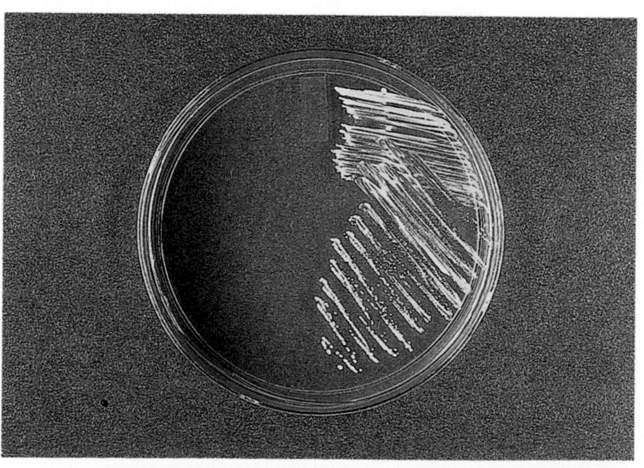

Figure 1-13 Mannitol salt agar containing oxacillin. Mannitol salt agar with oxacillin can be used to screen for the presence of MRSA in nasal specimens since the 7.5% salt and 6 μg of oxacillin in this medium inhibit most other organisms that normally colonize the nares. MRSA turns the medium yellow as a result of the fermentation of mannitol. Pictured here is a plate inoculated with a methicillin-susceptible *S. aureus* strain (left) and a MRSA strain (right). The methicillin-susceptible *S. aureus* strain failed to grow. As with most in vitro testing for methicillin susceptibility, oxacillin (not methicillin) is used because of its higher stability.

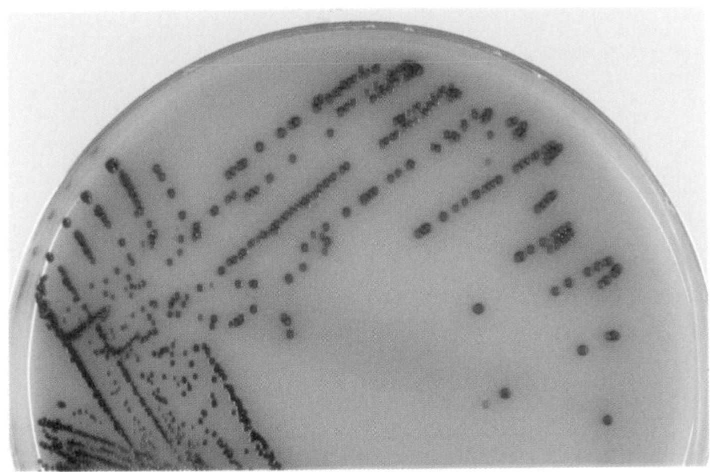

Figure 1-14 Spectra MRSA. Shown is a chromogenic medium, Spectra MRSA (Thermo Scientific Remel Products, Lenexa, KS), that is both selective and differential that can be used to detect MRSA. When the chromogenic substrate incorporated into the inhibitory agar is degraded by the enzymatic action of MRSA, the colony takes on a denim blue color. Shown here is an overnight nasal culture from which MRSA was isolated.

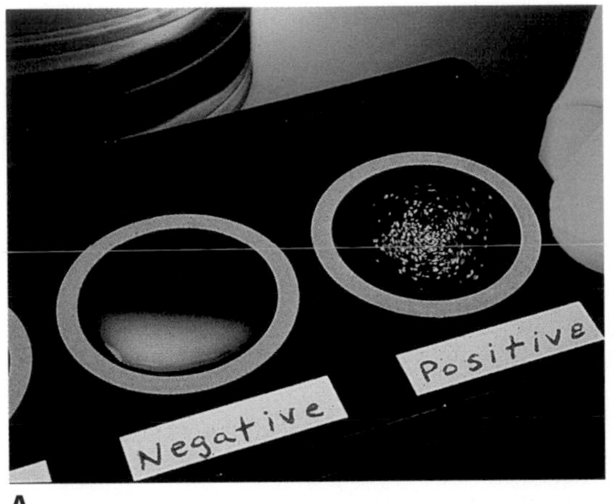

A

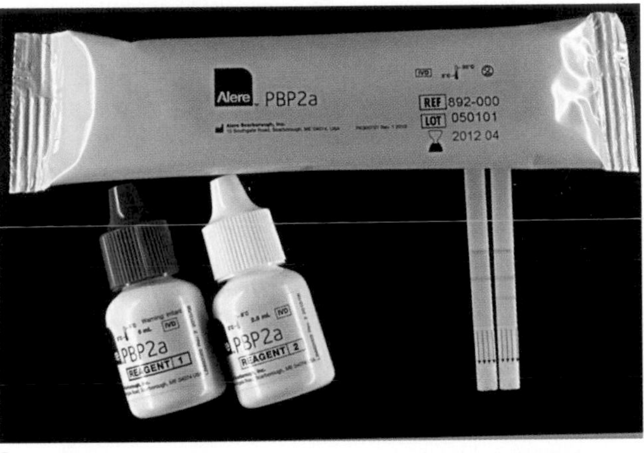

B

Figure 1-15 Assays to detect PBP2a protein found in MRSA. (A) The product of the *mecA* gene, which results in methicillin resistance, is an altered penicillin binding protein, PBP2a. Monoclonal antibody to this altered protein has been used to coat latex particles, which are then used in the Oxoid agglutination assay to detect PBP2a. (B) Shown is the Alere PBP2a lateral flow assay (Alere Inc., Waltham, MA) also utilizing monoclonal antibodies for the detection of PBP2a protein. Both formats are rapid tests that are used once the organism is isolated on solid media.

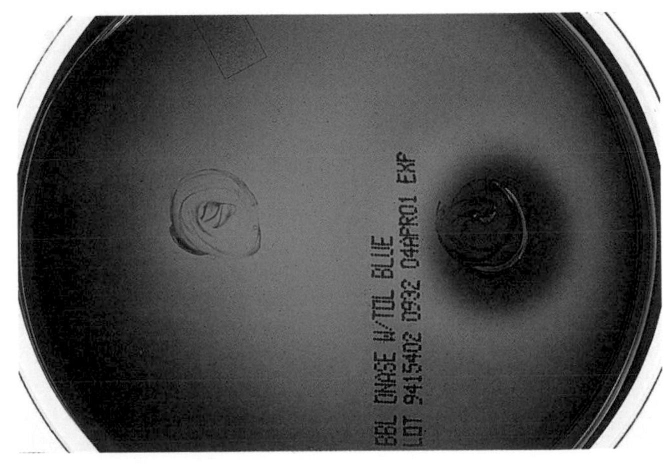

Figure 1-16 DNase plate to differentiate *Staphylococcus aureus* from CNS. *S. aureus* produces DNase, which can degrade DNA. This property is used to aid in the differentiation of *S. aureus* (right) from CNS (left). This is particularly useful for identification of *S. aureus* strains that produce a small amount of coagulase, thus giving an equivocal or weakly positive coagulase test. The only CNS species that shares this property with *S. aureus* is *S. schleiferi*. In this test, a heavy inoculum of the organism is used to spot an agar plate that contains DNA and toluidine blue. If the organism produces DNase, the DNA is degraded, resulting in the agar turning pink in the area surrounding the inoculum due to the metachromatic qualities of toluidine blue.

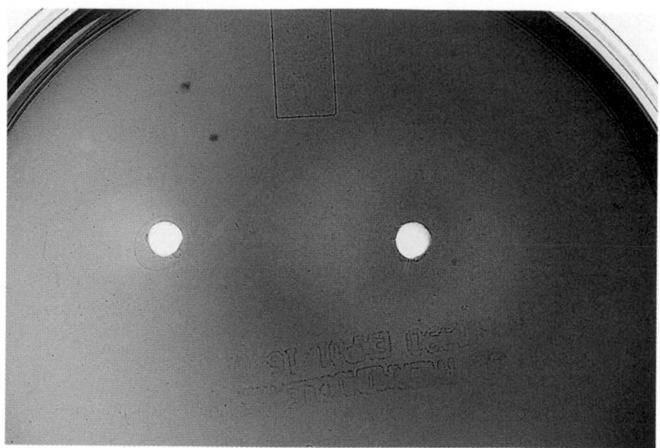

Figure 1-17 Thermostable endonuclease activity. In addition to DNase, *S. aureus* produces a thermostable endonuclease that can also cleave DNA. To test for this activity, a heavy suspension of the organism is boiled and then used to fill a well that is cut in the DNA plate containing toluidine blue. As described in the legend to Fig. 1-16, if the DNA is degraded there is a change in the color of the agar from blue to pink, as shown for the *S. aureus* strain (right). *S. epidermidis* does not produce a heat-stable endonuclease (left).

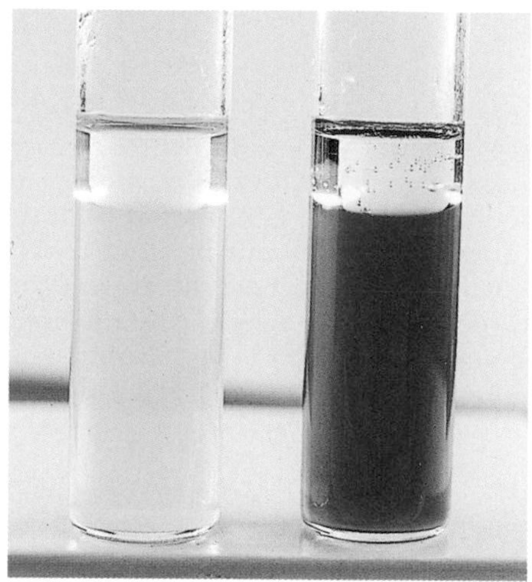

Figure 1-18 Ornithine decarboxylase test for the identification of *Staphylococcus lugdunensis*. Unlike most other CNS species, *S. lugdunensis* is ornithine decarboxylase positive. The decarboxylase medium containing 1% ornithine is inoculated and incubated overnight. Since some strains of *S. epidermidis* can also be positive at 24 h, the specimen should be examined at 8 h, a time at which *S. lugdunensis* is positive but *S. epidermidis* is still negative. The isolate on the left, *S. saprophyticus*, is negative since it is yellow, indicating only fermentation of glucose; however, *S. lugdunensis* (shown on the right) is positive due to the violet color resulting from the alkalinization of the medium.

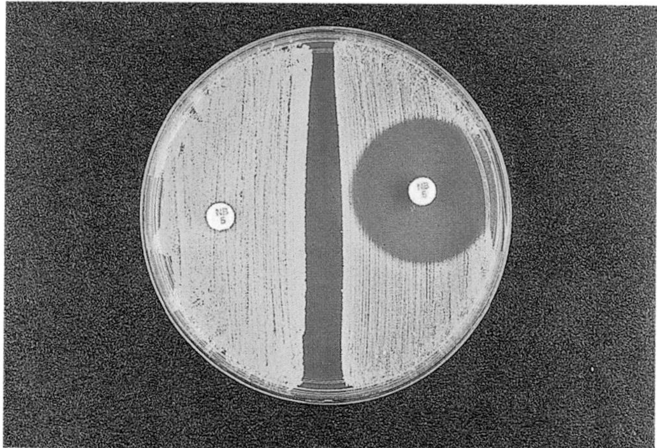

Figure 1-19 Novobiocin susceptibility. *S. saprophyticus* can be differentiated from other clinically significant CNS isolates by its resistance to the antibiotic novobiocin. As pictured, Mueller-Hinton agar was inoculated with a suspension equivalent to a 0.5 McFarland standard of *S. epidermidis* (right) and *S. saprophyticus* (left). Novobiocin disks (5 µg) were placed on the agar surface, which was incubated for 24 h at 35°C. Zones of inhibition measuring ≤16 mm indicate novobiocin resistance, as seen with this isolate of *S. saprophyticus*, which has no zone of inhibition. In contrast, the susceptible *S. epidermidis* isolate has a large zone of inhibition around the novobiocin disk.

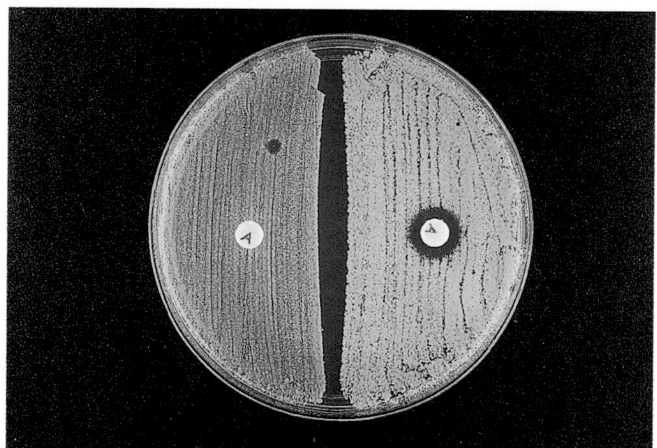

Figure 1-20 Bacitracin susceptibility. The same procedure used to test for the bacitracin susceptibility of *Streptococcus pyogenes* can be used to differentiate *Staphylococcus* spp., which are bacitracin resistant, from *Micrococcus* spp., which are susceptible. Here *M. luteus* (right) exhibits a zone of inhibition around a 0.04-U bacitracin disk, in contrast to *S. epidermidis* (left), which is not inhibited.

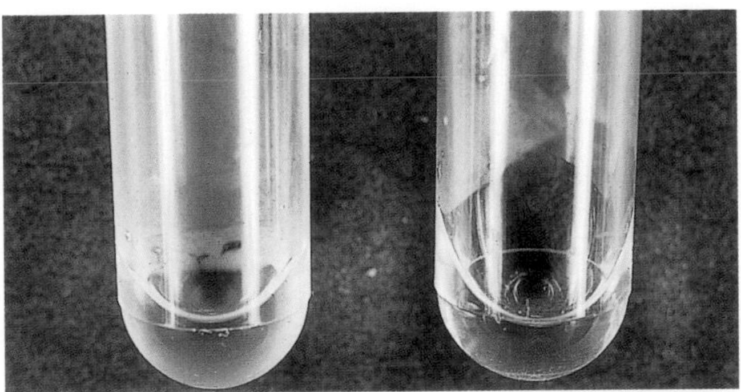

Figure 1-21 Lysostaphin susceptibility. Several species of *Staphylococcus* are susceptible to the endopeptidase lysostaphin, which cleaves the glycine-rich pentapeptide that is essential for cross bridging the cell wall. Cleavage of these basic units weakens the cell wall, making it susceptible to lysis. Depending on the makeup of this pentapeptide, specifically the glycine content, susceptibility to lysostaphin can vary. For example, while *S. aureus* is very susceptible, *S. saprophyticus* is less susceptible due to the serine content of its pentapeptide bridge. *Micrococcus* and related species are not susceptible to lysostaphin. As shown here, the test is performed by making a heavy suspension of the unknown organism in saline and then adding an equal volume of lysostaphin reagent. Clearing of the suspension after 2 h at 35°C indicates lysis of the organisms. In the example shown here, the lysostaphin test medium inoculated with *S. aureus* (right) was positive and the one inoculated with *M. luteus* (left) remained turbid and thus was negative. This assay can also be performed as a disk diffusion test.

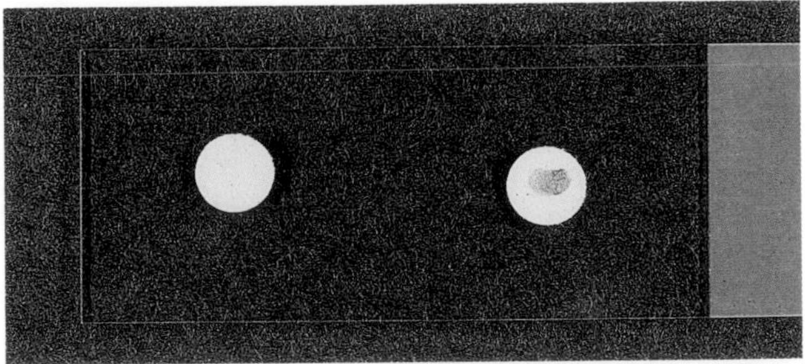

Figure 1-22 Modified oxidase test. A modified oxidase test, the Microdase test (Thermo Scientific Remel Products), is available for differentiating *Micrococcus* from *Staphylococcus*. *Micrococcus* spp. possess cytochrome *c*, which is essential for producing a positive oxidase reaction, whereas clinically relevant *Staphylococcus* spp. are microdase negative since they lack cytochrome *c*. In the example shown, a colony of *S. epidermidis* (left) and a colony of *M. luteus* (right) were rubbed onto a disk impregnated with tetramethyl-*p*-phenylenediamine (TMPD) dissolved in dimethyl sulfoxide. Development of a purple-blue color within 2 min indicates a positive test due to the reaction of the enzyme oxidase with cytochrome *c* and TMPD.

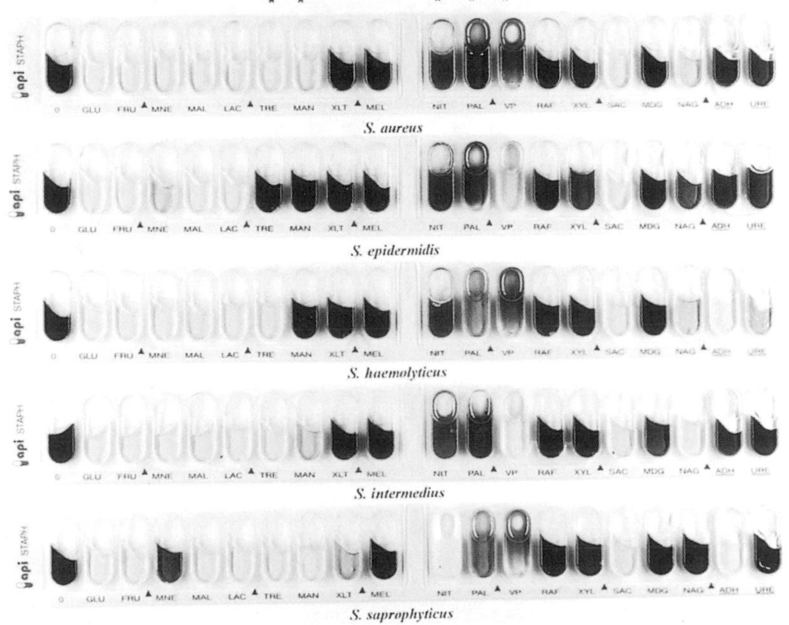

Figure 1-23 API Staph identification system. API Staph (bioMérieux, Inc., Durham, NC) is a commercial system that can differentiate among several *Staphylococcus* species. Each test strip consists of 20 microtubes, including the negative control well. Key reactions that aid in the differentiation and identification of the five *Staphylococcus* species shown are indicated by an asterisk at the top.

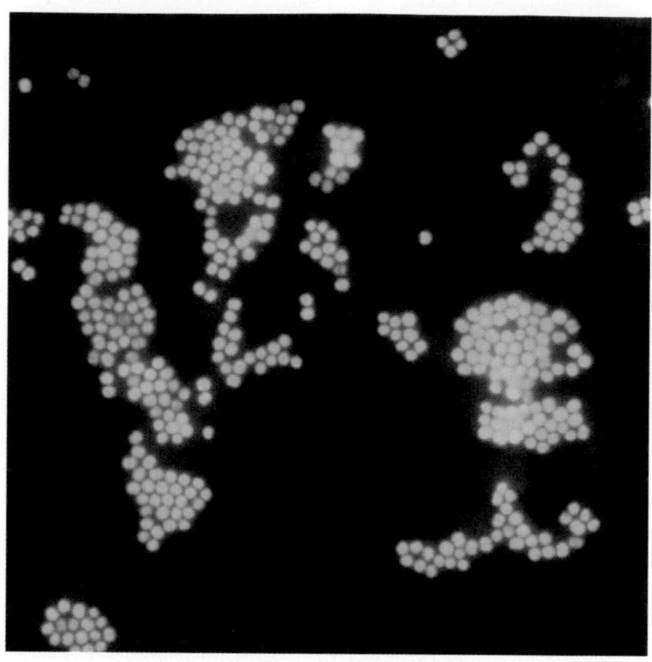

Figure 1-24 PNA FISH for the differentiation of *Staphylococcus aureus* from CNS in blood cultures. PNA FISH (AdvanDx, Woburn, MA) is a 90-min FISH utilizing fluorescent-labeled PNA. It is performed directly from blood culture bottles that are positive for gram-positive cocci in clusters. In the example shown, the gram-positive cocci are *S. aureus*, which hybridized with a green fluorescent probe. (Photo courtesy of AdvanDX.)

Streptococcus 2

The genus *Streptococcus* is characterized as consisting of gram-positive cocci in pairs and/or chains. Members of this genus commonly colonize mucosal membranes and are a predominant component of the respiratory, gastrointestinal, and genital tracts. Streptococci are catalase-negative facultative anaerobes that metabolize carbohydrates by fermentation, producing mainly lactic acid.

Traditionally, streptococci have been grouped by the phenotypic characteristics of hemolysis and Lancefield antigen composition as well as by pathogenic potential. While these are still useful ways to group organisms, there are many exceptions and overlapping characteristics with each grouping system; therefore, genetic analysis is a more definitive method for classifying these organisms. However, from a practical standpoint, phenotypic characteristics are very useful in identification algorithms. Streptococci can be either beta-hemolytic (complete hemolysis), alpha-hemolytic (incomplete hemolysis resulting in a green zone around the colony), or gamma-hemolytic (no hemolysis) on blood agar. With the Lancefield system, depending on the cell wall carbohydrate (Lancefield antigen) or lipoteichoic acid (group D), some of the streptococci have been placed in groups A, B, C, D, F, and G. Most members of the Lancefield groups are beta-hemolytic, the exception being group D, which is composed of alpha-hemolytic or nonhemolytic organisms.

STREPTOCOCCUS PYOGENES (GROUP A BETA-HEMOLYTIC STREPTOCOCCI)

S. pyogenes organisms are beta-hemolytic streptococci possessing the group A Lancefield antigen. *S. pyogenes* is one of the more virulent *Streptococcus* species and is responsible for a wide range of clinical entities, the most common being pharyngitis. Complications resulting from infection include rheumatic fever, glomerulonephritis, the scarlatiniform rash of scarlet fever, and toxic shock-like syndrome. This organism can also cause necrotizing fasciitis, although it is not considered a common complication.

Direct detection of *S. pyogenes* based on the Lancefield group A antigen is commonly performed on throat specimens. There are several commercial kits available for direct detection that have high specificity but vary in sensitivity. Therefore, especially with children, for whom the incidence of infection and potential to develop sequelae are greater, it is recommended that negative direct tests be followed up by culture. *S. pyogenes* is commonly isolated using blood agar incubated in 5% CO_2. Trimethoprim-sulfamethoxazole can be incorporated into the blood agar to increase the selection of *S. pyogenes*. Antibodies specific for the group A Lancefield carbohydrate antigen can be used to identify *S. pyogenes*. Bacitracin susceptibility has also traditionally been used to identify large-colony beta-hemolytic organisms. Here, a 0.04-U bacitracin disk is applied to a lawn of the organism and the formation of any zone of inhibition is considered a positive result. Another useful rapid biochemical test for identification of *S. pyogenes* is the PYR test, in which the enzyme pyrrolidonyl arylamidase is detected.

Small-colony beta-hemolytic organisms can also possess the Lancefield group A antigen; however, these isolates are classified as members of the viridans streptococci, anginosus group. Small-colony (*Streptococcus anginosus*) and large-colony (*S. pyogenes*) group A streptococci can be differentiated biochemically in that *S. pyogenes* is PYR positive and Voges-Proskauer (VP) negative while the opposite is true of *S. anginosus*.

Serological tests are available to detect the host response to the group A antigen and M protein as well as extracellular products associated with *S. pyogenes*, e.g., streptolysin O (ASO test) and DNase B. These tests are used to aid in the diagnosis of patients with sequelae consistent with a past infection with *S. pyogenes*.

STREPTOCOCCUS AGALACTIAE

Beta-hemolytic streptococci that possess the Lancefield group B antigen are classified as *S. agalactiae*. While these organisms can cause a variety of human infections, particularly in compromised hosts, they are best known as the leading infectious cause of neonatal morbidity and mortality in the United States.

In an effort to reduce the exposure of newborns, screening of pregnant females at 35 to 37 weeks of gestation by culture for *S. agalactiae* is currently recommended. Direct rapid nucleic acid amplification techniques are also available and have been found to be very sensitive, thus presenting an alternative to culture. Tests for the rapid direct detection of the group B antigen are available but, due to their low sensitivity, are not recommended for screening pregnant females. For detection of colonization of the female genital tract, it is recommended that a swab or swabs from the distal vagina and anorectum be collected. These swabs are then used to inoculate blood agar and placed in an enrichment broth containing antibiotics, e.g., colistin (10 μg/ml) or gentamicin (8 μg/ml) and nalidixic acid (15 μg/ml). In the event the primary plate is negative for *S. agalactiae*, the enrichment broth is subcultured to blood agar after 18 to 24 h of incubation. In general, colonies of *S. agalactiae*, in comparison to *S. pyogenes*, produce a narrow zone of beta-hemolysis on blood-based agar. Alternatively, carrot broth or Granada media, which will turn orange in the presence of *S. agalactiae*, have been used to detect the presence of this organism; however, nonhemolytic strains may not be detected with pigment-dependent differential media.

S. agalactiae can be identified by Lancefield typing using antibodies to detect the group B antigen. In addition, a CAMP (Christie, Atkins, Munch-Petersen) test can be performed to detect a protein, CAMP factor, produced by *S. agalactiae*. To detect the CAMP factor, *S. agalactiae* is streaked at right angles to a strain of *Staphylococcus aureus* that produces a beta-hemolysin that synergistically interacts with the CAMP factor. If *S. agalactiae* is present, hemolysis in the shape of an arrowhead is seen where the two lines of bacterial growth intersect. Commercially available disks impregnated with the *Staphylococcus* hemolysin are available that also enable the detection of enhanced hemolysis in the presence of the CAMP factor produced by *S. agalactiae*. Alternatively, *S. agalactiae* can be presumptively identified by its ability to hydrolyze hippurate. Both rapid (2-h) and overnight versions of this test are based on the hydrolysis of hippurate to glycine, which can subsequently be detected with the ninhydrin reagent.

STREPTOCOCCUS DYSGALACTIAE SUBSP. *EQUISIMILIS* (LARGE-COLONY BETA-HEMOLYTIC LANCEFIELD GROUPS C AND G)

Human isolates of large-colony beta-hemolytic streptococci that possess either the Lancefield group C or G antigen, and occasionally Lancefield group A and L antigens, are genetically related and have been placed into the same species, *S. dysgalactiae* subsp. *equisimilis*. These organisms cause an acute disease spectrum similar to that of *S. pyogenes*; however, they are not generally associated with sequelae, although there are reports of exceptions. *S. dysgalactiae* subsp. *equisimilis* strains are not the only streptococci possessing the Lancefield C and G antigens. Other large-colony strains possessing the group C or G antigen, which may be alpha- or beta-hemolytic or nonhemolytic, are found primarily in animals and can cause zoonoses.

Human isolates are generally identified by typing large-colony beta-hemolytic strains with antibodies to the Lancefield groups. However, small-colony beta-hemolytic organisms can also type as group C or

G but are members of the viridans streptococci, belonging to the anginosus group. Large- and small-colony beta-hemolytic group C and G streptococci can be differentiated from one another by a VP test for acetoin or a rapid test to detect β-D-glucuronidase (BGUR), since large-colony isolates are positive by this test but negative by the VP test. This enzyme can also be rapidly detected using methylumbelliferyl-β-D-glucuronide containing MacConkey agar.

STREPTOCOCCUS PNEUMONIAE

S. pneumoniae is part of the normal respiratory flora, and carriage of this organism is common. It is one of the leading causes of community-acquired pneumonia. In addition, it can cause bacteremia, endocarditis, meningitis, sinusitis, and otitis media. Traditionally this organism was universally susceptible to penicillin; however, increasing numbers of strains have developed decreased susceptibility to this first-line antimicrobial agent. A key characteristic of this gram-positive organism is its lancet-shaped appearance in a Gram stain. Encapsulated strains, often the more pathogenic strains due to the antiphagocytic characteristics of the capsule, can be detected by Gram staining when the combination of a proteinaceous background and correct illumination allows a halo (i.e., capsule) around the organism to be visible.

S. pneumoniae belongs to the *Streptococcus mitis* group of the viridans streptococci; however, due to their unique phenotypic and clinical manifestations, they will be discussed separately. Strains that once were considered *S. pneumoniae* that were not bile soluble or optochin (ethylhydrocupreine hydrochloride) susceptible have recently been included in the species *Streptococcus pseudopneumoniae*, which is also included in the *S. mitis* group.

S. pneumoniae grows on blood agar and often needs incubation in 5% CO_2 for optimal growth. Colonies are alpha-hemolytic and can be mucoid in appearance due to a capsule. As the colonies age, they tend to be described as concave and can appear to have a "punched-out" center. Strains of *S. pneumoniae* have been defined by their capsular antigens, and currently over 80 serotypes have been identified. Swelling of the capsule in the presence of type-specific antibodies is referred to as a quellung reaction. Alternatively, strains can be typed using commercially available agglutination tests.

The two tests that are most widely used to identify *S. pneumoniae* are bile solubility and optochin susceptibility. "Bile," or sodium deoxycholate, when added to *S. pneumoniae* growing in broth or on solid media, will cause lysis of the organisms. Zones of inhibition of ≥14 mm with a 6-mm, 5-μg optochin disk can also be used to distinguish *S. pneumoniae* from other alpha-hemolytic streptococcal organisms.

VIRIDANS STREPTOCOCCI

Members of the viridans streptococci are normal inhabitants of the mucosal membranes and therefore are commonly found in the gastrointestinal and urogenital tracts as well as the oral cavity. Several viridans species are associated with dental caries and subacute bacterial endocarditis, particularly in patients with damaged or prosthetic heart valves. It is not uncommon to isolate them from polymicrobic abscesses. *Streptococcus intermedius* can be found in deep abscesses, particularly of the brain and liver. Infections with the viridans group are becoming more frequent in neutropenic patients, probably due to the oral mucosal damage from some of the chemotherapeutic agents used.

It has traditionally been difficult to determine the species identity of the viridans group in the clinical laboratory setting. This is in part because they lack characteristic hemolytic reactions in that they can be alpha-hemolytic or nonhemolytic and occasional strains are beta-hemolytic. With the exception of members of the *Streptococcus bovis* group, which possess the group D antigen, most viridans streptococci lack distinct Lancefield antigens. In addition, several nomenclature systems have evolved to describe members within this group. Commercial systems that can identify species in this group are available, and with continued refinement of databases and consolidation of nomenclature they should prove very useful. Several conventional tests can be used to group and sometimes identify species of the viridans streptococci. Key tests include urea hydrolysis, which is performed on Christensen urea agar incubated at 35°C for 7 days; the VP test for acetoin production; arginine hydrolysis, which can be tested by different methods (depending on the method and the species, results of this test can vary); esculin hydrolysis, which can be performed using commercially available slants that are observed for blackening for up to 1 week; fermentation using 1% (wt/vol) carbohydrate in thioglycolate broth containing purple broth base (1.6% [wt/vol]), which is inoculated and incubated anaerobically for 24 h; and hyaluronidase production, which can be detected on agar plates containing 400 μg of hyaluronic acid. The use of fluorogenic substrates has also aided in the differentiation of species of viridans streptococci; by this method, 4-methylumbelliferyl-linked substrates are degraded and the by-product can be visualized under UV illumination.

The main species of the viridans streptococci can be placed in either the bovis, mitis, anginosus, mutans, or salivarius groups (Table 2-1).

Bovis Group (Group D Streptococci)

The *S. bovis* group has been subdivided based on DNA studies. Strains of *S. bovis* causing human infections belong mainly to two biotypes, I and II. The revised nomenclature for this group of organisms replaces *S. bovis* biotype I with *Streptococcus gallolyticus* subsp. *gallolyticus* (*S. gallolyticus*). Most importantly, there is a strong association of this organism with colorectal cancer. *S. bovis* biotype II organisms, which can also cause a variety of human infections including endocarditis, septicemia, meningitis, and gall bladder disease, are now designated *Streptococcus infantarius* subsp. *infantarius* (*S. infantarius*; *S. bovis* biotype II/1); *Streptococcus infantarius* subsp. *coli*, also referred to as *Streptococcus lutetiensis* (*S. bovis* biotype II/1); and *Streptococcus gallolyticus* subsp. *pasteurianus*, also referred to as *Streptococcus pasteurianus* (*S. bovis* biotype II/2). In order to more firmly establish the disease association of each of these organisms, it is important that microbiologists and clinicans adopt the new nomenclature.

Table 2-1 Grouping of the viridans streptococci associated with human disease

Group	Species within groups
Bovis	*S. gallolyticus* subsp. *gallolyticus* (*S. gallolyticus*; *S. bovis* biotype I)
	S. infantarius subsp. *infantarius* (*S. infantarius*; *S. bovis* biotype II/1)
	S. infantarius subsp. *coli* (*S. lutetiensis*; *S. bovis* biotype II/1)
	S. gallolyticus subsp. *pasteurianus* (*S. pasteurianus*; *S. bovis* biotype II/2)
Mitis	*S. mitis*
	S. pneumoniae
	S. pseudopneumoniae
	S. crista
	S. gordonii
	S. oralis
	S. parasanguis
	S. sanguis
Anginosus (milleri)	*S. anginosus*
	S. constellatus
	S. intermedius
Mutans	*S. mutans*
	S. cricetus
	S. downei
	S. rattus
Salivarius	*S. salivarius*
	S. vestibularis

Members of the *S. bovis* group are alpha-hemolytic or nonhemolytic on blood agar, which is commonly used to isolate these organisms. They can be differentiated from other alpha-hemolytic and nonhemolytic streptococci primarily by biochemical reactions. Key characteristics of the *S. bovis* group, along with possession of the group D Lancefield antigen, that can be used to distinguish *S. bovis* from other viridans streptococci are the ability to grow in the presence of 40% bile and hydrolyze esculin; the lack of sorbitol fermentation; the ability to ferment mannitol, inulin, and starch; and the inability to produce urease. Biotypes I and II of *S. bovis* can be differentiated by mannitol fermentation and glucan production, both of which are seen with biotype I but not biotype II. *S. bovis* strains can be differentiated from *Enterococcus* spp., which are also bile-esculin positive, by their inability to grow at 45°C or in 6.5% NaCl at 35°C and by the fact that they are PYR negative.

Mitis Group

The nomenclature of the mitis group of streptococci, which includes *Streptococcus mitis*, *Streptococcus oralis*, *Streptococcus sanguis*, *Streptococcus parasanguis*, *Streptococcus gordonii*, and *Streptococcus crista*, has varied; therefore, depending on the criteria used for identification, different species names have been assigned to similar organisms, making disease associations difficult. Members of this group are associated with endocarditis and with dental plaque. *S. mitis* has been isolated from the blood more frequently in patients undergoing chemotherapy and radiation treatment, most probably due to the oromucositis in these patients.

Members of this group are alpha-hemolytic. Some of the key biochemical reactions for the viridans group, notably production of acetoin (VP test), urease, and hyaluronidase, are negative for members of the mitis group. Arginine hydrolysis can be used to differentiate *S. oralis* and *S. mitis* from the other members of the group since these two species are negative. The majority of strains of *S. sanguis* and *S. gordonii* form hard, adherent, smooth colonies due to the extracellular production of dextran.

Anginosus Group

Three species, *Streptococcus anginosus*, *Streptococcus constellatus*, and *Streptococcus intermedius*, compose the anginosus group, which has also been referred to as the milleri group. These organisms are known to cause endocarditis and purulent infections of the liver, brain, abdomen, pleural cavity, and head and neck region.

Members of this group generally form small colonies and can be alpha- or beta-hemolytic or nonhemolytic. However, *S. constellatus* is commonly beta-hemolytic whereas strains of *S. intermedius* are often nonhemolytic. They are not characterized by a particular Lancefield antigen, since strains are unable to be placed in a group that can be easily tested. However, *S. intermedius* strains seem more homogenous in this regard in that they possess the Lancefield group F antigen. Growth of this group is often enhanced by the presence of CO_2 or anaerobic conditions. Many strains, due to the production of diacetyl, produce a butterscotch-type sweet odor when growing on solid media.

Members of this group are arginine positive, VP positive, and urease negative. The three species can be difficult to differentiate from one another, but tests that can be used are hyaluronidase (*S. anginosus* is negative), β-D-fucosidase activity (*S. intermedius* is positive), and β-D-glucosidase (*S. constellatus* is negative and *S. intermedius* is variable).

Mutans Group

The mutans group, especially *Streptococcus mutans*, is known for its association with dental caries. Of the species in this group, *S. mutans* and *Streptococcus sobrinus* are the most frequently isolated from human dental plaque whereas *Streptococcus criceti*, *Streptococcus downei*, and *Streptococcus rattus* are seldom found in humans. The other species in this group are isolated primarily from animals and therefore are not discussed here. *S. mutans* in general is alpha-hemolytic, with a few strains exhibiting beta-hemolysis, while *S. cricetus* is nonhemolytic with a few alpha-hemolytic strains. By Gram stain, *S. mutans* occasionally appears as short bacilli. Members of this group are arginine negative, esculin positive, VP positive, urease negative, and hyaluronidase negative.

Salivarius Group

The two species in the salivarius group associated with human disease, *Streptococcus salivarius* and *Streptococcus vestibularis*, are inhabitants of the oral cavity, whereas the third species, *Streptococcus thermophilus*, is found primarily in dairy products. Members of this group do not appear to be virulent, but *S. salivarius* can cause septicemia in neutropenic patients. Most strains are alpha-hemolytic, with occasional strains being nonhemolytic. *S. salivarius* occasionally types as Lancefield group K. Production of extracellular polysaccharide on sucrose agar gives *S. salivarius* colonies a large, mucoid appearance; alternatively, they can appear as large, hard colonies that pit the agar. *S. vestibularis* is urease positive and does not produce extracellular polysaccharides like *S. salivarius*.

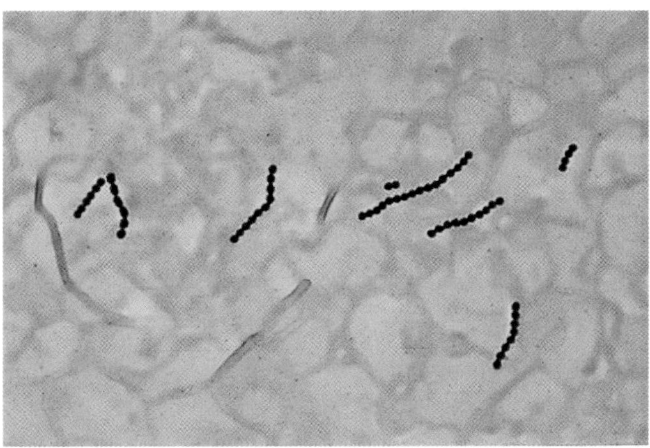

Figure 2-1 Gram stain of *Streptococcus pyogenes*. *S. pyogenes* (group A streptococcus) is a gram-positive coccus that is usually seen in pairs and chains. The Gram stain shown is from a blood culture.

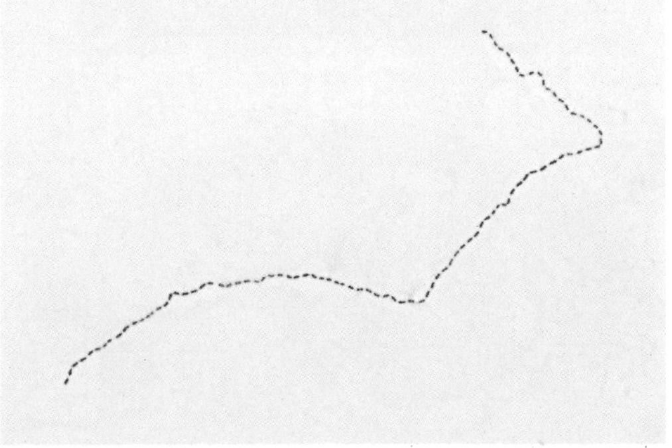

Figure 2-2 Gram stain of viridans streptococci. Viridans streptococci tend to form long chains of gram-positive cocci, as seen in this Gram stain of a blood culture. They often do not stain well, giving the impression they are not as "healthy" as other streptococci.

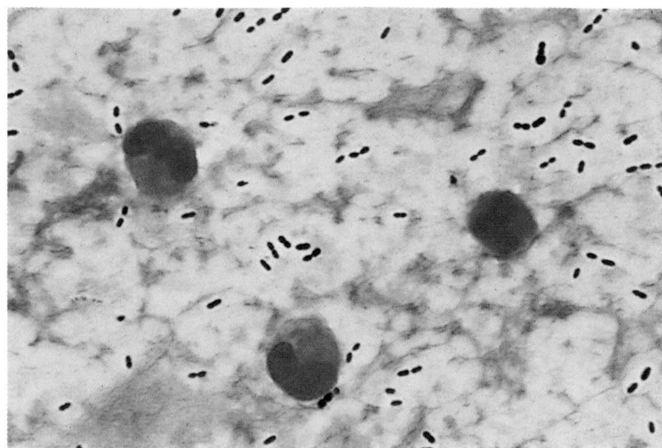

Figure 2-3 Gram stain of *Streptococcus pneumoniae*. This direct smear of a sputum specimen that grew predominantly *S. pneumoniae* shows the typical morphology of lancet-shaped, gram-positive cocci in pairs. Against the pink proteinaceous background of the specimen, the capsule of *S. pneumoniae* can be seen as a clear halo around the organisms.

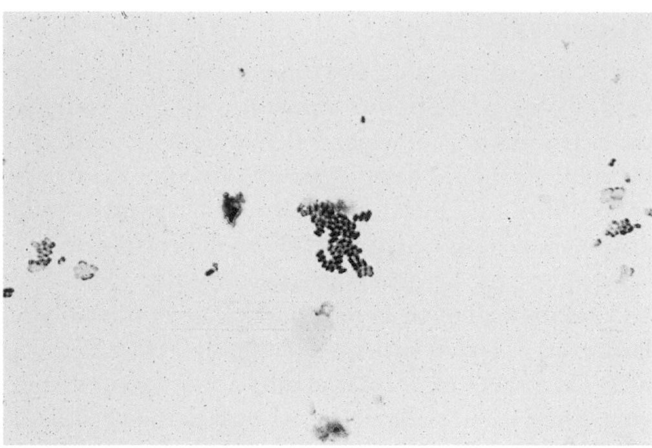

Figure 2-4 Gram stain of *Streptococcus mutans*. *S. mutans* can appear as cocci or even elongate to resemble bacilli, as demonstrated by the Gram stain shown here. The organisms shown were grown on blood agar overnight; however, growth in acidified broth is reported to also produce elongated forms of this organism.

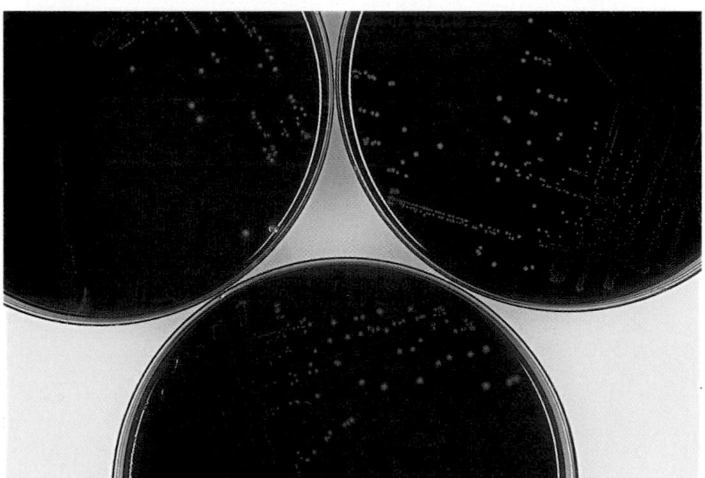

Figure 2-5 Beta-, alpha-, and gamma-hemolysis on blood agar. A key characteristic commonly used in identifying *Streptococcus* spp. is the type of hemolysis produced on blood agar. The three types of hemolysis are gamma-hemolysis (or no hemolysis); alpha-hemolysis, which appears as a greening of the agar around the bacterial colony; and beta-hemolysis, in which the red cells surrounding the colony are completely lysed, which results in a clear zone around the colony. Pictured are streptococci on blood agar that produce beta-hemolysis (top left), alpha-hemolysis (top right), or gamma-hemolysis (bottom).

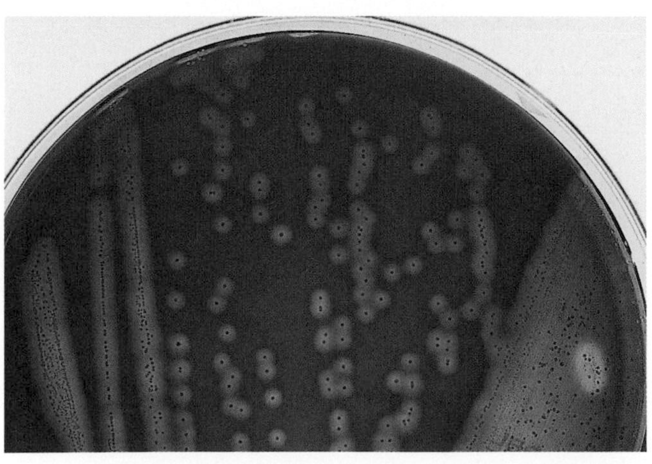

Figure 2-6 *Streptococcus pyogenes* on blood agar. *S. pyogenes* (group A streptococcus) produces a large zone of beta-hemolysis around a relatively small colony. This organism typically is translucent and has the appearance of a small water drop on a larger zone of beta-hemolysis. Colonies have a defined, smooth edge. Undercutting the agar, as shown in the lower right corner of this plate, often results in an "exaggerated" hemolytic reaction, due to reduced oxygen and the resulting contribution of both the oxygen-stable and -labile hemolysins.

Figure 2-7 *Streptococcus pyogenes* and *Streptococcus constellatus* on blood agar. *S. pyogenes* (right), referred to as large-colony group A streptococcus, can be confused with *S. constellatus* (*S. milleri*) (left), small-colony group A streptococcus, because both type with Lancefield group A antisera and are beta-hemolytic on blood agar. The blood agar plates shown were incubated for 48 h, and there is a marked difference in the colony size, with colonies of *S. constellatus* being smaller.

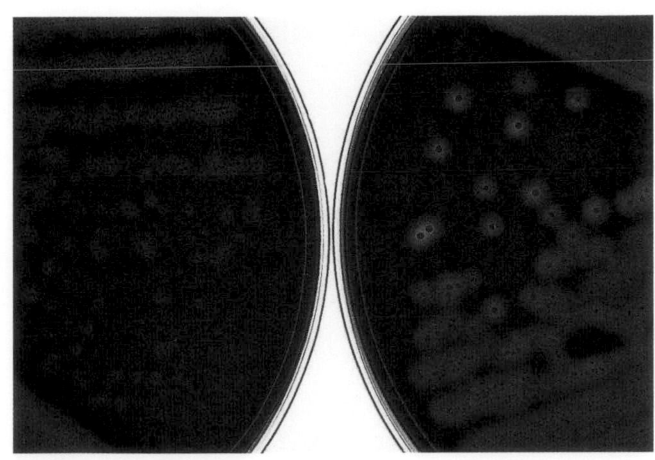

Figure 2-8 *Streptococcus agalactiae* on blood agar. In contrast to *S. pyogenes* (right), which produces a large zone of beta-hemolysis relative to the colony size, *S. agalactiae* (left), or group B streptococcus, produces a smaller zone of beta-hemolysis relative to the larger colony. The blood agar plate shown here was incubated for 24 h.

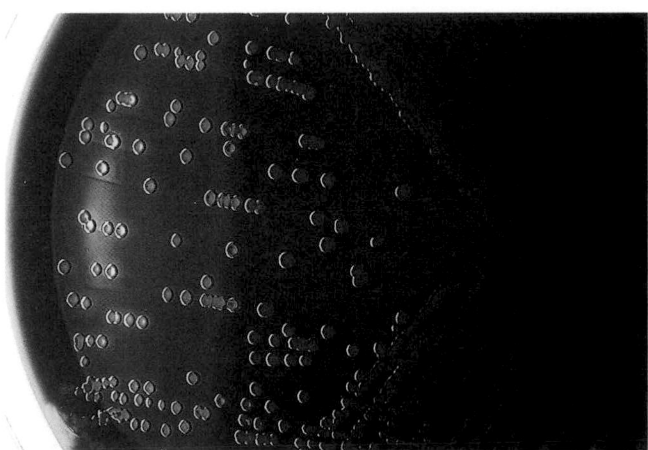

Figure 2-9 *Streptococcus pneumoniae* on blood agar. When grown on blood agar, *S. pneumoniae* produces a zone of alpha-hemolysis and the middle of the colony often appears to be indented or "punched out" due to autolysis of organisms in the center of the growing colony.

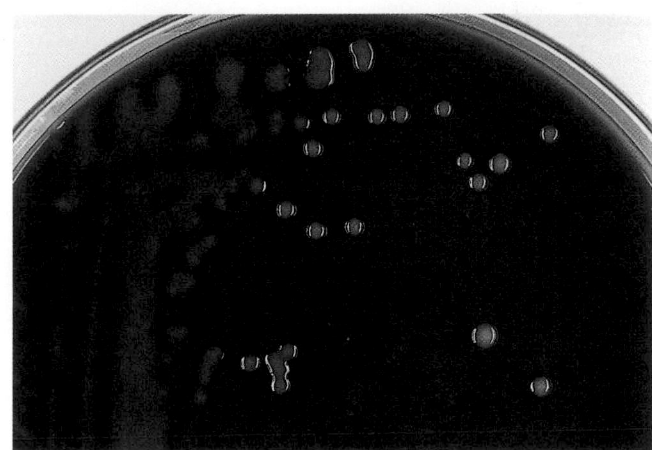

Figure 2-10 *Streptococcus pneumoniae* with a large capsule grown on chocolate agar. This strain of *S. pneumoniae*, in contrast to the *S. pneumoniae* strain in Fig. 2-9, appears mucoid when grown on chocolate agar. The mucoid appearance is related to capsule production.

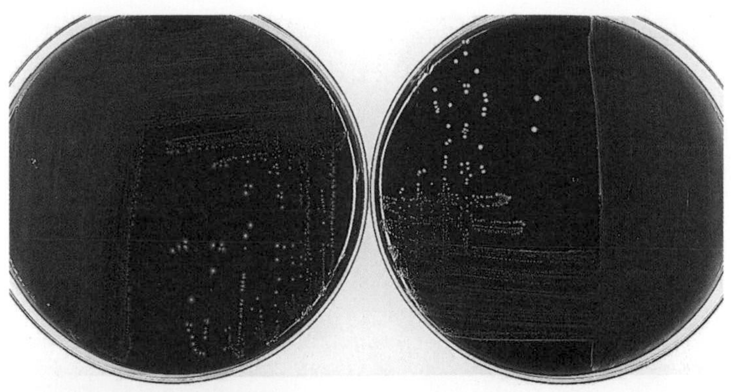

Figure 2-11 *Streptococcus bovis* group (group D) and *Enterococcus faecium* on blood agar. In general, on blood agar, members of the bovis group (left) produce alpha-hemolytic colonies that, as shown, can be confused with *E. faecium* (right).

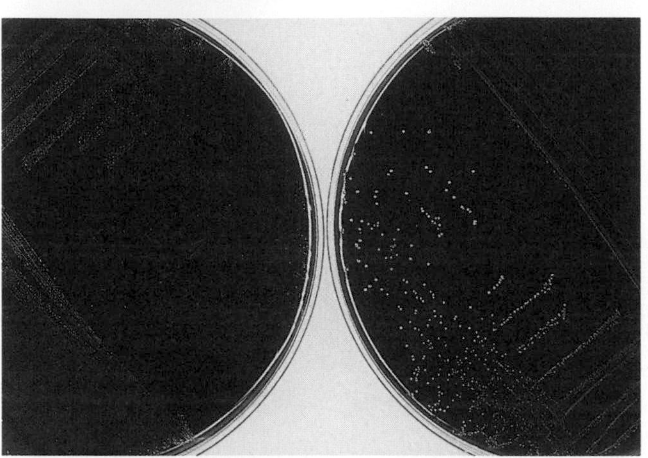

Figure 2-12 Growth enhancement of *Streptococcus constellatus* in the presence of 5% CO_2. Viridans streptococci belonging to the anginosus group frequently grow better in 5% CO_2 or under anaerobic conditions than under aerobic conditions. This is demonstrated here for *S. constellatus*, which was grown on blood agar and incubated overnight in air (left) or in the presence of 5% CO_2 (right).

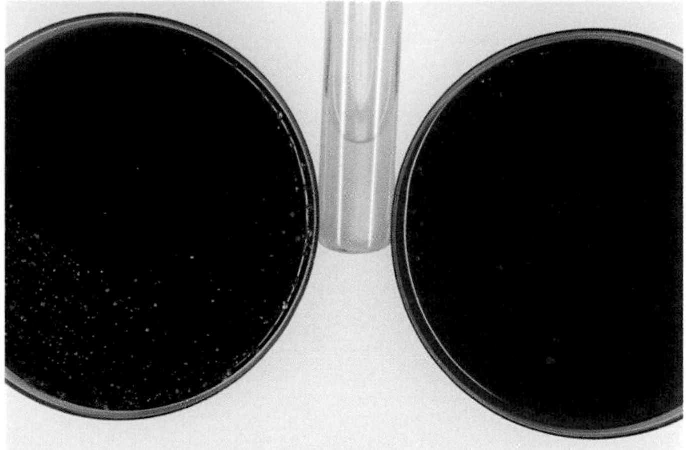

Figure 2-13 Selection for *Streptococcus agalactiae* (group B streptococcus). Pregnant females are screened for the presence of *S. agalactiae* at 35 to 37 weeks of gestation by obtaining a vaginal-anorectal swab. Specimens are plated onto blood agar and placed in a selective broth containing antibiotics such as the LIM broth shown here. If *S. agalactiae* is not isolated from blood agar after overnight incubation, the enhancement broth is subcultured to blood agar and incubated overnight. In the culture shown, *S. agalactiae* was not isolated from the primary blood plate (left); however, in the subculture (right) of the LIM broth (center), there was marked enhancement in the growth of *S. agalactiae*.

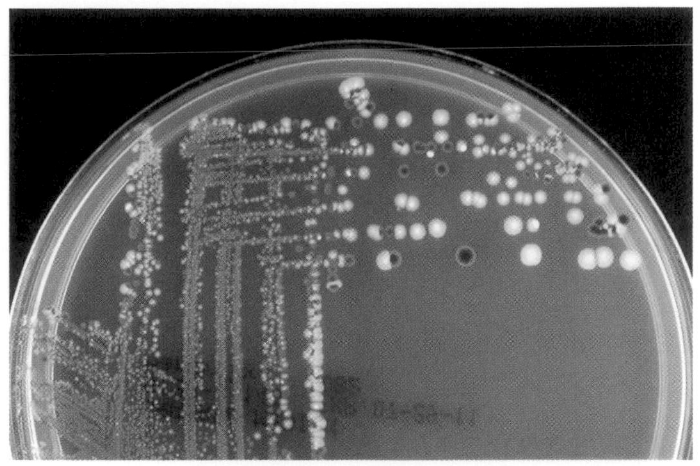

Figure 2-14 Granada agar for the detection of *Streptococcus agalactiae* from clinical specimens. An alternate method to that described in Fig. 2-13 for detection of *S. agalactiae* (group B streptococcus) in vaginal-anorectal swabs from pregnant females is to plate specimens directly onto Granada agar and incubate overnight. Colonies that appear orange, as shown, can be reported as *S. agalactiae*.

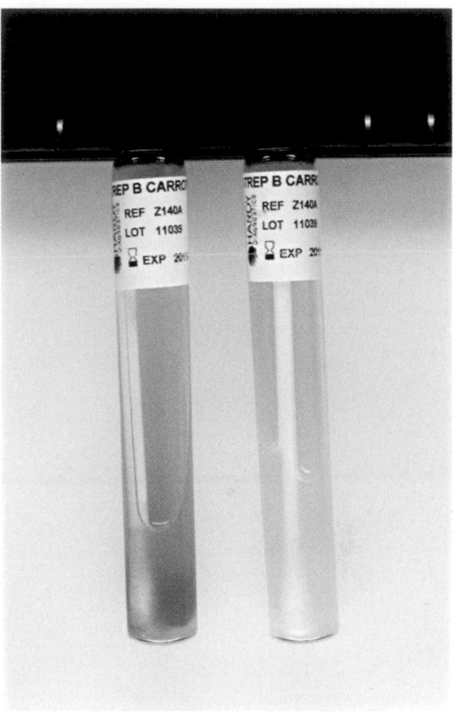

Figure 2-15 Carrot broth for the direct detection of *Streptococcus agalactiae*. Carrot broth can be used to both enrich for and identify *S. agalactiae* (group B streptococcus). Vaginal-anorectal swabs from pregnant females are placed in the broth and incubated overnight. Development of an orange color indicates the presence of *S. agalactiae*. If no orange color develops, yet there is growth in the broth, it is subcultured to rule out the presence of *S. agalactiae*.

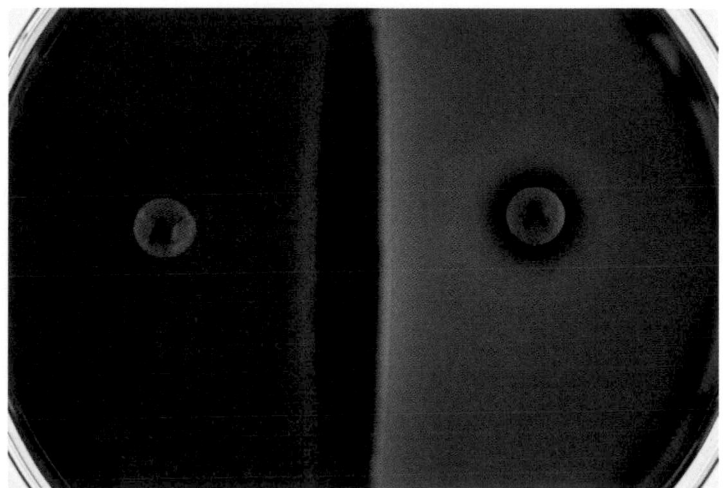

Figure 2-16 Bacitracin susceptibility test for the presumptive identification of *Streptococcus pyogenes* (group A streptococcus). The bacitracin susceptibility test is a common test used to presumptively distinguish group A streptococci from other beta-hemolytic streptococci. As shown, a paper disk impregnated with 0.04 U of bacitracin is able to inhibit the growth of *S. pyogenes* (right), in contrast to *S. agalactiae* (left), which is not inhibited and grows up to the disk. The formation of any zone of inhibition is considered a positive test. This test is an inexpensive way to identify *S. pyogenes* but is not highly specific or rapid, since 5 to 10% of other beta-hemolytic streptococci can also be inhibited and overnight incubation is required.

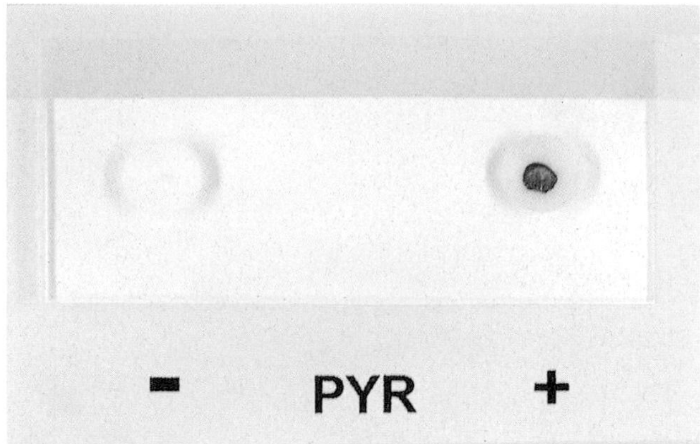

Figure 2-17 PYR test. The PYR test is a rapid, sensitive test for the identification of *S. pyogenes*. Many laboratories have replaced the bacitracin test with the PYR test for the presumptive identification of *S. pyogenes*. To perform this test, the isolate is rubbed onto a paper disk containing L-pyroglutamic acid β-naphthylamide. If the organism possesses the enzyme pyrrolidonyl arylamidase, it is able to degrade the substrate and β-naphthylamide is produced, which can be detected by the addition of *p*-dimethylamino-cinnamaldehyde (the PYR reagent). The isolate on the right is PYR positive (*S. pyogenes*), and the one on the left is negative.

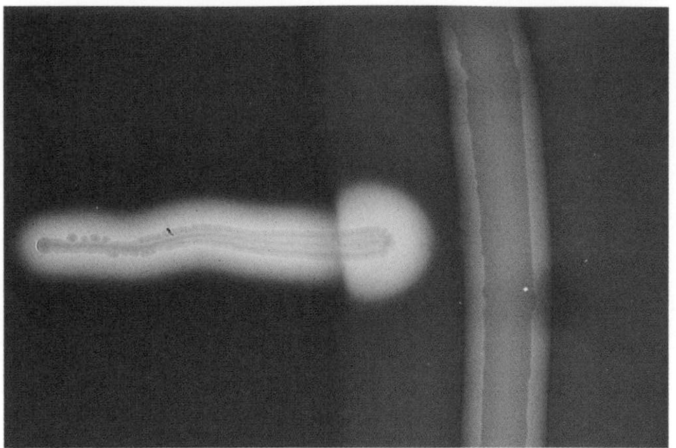

Figure 2-18 CAMP test for the identification of *Streptococcus agalactiae* (group B streptococcus). The CAMP test can be used to presumptively identify *S. agalactiae*. To perform the test, a beta-lysin-producing *Staphylococcus aureus* strain is inoculated in a thin line onto a blood agar plate. The isolate to be identified is inoculated at right angles to the *S. aureus* line, taking care that the two streak lines do not touch. After overnight incubation, if the isolate is *S. agalactiae*, the area of beta-hemolysis where the two organisms have grown in proximity to one another should take the shape of an arrowhead due to the synergistic action of the hemolysins produced by both organisms.

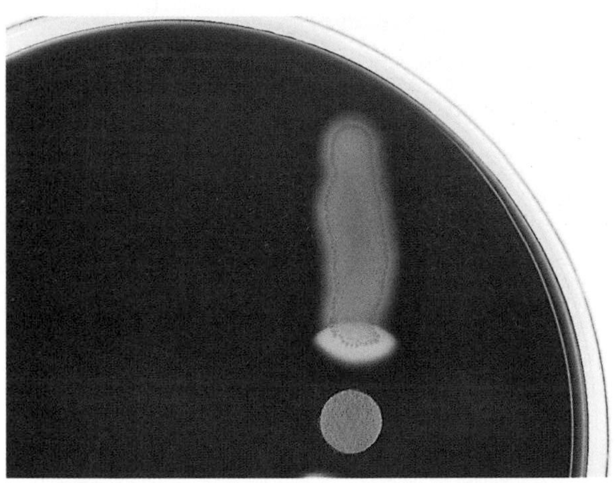

Figure 2-19 CAMP test using a beta-lysin disk. The CAMP test, as shown in Fig. 2-18, can also be performed with disks that have been impregnated with beta-lysin (Thermo Scientific Remel Products, Lenexa, KS). Here the organism to be identified is inoculated in a straight line within 5 mm of the disk and the culture is incubated overnight. If the isolate is *S. agalactiae*, as shown here, beta-hemolysis can be seen in the shape of a football or a crescent.

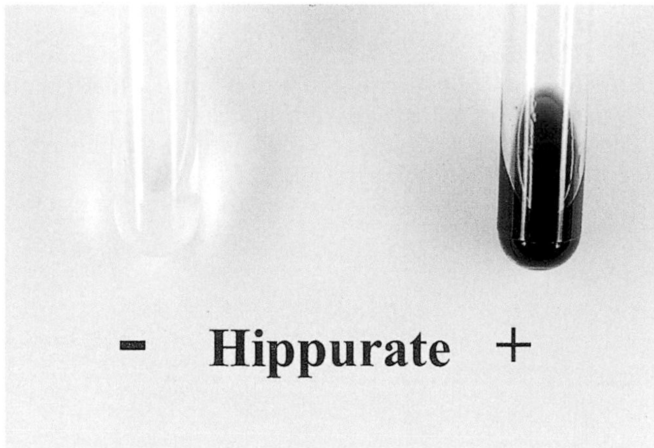

Figure 2-20 Hippurate test for the identification of *Streptococcus agalactiae*. As shown, *S. agalactiae* (right) is hippurate positive, in contrast to other beta-hemolytic streptococci (left).

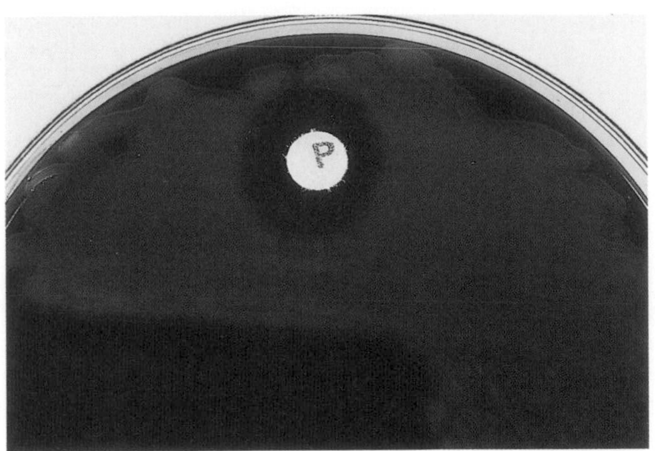

Figure 2-21 Optochin susceptibility for the identification of *Streptococcus pneumoniae*. Growth of *S. pneumoniae* is inhibited in the presence of optochin. On inoculation of blood agar with *S. pneumoniae*, a paper disk impregnated with 5 μg of optochin is placed firmly on the plate. After overnight incubation at 35°C in the presence of 5% CO_2, the formation of a zone of growth inhibition of >14 mm in diameter is considered presumptive identification of *S. pneumoniae*.

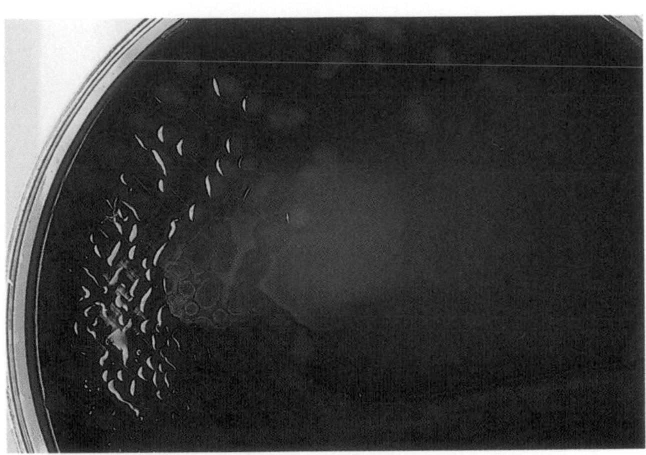

Figure 2-22 Bile solubility test for the identification of *Streptococcus pneumoniae*. The bile solubility test can be used to differentiate *S. pneumoniae* from other alpha-hemolytic streptococci. Here, colonies of *S. pneumoniae* on blood agar disappear or dissolve when a drop of 2% sodium deoxycholate is placed on the colonies and the plate is incubated for 30 min at 35°C.

Figure 2-23 Production of BGUR. Beta-hemolytic members of the anginosus (milleri) group can be confused with streptococci belonging to groups C and G. The BGUR test can help to distinguish between them. In this test, the substrate, methylumbelliferyl-β-D-glucuronide, can be broken down by β-D-glucuronidase to produce a fluorescent compound. As shown here, a heavy inoculum of both an isolate of group C and one belonging to the anginosus group was placed on a MacConkey agar plate containing methylumbelliferyl-β-D-glucuronide (BD Diagnostic Systems, Franklin Lakes, NJ). The plates were incubated for 30 min at 35°C and viewed under long-wave UV light. Fluorescence produced by the group C isolate (upper right quadrant) distinguished it from the nonfluorescent anginosus isolate (lower left quadrant).

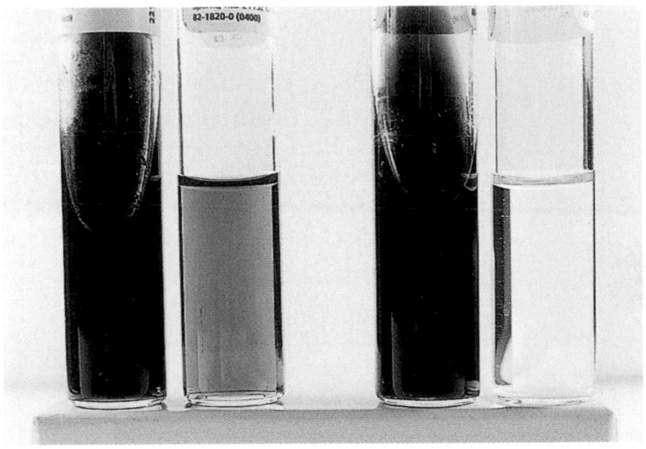

Figure 2-24 Differentiation of the *Streptococcus bovis* group from *Enterococcus faecium*. Bile esculin agar slants and 6.5% salt broth are often used in the differentiation and identification of alpha-hemolytic streptococci. In the example shown here, it can be difficult to distinguish the *S. bovis* group from *E. faecium* because colonies of these two organisms appear similar (Fig. 2-11) and because, when inoculated on a bile esculin slant, both organisms are able to grow in the presence of 40% bile and hydrolyze esculin, which results in blackening of the medium. However, *E. faecium* (right) can grow in the high-salt (6.5%) solution, as demonstrated by the color change of the broth from purple to yellow, in contrast to the *S. bovis* group isolate (left).

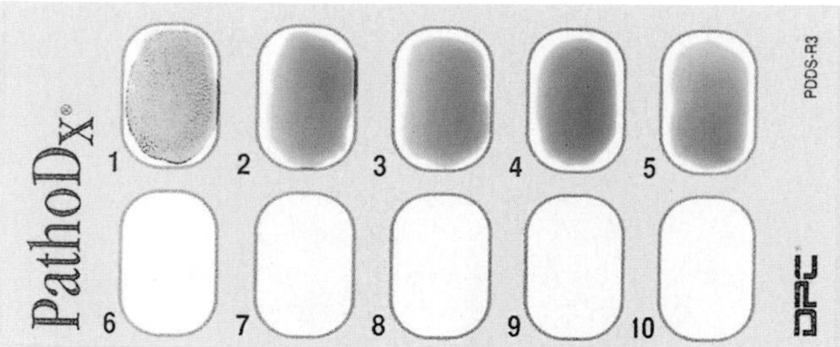

Figure 2-25 Latex agglutination test for the identification of Lancefield groups. Beta-hemolytic streptococci can be grouped on the basis of their Lancefield antigen. A common method to accomplish this involves latex agglutination using monoclonal antibodies coupled to latex particles. In the test shown here (PathoDX; Thermo Scientific Remel Products), a dye is incorporated into the latex reagent to facilitate visualization of the agglutination reaction. Most commercial kits contain reagents for groups A, B, C, F, and G, which are displayed in wells 1 through 5, respectively, in this typing reaction. The isolate shown is *S. pyogenes* (group A streptococcus).

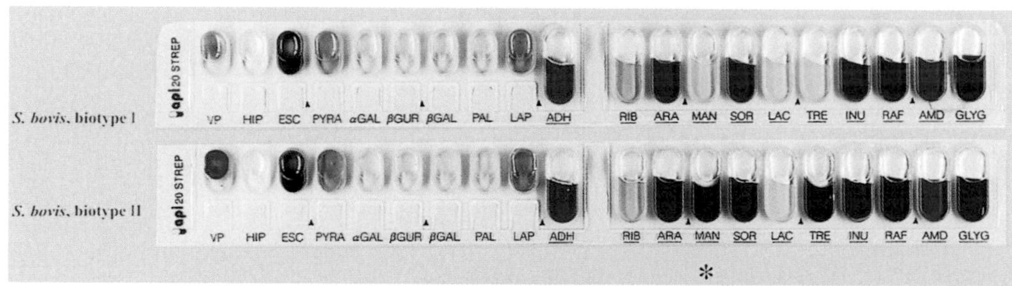

Figure 2-26 API 20 Strep test for the identification of streptococci. The API 20 Strep strip (bioMérieux, Inc., Durham, NC) can be used to identify or group more common clinically relevant streptococci. It consists of microtubes, enabling the simultaneous determination of 20 biochemical reactions. In the example shown, *S. bovis* I is differentiated from *S. bovis* II, a key reaction being mannitol fermentation (*).

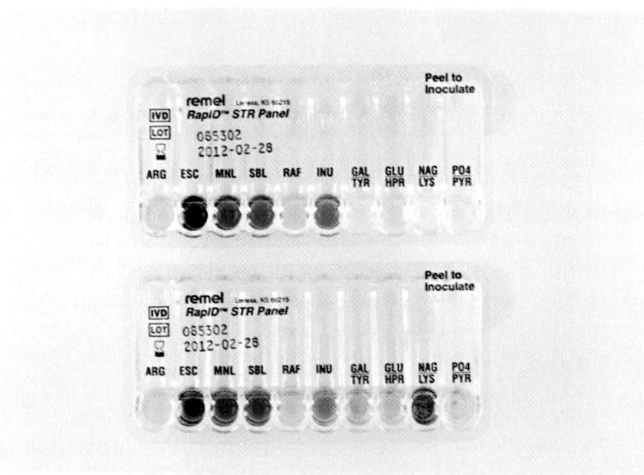

Figure 2-27 RapID STR system for the identification of streptococci. The RapID STR system (Thermo Scientific Remel Products) utilizes conventional and chromogenic substrates for the identification of streptococci. This system has 10 reaction wells. However, since the last four wells are bifunctional, in that a second reaction can be read when reagents are added to the wells, a total of 14 biochemical reactions are available. Along with the hemolysis reaction of the organisms, this system has the ability to identify most medically relevant streptococci. As with most commercial systems, not all identifications correlate with those obtained by a conventional biochemical battery. In the example shown, the isolate is identified as *S. salivarius*. The test shown in the upper panel was read before the reagents were added to the bifunctional wells as shown in the lower panel.

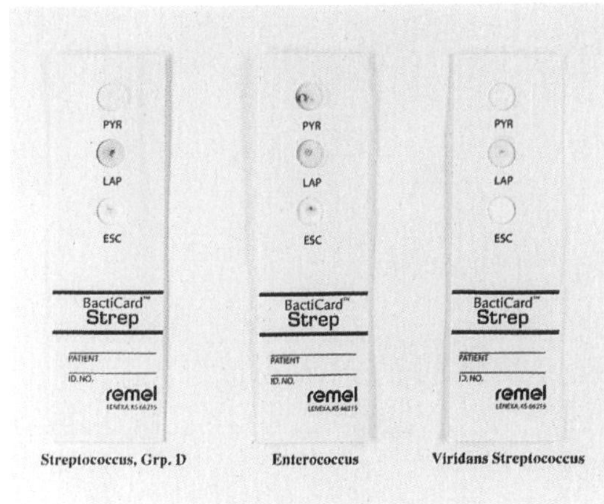

Figure 2-28 The BactiCard. The BactiCard (Thermo Scientific Remel Products) is a rapid system for the presumptive identification of streptococci. It tests for pyrrolidonyl arylamidase (PYR), leucine arylamidase (LAP), and esculin hydrolysis activity (ESC). Colonies of catalase-negative, gram-positive cocci are inoculated directly onto the three moistened sections of the strip, which is then incubated for 10 min at room temperature. Examples of typical reaction patterns for the following three organisms are shown: group D streptococcus (*S. bovis* group), LAP and ESC positive; *Enterococcus* spp., PYR, LAP, and ESC positive; viridans streptococci, LAP positive.

Enterococcus 3

Members of the genus *Enterococcus* are gram-positive cocci that can survive harsh conditions in nature and thus are ubiquitous, being found in soil, water, and plants. They colonize the gastrointestinal and genital tracts of humans. While there are more than 15 species in this genus, 80 to 90% of clinical isolates are *Enterococcus faecalis*, with the majority of the remainder made up of *Enterococcus faecium*. Less frequently encountered clinical species include *Enterococcus gallinarum*, *Enterococcus casseliflavus*, *Enterococcus avium*, and *Enterococcus raffinosus*. Other enterococcal species are rarely recovered from human specimens.

It is often difficult to establish whether an *Enterococcus* strain is contributing to the infection or is colonizing a site. However, enterococci are now one of the three leading causes of nosocomial bloodstream infections and can be the cause of nosocomially acquired urinary tract infections. Enterococci also play a role in wound infections and endocarditis. They only rarely cause infections of the central nervous system and respiratory tract. They have been an increasingly important cause of infection in elderly and immunocompromised individuals, in part due to the emerging resistance of these organisms to antimicrobial agents.

In the last decade, the nosocomial spread of vancomycin-resistant enterococci (VRE) has become a major challenge. In general, enterococcal isolates with reduced susceptibility to vancomycin can be categorized as *vanA*, *vanB*, and *vanC*. *vanA* and *vanB* strains pose the greatest threat because they are more resistant and the resistance genes are carried on a plasmid or by a transposon and thus are readily transferable. *vanA* isolates, predominantly *E. faecium* and occasionally *E. faecalis* strains, are typically associated with vancomycin MICs of ≥256 μg/ml and are also resistant to teicoplanin. The *vanC* strains, predominantly *E. gallinarum* and *E. casseliflavus*, are associated with lower vancomycin MICs (2 to 32 μg/ml), and the resistance appears to be constitutive and chromosomally mediated. *vanC* strains do not seem to contribute to the spread of vancomycin resistance. Occasional enterococcal strains that are vancomycin dependent have been reported. These strains grow only on media that provide a source of vancomycin.

Due to the growing importance of VRE, selective and differential media as well as molecular assays have been developed that have facilitated the rapid detection of these organisms. Selective media, e.g., *Camplyobacter* agar, and selective chromogenic media containing vancomycin have been employed to detect this organism in rectal swabs and feces. Molecular assays have been described that enable the identification of VRE directly from specimens or after broth enrichment from fecal specimens. One limitation is the specificity of the direct molecular assays, since some of the *van* genes can be found in other genera.

Enterococci typically are arranged in pairs and short chains; however, under certain growth conditions they elongate and appear coccobacillary. In general, enterococci are alpha-hemolytic or nonhemolytic; however, depending on the type of blood agar used, they may be beta-hemolytic. Some strains possess the group D Lancefield antigen and can be detected using monoclonal antibody-based agglutination tests. Enterococci are typically catalase negative, grow over a wide temperature range from 10 to 42°C, and are facultatively anaerobic.

Characteristically they are able to grow in 6.5% NaCl, hydrolyze esculin in the presence of 40% bile salts, and are pyrrolidonyl arylamidase and leucine arylamidase positive.

While different schemes for identification of enterococcal species have been proposed, the more common enterococcal isolates can be differentiated by a few key biochemical reactions. Utilization of arabinose, motility, acidification of methyl-α-D-glucopyranoside, and pigment can be used to identify most *E. faecalis*, *E. faecium*, *E. gallinarum*, and *E. casseliflavus* strains to the species level. Addition of sorbase and raffinose allows species identification of the less frequently isolated *E. avium* and *E. raffinosus*. Commercial identification systems to differentiate among the species are available. While these systems can identify the more frequently isolated species, they are not as reliable with the less common isolates.

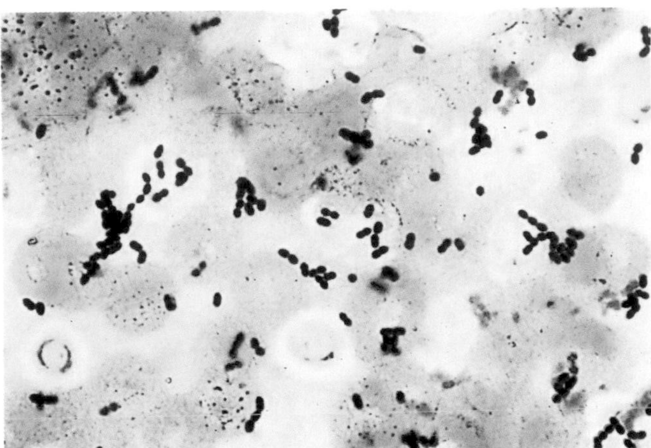

Figure 3-1 Gram stain of *Enterococcus faecalis*. Shown is *E. faecalis* obtained from a blood culture. This organism is described as gram-positive cocci in pairs and short chains.

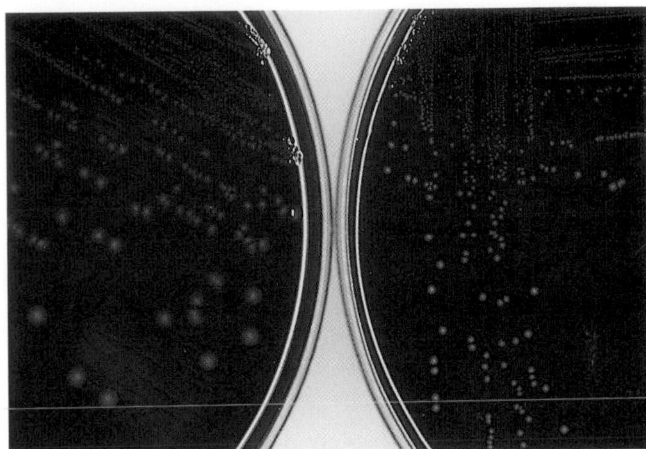

Figure 3-2 *Enterococcus faecium* and *Enterococcus faecalis* on blood agar. *E. faecalis* (left) forms a nonhemolytic, flat, gray colony with a smooth, translucent edge. In comparison, colonies of *E. faecium* (right) are surrounded by a small zone of alpha-hemolysis and have a defined opaque edge.

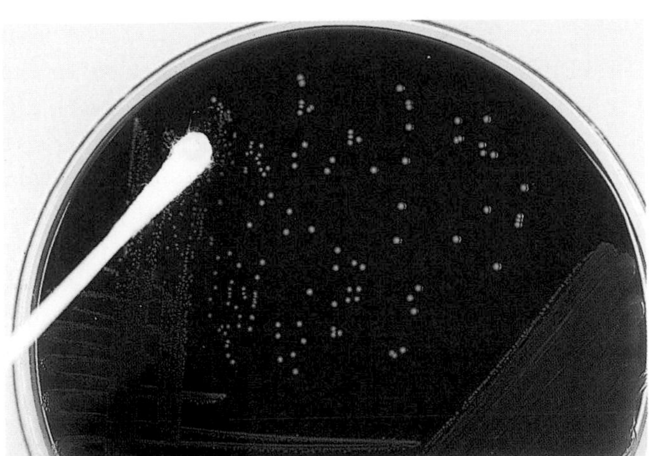

Figure 3-3 *Enterococcus casseliflavus* on blood agar. The typical yellow pigment of *E. casseliflavus* is most easily seen by picking up colonies with a cotton swab.

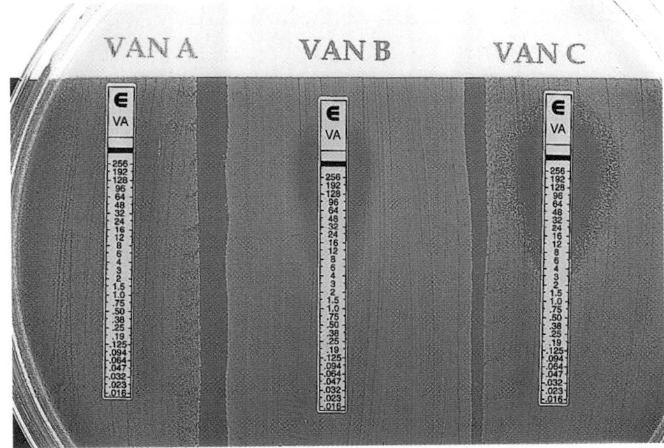

Figure 3-4 Comparison of vancomycin susceptibility of *vanA*, *vanB*, and *vanC Enterococcus* strains. In general, the E-test can be used to categorize enterococci into three main groups, *vanA*, *vanB*, and *vanC*, based on the vancomycin MIC. The *vanA* phenotype shown here is an *E. faecium* isolate with a high level of resistance to vancomycin. The *vanB* strain is an *E. faecalis* isolate for which the vancomycin MIC is 32 μg/ml. The *vanC* strain is an *E. gallinarium* isolate for which the vancomycin MIC is 16 μg/ml.

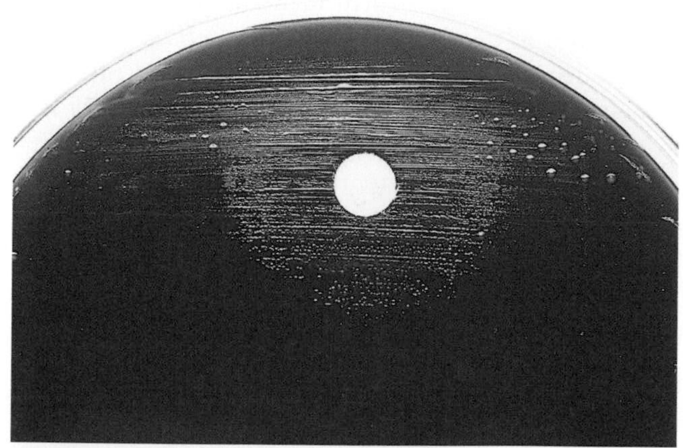

Figure 3-5 Vancomycin-dependent *Enterococcus faecalis* strain. This strain, isolated from a rectal culture, initially grew on *Campylobacter* medium containing 10 μg of vancomycin per ml but upon subculture failed to grow on blood agar. As seen here, the vancomycin (30 μg) in the disk supports the growth of this isolate on blood agar.

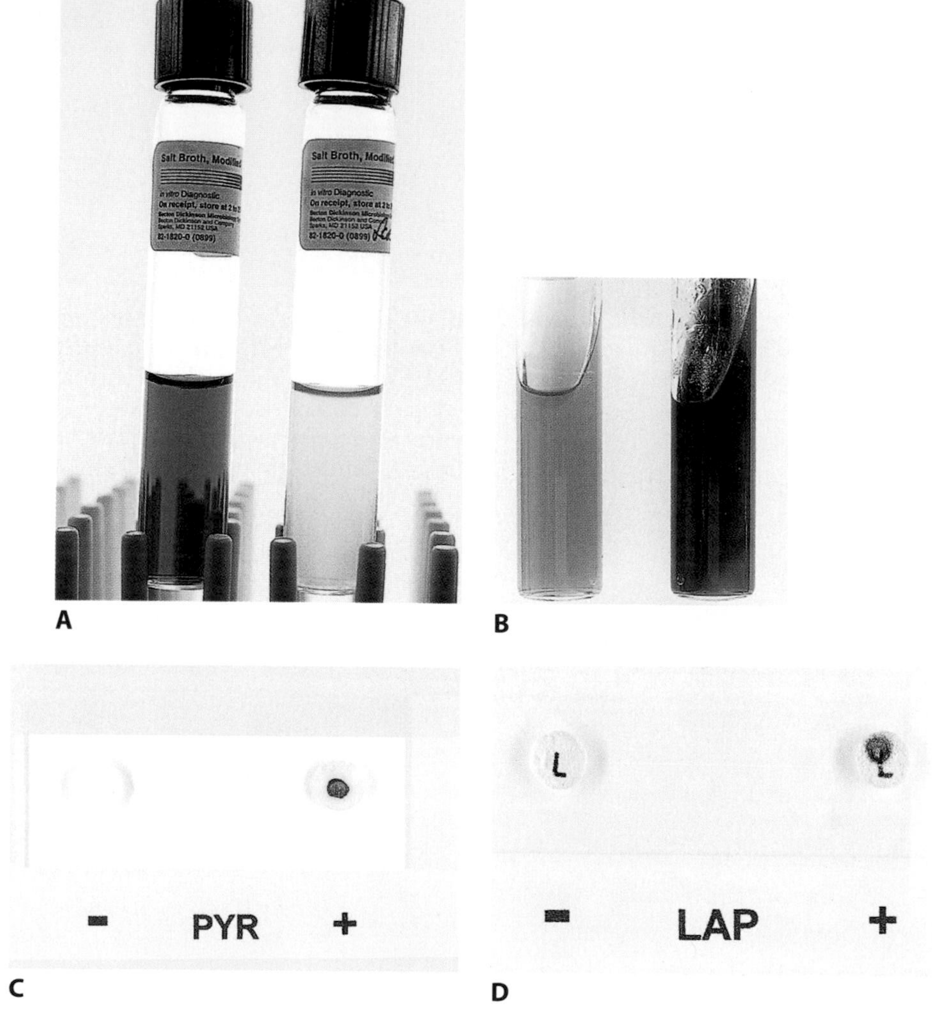

Figure 3-6 Biochemicals used to identify *Enterococcus* spp. A typical biochemical profile of the genus *Enterococcus* is growth in the presence of 6.5% NaCl (A), growth on media containing 40% bile salts and the ability to hydrolyze esculin (B), pyrrolidonyl arylamidase (PYR) positive (C), and leucine arylamidase (LAP) positive (D). A nonenterococcal isolate negative for each reaction is shown on the left, and the positive reactions typical of *Entercoccus* spp. are shown on the right.

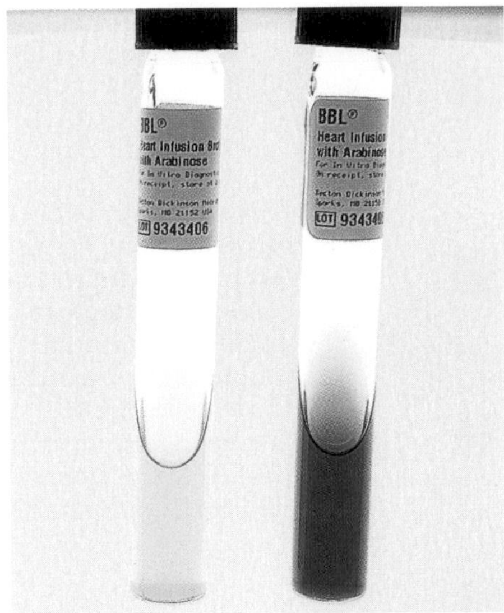

Figure 3-7 Arabinose utilization. Arabinose utilization can be used to separate *E. faecalis* from *E. faecium*. Brain heart infusion broth containing arabinose with a bromcresol purple indicator was inoculated with *E. faecium* (left) and *E. faecalis* (right). A positive reaction, as seen here with *E. faecium*, is yellow, and a negative reaction, with *E. faecalis*, is the original purple color of the medium.

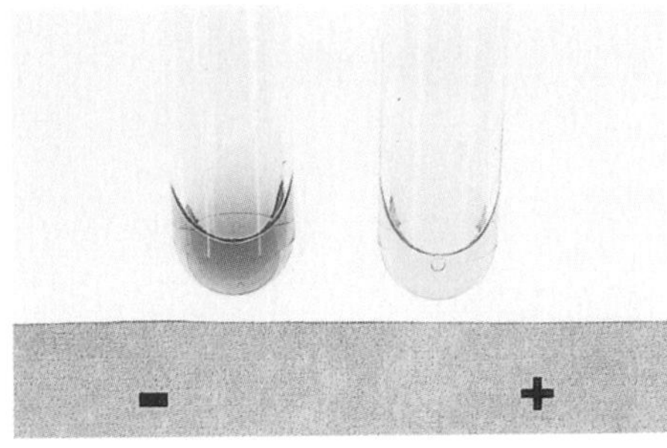

Figure 3-8 Acidification of methyl-α-D-glucopyranoside. A test that can distinguish *E. faecium* from *E. gallinarum* and *E. casseliflavus* is acidification of 1% methyl-α-D-glucopyranoside. *E. faecium* (left) does not utilize this compound, as demonstrated by the lack of change of color of the phenol red indicator. The other two species can utilize this compound, as illustrated by the yellow color of the broth inoculated with *E. gallinarum* (right), indicating acidification of the medium. The broths were incubated overnight at 35°C.

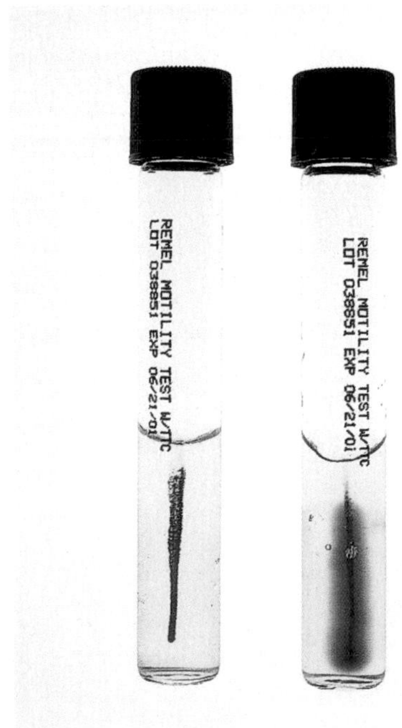

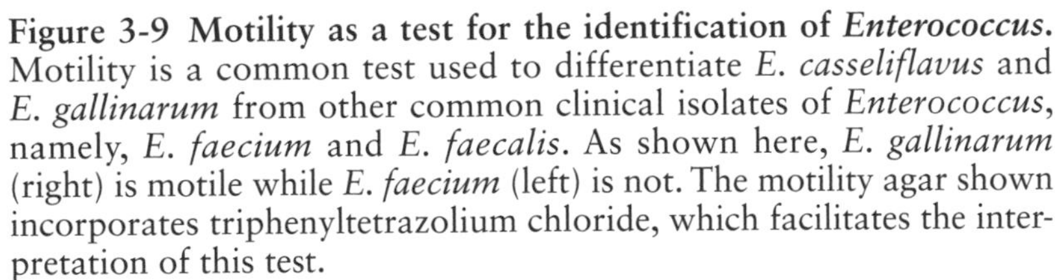
Figure 3-9 Motility as a test for the identification of *Enterococcus*. Motility is a common test used to differentiate *E. casseliflavus* and *E. gallinarum* from other common clinical isolates of *Enterococcus*, namely, *E. faecium* and *E. faecalis*. As shown here, *E. gallinarum* (right) is motile while *E. faecium* (left) is not. The motility agar shown incorporates triphenyltetrazolium chloride, which facilitates the interpretation of this test.

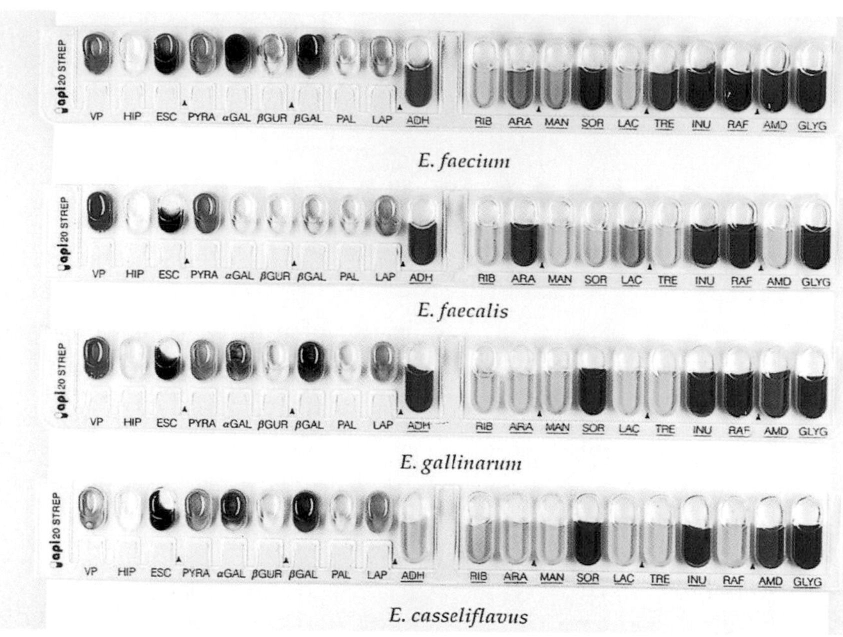

Figure 3-10 Identification of enterococci by the API 20 Strep test. Kits for the identification of streptococci can be used to differentiate the more common enterococcal isolates. Shown here are four species of *Enterococcus* inoculated into API 20 Strep strips (bioMérieux, Inc., Durham, NC).

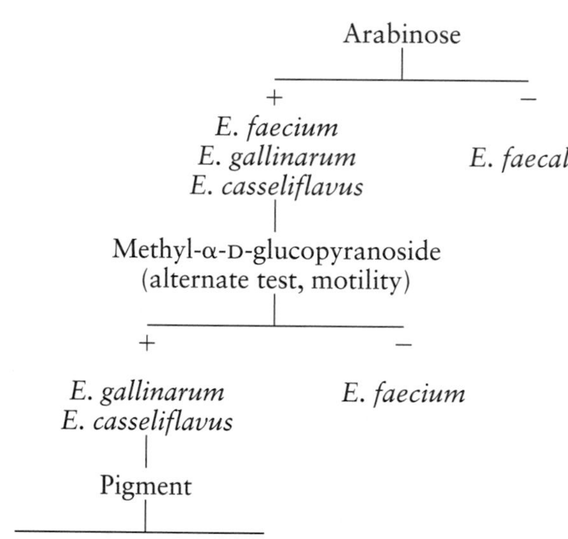

Figure 3-11 Simplified algorithm for identification of the more common clinical isolates of enterococci. Reactions with some of the biochemicals and tests may vary, depending on the species and strain.

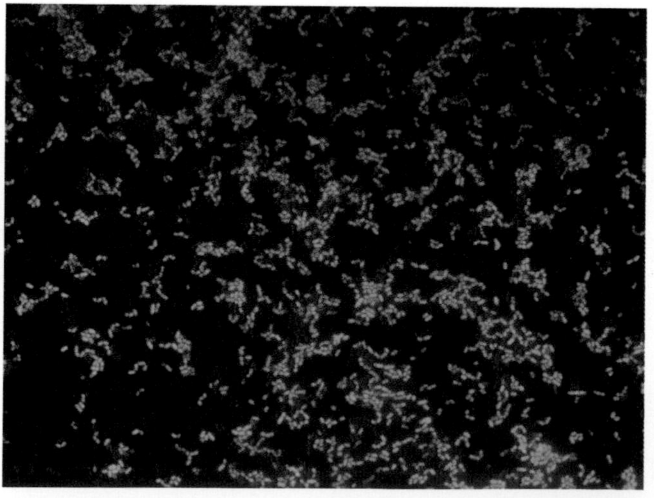

Figure 3-12 PNA FISH for the direct identification of *Enterococcus*. A blood culture positive for gram-positive cocci in short chains and pairs was tested by PNA FISH (AdvanDx, Woburn, MA). This is a 90-min fluorescent in situ hybridization (FISH) assay that utilizes fluorescent-labeled peptide nucleic acid (PNA). PNA FISH can detect *E. faecalis* (green) and other *Enterococcus* spp. (red). These probes target the species-specific rRNA in these organisms and can easily penetrate the bacterial cell wall and membrane. Shown is a mixed culture positive for both *E. faecalis* (green) and *E. faecium* (red). (Photo courtesy of AdvanDX.)

Aerococcus, *Abiotrophia*, and Other Miscellaneous Gram-Positive Cocci That Grow Aerobically

4

The organisms discussed in this chapter are catalase-negative, gram-positive cocci that can be found as members of the normal flora throughout the body and that, for the most part, cause opportunistic infections. They resemble, and as a result can be misidentified as, staphylococci and streptococci because of their microscopic and culture characteristics. In certain instances they are recognized only when presumptive streptococci are found to be resistant to vancomycin. The genera and species that are microscopically similar to *Staphylococcus* are *Aerococcus*, *Dolosigranulum*, *Gemella haemolysans*, *Helcococcus*, and *Pediococcus*. Those that resemble *Streptococcus* include *Abiotrophia*, *Dolosicoccus*, *Facklamia*, *Gemella* spp. other than *G. haemolysans*, *Globicatella*, *Granulicatella*, *Ignavigranum*, *Lactococcus*, *Leuconostoc*, *Vagococcus*, and *Weissella*. *Globicatella*, *Facklamia*, *Ignavigranum*, and *Dolosicoccus* are related genera that are infrequently isolated from clinical specimens.

The genus *Lactococcus* is composed of nonmotile organisms previously classified as Lancefield group N streptococci. However, the motile *Lactococcus*-like organisms with Lancefield group N antigen belong to the genus *Vagococcus*. Organisms previously classified as nutritionally deficient or satelliting streptococci are in the genera *Abiotrophia* and *Granulicatella*.

Although these organisms have low virulence, they can cause infections in immunocompromised patients. Infections usually occur following prolonged hospitalizations, invasive procedures, damage to tissues, entry of foreign bodies, and antimicrobial therapy. *Aerococcus*, *Abiotrophia*, *Gemella*, *Pediococcus*, *Globicatella*, *Lactococcus*, and *Leuconostoc* have been isolated from patients with bacteremia and/or endocarditis, while *Helcococcus* has been isolated from wound cultures of the lower extremities, e.g., foot ulcers. *Aerococcus urinae* has been implicated in urinary tract infections, primarily in the elderly, and can cause lymphadenitis, endocarditis, and peritonitis. *Aerococcus sanguinicola* and *Aerococcus urinaehominis* have also been isolated from urine.

As expected, the *Staphylococcus*-like organisms appear in pairs, tetrads, and clusters and the *Streptococcus*-like bacteria are arranged in pairs and chains. However, *Gemella* can appear gram variable or gram negative, and *Abiotrophia*, along with *Granulicatella*, may form coccobacilli in pairs and chains or may be pleomorphic if grown on nutritionally deficient media. Microscopic morphologic assessment should be made from cells grown in a broth medium such as thioglycolate.

These organisms are facultative anaerobes with the exception of *Aerococcus viridans*, which is microaerophilic because it grows poorly or not at all under anaerobic conditions. Most of these organisms grow well on chocolate agar and blood agar; the exceptions are *Abiotrophia* and *Granulicatella*. A test for satelliting is important for identification of these two genera. The organism is inoculated for confluent growth onto sheep blood agar. A single cross streak of *Staphylococcus aureus* (ATCC 25923) is applied to the inoculated area. Following incubation at 35°C in CO_2, strains of *Abiotrophia* and *Granulicatella* grow only in the area of staphylococcal growth. Alternatively, media can be supplemented with pyridoxal, which can be supplied in the form of a disk. *Helcococcus* grows slowly, requiring 48 to 72 h of incubation before visible colonies can be detected. These organisms grow best when incubated anaerobically and growth is stimulated by addition of 1% horse blood or 0.1% Tween 80 to the medium. Thayer-Martin medium may be used for the selective isolation of pyrrolidonyl aminopeptidase (pyrrolidonyl arylamidase) (PYR)-negative, vancomycin-resistant *Leuconostoc*, *Pediococcus*, and *Weissella* strains. Growth temperature characteristics are also important in differentiating *Lactococcus* from streptococci and enterococci. *Lactococcus* grows at 10 and 35°C, streptococci grow at 35°C, and some strains grow at 45°C, while enterococci grow at all three temperatures.

A few key tests that aid in the identification of these organisms include catalase production, esculin hydrolysis, growth in 6.5% NaCl, leucine aminopeptidase (LAP) and PYR production, and vancomycin susceptibility (Table 4-1). While most of these organisms are catalase negative and PYR positive, *Aerococcus viridans* may have a weak catalase-positive reaction, and *Aerococcus*, *Pediococcus*, *Leuconostoc*, and some strains of *Lactococcus* are PYR negative. LAP-negative genera include *Dolosicoccus*, *Globicatella*, *Helcococcus*, and *Leuconostoc*. Two species of *Aerococcus*, *A. urinaehominis* and *A. viridans*, are also LAP negative.

Table 4-1 Identification of miscellaneous gram-positive cocci that grow aerobically and have catalase-negative or weak reactions[a]

Organism	Esculin hydrolysis	LAP	PYR	Growth in 6.5% NaCl	VAN
Abiotrophia	V	+	+	0	S
Aerococcus viridans[b]	V	0	+	+	S
Aerococcus christensenii	ND	0	0	+	S
Aerococcus sanguicola	+	+	+	+	ND
Aerococcus urinae	V	+	0	+	S
Aerococcus urinaehominis	ND	0	0	ND	ND
Dolosicoccus	ND	0	+	0	S
Dolosigranulum	+	+	+	+	S
Facklamia	0	+	+	+	S
Gemella	0	+	+	0	S
Globicatella	+	0	V	+	S
Granulicatella	ND	+	+	0	S
Helcococcus	+	0	+	V	S
Inavigranum	0	+	+	+	S
Lactococcus	+	+	V	V	S
Leuconostoc	V	0	0	+	R
Pediococcus	V	+	0	V	R
Vagococcus	+	+	+	V	S
Weissella	V	0	0	+	R

[a]LAP, leucine aminopeptidase production; PYR, pyrrolidonyl aminopeptidase (pyrrolidonyl arylamidase) production; VAN, vancomycin susceptibility; +, positive; V, variable reaction; 0, negative; S, susceptible; R, resistant; ND, no data.

[b]Rare strains may be weakly catalase positive.

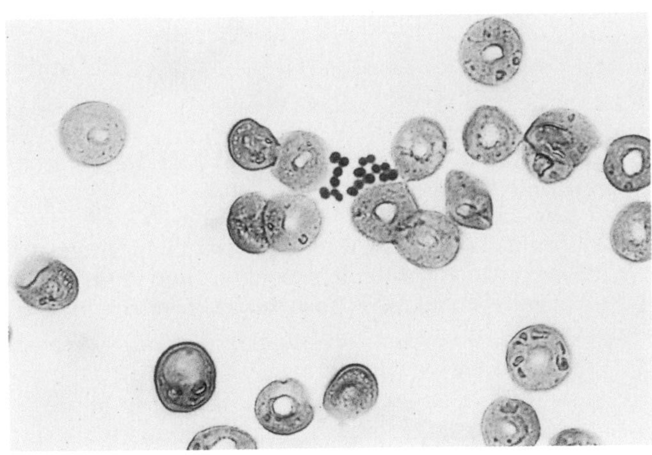

Figure 4-1 Gram stain of *Aerococcus viridans* from a blood culture. Microscopically *Aerococcus* strains resemble staphylococci, appearing as gram-positive cocci measuring approximately 1.0 to 2.0 μm in diameter. They are usually arranged in pairs, as shown here, or in tetrads when grown in liquid media.

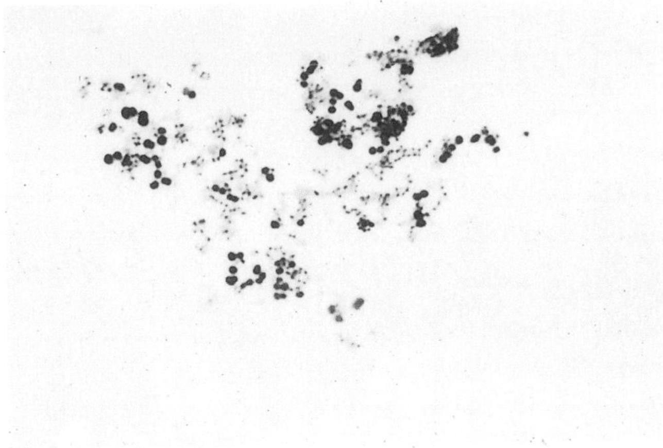

Figure 4-2 Gram stain of *Gemella*. Cells of *Gemella* can be spherical or elongated, measuring 0.5 to 0.8 μm by 0.5 to 1.4 μm. However, *G. haemolysans*, originally classified as *Neisseria* species due to its gram-variable or gram-negative nature, usually appears as diplococci that occur in pairs with adjacent flattened sides.

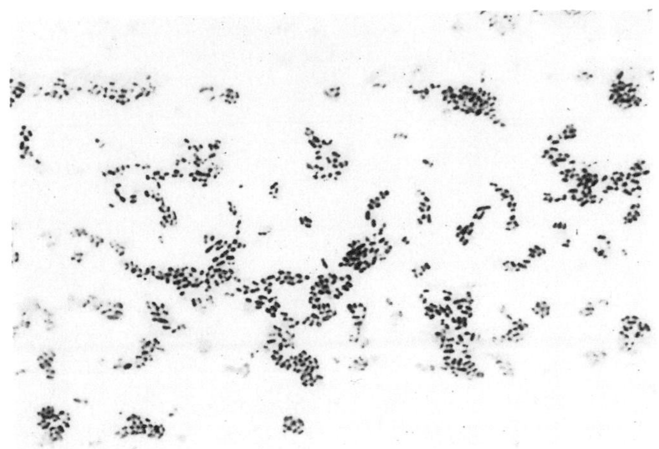

Figure 4-3 Gram stain of *Leuconostoc*. *Leuconostoc* cells are coccoid or coccobacillary with rounded ends, measuring 0.5 to 0.7 μm by 0.7 to 1.2 μm, and can form pairs and chains.

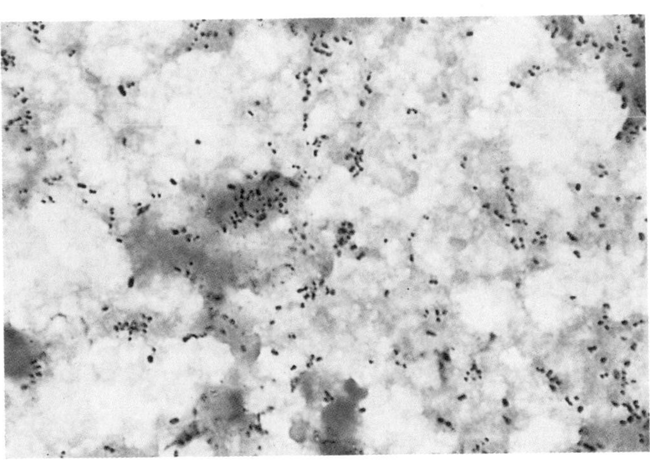

Figure 4-4 Gram stain of *Abiotrophia*. Microscopically, *Abiotrophia* spp. are tiny cocci or coccobacilli, measuring approximately 0.1 to 0.2 μm in diameter, arranged in pairs and/or long chains.

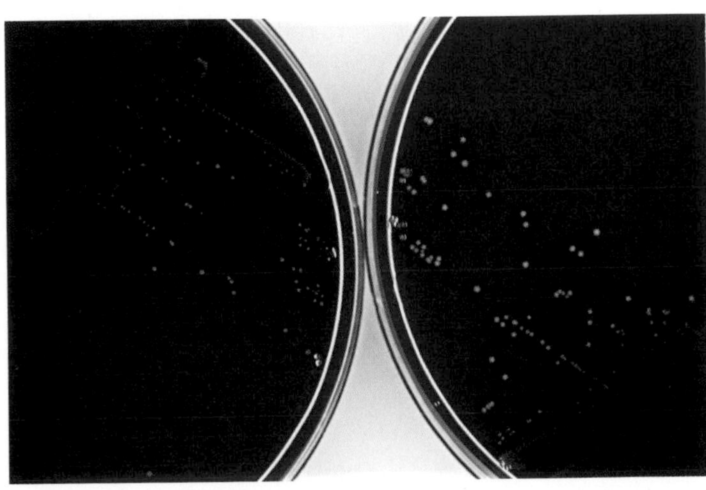

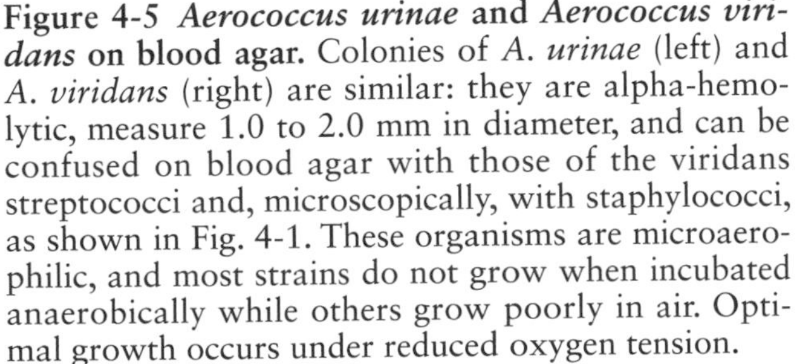

Figure 4-5 *Aerococcus urinae* and *Aerococcus viridans* on blood agar. Colonies of *A. urinae* (left) and *A. viridans* (right) are similar: they are alpha-hemolytic, measure 1.0 to 2.0 mm in diameter, and can be confused on blood agar with those of the viridans streptococci and, microscopically, with staphylococci, as shown in Fig. 4-1. These organisms are microaerophilic, and most strains do not grow when incubated anaerobically while others grow poorly in air. Optimal growth occurs under reduced oxygen tension.

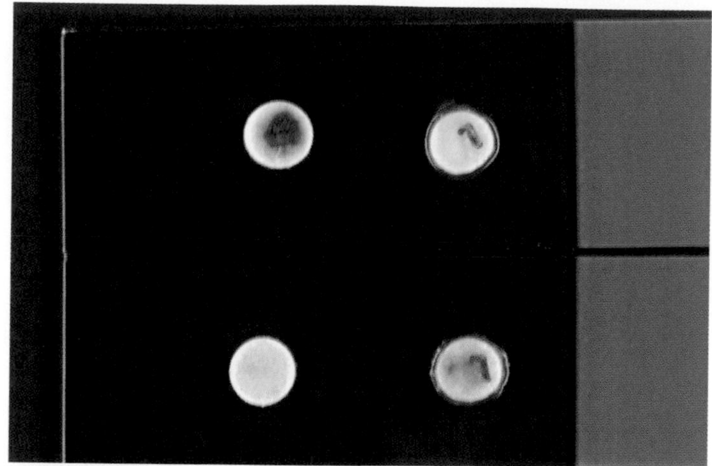

Figure 4-6 Production of PYR and LAP by *Aerococcus urinae* and *Aerococcus viridans*. *A. urinae* and *A. viridans* can be differentiated based on PYR (left) and LAP (right) reactions. *A. viridans* is PYR positive and LAP negative (top row, left to right), and *A. urinae* is PYR negative and LAP positive (bottom row, left to right).

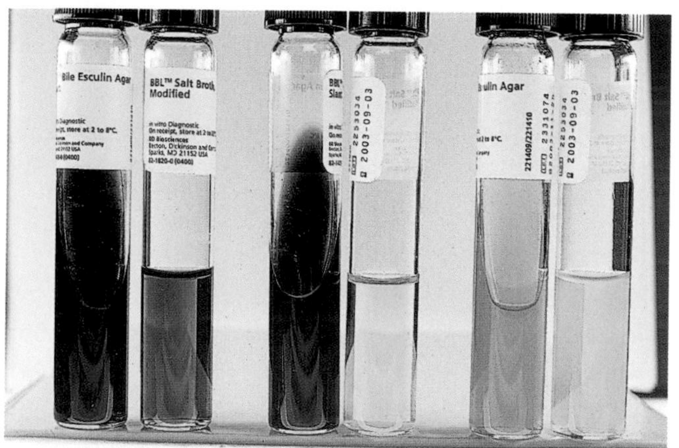

Figure 4-7 *Streptococcus bovis*, *Enterococcus faecalis*, and *Aerococcus viridans* on bile-esculin agar slants and in 6.5% NaCl broth. *S. bovis* (tubes on the left), *E. faecalis* (tubes in the center), and *A. viridans* (tubes on the right) may be differentiated based on their reactions on bile-esculin agar and in 6.5% NaCl broth. As shown here, *S. bovis* grows in the presence of 40% bile and hydrolyzes esculin, as indicated by the blackening of the slant, but does not grow in 6.5% NaCl, while *E. faecalis* is positive in both media. A positive reaction in the 6.5% NaCl broth is indicated by growth or turbidity and a color change from purple to yellow. The reaction of *A. viridans* on bile-esculin agar can vary. In this example, *A. viridans* did not hydrolyze esculin, but did grow in the 6.5% NaCl broth.

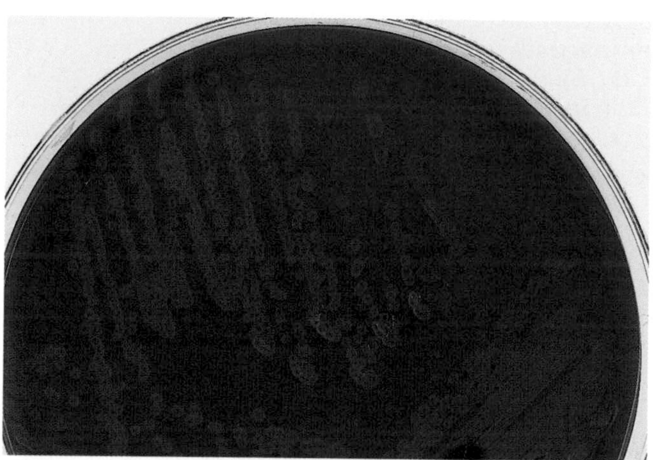

Figure 4-8 *Leuconostoc* on blood agar. Colonies of *Leuconostoc* spp. are alpha-hemolytic and small, measuring 1.0 to 2.0 mm in diameter, and can be confused with those of the viridans streptococci.

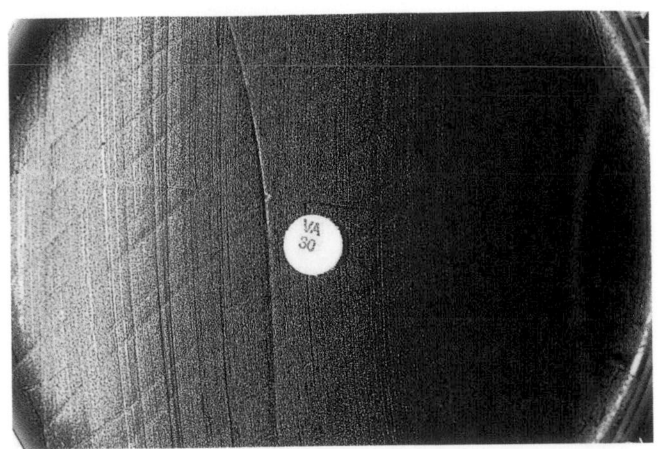

Figure 4-9 Vancomycin-resistant *Leuconostoc* on blood agar. Vancomycin resistance is used to differentiate *Leuconostoc* spp. from the viridans streptococci. A heavy inoculum of the organism is spread over blood agar, and a 30-μg vancomycin disk is placed in the center of the inoculum. The plate is incubated overnight at 35°C in CO_2. Any zone of inhibition indicates susceptibility, while resistant strains exhibit no zone of inhibition, as shown in this figure. Other vancomycin-resistant, catalase-negative, gram-positive cocci include *Pediococcus* and vancomycin-resistant strains of *Enterococcus*.

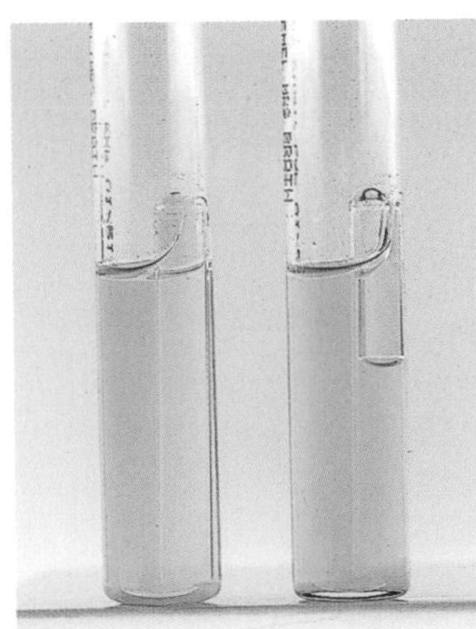

Figure 4-10 Gas production from glucose by *Leuconostoc*. Gas production from the fermentation of glucose is used to differentiate *Leuconostoc* spp. from other vancomycin-resistant organisms. In this example, *Pediococcus* was inoculated into the glucose broth on the left and *Leuconostoc* was inoculated into the tube on the right. No gas appears in the tube on the left, while there is gas in the top half of the tube inoculated with *Leuconostoc*. *Weissella* also produces gas and can be confused with *Leuconostoc*. The difference is that *Leuconostoc* is arginine negative while *Weissella* hydrolyzes arginine.

Figure 4-11 *Gemella* on blood agar. Colonies of *Gemella* spp. are alpha-hemolytic and small, measuring approximately 1.0 mm in diameter, and can be confused with those of the viridans streptococci. Some strains may be beta-hemolytic. The colonies are also similar to those of *A. viridans* and *Leuconostoc*, although they are slightly smaller and may grow more slowly.

Figure 4-12 *Abiotrophia* on chocolate agar. Colonies of *Abiotrophia* are small, measuring 1.0 mm in diameter; are either alpha- or nonhemolytic; and can be confused with those of the viridans streptococci. *Abiotrophia* grows on chocolate agar, as shown here, but does not grow on blood agar unless the medium is supplemented with pyridoxal or an inoculum of *S. aureus*, as shown in Fig. 4-13.

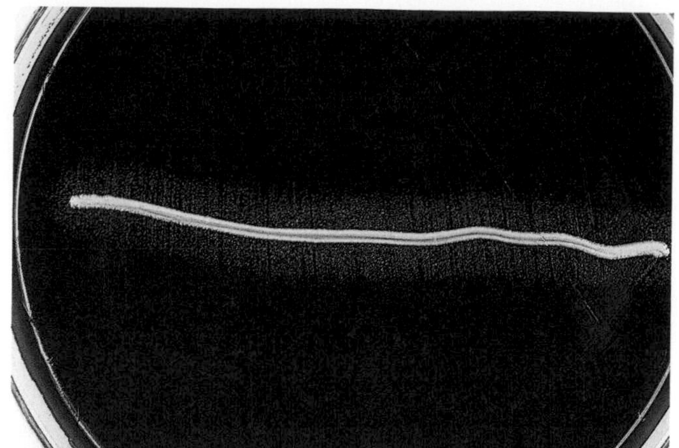

Figure 4-13 Satellite growth of *Abiotrophia* on blood agar. Colonies of *Abiotrophia*, formerly known as nutritionally variant streptococci, form satellite growth around a beta-hemolytic strain of *S. aureus* when grown on a medium that otherwise fails to support its growth. To perform this test, colonies of *Abiotrophia* are inoculated over the surface of the medium and *S. aureus* is then inoculated in a single streak, as shown in this figure. After incubation at 35°C in the presence of CO_2, colonies of *Abiotrophia* grow only in the area surrounding the staphylococcal streak.

Figure 4-14 Satellite growth of *Abiotrophia* on blood agar containing pyridoxal. An alternate method for demonstrating satellitism by *Abiotrophia* involves supplementing the medium with 0.001% pyridoxal. This can be done by using an aqueous solution of pyridoxal hydrochloride or applying a disk containing the reagent, as shown in this figure. Growth occurs only in the area surrounding the disk into which pyridoxal has diffused.

Coryneform Gram-Positive Bacilli

5

The organisms discussed in this chapter include aerobic, gram-positive, non-spore-forming, irregularly shaped bacilli called coryneforms. The term "coryneform" is derived from the Greek word *coryne*, meaning "club." Although the *Corynebacterium* spp. are the only true club-shaped bacteria, the other genera may have irregular morphologies as well. The more common genera include *Corynebacterium*, *Arcanobacterium*, *Rothia*, and *Gardnerella*. There are several less frequently isolated genera, and in general, they are usually acquired from the environment or are part of the indigenous bacterial flora of humans. Their pathogenic potential appears to be low. However, coryneform bacteria should be identified to the species level if they are isolated from normally sterile body sites, from adequately collected clinical material if they are predominant organisms, or from urine if they are isolated in pure culture at $>10^4$ CFU/ml or are the predominant organisms with a total count of 10^5 CFU/ml. The clinical significance of these organisms is strengthened if they are isolated from multiple specimens and if they are observed on a direct Gram stain along with leukocytes.

Table 5-1 includes organisms that have been isolated from blood and other sites and are related to the more frequently isolated coryneforms. The species most likely to be encountered in the clinical laboratory are the opportunistic pathogens, along with *Corynebacterium diphtheriae*, the causative agent of diphtheria. However, *Corynebacterium ulcerans* and *Corynebacterium pseudotuberculosis* may also harbor the bacteriophage that carries the diphtheria toxin gene. Some of the more frequently isolated opportunists in the *Corynebacterium* genus are *Corynebacterium amycolatum*, *Corynebacterium durum*, *Corynebacterium imitans*, *Corynebacterium jeikeium*, *Corynebacterium macginleyi*, *Corynebacterium pseudodiphtheriticum*, *C. pseudotuberculosis*, *Corynebacterium riegelii*, *C. ulcerans*, *Corynebacterium urealyticum*, and *Corynebacterium xerosis*. Other related species that were previously classified in the genus *Corynebacterium* but have been placed in new genera are *Arcanobacterium haemolyticum*, *Arcanobacterium pyogenes*, *Arcanobacterium bernardiae*, and *Gardnerella vaginalis*.

Microscopically, the corynebacteria vary in shape and size, ranging from coccoid forms approximately 1 to 2 μm in diameter to definite rod forms up to 6 μm long. They often stain unevenly with the Gram stain. The arrangement of cells is characteristic for the corynebacteria. They have been described as V forms, Chinese letters, and rods in a parallel or palisade formation.

C. diphtheriae is the most pathogenic of the corynebacteria. The diagnosis is usually based on clinical symptoms followed by culture confirmation. The preferred specimen is a nasopharyngeal swab. It is important to inoculate blood agar when investigating suspected cases of diphtheria, although it is difficult to distinguish *C. diphtheriae* from other corynebacteria. Although corynebacteria grow on blood agar, a selective medium, such as tellurite medium (Tinsdale or cystine-tellurite blood agar), should be inoculated if *C. diphtheriae* is suspected. *C. diphtheriae* can easily be distinguished from other corynebacteria by the brown halo surrounding the black colonies, an important differentiating characteristic. However, if the strain is sensitive to potassium tellurite,

Table 5-1 Identification of *Arcanobacterium*, *Corynebacterium*, *Gardnerella*, and *Rothia* spp.[a]

Species	Catalase	Nitrate	Urease	Oxidation or fermentation	Glucose	Maltose	Sucrose	Mannitol	Xylose
Arcanobacterium									
A. haemolyticum	0	0	0	F	+	+	V	0	0
A. pyogenes	0	0	0	F	+	V	V	V	+
A. bernardiae	0	0	0	F	+	+	0	0	0
Corynebacterium									
C. amycolatum	+	V	V	F	+	V	V	0	0
C. diphtheriae	+	+	0	F	+	+	0	0	0
C. jeikeium	+	0	0	OX	+	V	0	0	0
C. macginleyi	+	+	0	F	+	0	+	V	0
C. pseudodiphtheriticum	+	+	+	OX	0	0	0	0	0
C. pseudotuberculosis	+	V	+	F	+	+	V	0	0
C. reigelii	+	0	+	F	0	(+)	0	0	0
C. ulcerans	+	0	+	F	+	+	0	0	0
C. urealyticum	+	0	+	OX	0	0	0	0	0
C. xerosis	+	V	0	F	+	+	+	0	0
Other coryneform bacteria									
Gardnerella vaginalis	0	0	0	F	+	+	V	0	0
Rothia dentocariosa	V	+	0	F	+	+	+	0	0

[a]+, positive reaction (≥90% positive); V, variable reaction (11 to 89% positive); 0, negative reaction (≤10% positive); parentheses, delayed or weak reaction; F, fermentation; OX, oxidation.

it may not grow on tellurite-containing medium but will grow on blood agar. Even though Loeffler's serum medium is no longer recommended for primary plating because many organisms grow on it and it is difficult to distinguish the corynebacteria, it is the preferred medium to demonstrate the presence of metachromatic granules characteristic of *C. diphtheriae*.

A variety of carbohydrates and other tests can be used to identify the various corynebacteria (Table 5-1). Some of the important tests for identification include catalase, oxidation/fermentation in cystine Trypticase agar medium, motility, nitrate reduction, esculin production, urea hydrolysis, and acid production from glucose, maltose, sucrose, mannitol, and xylose. API Coryne (bioMérieux, Inc., Durham, NC) and RapID CB Plus (Thermo Scientific Remel Products, Lenexa, KS) are two examples of commercial identification systems for the corynebacteria.

The toxigenicity test is the most important method to determine the pathogenicity of *C. diphtheriae*. The in vitro diphtheria antitoxin test, also known as the modified *Elek* method, is the most useful and is performed by reference laboratories. Commercially available antitoxins applied to blank filter paper disks at 10 IU/disk have been successfully used with the modified *Elek* test, and precipitin lines can be read as early as 24 h. Also, PCR-based methods for detection of diphtheria toxin gene (*tox*) have been developed.

Since other corynebacteria cause infections in humans, *Corynebacterium* spp. other than *C. diphtheriae* should be considered probable pathogens. They should be identified to the species level if they are isolated from adequately collected specimens obtained from normally sterile sites, if multiple specimens are positive, or if they appear in the direct Gram stain with leukocytes.

C. amycolatum is a member of the normal flora of the skin and is often isolated from clinical specimens. It can cause bacteremia and wound, urinary and respiratory tract, and foreign body-mediated infections. Colonies are small (1 to 2 mm in diameter) and appear dry and grayish white with irregular edges. Because of its characteristic microscopic coryneform morphology and its appearance on blood agar, *C. amycolatum* is usually reported as a "diphtheroid." The API Coryne system identifies this species; however, additional tests may be needed to confirm the identification.

C. jeikeium, a common corynebacterium isolated from clinical specimens, is known to cause bacteremia and endocarditis. It is a strict aerobe, like many of the other corynebacteria, and its colony morphology is similar to that of other corynebacteria, with tiny grayish white colonies. It oxidizes glucose and sometimes maltose. Because it is one of the lipophilic corynebacteria, it usually grows better when blood agar is supplemented with Tween 80. It is often resistant to multiple antibiotics. *C. jeikeium* can also be identified by the API Coryne and the RapID CB Plus systems.

C. macginleyi, another lipophilic *Corynebacterium* species, ferments mannitol, which distinguishes it from most other corynebacteria. It is known to cause eye infections.

C. pseudodiphtheriticum is part of the normal flora of the oropharyngeal cavity and is probably the most common corynebacterium isolated from respiratory specimens. It has been associated with respiratory tract infections and endocarditis. Colonies are 1 to 2 mm in diameter, white, and dry. This species reduces nitrate and hydrolyzes urea.

Both *C. pseudotuberculosis* and *C. ulcerans* are closely related to *C. diphtheriae*. Both species can easily be differentiated from *C. diphtheriae* because they hydrolyze urea and produce a positive reverse CAMP reaction. *C. ulcerans* is also glycogen positive.

C. riegelii has been associated with urinary tract infections in women. Like *C. urealyticum*, it hydrolyzes urea within 5 min at room temperature. Unlike other corynebacteria, it ferments maltose but not glucose.

C. urealyticum is usually isolated from urine specimens with an alkaline pH and is associated with struvite crystals. Its colony morphology is similar to that of other lipophilic corynebacteria: pinpoint and grayish white on blood agar. This organism is often resistant to multiple antibiotics.

C. xerosis has been isolated from vaginal specimens. Colonies are small, measuring 1 to 1.5 mm in diameter; have irregular edges; and appear dry and slightly yellow. In the past, isolates of *C. xerosis* have been misidentified as *C. amycolatum* because of their biochemical similarities. The exception to this is that *C. amycolatum* strains produce propionic acid as the major end product of glucose metabolism while *C. xerosis* strains produce lactic acid.

There are three *Arcanobacterium* spp. that are known to cause infection in humans: *A. haemolyticum*, *A. pyogenes*, and *A. bernardiae*. They are all beta-hemolytic on blood agar. *A. haemolyticum* has been associated with pharyngitis in older children, wound and soft tissue infections, endocarditis, and osteomyelitis. Colonies of *A. haemolyticum* are tiny (<0.5 mm in diameter) (like *C. ulcerans*) even after incubation for 48 h at 37°C. *A. haemolyticum* is also positive for the reverse CAMP reaction and can be identified by both the API Coryne and the RapID CB Plus systems. Colonies of *A. pyogenes* are larger than those of *A. haemolyticum* but still small (1 mm in diameter) in comparison to some of the corynebacteria. These colonies exhibit the clearest beta-hemolysis of all the arcanobacteria on blood agar. *A. pyogenes* ferments xylose whereas the other two species do not. Microscopically, this species may appear as branching gram-positive bacilli. Colonies of *A. bernardiae* are pinpoint (<0.5 mm in diameter) and may have a creamy or sticky consistency. On Gram stain, they appear as gram-positive bacilli without branching. Another distinguishing characteristic of *A. bernardiae* is its ability to produce acid more quickly in maltose than in glucose.

G. vaginalis was previously classified in the genus *Corynebacterium*. However, it has no phylogenetic relationship to the corynebacteria. On Gram stain, it appears as gram-variable bacilli or coccobacilli. It is part of the anorectal flora of humans as well as the vaginal flora of women and is one of the organisms associated with bacterial vaginosis. Routine cultures for *G. vaginalis* are not recommended for the diagnosis of bacterial vaginosis because the organism can also be found in women without infection. However, a smear of vaginal discharge showing "clue cells" is suggestive of bacterial vaginosis. If a culture for *G. vaginalis* is requested, vaginal swabs should be inoculated onto vaginalis agar (V agar) or bilayer Tween agar with human blood (HBT agar) and incubated at 37°C in an atmosphere containing 5 to 7% CO_2. Colonies on these media are tiny and usually beta-hemolytic when incubated for 48 h. Hemolysis can be detected on media containing either human or horse blood but not sheep blood. Identification of *G. vaginalis* is based on the following reactions: catalase and oxidase negative; sodium hippurate hydrolysis positive; and acid production from glucose, maltose, and sucrose.

Rothia dentocariosa is part of the normal flora of the oropharyngeal cavity of humans and has been associated with dental caries and periodontal disease, as well as with endocarditis and pneumonia in immunodeficient hosts. On Gram stain, it appears as a pleomorphic, gram-positive coccoid to rod-shaped organism that can form branches. Colonies of *R. dentocariosa* are 1 to 2 mm in diameter, whitish, raised, and smooth and may have a spoke-wheel form when grown on blood agar and incubated under 5 to 10% CO_2 for 48 h at 37°C. This organism is catalase positive when tested on media without hemin and can be confused with *Actinomyces viscosus* because both are catalase positive. However, *A. viscosus* ferments lactose whereas *R. dentocariosa* does not.

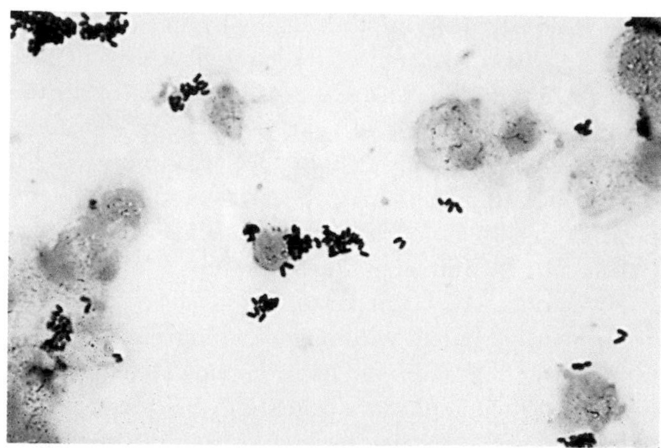

Figure 5-1 Gram stain of *Corynebacterium* spp. The small, gram-positive bacilli, 1 by 3 μm in size, appear in palisade, V, and L forms, resembling Chinese letters, and are usually referred to as diphtheroids. This arrangement is the result of cell division referred to as "snapping," which causes the cells to arrange themselves in both parallel and perpendicular formations.

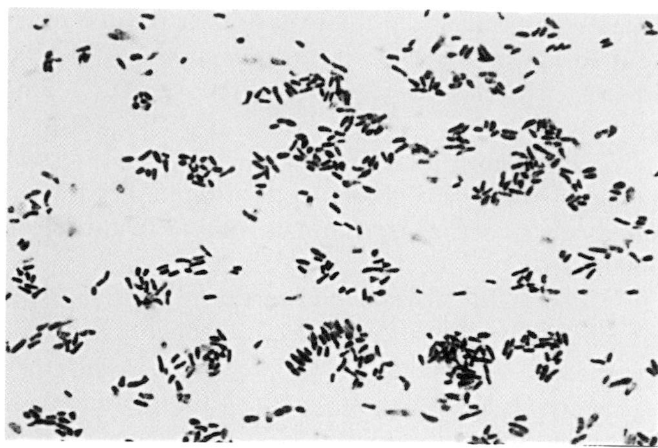

Figure 5-2 Gram stain of *Corynebacterium diphtheriae*. *C. diphtheriae* appears similar to other *Corynebacterium* spp. on Gram stain. The arrangement of these small, gram-positive bacilli, 1 by 3 μm in size, resembles that shown in Fig. 5-1. Another recommended stain is methylene blue. However, although metachromatic granules are in cells of *C. diphtheriae* when grown on Loeffler's medium and stained with methylene blue, these granules can occur in the cells of other corynebacteria.

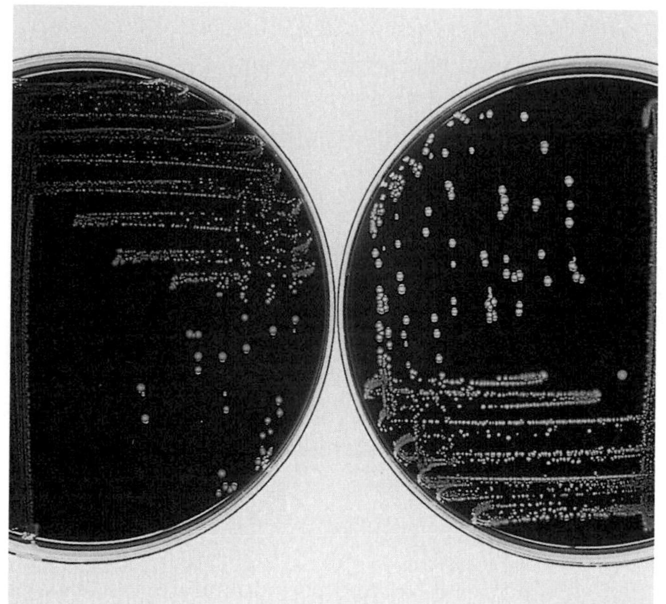

Figure 5-3 *Corynebacterium diphtheriae* on blood agar and colistin-nalidixic acid blood agar (CNA). *C. diphtheriae* grows well as nonhemolytic, whitish, opaque colonies after overnight incubation on blood agar under 5 to 10% CO_2. Although blood agar is a primary isolation medium, CNA is recommended as a selective medium for the isolation of *C. diphtheriae* and other corynebacteria if tellurite medium is not available. In this figure, *C. diphtheriae* cells are shown on blood agar (left) and CNA (right). If CNA is used as the selective medium for the isolation of *C. diphtheriae*, several colonies should be picked for stains and biochemical tests because other organisms can also grow on this medium.

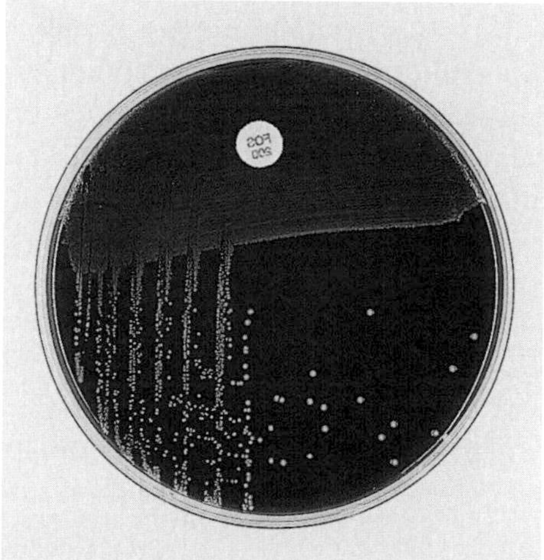

Figure 5-4 *Corynebacterium diphtheriae* on blood agar with 200-μg fosfomycin disk. Corynebacteria, including *C. diphtheriae*, are highly resistant to fosfomycin (>50 μg); therefore, a blood agar-based medium containing up to 100 μg of fosfomycin/ml can serve as a selective medium for the isolation of most corynebacteria. Alternatively, a fosfomycin disk can be placed on a blood agar plate. In this example, *C. diphtheriae* growth is not inhibited by 200 μg of fosfomycin.

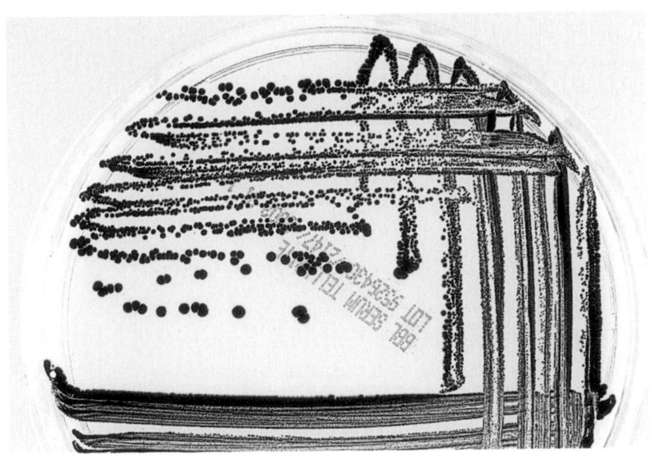

Figure 5-5 *Corynebacterium diphtheriae* on tellurite agar. Primary plating media for *C. diphtheriae* should include a blood agar plate and a selective medium, preferably containing potassium tellurite. On the selective tellurite medium, *C. diphtheriae* colonies have a gunmetal, gray-black appearance, as shown, while other corynebacteria grow but most do not reduce tellurite.

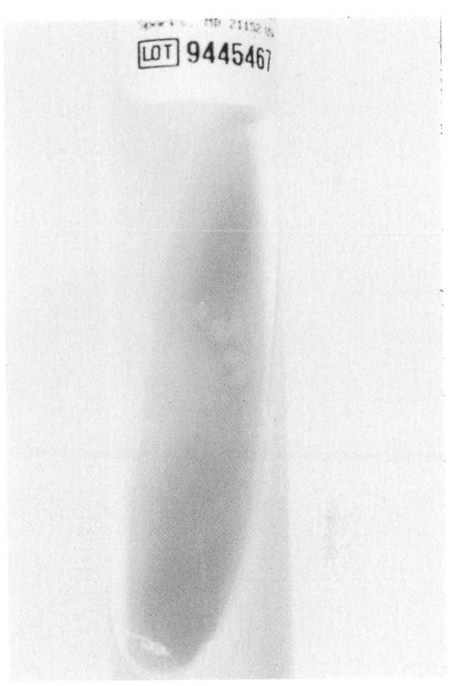

Figure 5-6 *Corynebacterium diphtheriae* on Loeffler's serum agar slant. Loeffler's serum agar slant is no longer recommended as a primary plating medium for the isolation of *C. diphtheriae* because of the overgrowth of other bacteria. On Loeffler's medium there is no characteristic appearance to distinguish the corynebacteria from other aerobic, gram-positive bacilli. However, it is important to inoculate suspected colonies of *C. diphtheriae* onto this medium to check for metachromatic granules detected by staining with methylene blue.

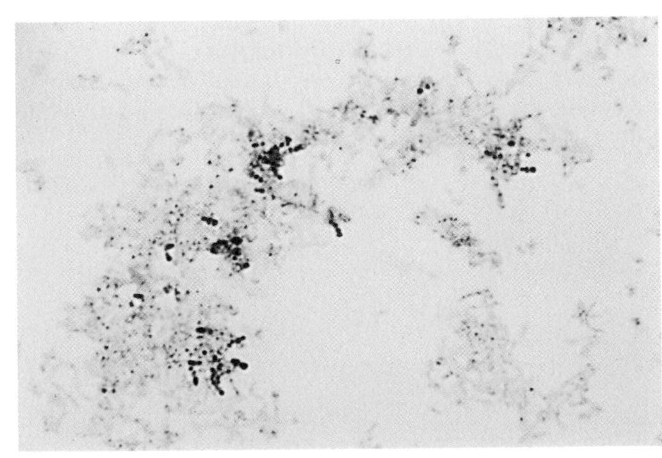

Figure 5-7 Methylene blue stain showing metachromatic granules. *C. diphtheriae* and other *Corynebacterium* spp. produce metachromatic granules (polar bodies) when grown on Loeffler's serum agar. These granules, also known as volutin granules, are an accumulation of inorganic polyphosphates. Methylene blue imparts a deeper blue or red hue to the metachromatic granules of *C. diphtheriae*. These are demonstrated microscopically in this figure.

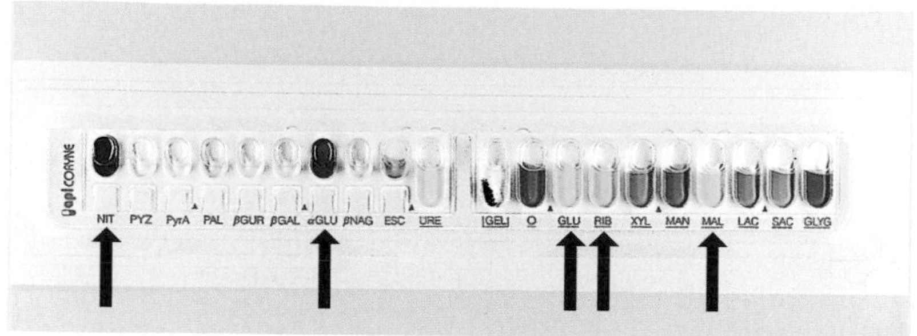

Figure 5-8 ***Corynebacterium diphtheriae*** **identified by the API Coryne system.** The API Coryne is a commercial test system that is designed for the identification of *Corynebacterium* spp. and related bacteria. It consists of 20 dehydrated substrates for the demonstration of enzymatic activity or the fermentation of carbohydrates. Following inoculation, the strip is incubated at 35 to 37°C for 24 h. Positive reactions, indicated by the arrows, are indicated by a color change. In this example, from left to right, positive reactions occur in nitrate (NIT), α-glucosidase (αGLU), glucose (GLU), ribose (RIB), and maltose (MAL). A catalase test was positive for this isolate. This combination of test reactions confirmed the identification of *C. diphtheriae*.

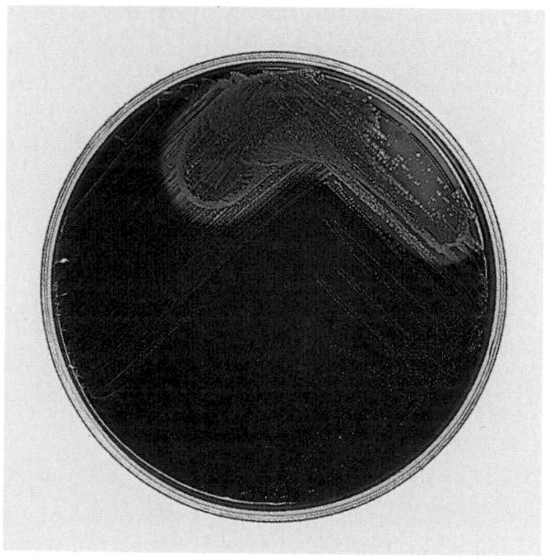

Figure 5-9 ***Corynebacterium jeikeium*** **on blood agar with Tween 80.** *C. jeikeium* is a lipophilic *Corynebacterium* species, and its growth is enhanced by the addition of 0.1 to 1.0% Tween 80. In this case Tween 80 has been added to the blood agar plate. This figure demonstrates the enhanced growth on the area of the plate where the Tween 80 has been added.

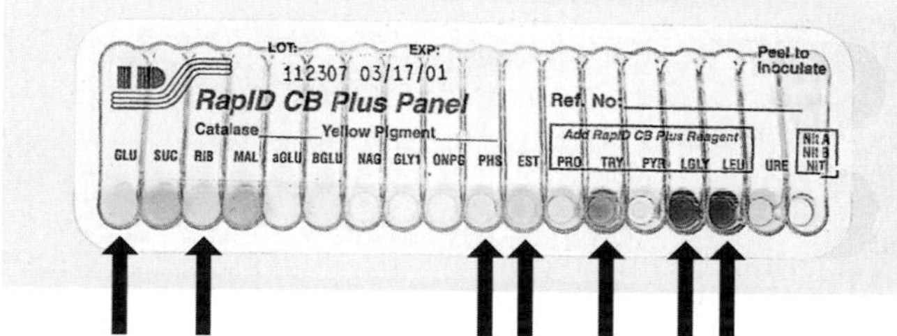

Figure 5-10 ***Corynebacterium jeikeium*** **identified by the RapID CB Plus system.** The RapID CB Plus system (Thermo Scientific Remel Products, Lenexa, KS) is an 18-well micromethod employing conventional and chromogenic substrates for the identification of medically important corynebacteria and related organisms. Inoculated panels are incubated for 4 to 6 h at 35 to 37°C in an atmosphere without CO_2. Reagents are added and the results are interpreted as specified by the manufacturer. For the first 11 wells, a yellow or yellow-orange color is interpreted as positive; for the remaining wells, purple, red, or pink colors indicate a positive reaction. In this example, glucose (GLU), ribose (RIB), *p*-nitrophenyl phosphate (PHS), fatty acid ester (EST), tryptophan-β-naphthylamide (TRY), leucyl-glycine-β-naphthylamide (LGLY), and leucine-β-naphthylamide (LEU) are positive, as indicated by the arrows. These reactions are consistent with *C. jeikeium*.

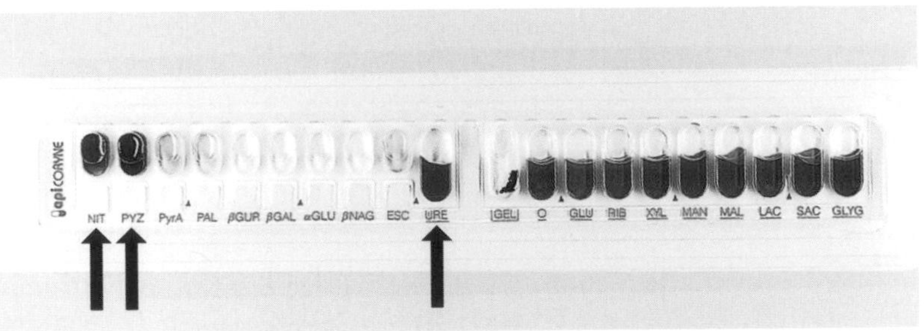

Figure 5-11 ***Corynebacterium pseudodiphtheriticum*** **identified by the API Coryne system.** Reactions are interpreted as described in the legend to Fig. 5-8. In this example, nitrate (NIT), pyrazinamidase (PYZ), and urease (URE) are positive, as indicated by the arrows. The catalase test was also positive for this organism. These reactions confirm the identification of *C. pseudodiphtheriticum*.

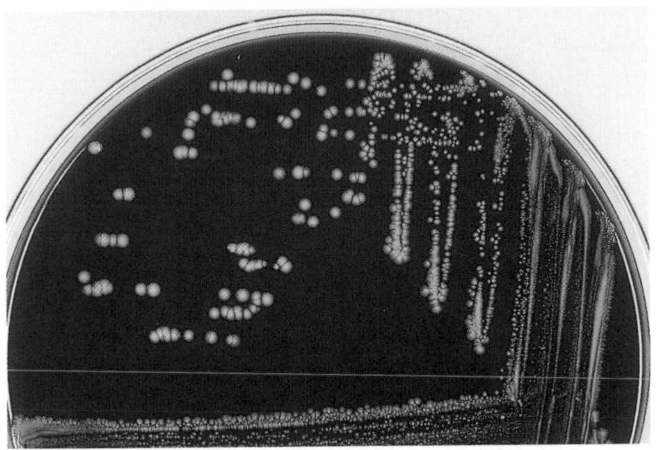

Figure 5-12 ***Corynebacterium pseudodiphtheriticum*** **on blood agar.** Colonies of *C. pseudodiphtheriticum* are white and slightly dry with entire edges and measure approximately 2 mm in diameter after 48 h of incubation.

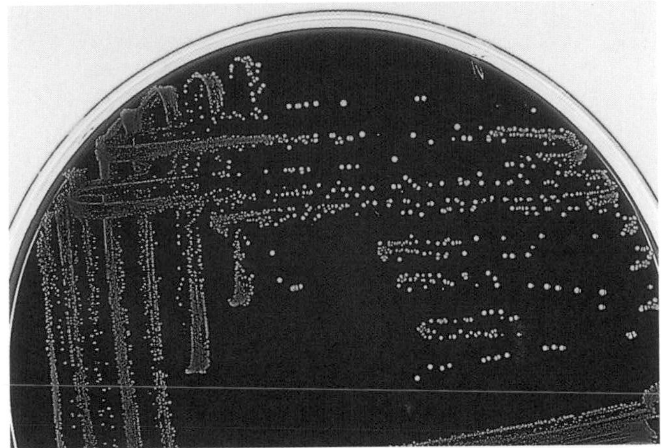

Figure 5-13 ***Corynebacterium urealyticum*** **on blood agar.** Colonies of *C. urealyticum* are pinpoint to small, approximately 0.5 to 1 mm in diameter, convex, smooth, and light gray on blood agar. Like *C. jeikeium*, *C. urealyticum* is a lipophilic species; therefore, growth is enhanced when it is grown in the presence of Tween 80.

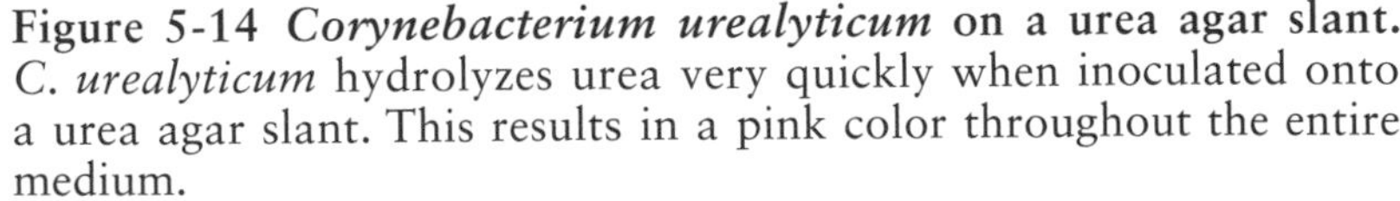

Figure 5-14 ***Corynebacterium urealyticum*** **on a urea agar slant.** *C. urealyticum* hydrolyzes urea very quickly when inoculated onto a urea agar slant. This results in a pink color throughout the entire medium.

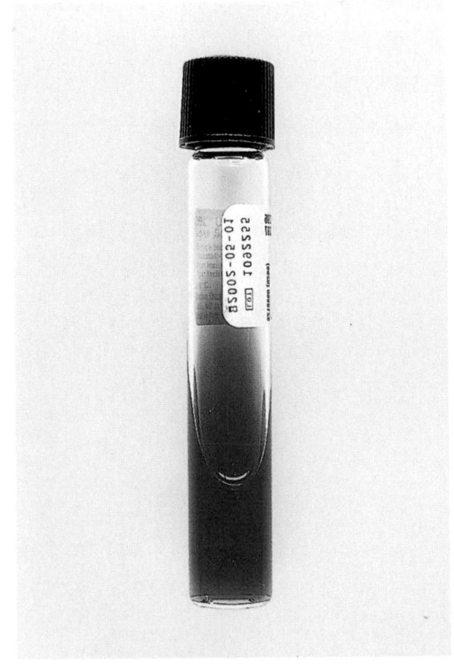

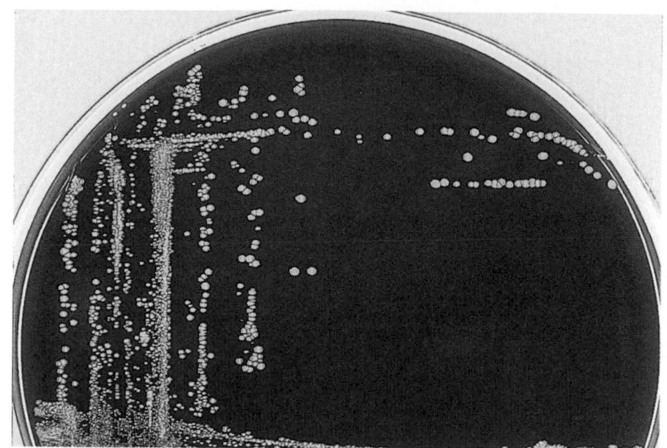

Figure 5-15 ***Corynebacterium xerosis*** **on blood agar.** Colonies of *C. xerosis* on blood agar are small to medium in size (1 to 3 mm in diameter), dry, pale yellow, and granular.

Figure 5-16 ***Arcanobacterium haemolyticum*** **on blood agar.** Colonies of *A. haemolyticum* are small (<0.5 to 1 mm in diameter) and beta-hemolytic on blood agar when incubated for 48 h at 35 to 37°C under CO_2. The colonies can be either smooth or rough. In general, the smooth form, shown here, is isolated from wound specimens and the rough form is isolated from respiratory specimens. Colonies of *A. pyogenes* have a similar appearance.

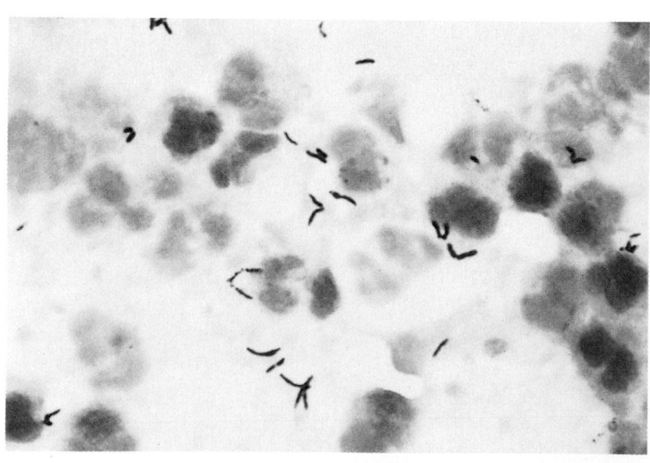

Figure 5-17 Gram stain of ***Arcanobacterium pyogenes.*** This Gram stain of *A. pyogenes* was prepared from a peritonsillar abscess. These gram-positive bacilli are longer than corynebacteria, measuring up to 6 μm in length. Both V formation and branching can be seen; both are characteristics of this organism.

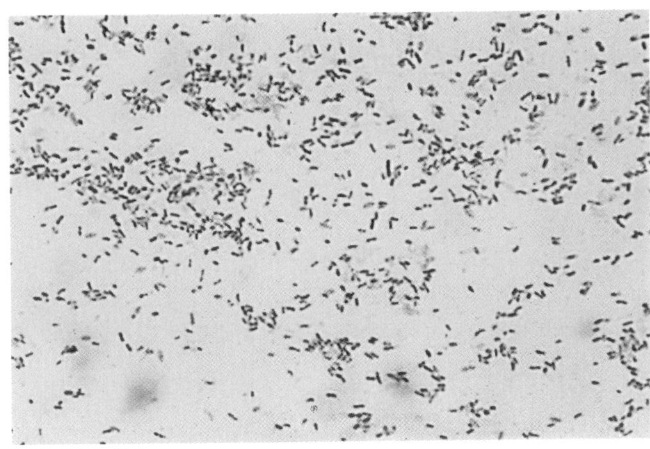

Figure 5-18 Gram stain of *Gardnerella vaginalis*. *G. vaginalis* appears as thin, gram-variable bacilli and coccobacilli, as shown here. Because of the variable Gram reaction, this organism was previously included in the genera *Corynebacterium* and *Haemophilus*.

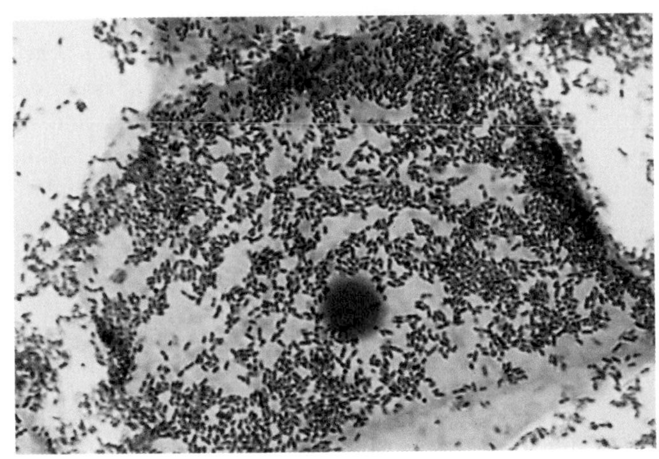

Figure 5-19 Gram stain of a clue cell. A clue cell is an epithelial cell covered with mixed bacteria collected from a vaginal discharge of a patient with bacterial vaginosis. The typical smear, as seen in the figure, shows the clue cell (epithelial cell) covered with small, gram-variable bacilli and coccobacilli.

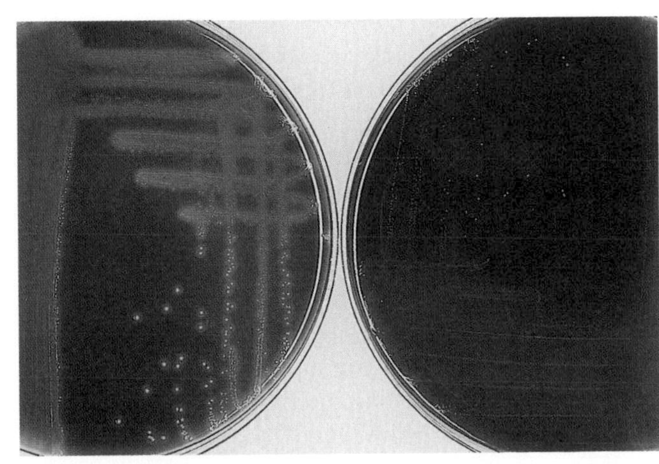

Figure 5-20 Colonies of *Gardnerella vaginalis* on blood agar and V agar. Shown here are colonies of *G. vaginalis* growing on 5% blood agar (right) and V agar (left). V agar is a nonselective enriched medium containing human blood that supports the isolation and beta-hemolytic reaction of *G. vaginalis*. Colonies growing on 5% sheep blood agar are barely visible after incubation for 48 h at 37°C in an atmosphere of 5 to 7% CO_2, while colonies grown on V agar with 5% human blood are opaque, measuring 1 mm in diameter and surrounded by zones of beta-hemolysis.

Listeria and *Erysipelothrix* 6

The genus *Listeria* includes several species; however, only *Listeria monocytogenes* and *Listeria ivanovii* are pathogenic to humans and animals. *Listeria innocua*, the species most frequently isolated from foods, is not a human pathogen. These organisms can be isolated from soil, water, and vegetation.

L. monocytogenes causes infections mainly during the summer months in pregnant women, newborns, patients with compromised cell-mediated immunity (such as individuals with AIDS, lymphomas, and transplants), and elderly persons. High mortality rates can occur in pregnant or immunocompromised patients. During gestation, *L. monocytogenes* can lead to amnionitis and infection of the fetus that can result in termination of the pregnancy. Both epidemics and sporadic cases have been described. Food, particularly dairy products and meat, is the most common vehicle of transmission. In addition to septicemia, infections of the central nervous system, including meningitis and encephalitis, are the most frequent clinical presentations. *L. ivanovii* is mainly a pathogen of ruminants, but human systemic infections can occur, particularly in patients with HIV-1.

Blood, amniotic fluid, and cerebrospinal fluid are frequently submitted for detection of *L. monocytogenes*. Cultures of specimens from nonsterile sites, such as the vagina or stool, are often not diagnostically useful since approximately 1 to 5% of healthy individuals are colonized. However, for studies of carriage, stool specimens rather than rectal swabs are preferred for isolating this organism from the gastrointestinal tract. Although *L. monocytogenes* grows well on blood and chocolate agars, cold enrichment, performed by storing the specimen in the refrigerator for several days, decreases contamination with rapidly growing bacteria and enhances recovery when plating specimens from nonsterile sites. Selective media for culturing *Listeria* spp. include lithium chloride-phenylethanol-moxalactam (LPM) and PALCAM agars. PALCAM is a highly selective medium due to the inclusion of polymyxin B, acriflavine hydrochloride, lithium chloride, and ceftazidime. Chromogenic media for the selective isolation of *Listeria* spp. are commercially available.

L. monocytogenes is an aerobic, non-spore-forming, short (0.4 to 0.5 μm by 0.5 to 2 μm), gram-positive bacillus, or coccobacillus, with rounded ends, occurring singly or in short chains. In cerebrospinal fluid, the organism may be intracellular or extracellular, and it can be confused with *Enterococcus* spp. or *Streptococcus pneumoniae* if the cells are coccoid and arranged in pairs. *L. monocytogenes* may also have a pleomorphic palisade structure resembling that of *Corynebacterium*. If the Gram stain is overdecolorized, this organism can also be confused with *Haemophilus*.

Identification of *L. monocytogenes* from clinical specimens is based on Gram stain morphology, a narrow zone of beta-hemolysis on blood agar, tumbling motility, esculin hydrolysis, positive catalase reaction, negative reaction for H_2S, acid production from D-glucose, and positive Voges-Proskauer and methyl red reactions. *L. ivanovii* produces large zones of beta-hemolysis while *L. innocua* is nonhemolytic. Molecular techniques are available for the identification and epidemiological characterization of *Listeria* spp.

Two species, *Erysipelothrix rhusiopathiae* and *Erysipelothrix tonsillarum*, are included in the genus *Erysipelothrix*. Only *E. rhusiopathiae* is known to be a human pathogen. *E. rhusiopathiae* is carried by a variety of animals and occasionally causes a human cutaneous infection called erysipeloid, which is localized on the hands. This lesion is acquired as a result of skin abrasion, injury, or bites from infected animals, particularly domestic swine and fish. Therefore, veterinarians, butchers, and fish handlers are frequently affected. Generalized cutaneous infections are rare. The infection can disseminate in immunocompromised patients, resulting in bacteremia and endocarditis.

E. rhusiopathiae is a gram-positive, nonsporulating, thin, short (0.2 to 0.4 μm by 0.8 to 2.5 μm) bacillus with rounded ends; it is usually found singly or in short chains but has a tendency to form slender, long filaments up to 60 μm in length.

Clinical specimens should be inoculated into nutrient broth with 1% glucose, incubated at 35°C under 5% CO_2, and subcultured daily. *Erysipelothrix* spp. are catalase and oxidase negative, do not hydrolyze esculin, and are methyl red and Voges-Proskauer negative. These organisms do not produce indole or hydrolyze urea, but they produce H_2S in triple sugar iron agar. This last characteristic helps to differentiate members of this genus from *Lactobacillus*, *Listeria*, *Brochothrix*, and *Kurthia*. In addition, *Erysipelothrix* does not grow at 4°C while *Listeria* can grow at low temperatures. Sucrose can be used to differentiate the two species of *Erysipelothrix*: *E. rhusiopathiae* is sucrose negative, whereas *E. tonsillarum* is positive.

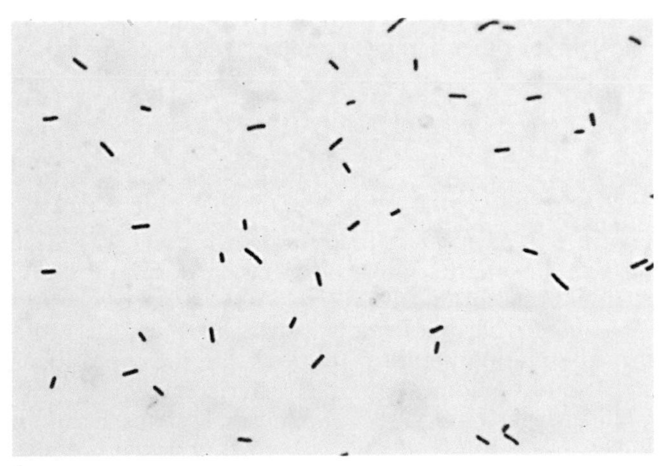
A

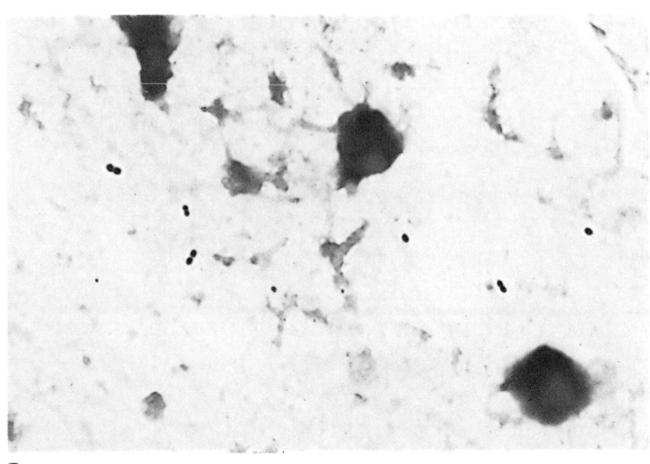
B

Figure 6-1 Gram stain of *Listeria monocytogenes*. (A) A Gram stain shows the typical morphology of *L. monocytogenes*, consisting of single or short chains of small, gram-positive bacilli. (B) Older cultures often appear as gram-variable with a coccoid morphology that can also occur in clinical specimens such as cerebrospinal fluid, as seen here. In this particular case, it is very important to differentiate *L. monocytogenes* from *Streptococcus pneumoniae*.

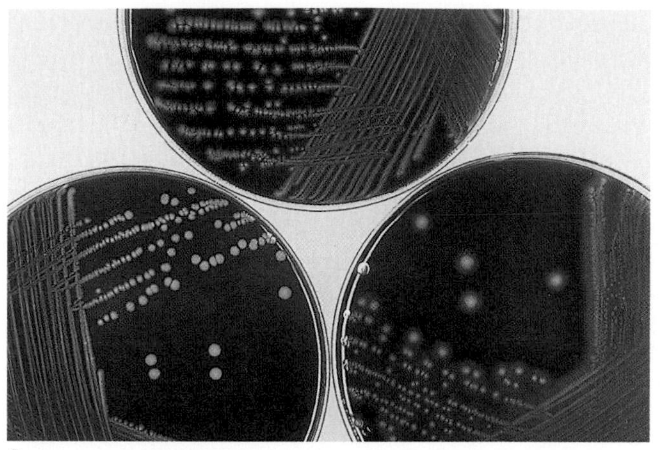

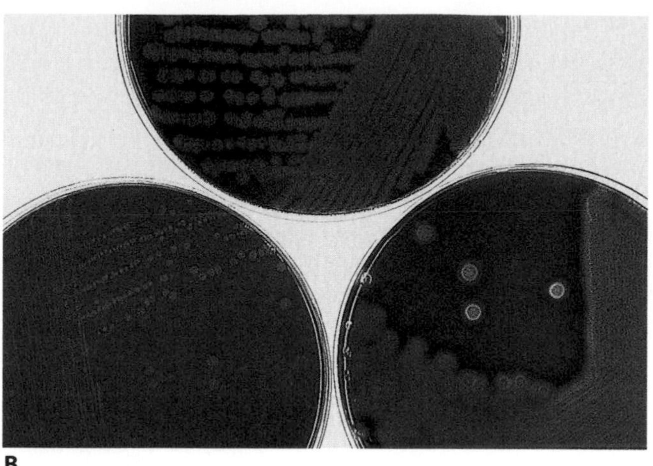

Figure 6-2 ***Listeria*** **spp. on blood agar.** (A) Front light; (B) back light. The colonies of *L. monocytogenes* (top) are small, translucent, or gray with a narrow zone of beta-hemolysis and can easily be confused with group B streptococci. Hemolysis is important for differentiating between *L. monocytogenes* and the other two species of *Listeria* that are beta-hemolytic: *L. monocytogenes* and *Listeria seeligeri* produce zones of hemolysis that frequently do not extend beyond the edge of the colony, while *Listeria ivanovii* (bottom right) produces large zones of hemolysis. Thus, in the case of *L. monocytogenes* and *L. seeligeri*, removal of the colony may be required to observe the hemolysis. *Listeria innocua* (bottom left), on the other hand, is nonhemolytic.

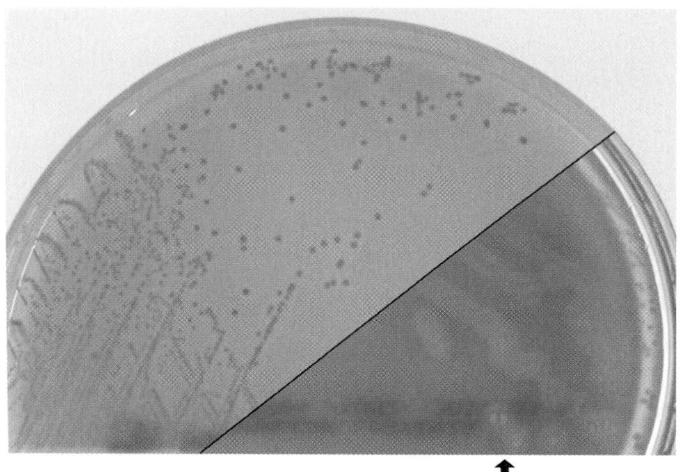

Figure 6-3 ***Listeria monocytogenes*** **on chromogenic media.** Phosphatidylinositol-specific phospholipase C is an enzyme produced only by *L. monocytogenes* and *L. ivanovii*. Chromogenic substrates are incorporated into the plating medium to allow for the rapid identification of colonies by a characteristic color. On BD CHROMagar Listeria (BD Diagnostic Systems, Franklin Lakes, NJ), *L. monocytogenes* and *L. ivanovii* produce blue-green colonies surrounded by an opaque, white halo; however, the colony size of *L. ivanovii* is smaller.

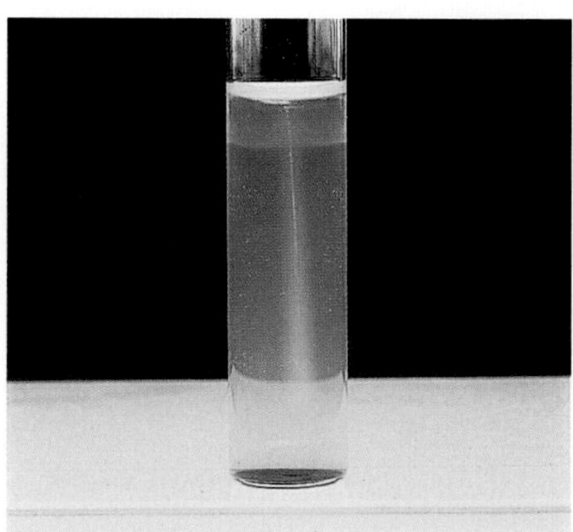

Figure 6-4 Motility of ***Listeria monocytogenes*** **on semisolid medium.** As shown here, in a tube of semisolid medium incubated overnight at room temperature, *L. monocytogenes* develops a typical umbrella-shaped pattern as a result of its motility, whereas when it is incubated at 37°C, this pattern does not occur. The end-over-end tumbling motility can be observed under a microscope after incubation for 1 to 2 h in nutrient broth at room temperature (not shown).

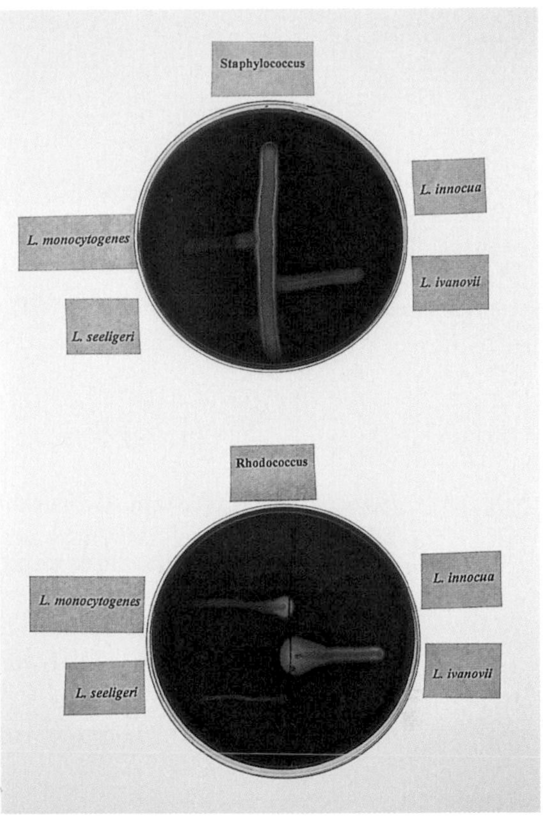

Figure 6-5 The CAMP test. The CAMP test is used to differentiate between species of *Listeria*. Here, *Staphylococcus aureus* and *Rhodococcus equi* were streaked in one direction on a blood agar plate and test cultures of the *Listeria* spp. were streaked at right angles to the *S. aureus* and *R. equi* streaks but without touching the streaks. *L. monocytogenes* and *L. seeligeri* hemolysis is enhanced in proximity to *S. aureus*; *L. ivanovii* hemolysis is enhanced near *R. equi*, giving the typical picture of a shovel. Depending on the strain, the hemolysis of *L. monocytogenes* may or may not be enhanced near *R. equi*. The CAMP factor is a diffusible extracellular protein, produced by certain organisms such as *L. monocytogenes*, *L. seeligeri*, and most group B streptococci, that acts synergistically with the staphylococcal beta-lysin.

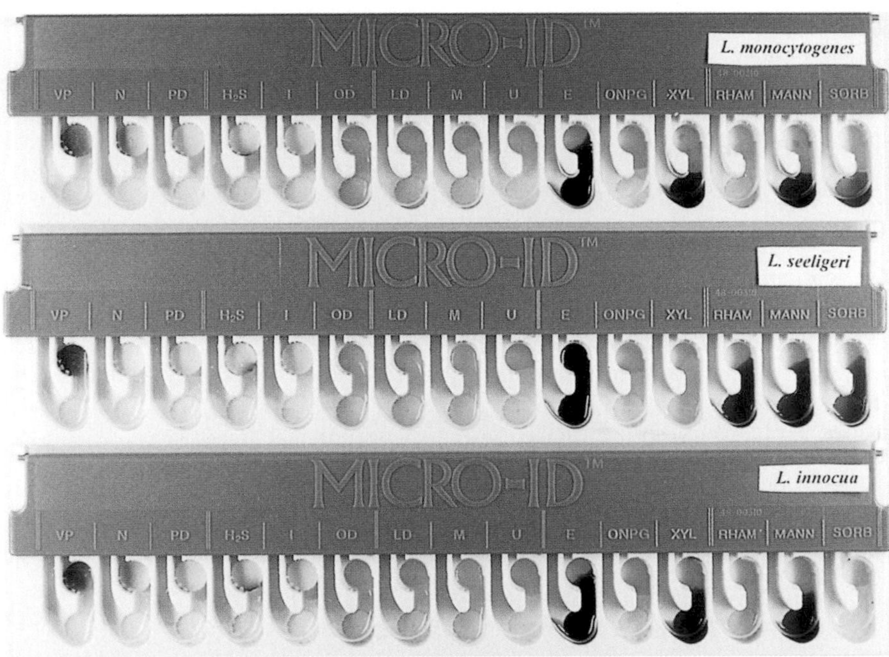

Figure 6-6 Micro-ID Listeria system. The Micro-ID Listeria assay (Thermo Scientific Remel Products, Lenexa, KS) includes 15 biochemical tests used to identify *Listeria* to the species level. An additional test for hemolytic activity is required to differentiate between *L. monocytogenes* and *L. innocua*. As shown here, *L. monocytogenes* and *L. innocua* are D-xylose and mannitol negative and L-rhamnose positive, while *L. seeligeri* is xylose positive.

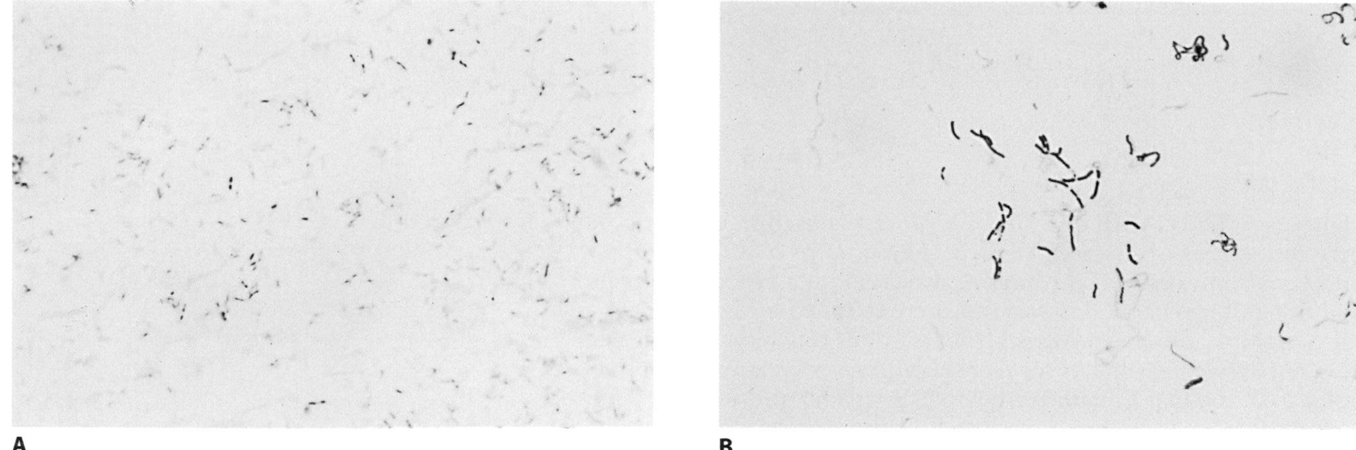

Figure 6-7 Gram stain of *Erysipelothrix rhusiopathiae*. *E. rhusiopathiae* is gram positive but can be easily decolorized, giving a beaded appearance. Bacteria stained from smooth colonies appear as bacilli or coccobacilli (A), while cells from rough colonies are long and filamentous (B).

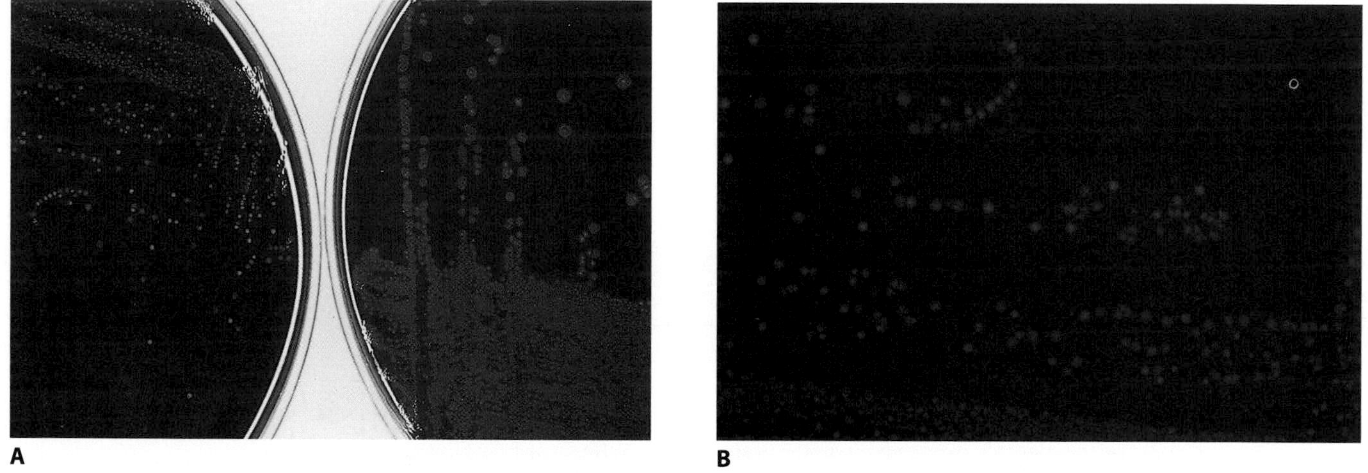

Figure 6-8 *Erysipelothrix rhusiopathiae* on blood agar. Colonies of *E. rhusiopathiae* at 24 h are small and pinpoint (A, left). By 72 h, two types can be recognized (A, right, and B): smooth, transparent, glistening, circular, convex colonies with entire edges, measuring approximately 1 mm in diameter; and larger, rough colonies that are flat and opaque, with a matte surface and an irregular edge. The colonies are nonhemolytic, although a greenish discoloration can be found under them.

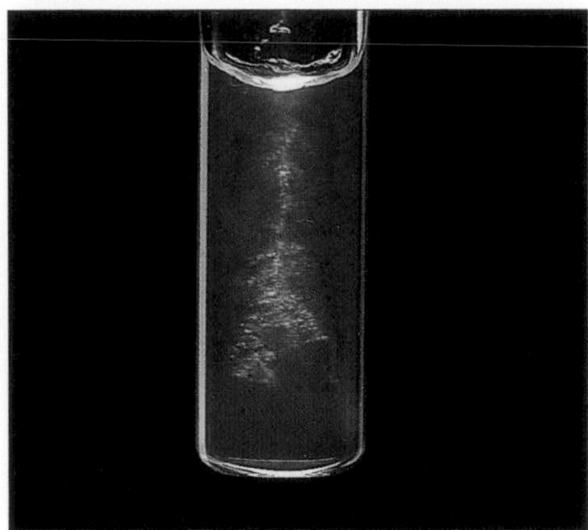

Figure 6-9 ***Erysipelothrix rhusiopathiae*** **in a gelatin stab culture.** A useful differential characteristic of *E. rhusiopathiae* is its "pipe cleaner" or "bottle brush" pattern of growth in gelatin stab cultures incubated at 22°C.

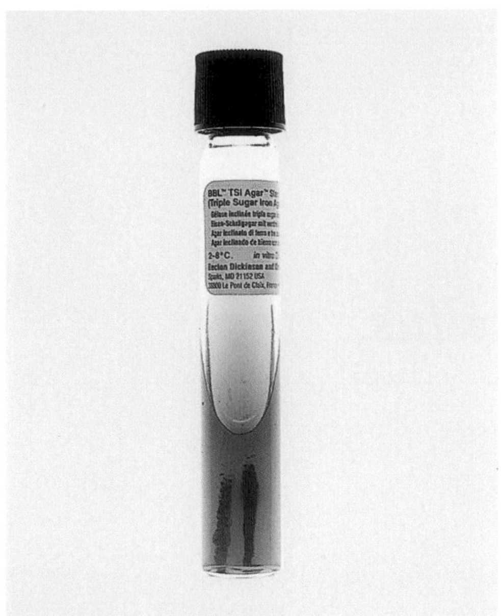

Figure 6-10 Production of H_2S by *Erysipelothrix*. As shown in this figure, *Erysipelothrix* species produce H_2S on a triple sugar iron agar slant.

Bacillus

7

The genus *Bacillus* belongs to the family *Bacillaceae*. There are more than 150 species of *Bacillus*; however, the most frequently isolated are *Bacillus anthracis*, *Bacillus cereus*, *Bacillus licheniformis*, *Bacillus megaterium*, *Bacillus mycoides*, *Bacillus pumilus*, *Bacillus subtilis*, and *Bacillus thuringiensis*. Another species with a familiar name has been transferred to a new genus and is now known as *Geobacillus stearothermophilus* (it is frequently used as an indicator organism in autoclave sterility testing). Most *Bacillus* spp. are saprophytes and are widely distributed in nature, but some are opportunists. The exception is *B. anthracis*, which is an obligate pathogen of humans and animals.

Microscopically, *Bacillus* spp. are gram-positive bacilli; however, it is not unusual for them to be gram variable or gram negative, especially in older cultures. They produce endospores and may be either aerobes or facultative anaerobes. Endospores are very resistant to heat, radiation, disinfectants, and desiccation and are frequent contaminants of otherwise clean environments such as operating rooms, pharmaceutical products, and food. They can germinate when hydrated and, in the case of food, can cause spoilage or result in food poisoning.

Bacillus spp. are catalase positive and hydrolyze gelatin, casein, and starch; most species, with the exception of *B. anthracis* and *B. mycoides*, are motile. Other tests that assist in the identification of *Bacillus* spp. are lecithinase production (egg yolk reaction), nitrate reduction, and the ability to grow anaerobically. Identification systems, e.g., API 20E (bioMérieux, Inc., Durham, NC), can be used to identify members of the *B. cereus* group (*B. cereus*, *B. anthracis*, *B. mycoides*, and *B. thuringiensis*).

B. anthracis is clinically the most important member of the genus since it is the causative agent of anthrax in animals and humans. Anthrax is primarily a disease of herbivores and humans and is contracted by direct or indirect contact with infected animals or their carcasses. Dissemination of toxigenic strains is a major public health concern. For this reason, diagnostic laboratories should be prepared to recognize *B. anthracis* from clinical specimens and refer suspicious isolates to the appropriate reference or public health laboratory. It is recommended that isolation and presumptive identification of *B. anthracis* be performed in a Biosafety Level 3 facility.

The three major clinical presentations of anthrax are cutaneous, respiratory (inhalation), and gastrointestinal (ingestion). Cutaneous anthrax presents with a nondescript painless papule that evolves from a vesicle with central necrosis and formation of a black eschar; it accounts for 99% of naturally acquired anthrax cases worldwide. Inhalation anthrax begins with a "flu-like" illness, and subsequently the patient develops wheezing, cyanosis, shock, and meningitis. X rays of the chest show widening of the mediastinum, pulmonary infiltrates, and pleural effusions. Ingestion anthrax occurs in two forms: oral or oropharyngeal and gastrointestinal. In oral or oropharyngeal infection, the lesion is in the buccal cavity or on the tongue, tonsil, or posterior pharyngeal wall. The symptoms can include sore throat with cervical edema, dysphagia, and respiratory difficulties. Intestinal anthrax causes nausea, vomiting, sepsis, and bloody diarrhea with ulcerations primarily in the mucosae of the terminal ileum or cecum. The three virulence factors of *B. anthracis*—edema toxin, lethal toxin, and a capsular antigen—contribute to the high mortality rate, especially in cases of intestinal and pulmonary anthrax.

If the microscopic and colony morphologies of the organism being studied are consistent with *B. anthracis* and the isolate is nonhemolytic, catalase positive, and nonmotile, the public health laboratory should be notified immediately and the isolate should be sent to that laboratory to rule out *B. anthracis*. Gram stain of the colonies reveals gram-positive bacilli in chains with oval spores that do not cause significant swelling of the cells. Spores may also be observed in a wet mount, phase microscopy, or a malachite green stain. Spores are not found in clinical material unless it is exposed to CO_2. Microscopically, *B. anthracis* cells are gram-positive bacilli measuring 1 to 1.5 µm by 3 to 5 µm. When seen in clinical specimens, the bacilli appear encapsulated and occur in short chains of two to four cells. India ink may be used to visualize the capsules by direct examination of peripheral blood, cerebrospinal fluid, or cells grown on medium supplemented with sodium bicarbonate. Both blood and chocolate agars support the growth of *B. anthracis*. After overnight incubation at 35 to 37°C on blood agar, colonies are 2 to 5 mm in diameter, nonhemolytic, and flat or slightly convex, with irregular or waxy borders and a ground-glass appearance. The colonies have a tenacious consistency, causing them to pull up, like a beaten egg white, when teased with an inoculating loop. Some of the tests that may be performed in reference laboratories to confirm *B. anthracis* include lysis by gamma phage, direct fluorescent-antibody (DFA) assay, time-resolved fluorescence, and molecular characterization, as well as antimicrobial susceptibility testing.

B. cereus is also an important pathogen in humans, causing food-borne illness. This organism causes two forms of food-borne illness: intoxication and true infection. Intoxication is caused by a heat-stable enterotoxin, resulting in an abrupt onset of nausea and vomiting within 1 to 5 h after ingestion of the contaminated food. True infection is caused by a heat-labile enterotoxin, resulting in abdominal pain and diarrhea within 8 to 16 h after the food ingestion. *B. cereus* can also cause serious eye and wound infections following trauma.

B. cereus colonies are large (4 to 7 mm in diameter) and beta-hemolytic and vary in shape from circular to irregular with a grayish to greenish color and a ground-glass appearance. The colonies may appear very similar to *B. anthracis*, except that *B. cereus* is hemolytic and usually motile and grows on phenylethyl alcohol blood agar. Other reactions that differentiate *B. cereus* from *B. anthracis* and other members of the *Bacillaceae* are that it is lecithinase positive and gelatin hydrolysis positive and produces acid from glucose, maltose, and salicin.

Other *Bacillus* spp. demonstrate a wide variety of colony morphologies ranging from smooth and glossy to granular and wrinkled. Colonies may range in color from creamy to greenish or orange. Overall, the *Bacillus* spp. are easily recognized despite their morphologic diversity. Identification of the various species of *Bacillus* should include the basic tests assessing spore and colony characteristics, motility, hemolysis, and the egg yolk reaction. If further identification is required for isolates other than *B. anthracis*, commercial identification systems may be used once the basic tests have been performed. Differentiating characteristics of *Bacillus* spp. are presented in Table 7-1.

Table 7-1 Differentiation of *Bacillus* species[a]

Species	Anaerobic growth	Motility	Lecithinase (egg yolk reaction)	Gelatin hydrolysis	Arginine dihydrolase	Nitrate reduction
B. anthracis	+	0	+	V	0	+
B. cereus	+	+	+	+	V	V
B. licheniformis	+	+	0	+	V	+
B. megaterium	0	+	0	+	0	0
B. mycoides	+	0	+	+	V	V
B. pumilis	0	+	0	+	0	0
B. subtilis	0	+	0	+	0	+
B. thuringiensis	+	+	+	+	+	+

[a]+, positive reaction (≥85% positive); V, variable reaction (15 to 84% positive); 0, negative reaction (<15% positive).

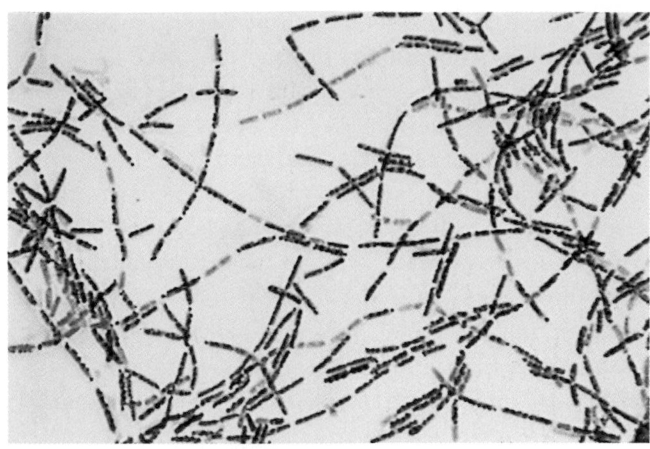

Figure 7-1 Gram stain of *Bacillus anthracis*. Gram stain of *B. anthracis*, showing cells approximately 1 to 5 μm in size occurring in long chains. The bacilli are primarily gram positive; however, a few gram-variable and gram-negative cells are also present. The spores are oval, and central to subterminal, and do not cause significant swelling of the cell.

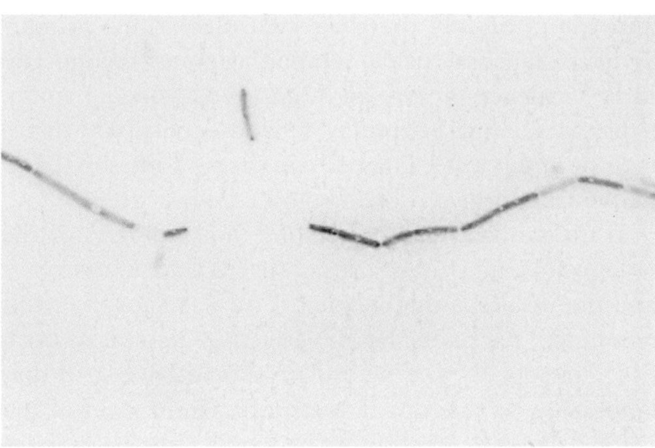

Figure 7-2 Gram stain of *Bacillus anthracis* grown on a urea agar slant. *Bacillus* spp. do not always stain gram positive, as demonstrated here. In this example, *B. anthracis* was grown on a urea agar slant to enhance the formation of spores. This Gram-stained smear shows gram-negative bacilli with bamboo-type joints and unstained areas suggestive of spores.

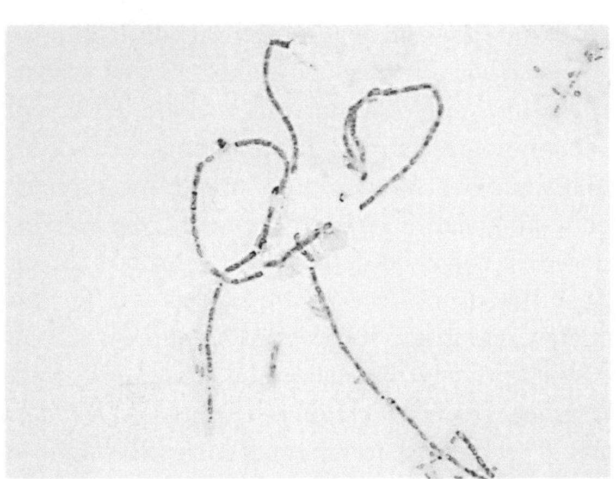

Figure 7-3 Spore stain of *Bacillus anthracis*. Spores are stained by flooding a heat-fixed smear with 10% aqueous malachite green for up to 45 min. The slide is then washed, and 0.5% aqueous safranin is applied as the counterstain for 30 s. Spores stain green and the vegetative cells are pinkish red, as shown in this figure. (Courtesy of Tamra Townsen, Orange County Health Department, Santa Ana, CA.)

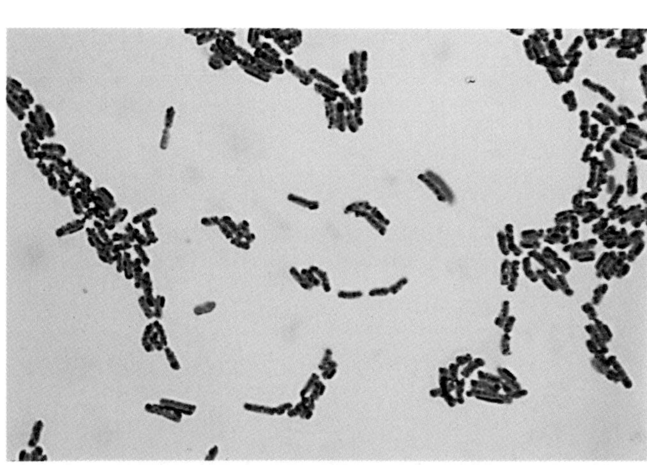

Figure 7-4 Gram stain of *Bacillus cereus*. A Gram stain of *B. cereus* showing cells similar to those of *B. anthracis* (Fig. 7-1); however, the *B. cereus* cells appear in a palisade formation rather than in long chains.

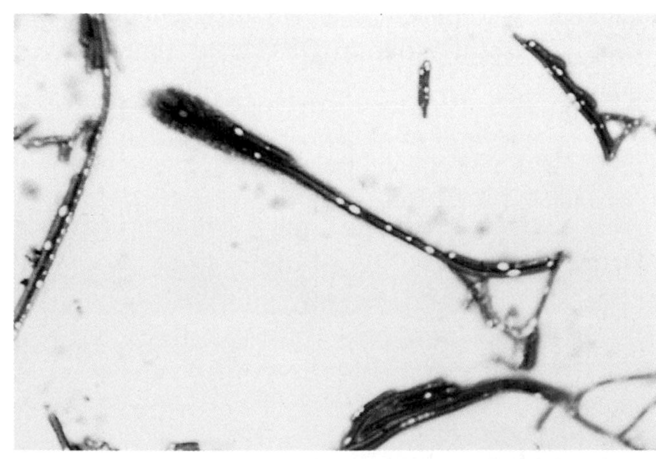

Figure 7-5 M'Fadyean stain of *Bacillus anthracis*. The M'Fadyean stain is a modification of the methylene blue stain developed for the detection of *B. anthracis* in clinical specimens. As shown here, the bacilli stain deep blue surrounded by a pink capsule; this is known as the M'Fadyean reaction.

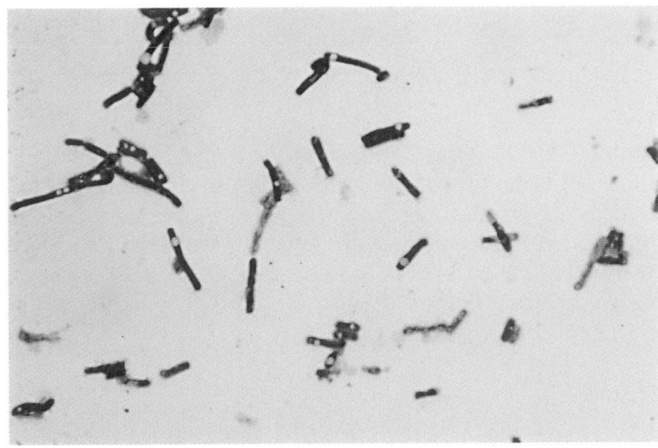

Figure 7-6 M'Fadyean stain of *Bacillus cereus*. In contrast to *B. anthracis*, cells of *B. cereus* stain deep blue but are not surrounded by a pink area because they are not encapsulated.

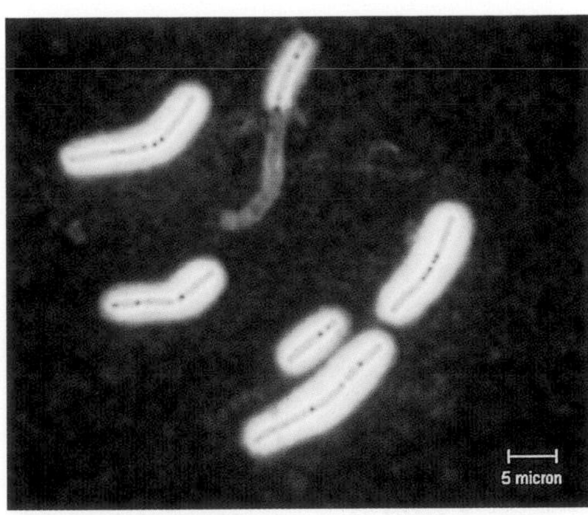

Figure 7-7 India ink stain of *Bacillus anthracis*. The India ink stain is used to improve visualization of encapsulated *B. anthracis* in clinical specimens, as shown here. (Courtesy of Tamra Townsen, Orange County Health Department, Santa Ana, CA.)

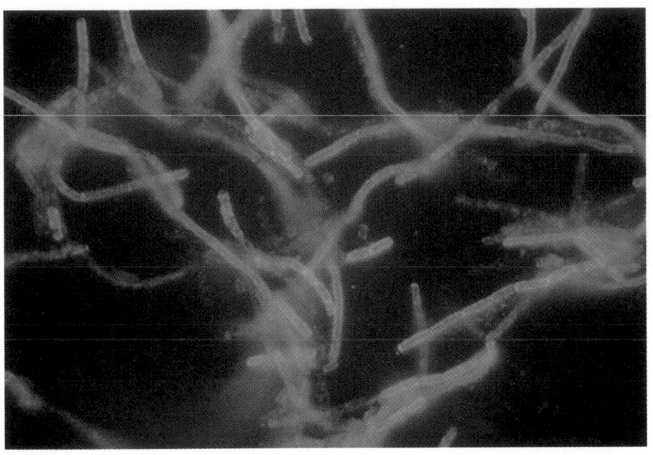

A

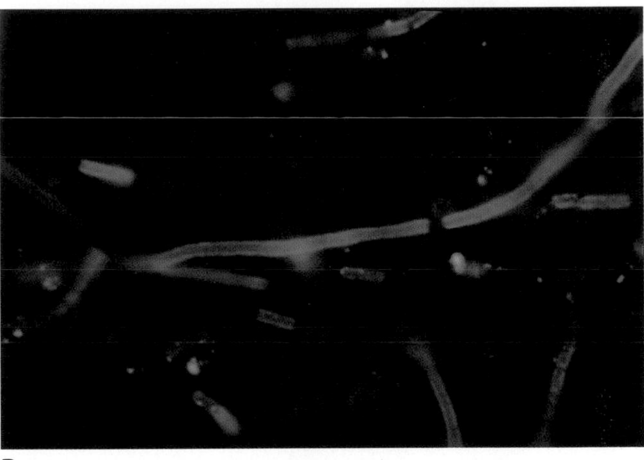

B

Figure 7-8 DFA assay of *Bacillus anthracis*. The DFA assay is used to detect the galactose/*N*-acetylglucosamine cell-wall-associated polysaccharide and capsule produced by vegetative cells of *B. anthracis*. The availability of monoclonal antibodies recognizing the cell wall polysaccharide (A) and capsule antigens (B) provides the ability to rapidly differentiate *B. anthracis* from other *Bacillus* spp. Concomitant demonstration of both antigens confirms the identification.

Figure 7-9 *Bacillus anthracis* on blood agar. After overnight incubation at 35°C on blood agar, colonies of *B. anthracis* measure approximately 2 to 5 mm in diameter. The flat or slightly convex nonhemolytic colonies may vary in shape from circular to irregularly round, with edges that are entire or irregular and with a matte, wavy, or ground-glass appearance. The colonies are tenacious and behave like beaten egg white when lifted with an inoculating loop, as shown above the arrow in the center of this figure. Colonies may also appear comma shaped or with "curled-hair" projections resembling a medusa head.

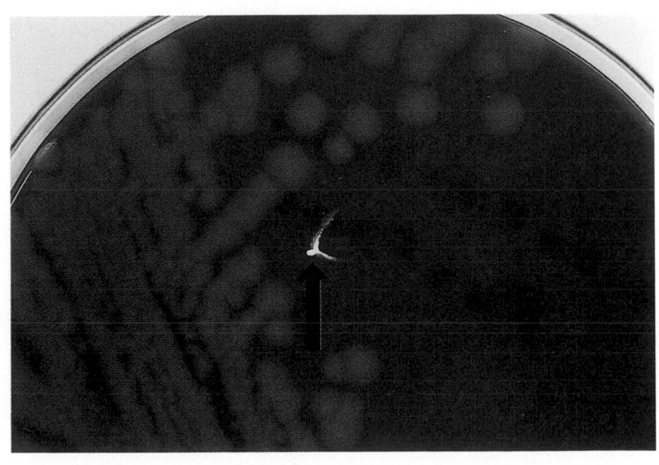

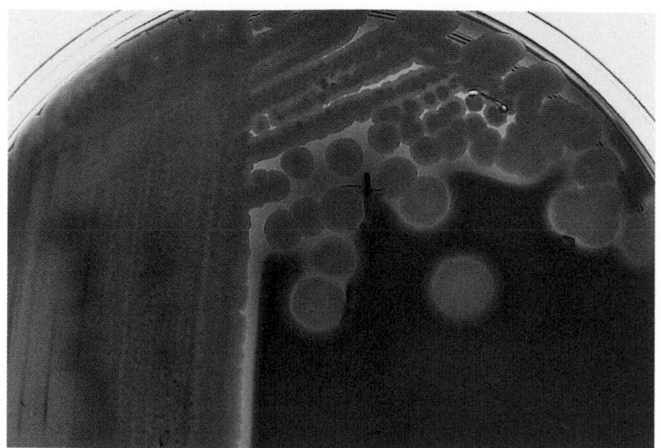

Figure 7-10 ***Bacillus cereus*** **on blood agar.** *B. cereus* colonies are large (approximately 7 mm in diameter), beta-hemolytic, circular, greenish, and with a ground-glass appearance. The colonies are very similar in appearance to those of *B. anthracis*; however, *B. anthracis* colonies are slightly smaller, nonhemolytic, and very tenacious.

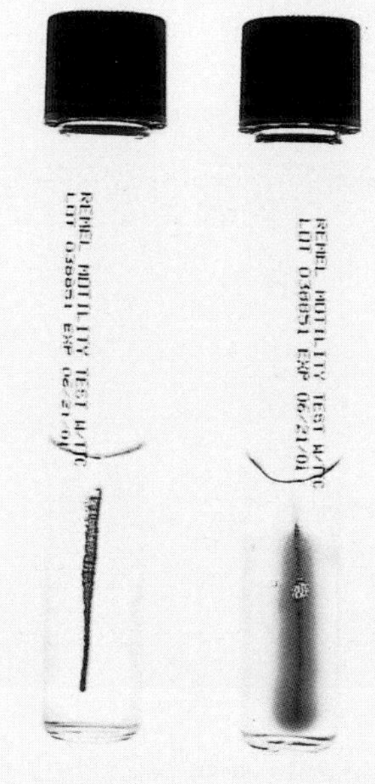

Figure 7-11 Motility test differentiating ***Bacillus anthracis*** **from other** ***Bacillus*** **spp.** Colony morphology, hemolysis, and motility are the key reactions that differentiate *B. anthracis* from other *Bacillus* spp. To determine motility, an agar deep containing tryptose and the dye triphenyltetrazolium is inoculated with an organism and incubated at 35°C overnight. If the organism is motile, it will migrate from the inoculation or stab line. This migration is visualized with the aid of triphenyltetrazolium, which is reduced by the organism to form an insoluble red pigment (formazan). In this example, *B. anthracis* is nonmotile (left) and *B. cereus* is motile (right).

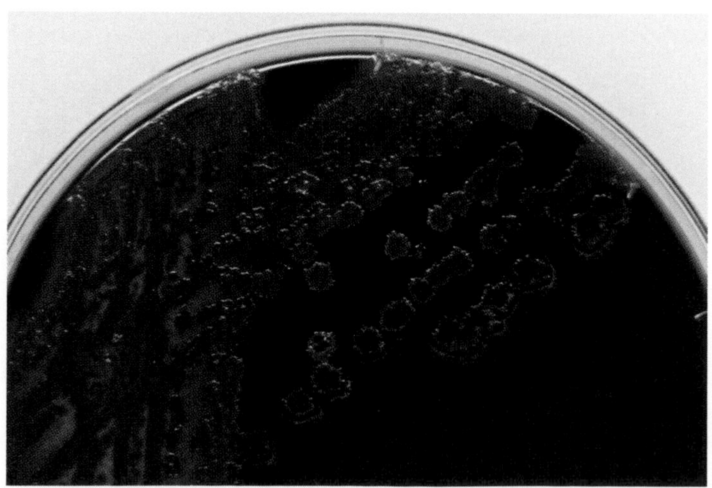

Figure 7-12 ***Bacillus licheniformis*** **on blood agar.** *B. licheniformis* derives its name from the formation of lichen-like colonies. The colonies are irregular in shape and 3 to 4 mm in size. Young colonies can appear moist, butyrous, and mucoid; they become dry, rough, and crusty as they age, giving them the licheniform appearance, as shown in this figure. Initially they can be confused with *B. subtilis* colonies; however, the licheniform appearance distinguishes them from other *Bacillus* spp.

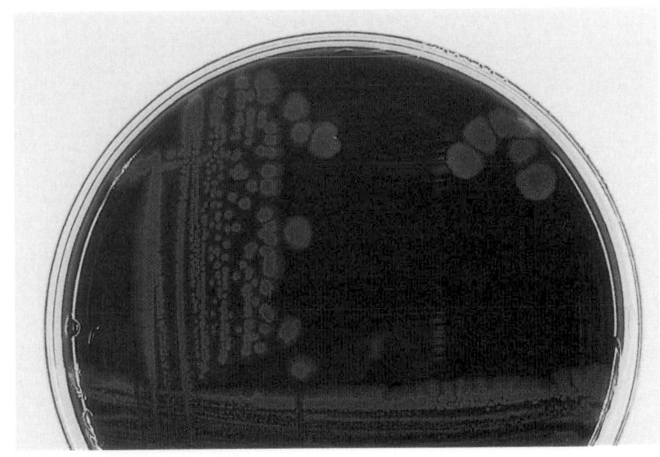

Figure 7-13 *Bacillus subtilis* on blood agar. *B. subtilis* colonies are approximately 4 to 5 mm in diameter, flat, dull, and somewhat dry with a ground-glass appearance. The beta-hemolysis distinguishes *B. subtilis* from *B. anthracis*. The colonies are similar to those of *B. cereus* (Fig. 7-10) but usually smaller.

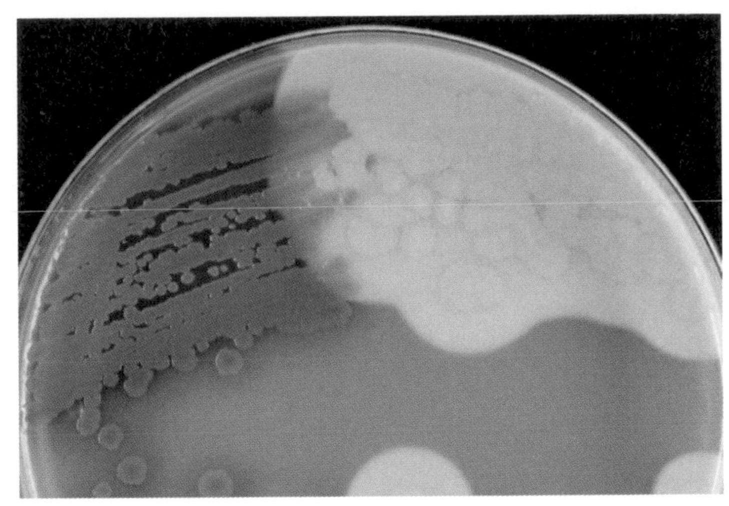

Figure 7-14 Egg yolk reaction of *Bacillus cereus* and *Bacillus subtilis*. *B. cereus* synthesizes lecithinases, forming opaque zones of precipitation around the colonies on egg yolk agar (right), while *B. subtilis* does not (left).

Figure 7-15 *Bacillus mycoides* on blood agar. Colonies of *B. mycoides* have a characteristic rhizoid or hairy-looking appearance, as shown in this figure. Eventually, these hairy, rhizoid, rootlike outgrowths spread across the entire plate. Unlike other *Bacillus* spp. (with the exception of *B. anthracis*), *B. mycoides* is nonmotile.

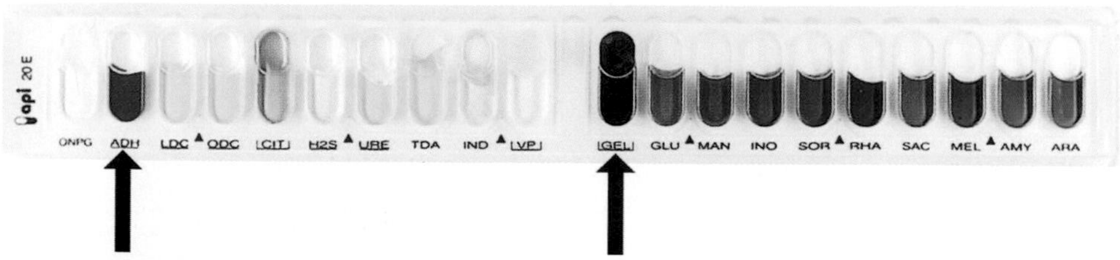

Figure 7-16 ***Bacillus cereus*** **identified by the API 20E system.** The API 20E system includes *Bacillus* spp. in its database. In this example, the arginine dihydrolase test is positive. This test rules out *B. anthracis*. Of the remaining reactions, gelatin is positive and the other tests are negative, confirming the identification of *B. cereus*. The positive reactions are indicated by the arrows.

Nocardia, *Rhodococcus*, *Actinomadura*, *Streptomyces*, and Other Aerobic Actinomycetes

8

More than 40 genera are classified as aerobic actinomycetes, of which approximately 10 are relevant to humans, including *Nocardia*, *Actinomadura*, *Streptomyces*, *Rhodococcus*, *Gordonia*, *Tsukamurella*, and *Tropheryma* (specifically, *Tropheryma whipplei*). These organisms are classified in this group mainly on the basis of microscopic characteristics. They are gram-positive and partially acid-fast bacilli and may have branched, filamentous hyphae that can form spores or can reproduce by fragmentation. The taxonomy of these organisms is currently undergoing significant changes based primarily on the application of molecular techniques. Until the new classification is established and accepted by the clinical laboratories, we have opted to use the classical nomenclature.

Nocardia spp. are found worldwide in the soil and water. Infections usually occur via the pulmonary and cutaneous routes in immunocompromised patients or those with an underlying pulmonary disease. The species most often isolated from humans include *Nocardia asteroides*, *Nocardia brasiliensis*, and *Nocardia otitidiscaviarum*. The *N. asteroides* complex includes *N. asteroides* sensu stricto type VI, *Nocardia abscessus*, *Nocardia farcinica*, and *Nocardia nova*.

Infection with *N. asteroides* via the pulmonary route usually results in a chronic bronchopneumonia that progresses in a matter of weeks or months and has a high mortality rate. Following a focus of pneumonitis, necrosis occurs with minimal inflammatory response. The organism may eventually disseminate to other organs including the brain, subcutaneous tissues, and kidneys. The sputum is thick and purulent, but unlike in infections due to anaerobic actinomycetes, sulfur granules or sinus tracts are observed only rarely.

Inoculation of *N. brasiliensis* in the skin or subcutaneous tissues of the foot may result in the formation of abscesses, termed actinomycotic mycetomas (in contrast to the eumycotic mycetomas produced by fungi), that can destroy the surrounding tissues including the bone. Sinuses are formed that drain in the skin, and the pus may contain sulfur granules that consist of groups of organisms and calcium sulfate and are yellow to orange with a granular appearance. Pus from draining sinuses can be used for direct examination using wet mounts. The granules can be broken between two glass slides, releasing the gram-positive branching, interwoven thin filaments.

Nocardia spp. are aerobic, gram-positive bacilli. However, they may appear gram negative with gram-positive beads and can form filamentous branches, similar to fungal hyphal forms. These hyphal forms can fragment into rod or coccoid, nonmotile elements. The cell wall of these organisms contains mycolic acid, and as a result they are partially acid fast. *Nocardia* spp. are catalase positive and utilize carbohydrates oxidatively.

Nocardia spp. grow relatively well on nonselective media including blood and chocolate agars, Sabouraud's dextrose agar without chloramphenicol, and Löwenstein-Jensen or Middlebrook media. However, *Nocardia* spp. grow slowly, and typically it takes 5 to 7 days for the colonies to appear at temperatures between 25° and 37°C. Nocardiae form aerial hyphae on culture media, and their hyphae may be visible under a dissecting microscope. The ability of *Nocardia* spp.

to utilize paraffin as an energy source is a characteristic that has been used to differentiate them from other aerobic bacteria.

The genus *Rhodococcus* (red-pigmented coccus) includes more than 20 species of gram-positive, partially acid-fast, coccobacillary, obligate aerobic actinomycetes. *Rhodococcus equi* is clinically the most important species and may cause granulomatous pneumonia in immunocompromised patients, particularly those infected with HIV type 1. Cavitating lesions in the lungs frequently occur, and the organisms may disseminate to other organs including the brain and subcutaneous tissues. This organism can be recovered from sputum, bronchoalveolar lavage fluid, lung biopsy specimens, and blood cultures. It grows well on nonselective media, although the typical salmon-pink pigment may take 3 to 5 days to appear. Biochemical characterization is difficult, and identification usually relies on colony morphology and the Gram stain showing gram-positive coccobacilli with traces of branching and the partial acid-fast properties.

In tropical and subtropical countries, *Actinomadura madurae*, *Actinomadura latina*, and *Actinomadura pelletieri* cause actinomycotic mycetomas, particularly in individuals who walk barefooted. Members of this species have very similar microscopic and colony characteristics to *Nocardia* spp. but can be differentiated on the basis of biochemical reactions.

Streptomyces anulatus (previously called *Streptomyces griseus*) and *Streptomyces somaliensis* are organisms usually found in immunocompromised patients. In certain parts of the world, particularly in Africa, *S. somaliensis* is a relatively frequent cause of actinomycotic mycetomas of the head and neck. Other *Streptomyces* spp. have recently been associated with a variety of infections, particularly in patients with AIDS. Colonies of *Streptomyces* spp. can produce a diverse range of pigments, which may result in coloration of the substrate, and aerial hyphae, although these are not produced by all the strains.

Nocardia, *Actinomadura*, and *Streptomyces* species may be differentiated on the basis of their ability to decompose casein, tyrosine, xanthine, and starch on the Nocardia ID Quad plate (BD Diagnostic Systems, Franklin Lakes, NJ) (Table 8-1).

Gordonia and *Tsukamurella* spp., which are closely related to *Rhodococcus* spp., are found in the soil and are considered opportunistic human pathogens. Members of these two genera have been associated with catheter-related sepsis and cutaneous, pulmonary, and central nervous system infections, particularly in immunocompromised patients. The colony morphology of *Gordonia* spp. ranges from smooth and mucoid to dry, and the colonies are beige to salmon pink. Rudimentary hyphae are produced by some strains, while others form aerial synnemata, which should not be confused with aerial hyphae. Synnemata or coremia are groups of erect conidiophores cemented together and producing conidia at the apex and/or the sides of the upper portion. Colonies of *Tsukamurella* measure 0.5 to 2 mm in diameter and are circular, with smooth to rhizoid edges; dry; and white to orange. On prolonged incubation the colonies have a cerebroid morphology but do not produce aerial hyphae.

Tropheryma whipplei causes Whipple's disease, which is characterized by diarrhea, weight loss, lymphadenopathy, fever, arthralgia, and skin pigmentation. Histologically the typical finding includes foamy macrophages infiltrating the lamina propria of the small intestine that stain positive with periodic acid-Schiff (PAS) stain. In the absence of histopathological findings, a positive nucleic acid amplification test for this organism should be interpreted cautiously if no clinical symptoms are present. *T. whipplei* has been cultured in some tissue culture systems but not on artificial media.

Table 8-1 Decomposition of substrates used for the differentiation of actinomycetes

Organism	Decomposition of[a]:				
	Casein	Tyrosine	Xanthine	Starch	Urea
Actinomadura madura	+	+	0	+	0
Actinomadura pelletieri	+	+	0	0	0
Nocardia asteroides	0	0	0	0	+
Nocardia brasiliensis	+	+	0	0	+
Nocardia otitidiscaviarum	0	0	+	0	+
Streptomyces somaliensis	+	+	0	V	0
Streptomyces anulatus	+	+	+	+	V

[a]+, positive reaction (>90% positive); V, variable reaction (11 to 89% positive); 0, negative reaction (<10% positive).

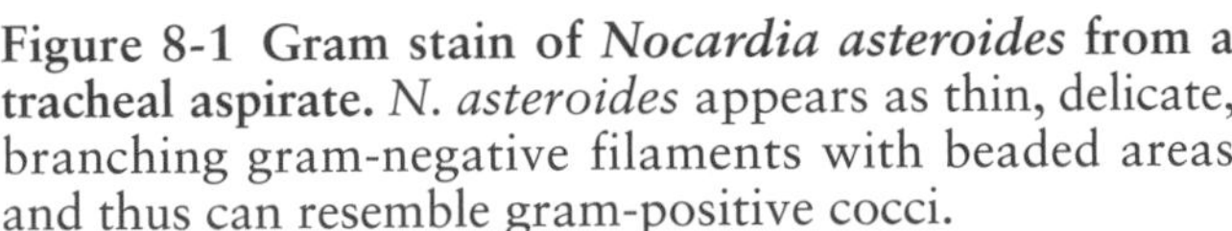

Figure 8-1 Gram stain of *Nocardia asteroides* from a tracheal aspirate. *N. asteroides* appears as thin, delicate, branching gram-negative filaments with beaded areas and thus can resemble gram-positive cocci.

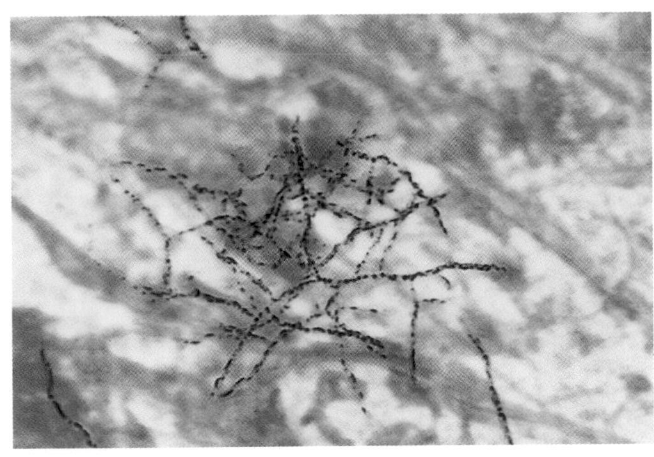

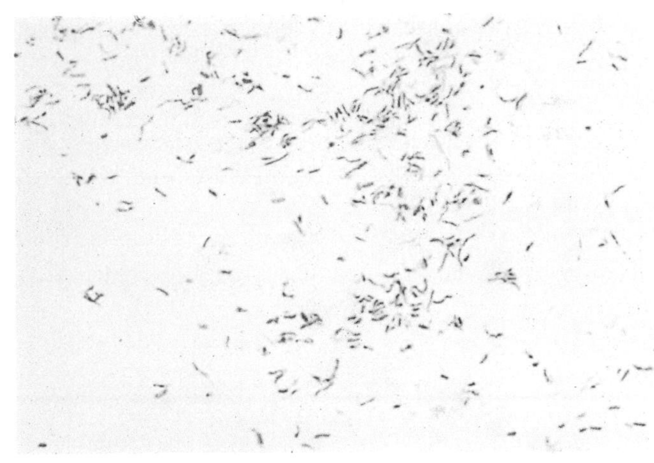

Figure 8-2 Acid-fast stain of *Nocardia asteroides*. *N. asteroides* produces long, thin, filamentous structures that are partially acid fast. In culture, the filaments fragment, as shown here.

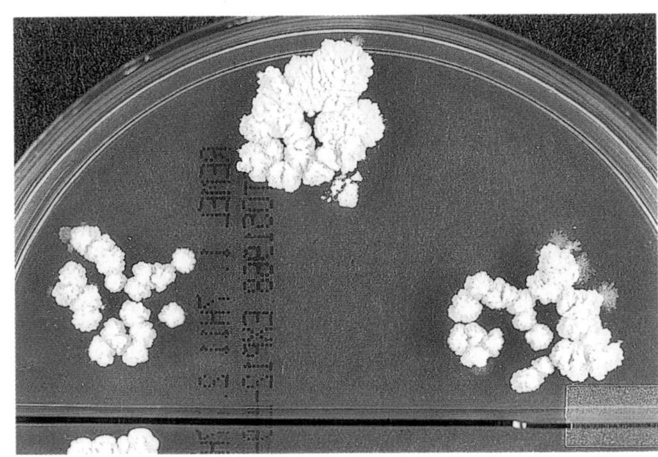

Figure 8-3 *Nocardia asteroides* on 7H11 medium. Colonies of *N. asteroides* are highly variable in morphology, depending on the culture conditions. The color can range from chalky white, as shown here, due to the growth of aerial hyphae, to orange and salmon pink.

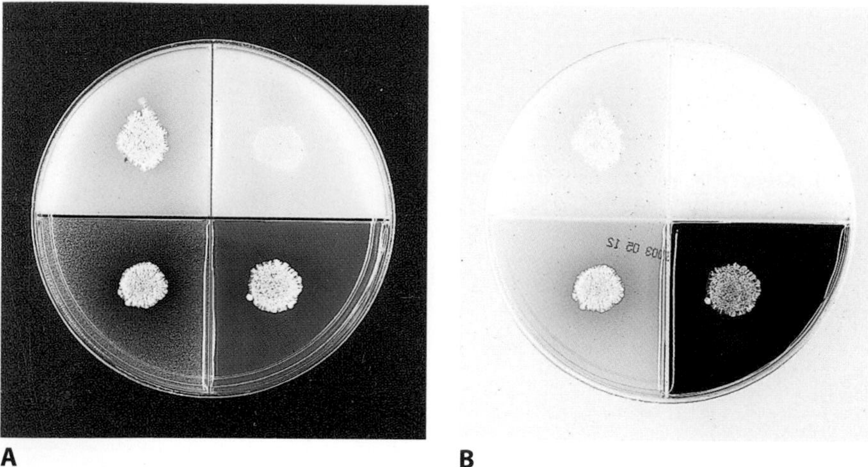

Figure 8-4 ***Nocardia asteroides*** **on a Nocardia ID Quad plate.** The Nocardia ID Quad plate is used to determine the ability of the organism to decompose casein (top right), starch (bottom right), tyrosine (bottom left), and xanthine (top left). (A) Organisms that can utilize these substrates produce a clear halo around the colonies. (B) Hydrolysis of starch is indicated by the presence of a colorless zone around the colonies after the quadrant is flooded with Gram's iodine. As shown here, *N. asteroides* does not decompose any of these four substrates. These plates should be observed weekly for 1 month because the organisms grow, and break down the substrates, at different rates. Production of a melanin-like pigment may occur in the quadrants containing the tyrosine and xanthine agars.

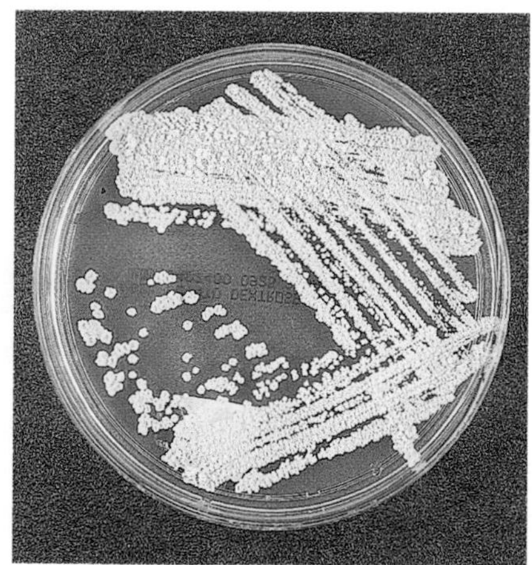

Figure 8-5 ***Nocardia brasiliensis*** **on Sabouraud dextrose agar.** Colonies of *N. brasiliensis* are typically orange-tan with a dry, crumbly consistency.

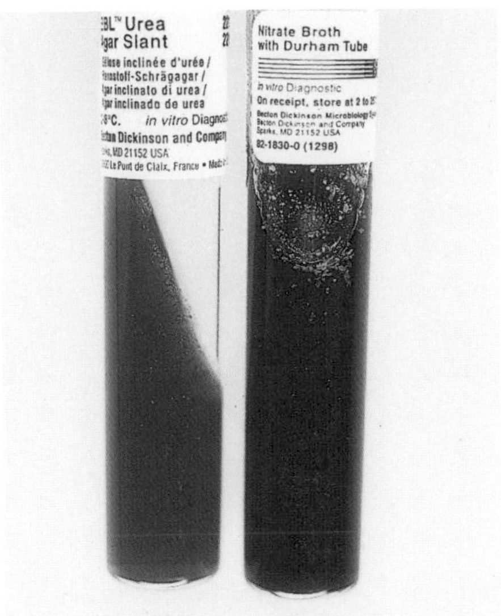

Figure 8-6 *Nocardia brasiliensis* in urea and nitrate broths. *N. brasiliensis* hydrolyzes urea (left) and reduces nitrates to nitrites or nitrogen gas (right). To perform the urease test, Christensen urea agar is inoculated and incubated at room temperature for several weeks. *Nocardia* spp. contain urease, which breaks down urea to form carbonic acid and ammonia, resulting in an increase in the pH that turns the medium red due to the phenol red present in the agar. Reduction of nitrate to nitrite results in the development of a red color due to the formation of a red diazonium dye. Negative reactions are confirmed by adding zinc dust; this should result in the appearance of a red color in 5 to 10 min, indicating that nitrate has not been reduced. If the broth remains clear after the addition of the zinc dust, it means that nitrate has been reduced to free nitrogen gas and the reaction should be considered positive.

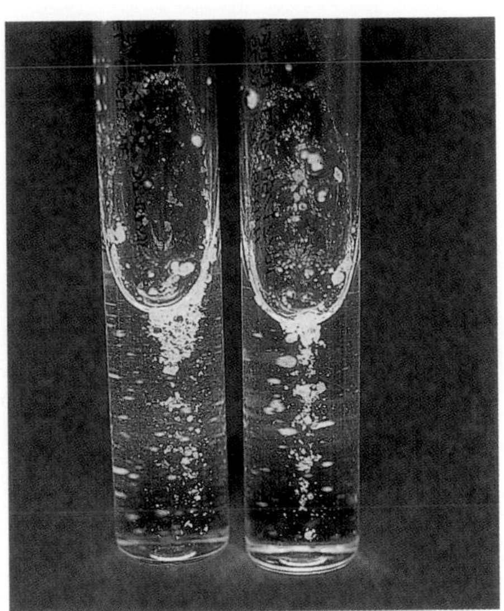

Figure 8-7 Lysozyme test for *Nocardia brasiliensis*. Practically all members of the genus *Nocardia* can grow in the presence of lysozyme. This is in contrast to anaerobic actinomycetes, which do not grow in the presence of lysozyme. To perform this test, two tubes of sterile glycerol broth, one with lysozyme (left) and one without (right), are inoculated with the organism to be identified. As shown here for *N. brasiliensis*, the test is considered positive if the bacteria grow equally well in both tubes. If there is no growth in the tube containing lysozyme, the test is considered negative.

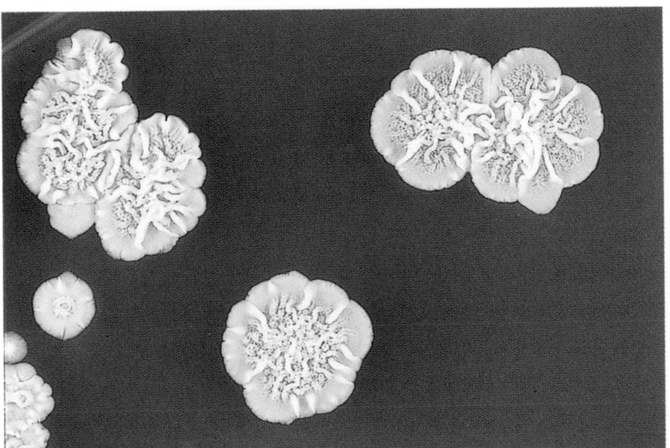

Figure 8-8 *Nocardia otitidiscaviarum* on Sabouraud dextrose agar. *N. otitidiscaviarum* usually produces pale tan colonies. This particular isolate has formed dried, cerebroid colonies after 2 weeks of incubation.

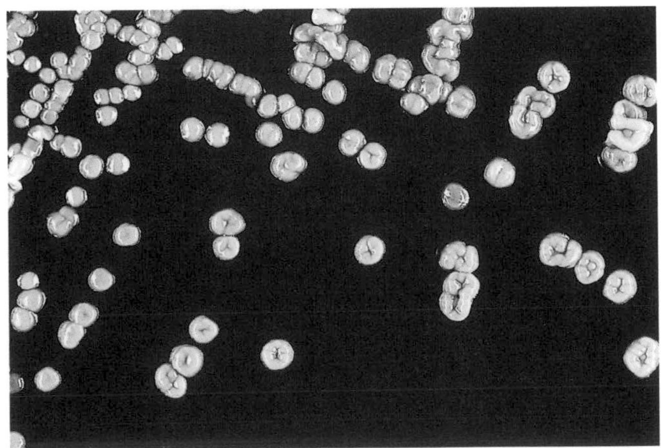

Figure 8-9 *Actinomadura madura* on Sabouraud dextrose agar. The colonies of *A. madura* can be white to pink, are usually mucoid, and, as shown here, have a molar-tooth appearance. *Actinomadura* spp. sometimes produce aerial hyphae.

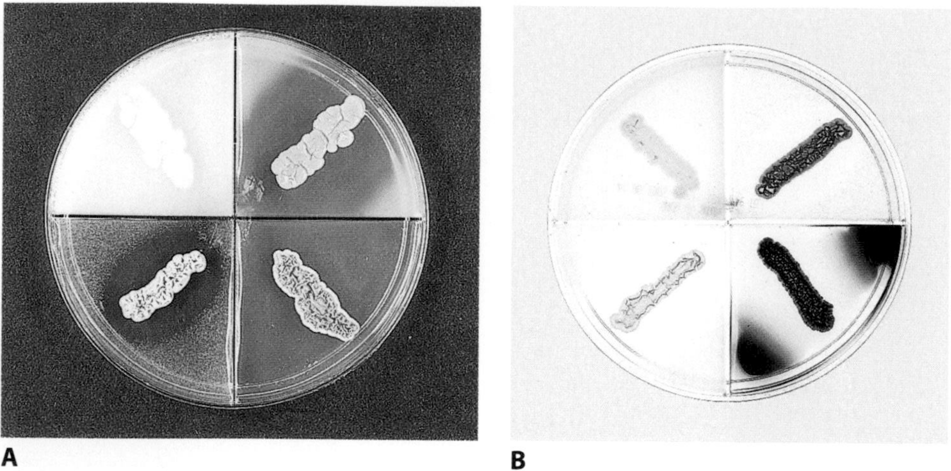

Figure 8-10 ***Actinomadura madura*** **on a Nocardia ID Quad plate.** *A. madura* breaks down casein (top right), starch (bottom right), and tyrosine (bottom left) but not xanthine (top left) (see Fig. 8-4 for details).

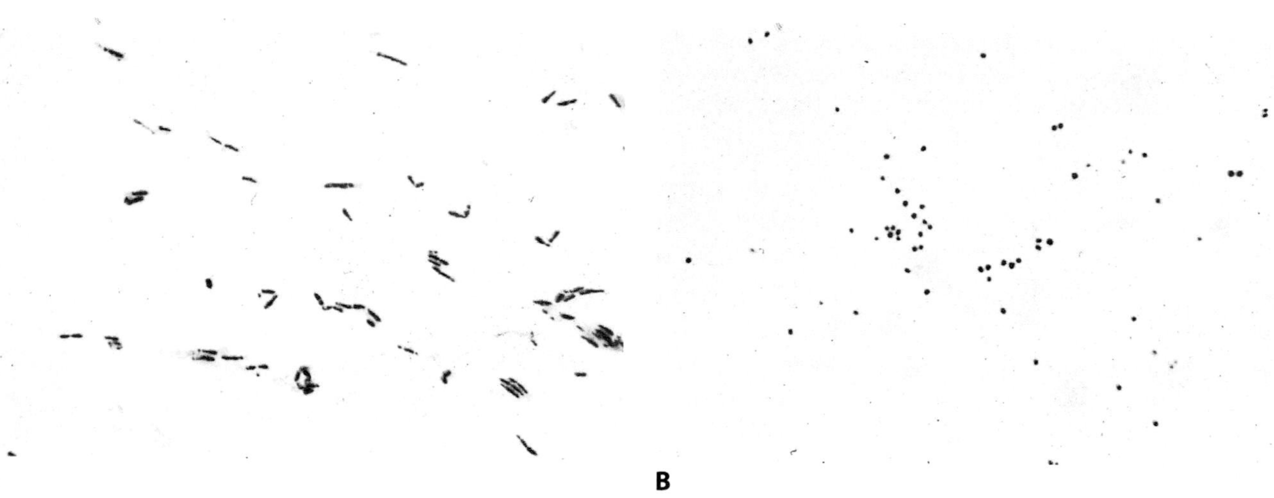

Figure 8-11 Gram stain of ***Rhodococcus equi.*** Depending on the culture conditions, the morphology of *R. equi* can range from bacillary to coccoid. (A) In a 24-h culture, the bacillary morphology of *R. equi* is evident. (B) After 72 h in culture, the same organism has a coccoid structure.

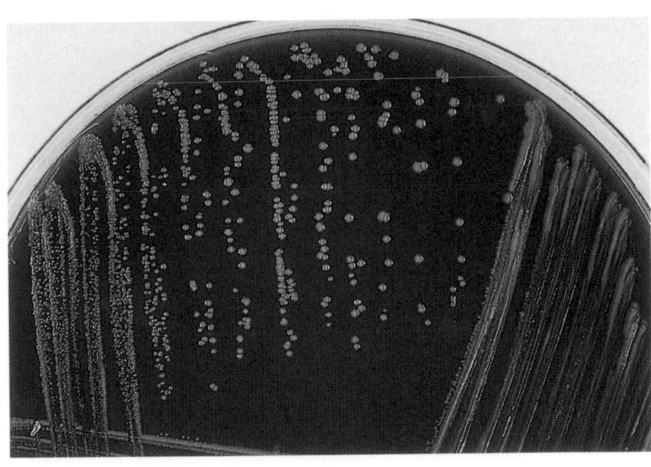

Figure 8-12 ***Rhodococcus equi*** **on blood agar.** Members of the genus *Rhodococcus* may have variable colony morphology, ranging from rough to smooth or mucoid. The color can also vary from buff to orange or deep rose. The isolate shown here has smooth, round colonies with a pink-orange color.

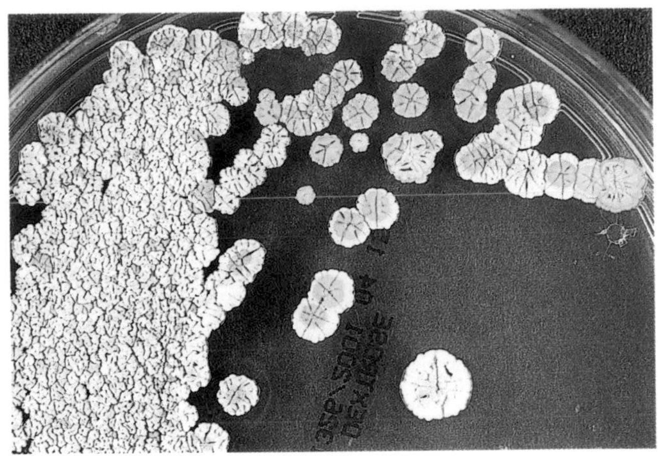

Figure 8-13 ***Streptomyces*** **spp.** on Sabouraud dextrose agar. There are many colony morphotypes due to the great variety of organisms included in this group. The colonies shown here are orange to tan, irregular, and with a smooth surface due to the growth of *Streptomyces anulatus*.

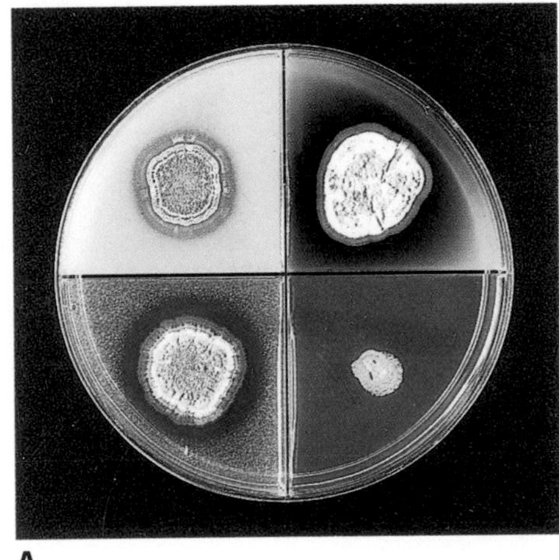

A

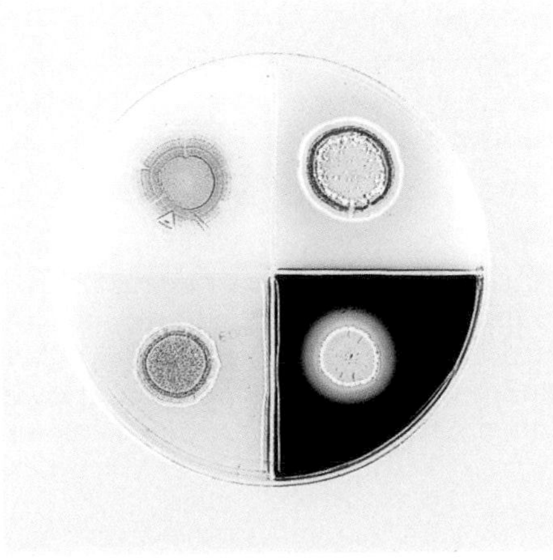

B

Figure 8-14 ***Streptomyces anulatus*** **on a Nocardia ID Quad plate.** *S. anulatus* can decompose the four substrates casein (top right), starch (bottom right), tyrosine (bottom left), and xanthine (top left), present in the Nocardia ID Quad plate (see Fig. 8-4 for details).

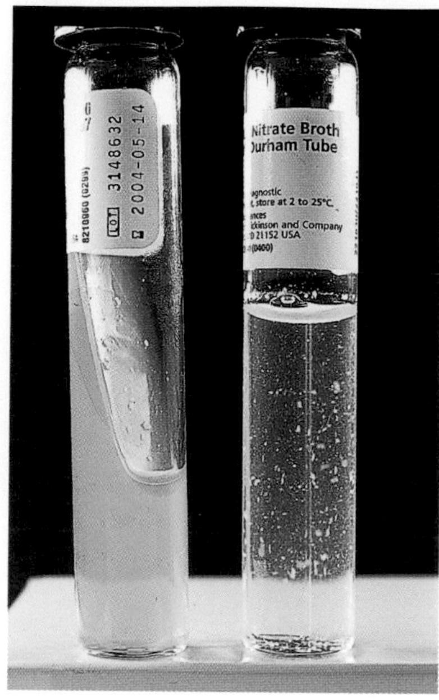

Figure 8-15 ***Streptomyces*** **spp.** in urea and nitrate broths. Most *Streptomyces* spp. do not produce urease and cannot reduce nitrates to nitrites, in contrast to *Nocardia* spp. (Fig. 8-6).

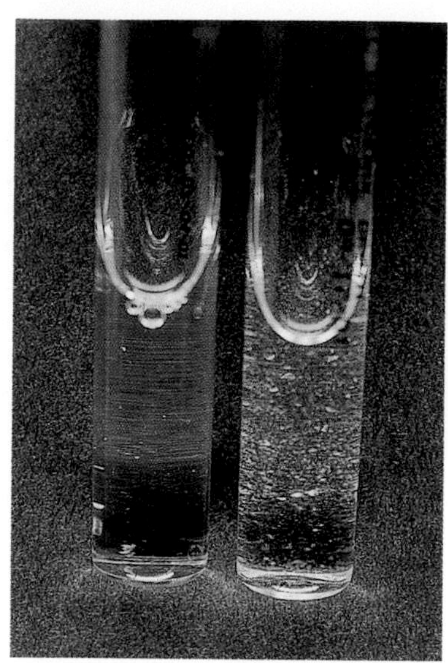

Figure 8-16 Lysozyme test for ***Streptomyces*** **spp.** *Streptomyces* spp. do not grow in the presence of lysozyme (left). The organism was able to grow only in the tube that did not contain lysozyme (right). This is in contrast to members of the genus *Nocardia*, which can grow in media containing lysozyme (Fig. 8-7).

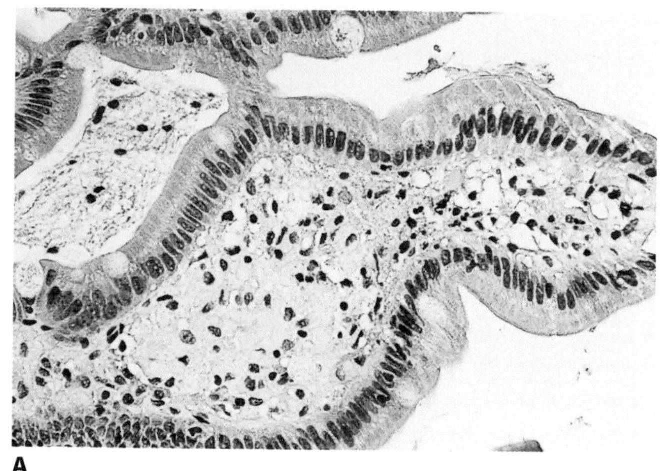

A

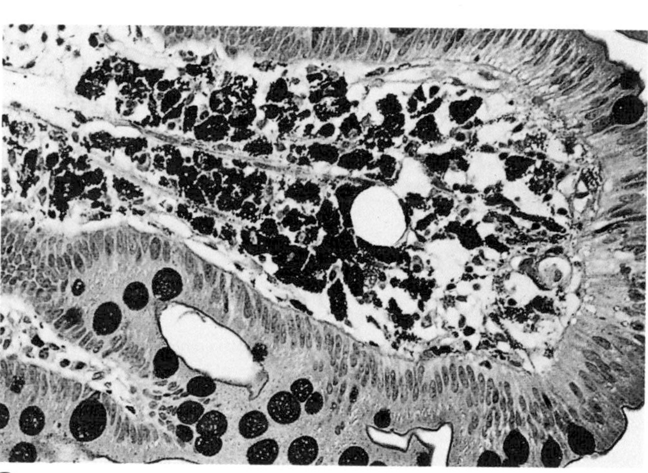

B

Figure 8-17 Small-intestine biopsy specimen from a patient with Whipple's disease. *T. whipplei* causes Whipple's disease, characterized by the presence of large quantities of histiocytes in the lamina propria of the intestinal mucosa, which contains numerous organisms. (A) Extracellular bacilli are also found below the basal lamina of the epithelial cells, and the number of organisms diminishes toward the submucosa. (B) Macrophages containing *T. whipplei* have a coarsely granular material that stains intensely with PAS. Hematoxylin and eosin (A) and PAS (B) stains. Magnification, ×250.

Mycobacterium 9

Mycobacterium is the only genus in the family *Mycobacteriaceae* and includes more than 100 species. Based on the epidemiology and disease presentation, isolates of human relevance are divided into the *Mycobacterium tuberculosis* complex (which includes *M. tuberculosis*, *Mycobacterium bovis*, *M. bovis* bacille Calmette-Guérin [BCG], *Mycobacterium africanum*, *Mycobacterium canettii*, *Mycobacterium caprae*, *Mycobacterium microti*, *Mycobacterium pinnipedii*, and *Mycobacterium mungi*), the nontuberculous mycobacteria, and the noncultivable nontuberculous mycobacteria. Culturable mycobacteria of clinical significance are listed in Table 9-1.

It is estimated that approximately one-third of the world's population is infected with *M. tuberculosis*, and approximately 2 million people die as a result of this infection on an annual basis. The appearance of multidrug-resistant and extensively drug-resistant isolates of *M. tuberculosis* and the increased risk of infection in patients infected with HIV have further augmented the awareness of this disease. *M. tuberculosis* is transported by airborne particles generated mainly by patients with a productive cough. Humans are exposed to *M. bovis* by ingesting contaminated milk from infected cows. *M. bovis* has a wide host range including nonhuman primates, cattle, buffalo, goats, pigs, dogs, cats, and some birds. The *M. bovis* BCG strain is an attenuated form of *M. bovis* that has been used extensively in many parts of the world as a vaccine to protect against tuberculosis. It is also used against certain tumors, e.g., those of the urinary bladder, due to its ability to stimulate the immune system. *M. africanum* and *M. canettii* are found mainly in Africa, and their epidemiology is not well characterized. *M. microti* has been found to cause infections in immunocompetent and immunocompromised humans. *M caprae*, formerly identified as *M. tuberculosis* subsp. *caprae* and *M. bovis* subsp. *caprae*, causes up to 30% of cases of human tuberculosis, most with pulmonary manifestations, in certain parts of Europe. Transmission of *M. pinnipedii* from sea lions to humans has been demonstrated and results in granulomatous lesions involving the lungs, pleura, lymph nodes, and spleen.

The nontuberculous bacteria are ubiquitous in the environment and can be found on the skin and in the respiratory and gastrointestinal tracts of healthy individuals. The route of transmission can include the respiratory and gastrointestinal tracts, and occasionally infections are iatrogenically or nosocomially acquired. Transmission from person to person is unusual, and pathogenicity is low. Gastrointestinal manifestations usually predominate in immunocompromised patients, and blood cultures are frequently positive in this group of individuals.

The *Mycobacterium avium* complex (MAC) includes two species, *M. avium* and *Mycobacterium intracellulare*, and multiple serovars. These mycobacteria are found readily in the environment, including water and soil, and in pigs, chickens, and cats. From the point of view of human infections, their importance has significantly increased with the HIV epidemic.

Mycobacterium ulcerans is, after *M. tuberculosis* and *Mycobacterium leprae*, the most common mycobacterial pathogen in humans. This organism is particularly prevalent in Africa, where the disease it causes is known as Buruli ulcer; in Australia, it is called Bairnsdale ulcer.

Table 9-1 Cultivable mycobacteria of clinical significance

Slow growers			Rapid growers	
M. tuberculosis complex	Nonchromogens	Chromogens	Nonchromogens	Chromogens
M. tuberculosis	*M. avium* complex	*M. asiaticum*	*M. abscessus*	*M. phlei*
M. africanum	*M. celatum*	*M. flavescens*	*M. chelonae*	*M. vaccae*
M. bovis	*M. gastri*	*M. gordonae*	*M. fortuitum* group	
M. bovis BCG	*M. genavense*	*M. kansasii*	*M. mucogenicum*	
M. canettii	*M. haemophilum*	*M. marinum*	M. *smegmatis*	
M. caprae	*M. malmoense*	*M. scrofulaceum*		
M. microti	*M. shimoidei*	*M. simiae*		
M. mungi	*M. terrae* complex	*M. szulgai*		
M. pinnipedii	*M. triviale*	*M. xenopi*		
	M. ulcerans			

The noncultivable nontuberculous mycobacteria include *M. leprae*, which causes leprosy (Hansen's disease), a chronic granulomatous disease that usually manifests with anesthetic skin lesions and peripheral neuropathy. *M. leprae* cannot be cultured in vitro, and thus the diagnosis is made based on the clinical presentation and skin biopsy. A skin test with lepromin, a preparation of the bacterial antigen, can help in the diagnosis.

Mycobacteria are straight or slightly curved bacilli that measure 1.0 to 10.0 μm by 0.2 to 0.6 μm, may branch, are nonmotile, and do not form spores. The large amount of lipids present in the wall of the mycobacteria makes these organisms difficult to stain. Arylmethane dyes, such as fuchsin and auramine O, are used as primary stains that in the presence of phenol can penetrate the cell wall and are complexed to mycolic acid. After exposure of the cells to acid-alcohol or to strong mineral acids, a counterstain is added. The ability of these organisms to resist decoloration with up to 3% hydrochloric acid is referred to as acid-fastness. Other microorganisms that are partially acid fast include species of *Nocardia* and *Rhodococcus*; *Legionella micdadei*; and the protozoa *Isospora*, *Cyclospora*, and *Cryptosporidium*.

Respiratory tract samples are the specimens most frequently submitted for culture. Biopsy specimens, gastric aspirates, cerebrospinal fluid, and urine are also often processed in the mycobacteriology laboratory. Blood and feces are usually obtained from immunocompromised patients. Optimal recovery of mycobacteria from clinical specimens requires the inoculation of both a broth and a solid medium. Broth media have the advantage of being more sensitive and provide more rapid detection than solid media. Semiautomated systems are available that utilize a broth medium. Solid media, on the other hand, allow preliminary identification of isolates on the basis of colony morphology and pigment production.

Löwenstein-Jensen medium can be used for the isolation of mycobacteria. It contains whole eggs, glycerol, potato flour, and salts to support the growth of mycobacteria and malachite green to inhibit the growth of contaminating bacteria. Some selective media contain additional antibiotics to minimize the growth of other bacteria. Middlebrook 7H10 and 7H11 are transparent agar-based media that, in comparison with Löwenstein-Jensen medium, have the advantages of allowing early detection of growth and microscopic examination of the morphology of the colonies by looking through the back of the plate. These media, in addition to defined salts, vitamins, and malachite green, contain some enrichment factors such as oleic acid, bovine albumin, glucose, and catalase; 0.1% casein hydrolysate is added to 7H11 to improve the recovery of isoniazid-resistant strains of *M. tuberculosis*.

Mycobacteria are classified as rapid growers if they produce visible colonies in less than 7 days and as slow growers if they form colonies in 2 to 8 weeks (Table 9-1). The growth rate depends on the species of mycobacteria and is influenced by the media and the temperature of incubation. According to their photoreactive characteristics, mycobacteria are categorized into three groups. Species that produce yellow to dark orange carotene pigment in response to light are called photochromogens, while those that produce pigment independent of the amount of light are termed scotochromogens. Species that do not produce pigment, such as *M. tuberculosis*, have a buff color and are classified as nonchromogens.

All cultures for mycobacteria should be incubated at 37°C under 5 to 10% CO_2 for at least 6 to 8 weeks.

Table 9-2 Useful tests for the identification of mycobacteria

Test[a] for:			
Nonchromogens	**Photochromogens**	**Scotochromogens**	**Rapid growers**
Arylsulfatase	Arylsulfatase at 28°C	Arylsulfatase at 42°C	Arylsulfatase
Catalase	Catalase	Catalase	Catalase
NaCl tolerance	Growth rate at 28°C	Growth rate at 42°C	Iron uptake
Niacin	Niacin	NaCl tolerance	NaCl tolerance
Nitrate reduction	Nitrate reduction	Nitrate reduction	Nitrate reduction
PZA	Pigment	Pigment at 25°C	MacConkey without CV
Tween 80 hydrolysis	Tween 80 hydrolysis	Tween 80 hydrolysis	Utilization of sodium citrate, inositol, and mannitol
Urease		Urease	
T2H			

[a]PZA, pyrazinamidase; CV, crystal violet; T2H, thiophene-2-carboxylic acid hydrazide.

In addition, specimens from skin lesions should be incubated at 30°C because pathogens such as *Mycobacterium marinum*, *Mycobacterium haemophilum*, *Mycobacterium chelonae*, and *M. ulcerans* grow better at lower temperatures. To recover *M. haemophilum*, a chocolate agar medium should also be included since this organism requires hemin or hemoglobin for growth.

DNA probes are commercially available to identify *M. tuberculosis* complex, *M. avium* complex, *M. avium*, *M. intracellulare*, *Mycobacterium gordonae*, and *Mycobacterium kansasii*. The probes for the *M. tuberculosis* complex cannot differentiate between *M. tuberculosis*, *M. bovis*, *M. bovis* BCG, *M. africanum*, *M. microti*, and *M. canettii*. Compared with culture and biochemicals, the probes for identification from culture have sensitivities and specificities greater than 99%. Nucleic acid amplification methods such as PCR are performed in some laboratories for the detection and identification of mycobacteria directly from clinical specimens. The specificity and sensitivity of these techniques, however, are still under investigation. Mass spectrometry for the identification of mycobacteria is being developed. Useful tests for the identification of mycobacteria are listed in Table 9-2.

The most frequently utilized immunodiagnostic test for the diagnosis of tuberculosis is the tuberculin skin test. This test has shortcomings, though, including the inability to distinguish active tuberculosis from past sensitization with BCG and cross-reactivity with nontuberculous mycobacteria. New gamma-interferon release assays may be able to overcome some of these shortcomings. These assays determine T-cell gamma-interferon responses to two or three antigens that are only found in *M. tuberculosis*, *Mycobacterium szulgai*, *M. kansasii*, and *M. marinum*. However, the performance characteristics of these assays in different populations and settings are still under investigation.

A

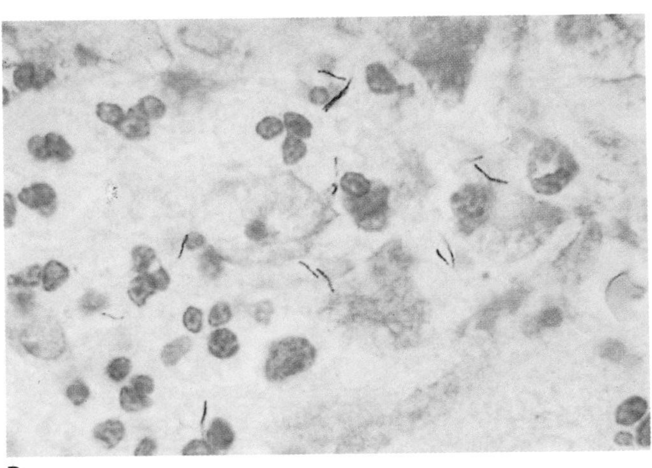
B

Figure 9-1 Kinyoun stain of *Mycobacterium tuberculosis*. In sputum (A) and tissue (B) specimens stained by the carbol fuchsin methods, such as those involving Ziehl-Nielsen and Kinyoun stains, *M. tuberculosis* appears as red-purple, curved, short or long bacilli, ranging from 1.0 to 10.0 μm by 0.2 to 0.6 μm, against a blue or a green background.

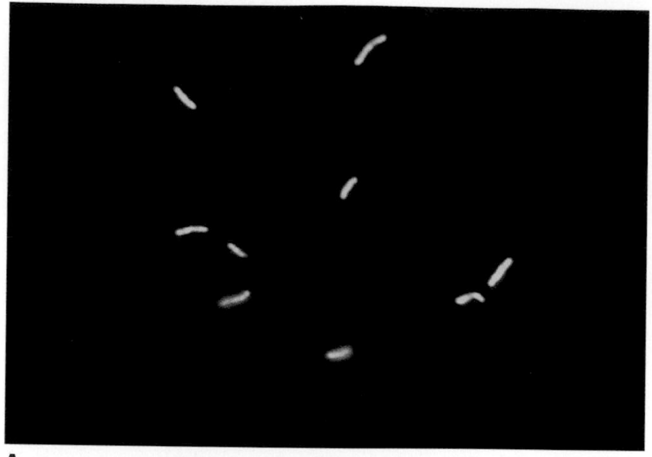

A

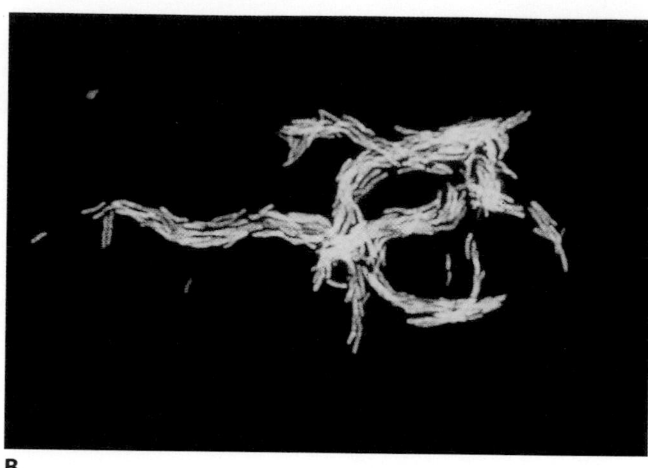

B

Figure 9-2 Auramine stain of *Mycobacterium tuberculosis*. (A) With the two fluorochromes commonly used, auramine O and auramine-rhodamine, *M. tuberculosis* fluoresces yellow to orange, depending on the microscope filters used. The fluorescent stains are more sensitive and have the advantage that the specimen can be screened at low magnification. According to some authors, one of the shortcomings of the fluorescence methods is that some of the rapid growers may not stain. For this reason, they recommend counterstaining the smear with the Ziehl-Nielsen or Kinyoun stain when rapid growers are suspected. (B) Following incubation in liquid medium, *M. tuberculosis* organisms form large cordae.

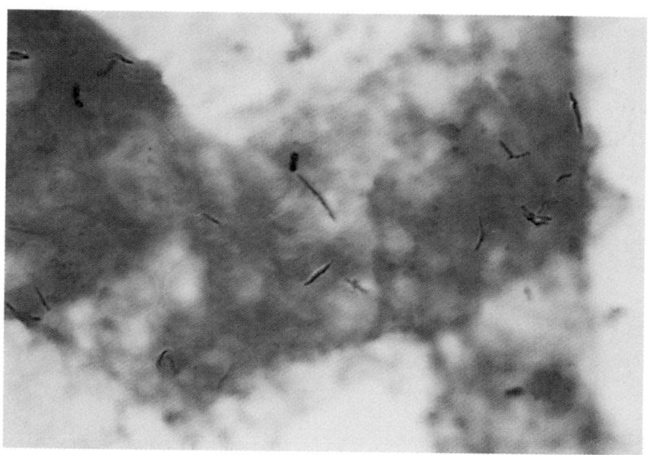

A

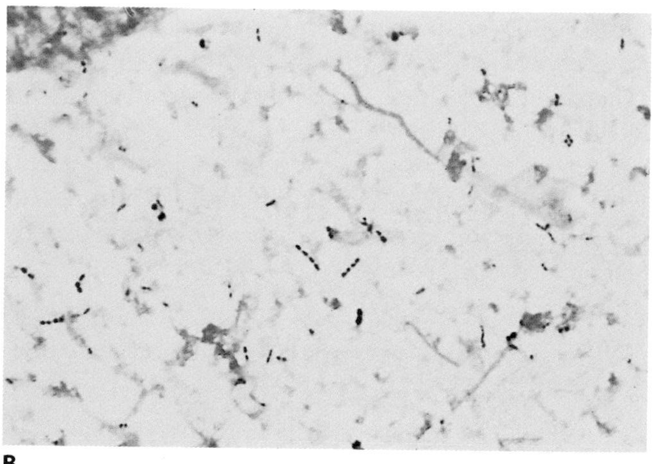

B

Figure 9-3 Gram stain of *Mycobacterium tuberculosis*. Mycobacteria are considered gram positive, although they are usually not easily stained by this method. (A) This Gram stain of a sputum sample shows that mycobacteria may stain faintly or not at all, producing a "ghost-like" image. (B) Sometimes, however, they appear as beaded gram-positive bacilli.

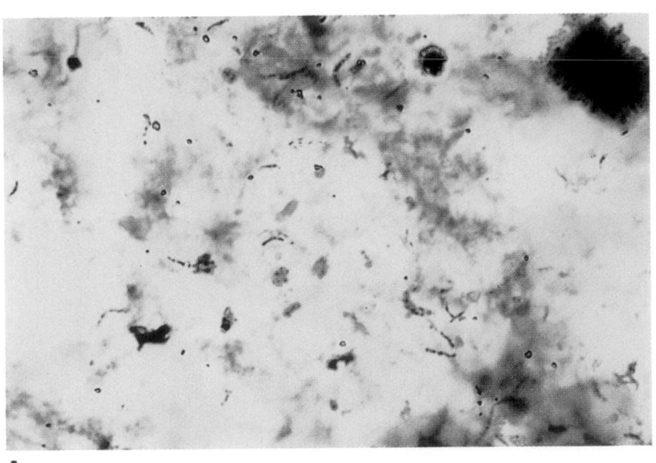

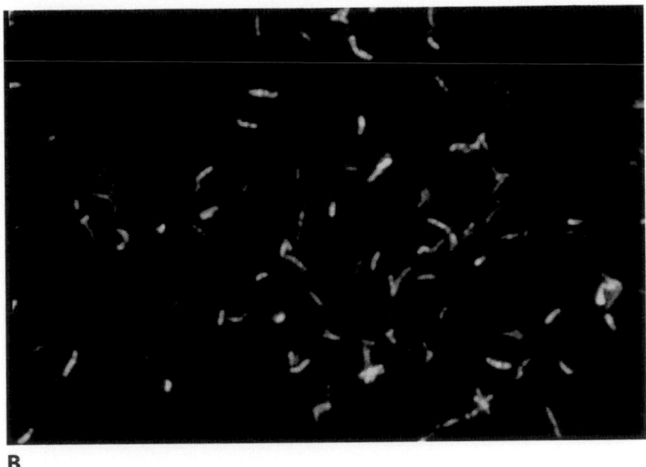

A B

Figure 9-4 Kinyoun and auramine stains of *Mycobacterium avium-intracellulare*. (A) *M. avium-intracellulare* has a beaded appearance when stained by the Kinyoun method. (B) In liquid medium, these organisms remain as single cells and do not form cordae as does *M. tuberculosis*.

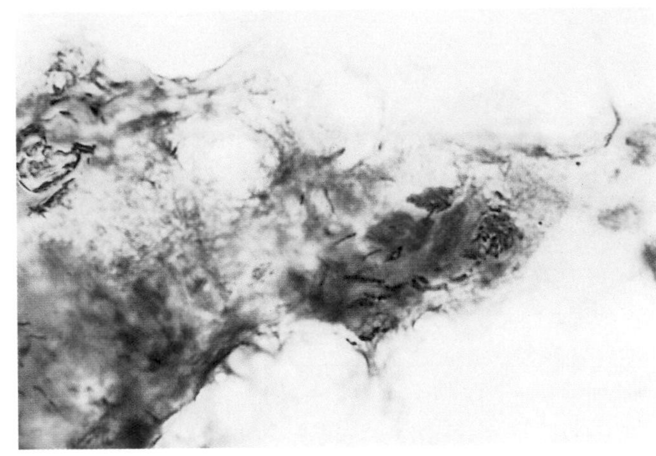

Figure 9-5 *Mycobacterium leprae* stained by the Fite-Faraco method. *M. leprae* is only partially acid fast and thus stains weakly, if at all, with the standard acid-fast stains. For this reason, it is recommended to use the Fite-Faraco stain.

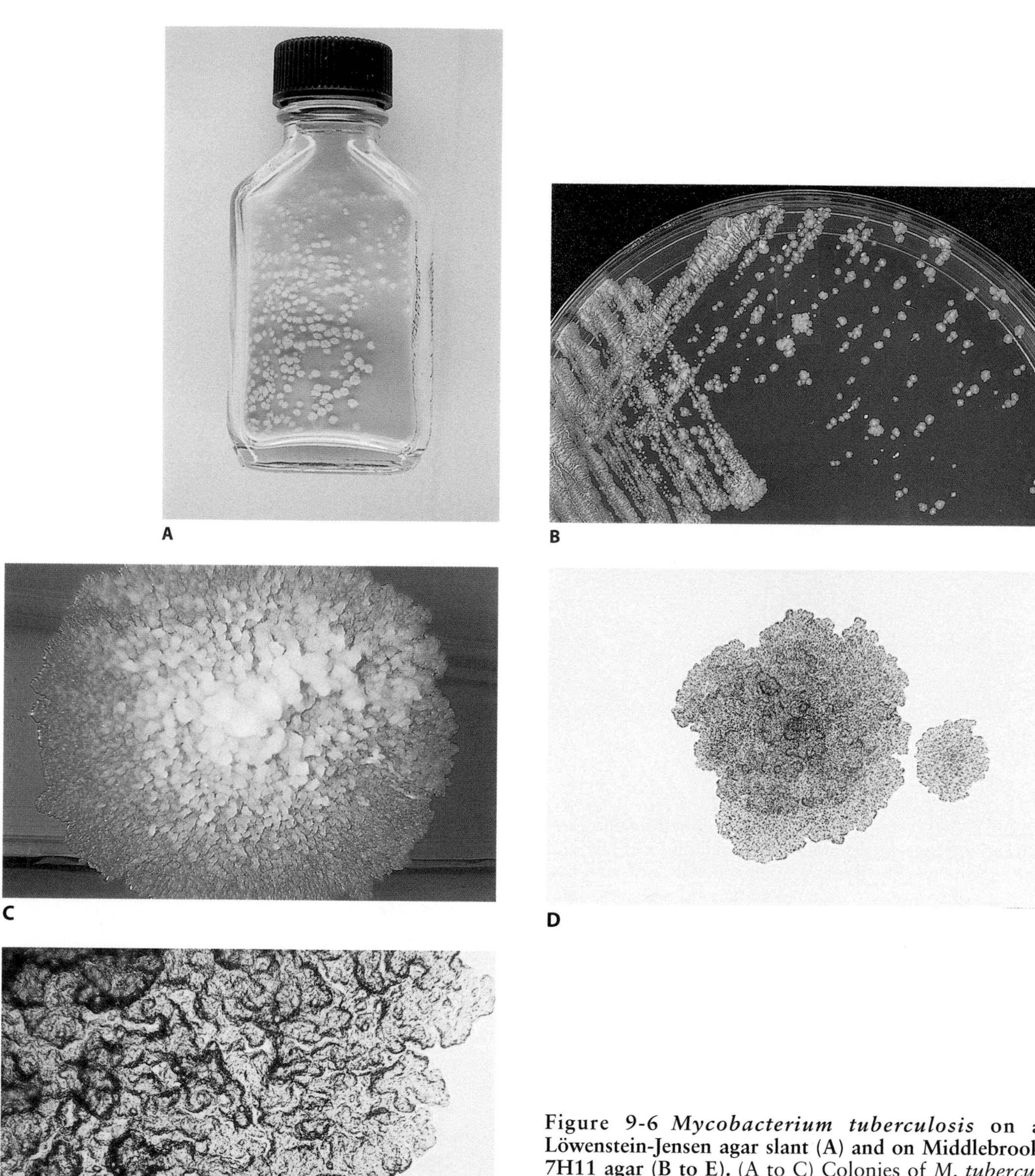

Figure 9-6 ***Mycobacterium tuberculosis*** **on a Löwenstein-Jensen agar slant (A) and on Middlebrook 7H11 agar (B to E).** (A to C) Colonies of *M. tuberculosis* are dry, wrinkled, rough, thin, and friable with an irregular periphery and buff color. (D and E) When the colonies on Middlebrook agar are examined from the reverse side with transmitted light, cording can be observed at low magnification and is more apparent in older colonies and at higher magnification.

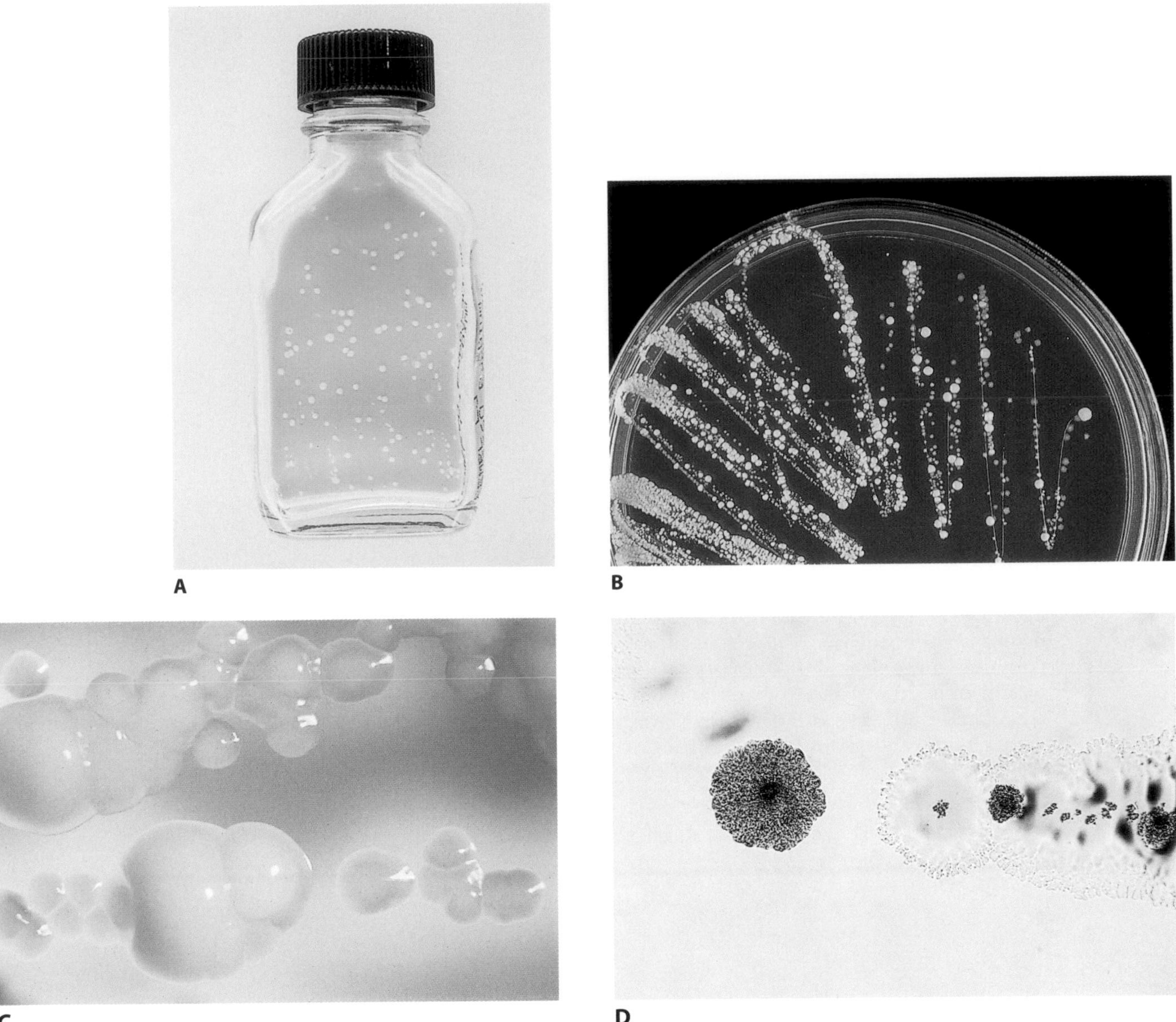

Figure 9-7 ***Mycobacterium avium-intracellulare*** **on a Löwenstein-Jensen agar slant (A) and on Middlebrook 7H11 agar (B to D).** (A) These organisms grow very slowly on Löwenstein-Jensen agar, and it usually takes 3 to 4 weeks before the colonies are clearly visible. (B) As shown in this Middlebrook 7H11 agar culture, most strains of *M. avium-intracellulare* grow with mixed colony morphology. Like *M. tuberculosis*, they are buff colored; however, they are significantly smaller than *M. tuberculosis*. (C) Smooth-domed, round, entire, transparent, nonpigmented, and glistening colonies can be observed. Rough and wrinkled colonies similar to those produced by *M. tuberculosis* are also frequently present. (D) When observed from the reverse side with transmitted light, colonies may have a rough, dry, wrinkled, "sunspot" appearance or smooth translucent edges with a buff-colored center.

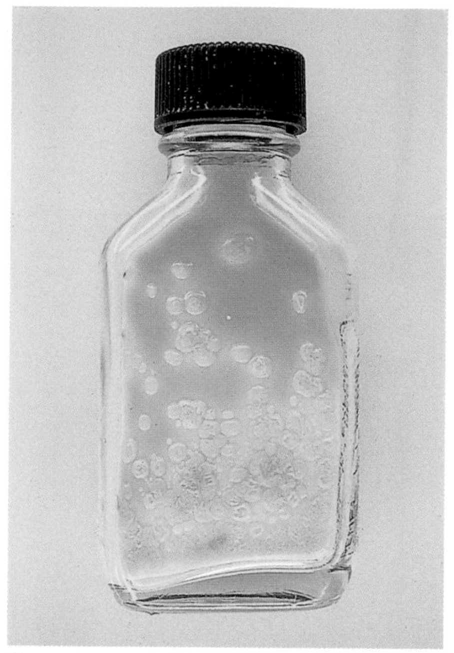

A

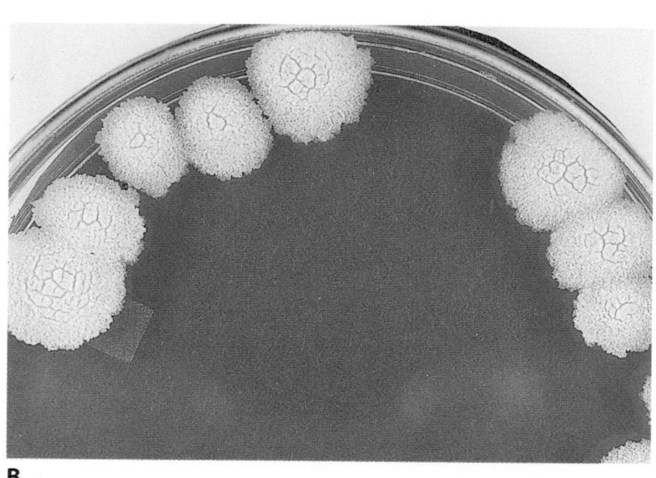

B

Figure 9-8 ***Mycobacterium abscessus*** **on a Löwenstein-Jensen agar slant (A) and on Middlebrook 7H11 agar (B).** *M. abscessus* rapidly forms large, rounded, entire or scalloped, smooth colonies with a dark buff color. Occasionally rough, wrinkled colonies are also found. This organism is present in tap water and has been associated with several injection- and catheter-related outbreaks of nosocomial infections. In addition, it can produce pulmonary and disseminated cutaneous lesions, particularly in immunosuppressed patients.

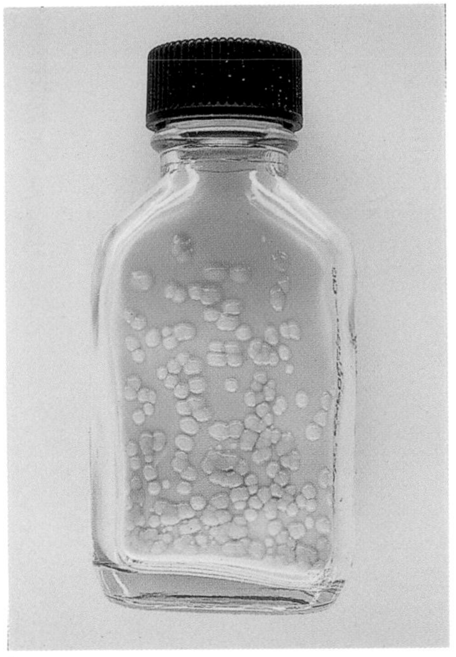

A

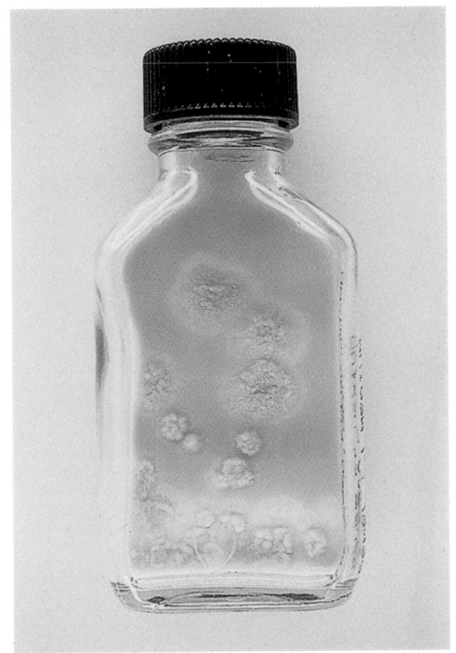

B

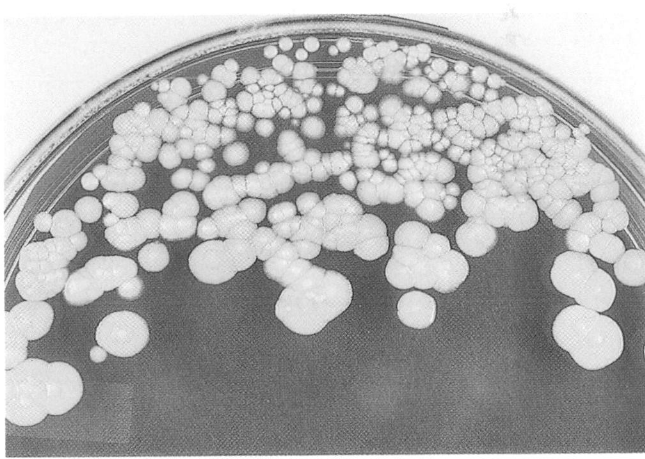

C

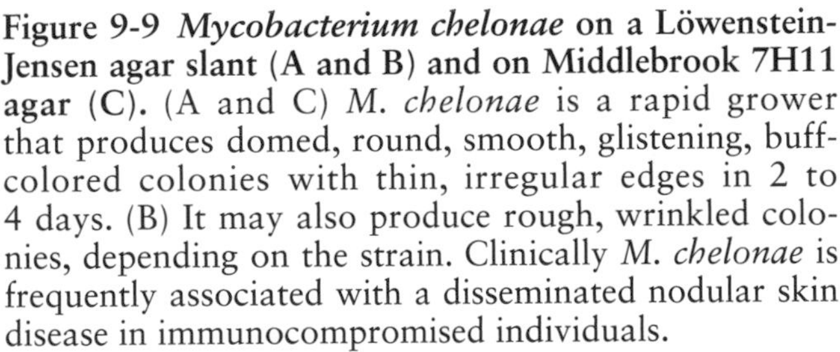

Figure 9-9 *Mycobacterium chelonae* on a Löwenstein-Jensen agar slant (A and B) and on Middlebrook 7H11 agar (C). (A and C) *M. chelonae* is a rapid grower that produces domed, round, smooth, glistening, buff-colored colonies with thin, irregular edges in 2 to 4 days. (B) It may also produce rough, wrinkled colonies, depending on the strain. Clinically *M. chelonae* is frequently associated with a disseminated nodular skin disease in immunocompromised individuals.

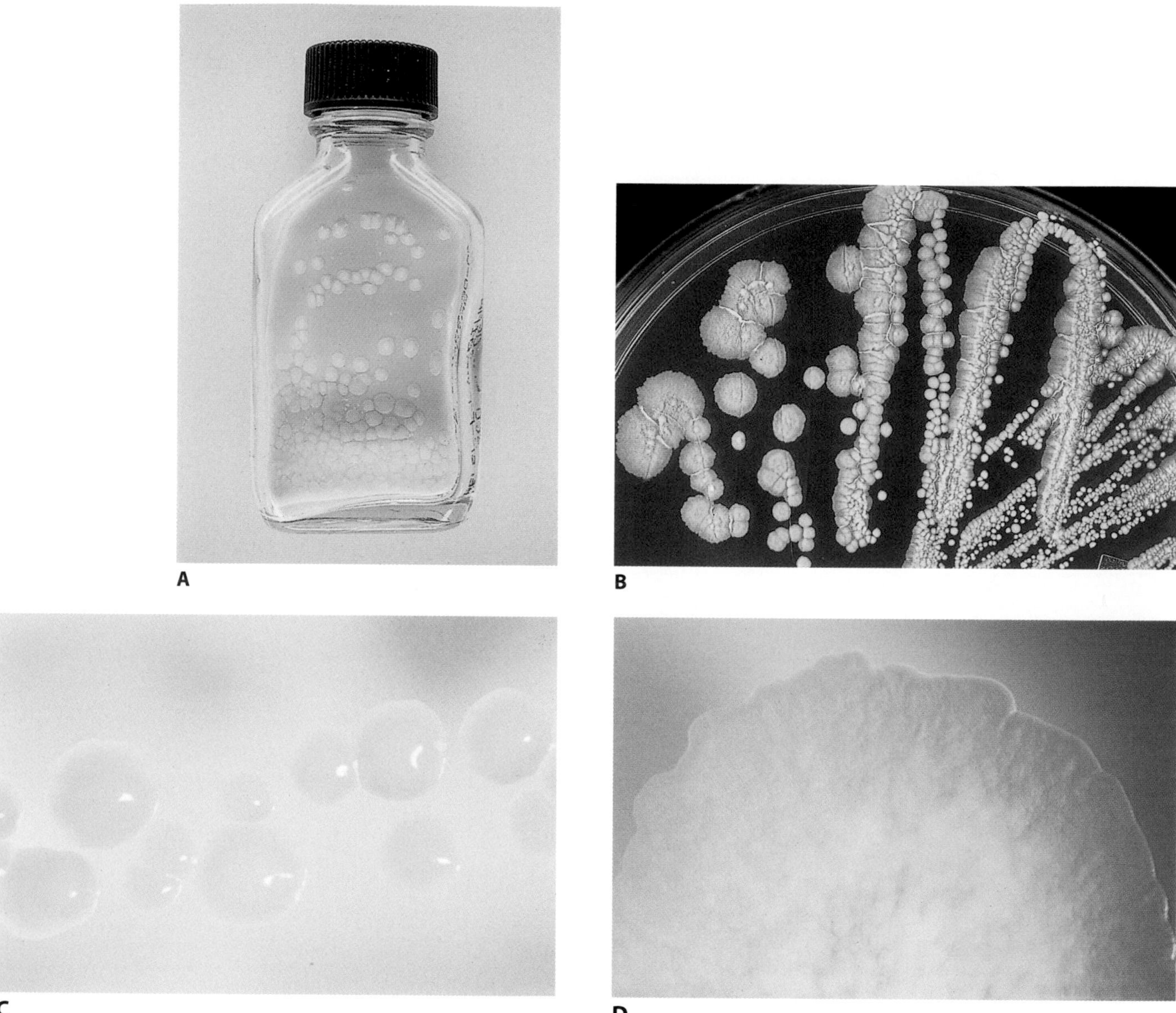

Figure 9-10 ***Mycobacterium fortuitum*** **on a Löwenstein-Jensen agar slant (A) and on Middlebrook 7H11 agar (B to D).** Depending on the strain, smooth or rough colonies of *M. fortuitum* may grow in 2 to 4 days on Middlebrook medium. (A and C) The smooth colonies shown here on the Löwenstein-Jensen agar slant and at higher magnification on the 7H11 agar are circular, convex, smooth, glistening, entire, and buff. (B and D) Rough, wrinkled colonies can also be observed on Middlebrook 7H11 agar. *M. fortuitum* usually causes infection secondary to a penetrating injury, such as trauma or surgical procedure, associated with contaminated water or soil.

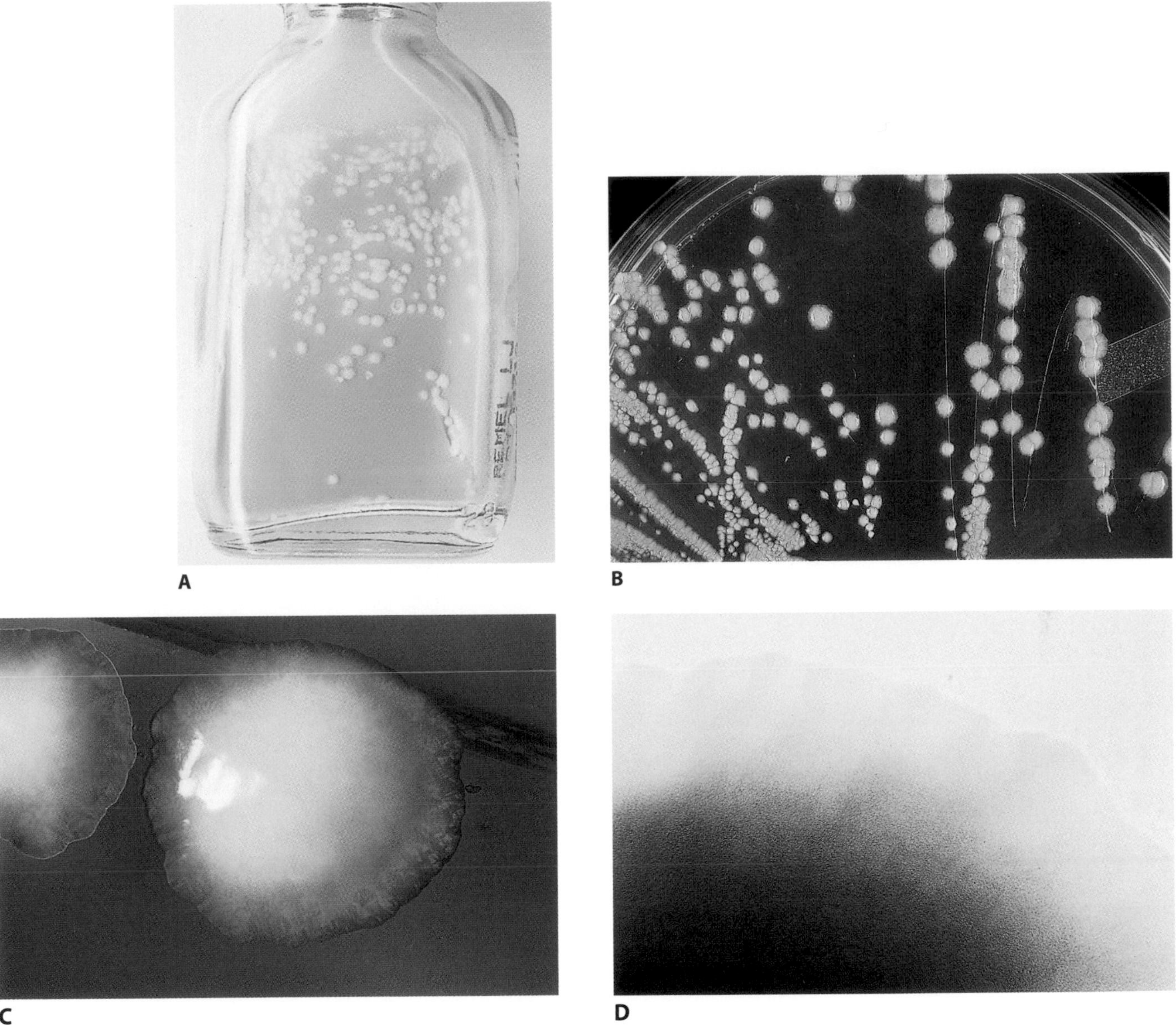

Figure 9-11 ***Mycobacterium gordonae*** **on a Löwenstein-Jensen agar slant (A) and on Middlebrook 7H11 agar (B to D).** (A and B) *M. gordonae* (referred to as the "tap water bacillus") produces round, smooth, convex, entire, glistening, yellow to orange colonies. Pigmentation appears in the absence of exposure to light. (C) Under higher magnification, the colonies are dense with a smooth edge. (D) Reverse side of a colony of *M. gordonae* illuminated with transmitted light. *M. gordonae* is frequently found in water and soil but rarely causes disease in humans.

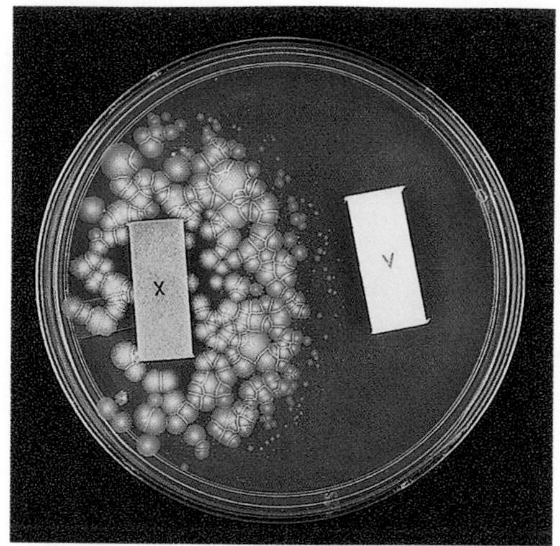

Figure 9-12 ***Mycobacterium haemophilum*** **on Middlebrook 7H11 agar.** A unique characteristic of *M. haemophilum* is that it requires hemin or hemoglobin for growth. On this plate the organism grows next to the strip containing X factor but does not grow next to the strip containing V factor. The colonies shown here are smooth, round, and nonpigmented. This mycobacterium is usually isolated from immunocompromised patients, particularly those with AIDS.

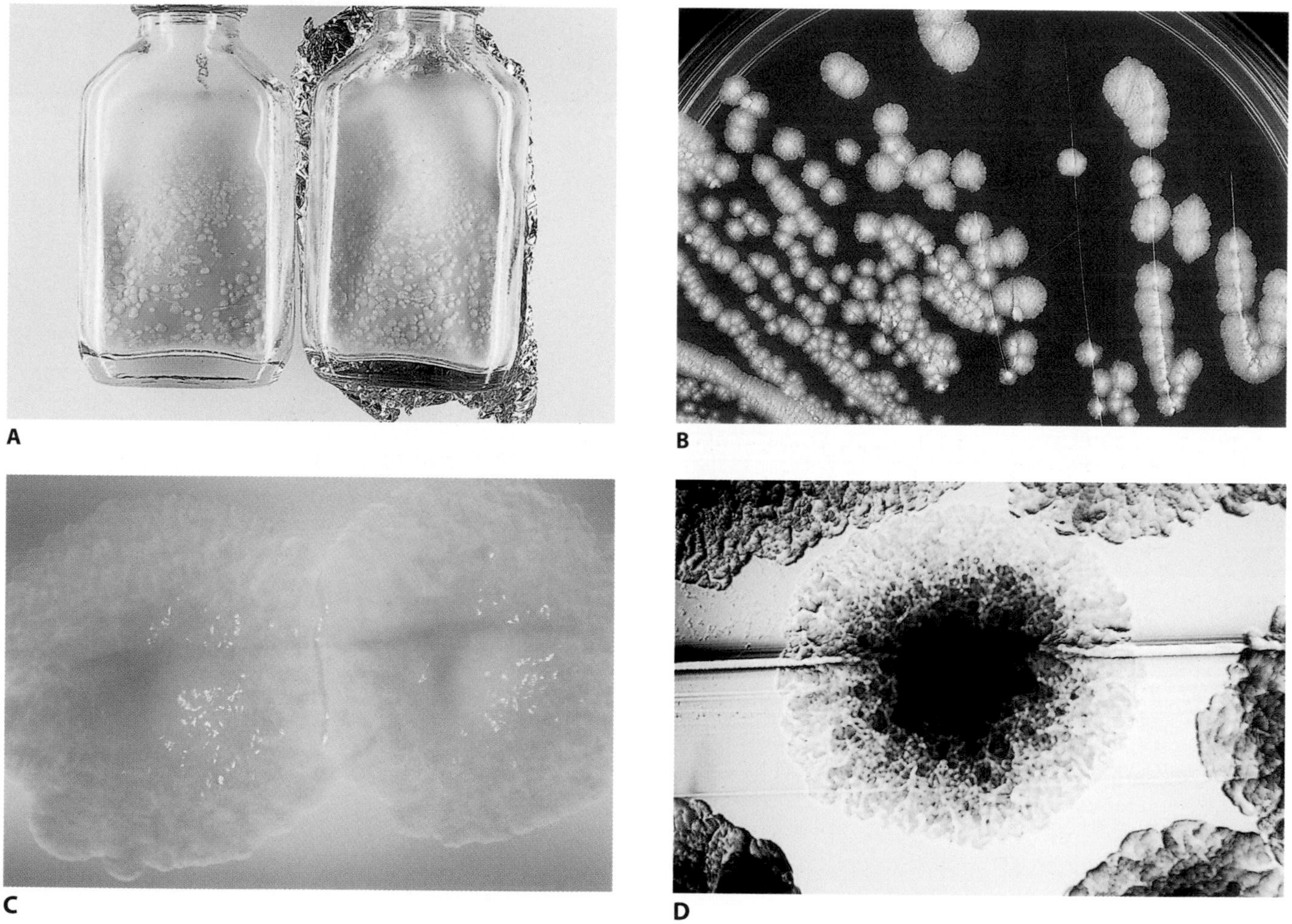

A **B**

C **D**

Figure 9-13 ***Mycobacterium kansasii*** **on a Löwenstein-Jensen agar slant (A) and on Middlebrook 7H11 agar (B to D).** (A) Colonies of *M. kansasii* are usually smooth, domed, and yellow when exposed to light (left) and buff with thin irregular edges when grown in the dark (right). (B and C) They can also be rough and wrinkled with wavy edges and a dark center containing β-carotene crystals. (D) The dark center can easily be seen by looking at the back of the plate with transmitted light. *M. kansasii* is one of the most common causes of nontuberculous mycobacterial pulmonary disease in humans and is isolated more frequently from individuals with AIDS or organ transplants than from the general population.

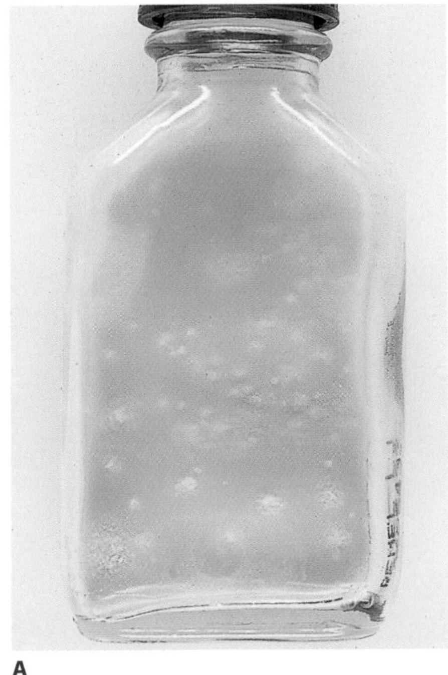

A

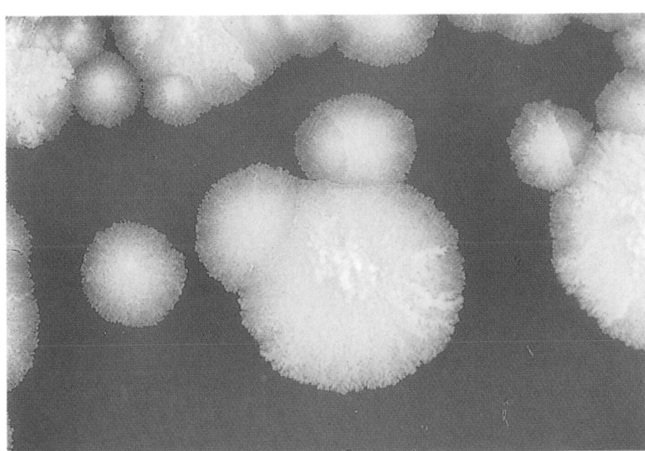

B

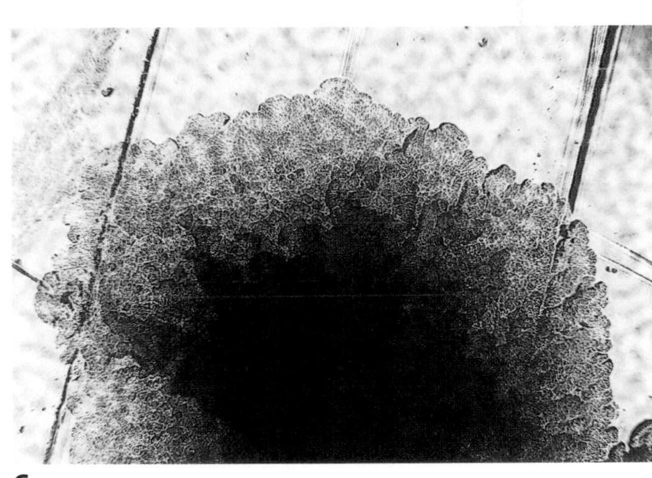

C

Figure 9-14 *Mycobacterium marinum* on a Löwenstein-Jensen agar slant (A) and on Middlebrook 7H11 agar (B and C). (A) Overall, the colonies of this microorganism are irregular, with thin, trailing edges and a buff color that turns yellow following exposure to light. (B and C) The colonies of *M. marinum* shown here are rough and wrinkled (front of colony [B] and back of transilluminated colony [C] are shown). Occasionally some strains produce smooth colonies. This organism should be suspected in individuals who have sustained skin trauma while in contact with freshwater ("swimming pool or fish tank granuloma") or salt water.

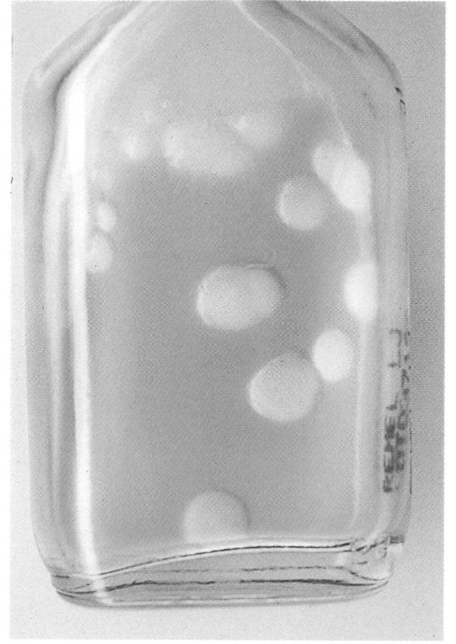

A

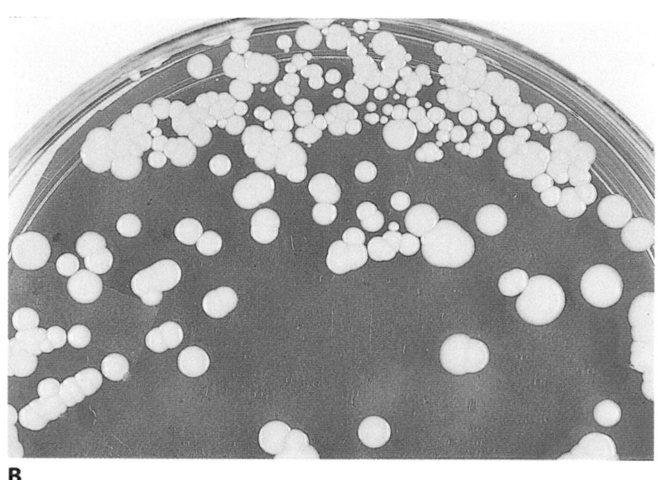

B

Figure 9-15 ***Mycobacterium mucogenicum*** **on a Löwenstein-Jensen agar slant (A) and on Middlebrook 7H11 agar (B).** This organism typically produces large, smooth, very mucoid colonies with a buff color, as shown here. It used to be known as *M. chelonae*-like organism and is frequently isolated from tap water. *M. mucogenicum* causes catheter-related sepsis and posttraumatic wound infections. Isolation of this organism from a single sputum sample is usually not clinically significant.

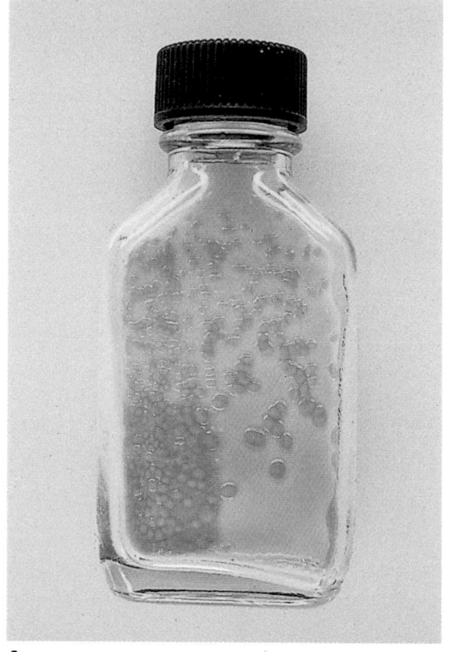

A

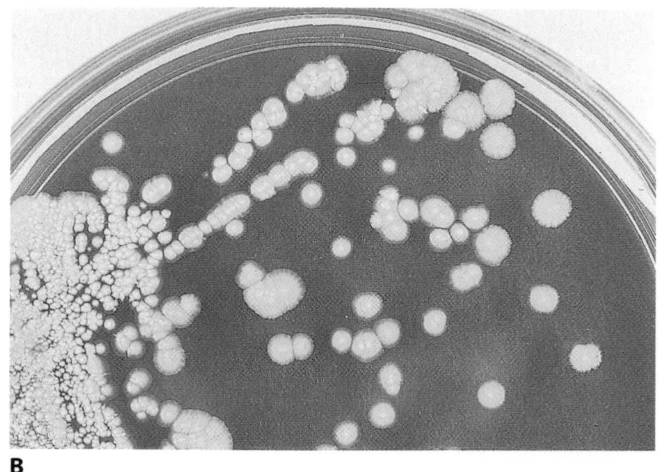

B

Figure 9-16 ***Mycobacterium scrofulaceum*** **on a Löwenstein-Jensen agar slant (A) and on Middlebrook 7H11 agar (B).** *M. scrofulaceum* produces smooth, round, moist, glistening colonies with elevated centers and a light yellow color that can become dark orange, depending on the strain. This organism is a slow grower and usually takes 3 to 4 weeks to form distinct colonies. It is most commonly isolated from children younger than 5 years with cervical lymphadenitis.

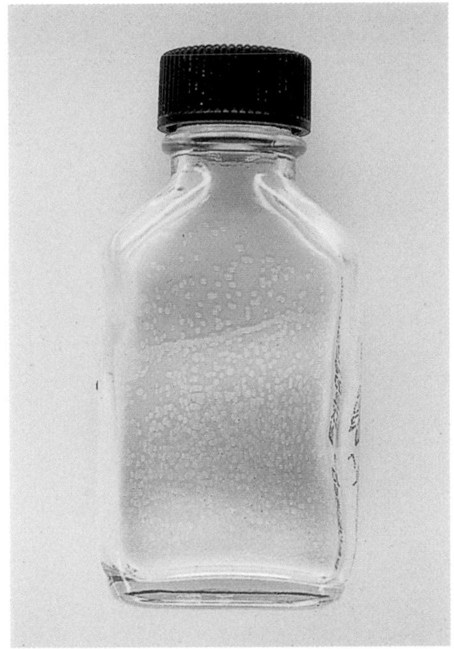

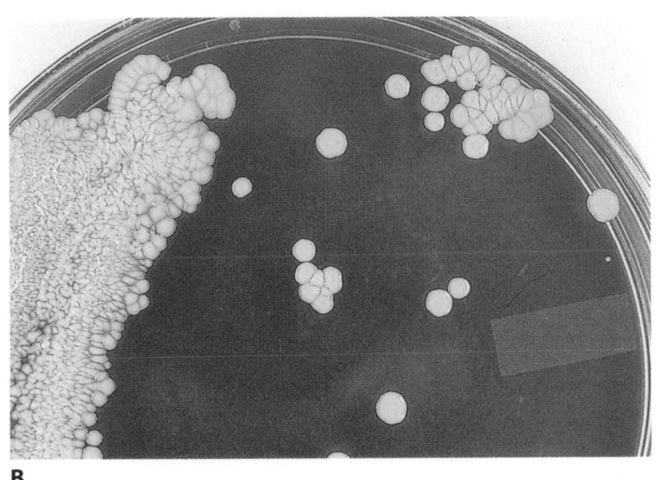

A B

Figure 9-17 ***Mycobacterium simiae*** **on a Löwenstein-Jensen agar slant (A) and on Middlebrook 7H11 agar (B).** *M. simiae* produces smooth, domed, round, glistening colonies that change from buff to light yellow when exposed to light. Originally isolated from monkeys, it has now been found in a few humans with a clinical presentation similar to that caused by *M. avium-intracellulare* complex in patients with AIDS.

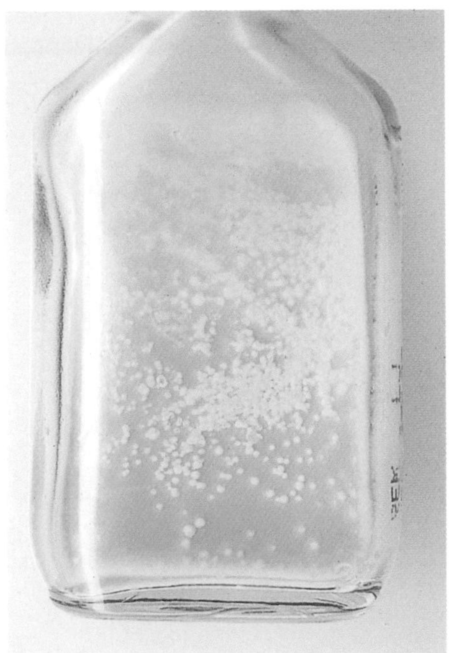

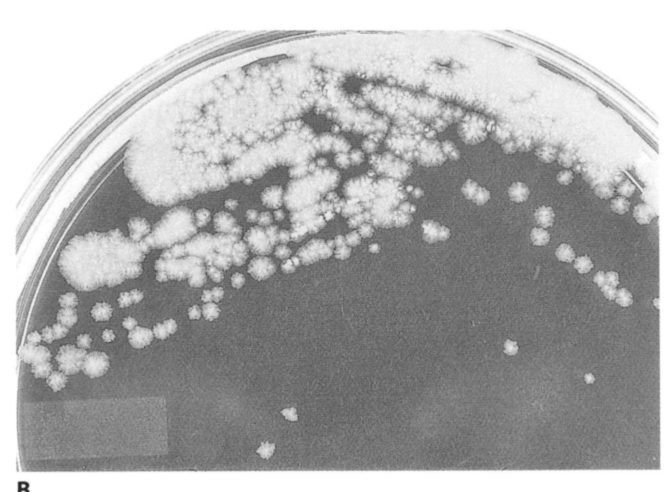

A B

Figure 9-18 ***Mycobacterium szulgai*** **on a Löwenstein-Jensen agar slant (A) and on Middlebrook 7H11 agar (B).** *M. szulgai* forms small, buff-colored colonies that range from smooth to rough. This organism is scotochromogenic when grown at 37°C and photochromogenic when grown at 25°C. It causes a chronic pulmonary disease similar to tuberculosis in middle-aged men.

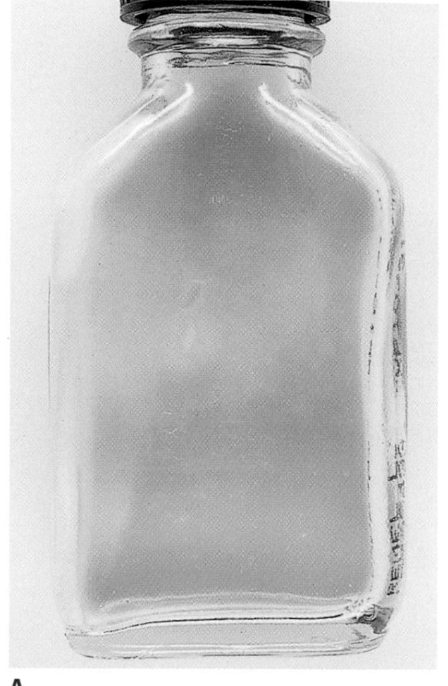

A

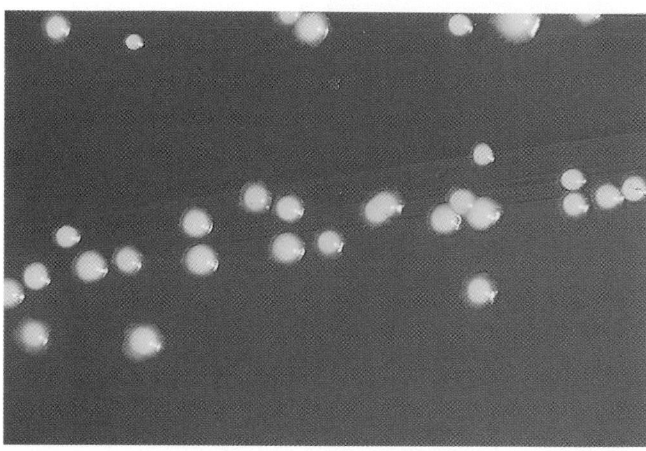

B

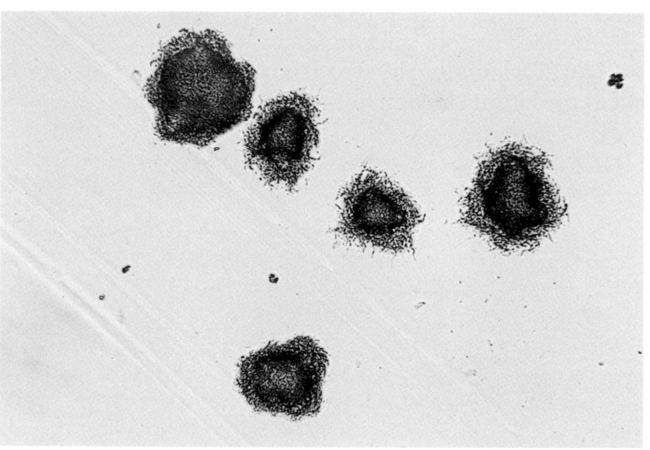

C

Figure 9-19 ***Mycobacterium xenopi*** **on Löwenstein-Jensen agar slant (A) and on Middlebrook 7H11 agar (B and C).** (A and B) *M. xenopi* produces small, round, smooth, yellow colonies. (C) Microscopic examination of the reverse side of a young colony on Middlebrook media with transmitted light reveals a typical "bird's nest" appearance, with stick-like projections. This is particularly evident when the organism is grown at 45°C. Originally isolated from the African toad *Xenopus laevis*, *M. xenopi* is now found all over the world in individuals with a predisposing condition such as diabetes mellitus, chronic lung problems, malignancy, or alcoholism.

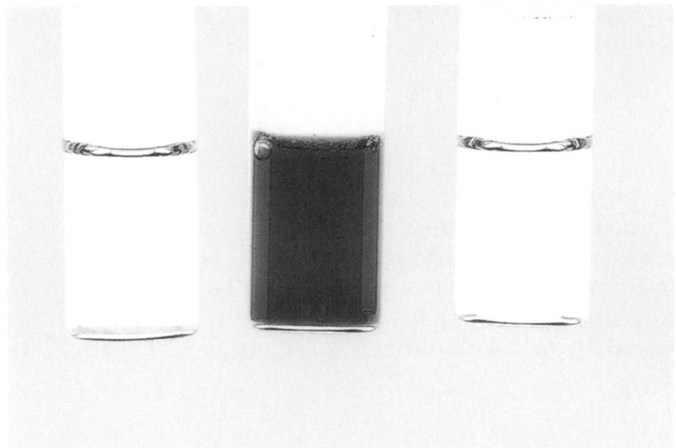

Figure 9-20 Arylsulfatase test. The enzyme arylsulfatase, present in most *Mycobacterium* species, breaks down tripotassium phenolphthalein disulfate into phenolphthalein, which in the presence of sodium carbonate, as a result of a pH change, yields a red color, as shown in the tube in the center of this figure. The 3-day test is used to identify rapid growers, while 14 days may be required for the identification of slow growers. *M. chelonae* and *M. fortuitum* give a positive reaction in less than 3 days, while *M. szulgai*, *Mycobacterium smegmatis*, *Mycobacterium asiaticum*, and *Mycobacterium flavescens* may be positive in the 14-day test. *M. xenopi* and *Mycobacterium triviale*, although slow growers, may give a positive reaction in 3 days. The tube on the left is a control uninoculated tube, the tube in the center contains *M. fortuitum* (positive), and the one on the right contains *M. avium* (negative).

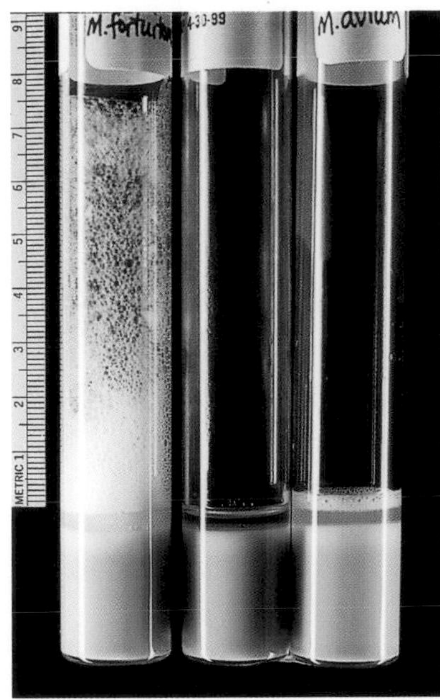

Figure 9-21 Catalase test. In general, mycobacteria possess catalase, except for *Mycobacterium gastri*, some isoniazid-resistant mutants of *M. tuberculosis* and *M. bovis*, and some nonpathogenic isoniazid-resistant strains of *M. kansasii*. In this test, catalase splits hydrogen peroxide to water and oxygen. The height of the oxygen bubbles produced allows mycobacteria to be classified into two groups: those that produce a column of bubbles less than 45 mm in height and those that produce one higher than 45 mm. This test can further help subdivide mycobacteria based on the thermostability of the catalase. Some mycobacteria have a catalase that is thermostable up to 68°C for 20 min, while other catalases are thermolabile under these conditions. Here, *M. fortuitum* (left) produced a column of bubbles higher than 45 mm, while *M. avium* generated a column less than 45 mm high (right). The tube in the center is an uninoculated control.

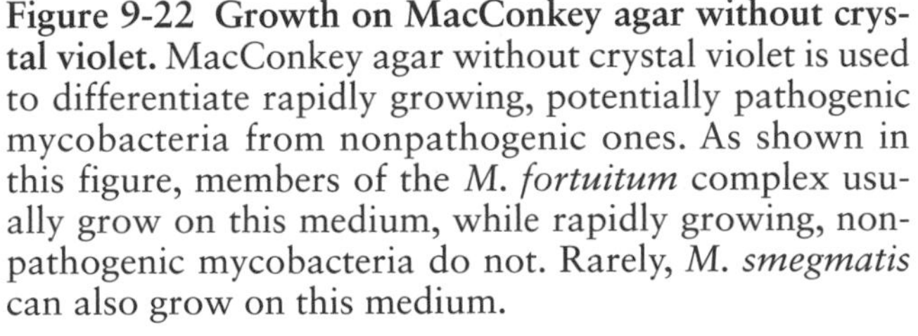

Figure 9-22 Growth on MacConkey agar without crystal violet. MacConkey agar without crystal violet is used to differentiate rapidly growing, potentially pathogenic mycobacteria from nonpathogenic ones. As shown in this figure, members of the *M. fortuitum* complex usually grow on this medium, while rapidly growing, nonpathogenic mycobacteria do not. Rarely, *M. smegmatis* can also grow on this medium.

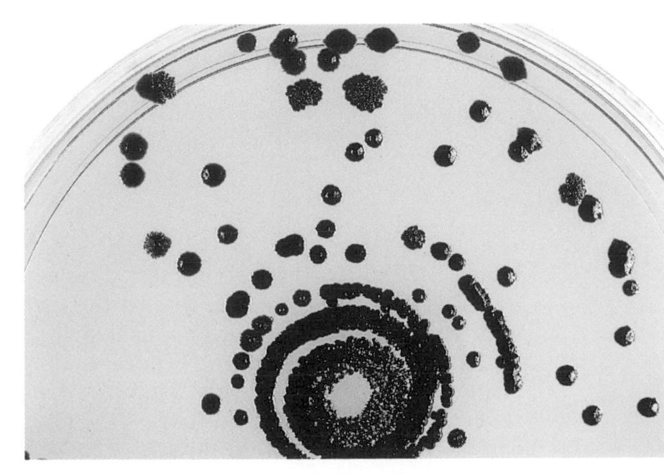

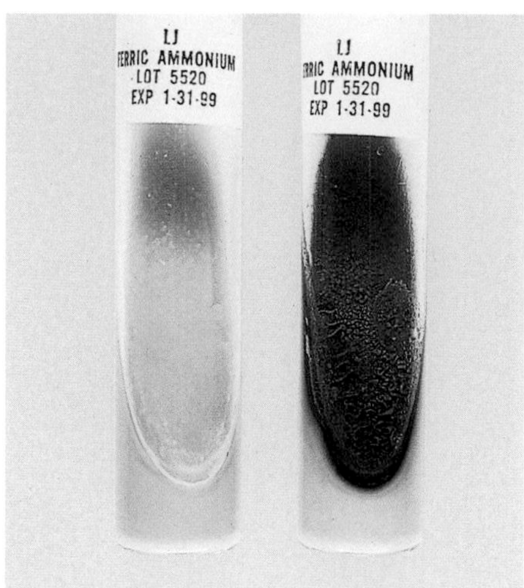

Figure 9-23 Iron uptake test. Mycobacteria able to convert ferric ammonium citrate to an iron oxide produce red-brown-rust colonies. This test is used to distinguish *M. chelonae*, which is usually negative (left), from *M. fortuitum* (right). Most rapid growers are positive, while slow growers are negative. The cultures should be incubated at 28°C for 2 weeks in tubes with the caps loose. They should be incubated for an additional 2 weeks before the test is considered negative.

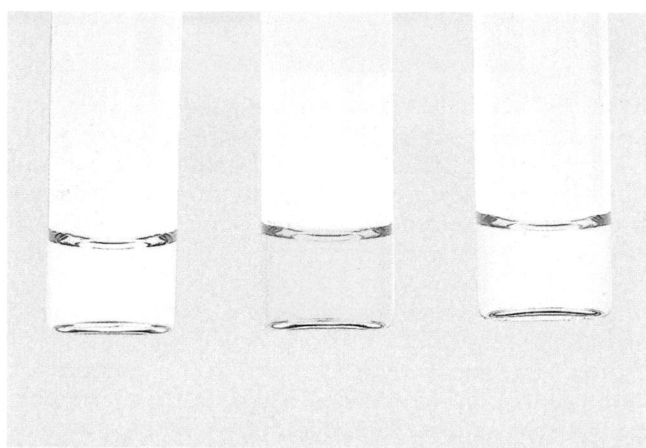

Figure 9-24 Niacin accumulation test. Certain mycobacteria including *M. tuberculosis*, *M. simiae*, and some strains of *M. marinum* and *M. bovis* BCG have a block in the metabolic pathway that converts free niacin to nicotinic acid. The niacin reacts with cyanogen bromide and a primary aromatic amine to produce a yellow color. *M. tuberculosis* (positive) is shown in the center of the figure, while an uninoculated control is shown on the left and *M. avium* (negative) is shown on the right.

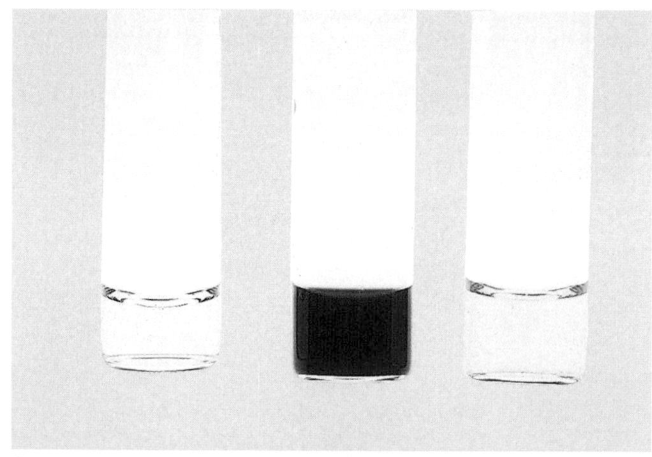

A

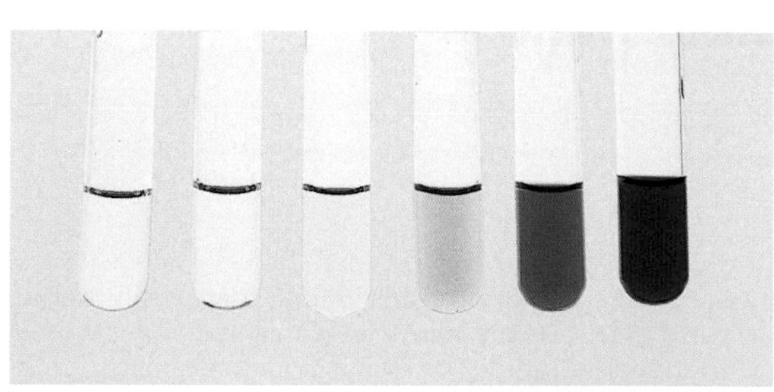

B

Figure 9-25 Nitrate reduction test. This assay is based on the ability of certain mycobacteria to reduce nitrate to nitrite due to the production of nitroreductase. It can be performed with chemical reagents or chemical strips. (A) In addition to *M. tuberculosis*, *M. kansasii*, *M. szulgai*, *M. ulcerans*, *M. fortuitum*, and the *Mycobacterium terrae* complex give positive results. The tube on the right contains *M. avium* (negative), the one in the center contains *M. tuberculosis* (positive), and that on the left is an uninoculated control. (B) A nitrate standard can be used to compare results.

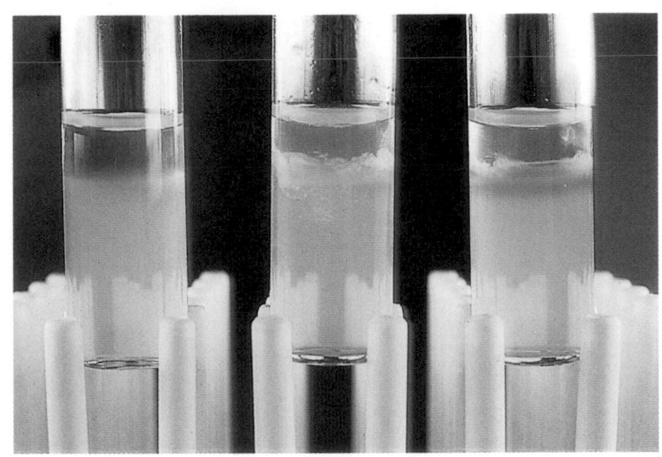

Figure 9-26 Pyrazinamidase test. Pyrazinamidase hydrolyzes pyrazinamide to pyrazinoic acid and ammonia. Pyrazinoic acid is detected in the presence of ferrous ammonium sulfate. *M. tuberculosis* gives positive results within 4 days (tube on the right), while *M. bovis* is negative even after 7 days (tube in the center). The tube on the left is an uninoculated control. The pyrazinamidase test is also useful to differentiate *M. kansasii* (negative) from *M. marinum* (positive in 4 days).

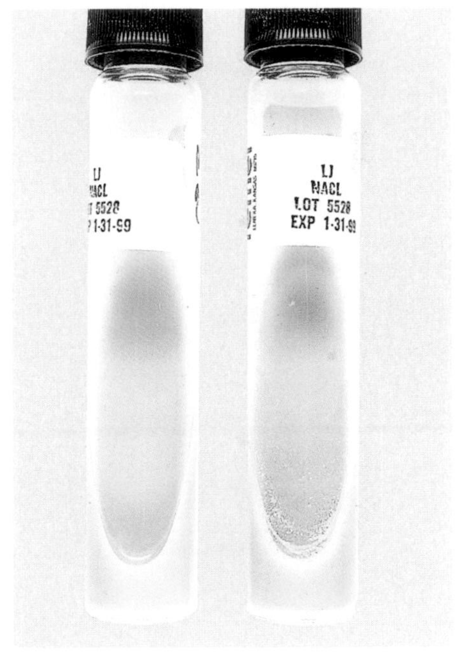

Figure 9-27 NaCl tolerance test. Most rapid growers, except *M. chelonae* and *M. mucogenicum*, and the slow-growing *M. triviale* can grow in the presence of 5% NaCl. Here, *M. gordonae* (negative) was inoculated in the left tube and *M. flavescens* (positive) was inoculated in the right tube.

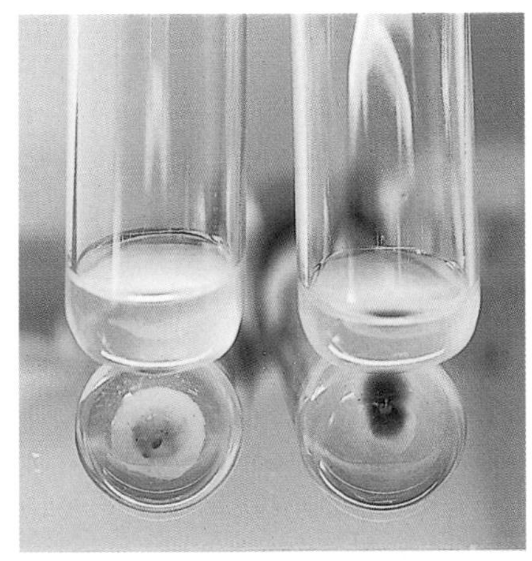

Figure 9-28 Tellurite reduction test. Certain mycobacteria contain tellurite reductase, which reduces colorless potassium tellurite to a black metallic tellurium precipitate. This is illustrated by the negative reaction of *M. gordonae* (left). Organisms in the *M. avium-intracellulare* complex group (right) reduce tellurite within 3 to 4 days, while other nonchromogens do not.

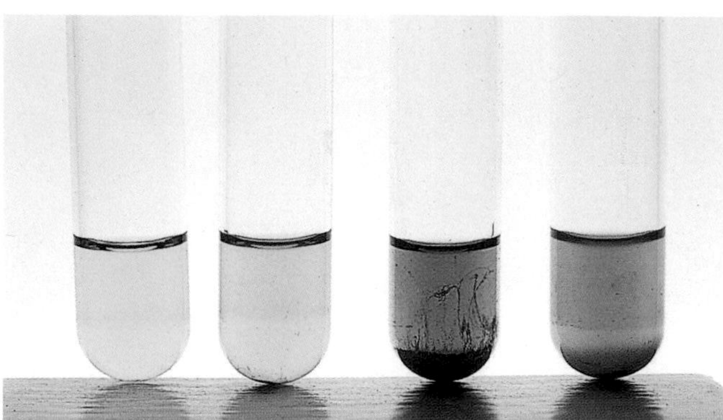

Figure 9-29 Tween 80 hydrolysis test. This assay helps to separate commonly saprophytic from potentially pathogenic, slow-growing scotochromogens and nonchromogens. *M. avium-intracellulare* complex, *M. xenopi*, and *M. scrofulaceum* are usually negative. Lipases produced by some mycobacteria hydrolyze Tween 80 (polyoxyethylene sorbitan monooleate) into oleic acid and polyoxyethylene sorbitol, resulting in a change in color of the medium. When bound by Tween 80, neutral red has an amber color at neutral pH as a result of the optical rotation of the transmitted light. Hydrolysis of Tween 80 releases the neutral red, which changes to a red color. Here, from left to right are an uninoculated tube and tubes containing *M. avium*, *M. kansasii*, and *M. gordonae*.

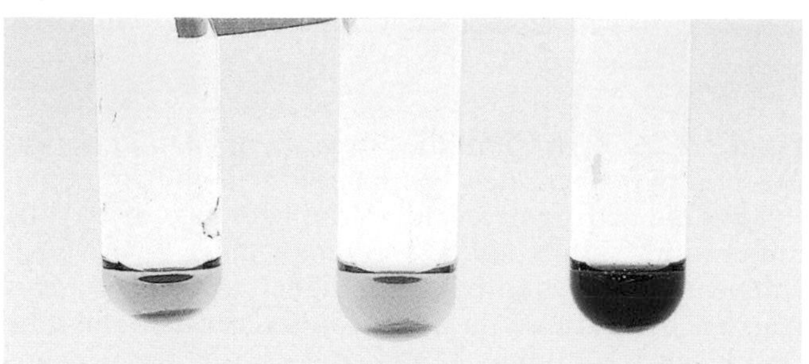

Figure 9-30 Urease test. Several methods are available for the detection of urease in mycobacteria. Hydrolysis of urea results in the production of ammonia and CO_2. This test is helpful in identifying scotochromogens and nonchromogens. Thus, pigmented strains of *M. avium-intracellulare* complex should be urease negative (middle tube), while *M. scrofulaceum* produces urease (right tube). The tube on the left was not inoculated.

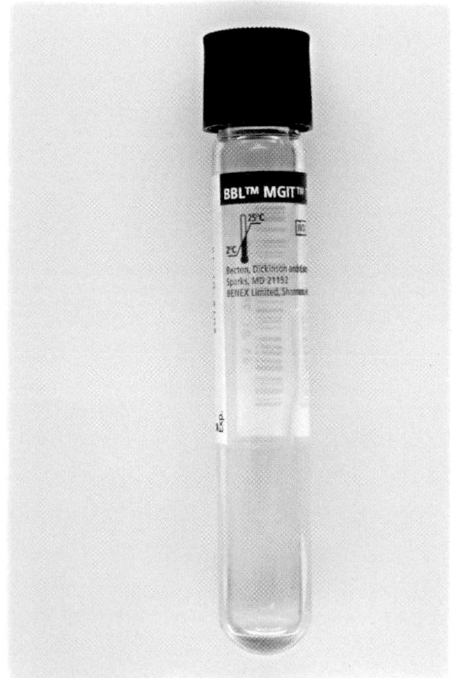

Figure 9-31 BD BACTEC MGIT. BD BACTEC MGIT (Mycobacteria Growth Indicator Tube) (BD Diagnostic Systems, Franklin Lakes, NJ) tubes use fluorometric technology to expedite the reading of results. Positive tests emit an orange fluorescent glow at the base of the tube and at the meniscus that can be read using a Wood's lamp or other long-wave UV light source, or they can be incubated and read in the BD BACTEC 960 Instrumented Mycobacterial Growth Systems.

Introduction to *Enterobacteriaceae* 10

The family *Enterobacteriaceae* is composed of numerous genera of gram-negative bacilli; however, fewer than 10 are responsible for the majority of clinical infections. These include *Escherichia*, *Enterobacter*, *Klebsiella*, *Proteus*, *Citrobacter*, *Serratia*, *Salmonella*, *Shigella*, and *Yersinia*.

Some strains of *Enterobacteriaceae* colonize the intestinal tract of humans. However, they can cause both gastrointestinal and extraintestinal infections, especially in compromised hosts. Four genera are known to cause intestinal infections: *Escherichia*, *Salmonella*, *Shigella*, and *Yersinia*. Other genera in the *Enterobacteriaceae* have occasionally been implicated, but their pathogenicity is uncertain. Urinary and respiratory tract, wound, and bloodstream infections are the most common extraintestinal infections.

Members of the family *Enterobacteriaceae* are gram-negative bacilli. They vary from short, measuring 2 to 3 μm in length, to long, slender bacilli, measuring 6 to 7 μm in length, and are 0.5 to 2 μm in width. Some species are motile by peritrichous flagella, while others are nonmotile. The *Enterobacteriaceae* do not form spores.

The *Enterobacteriaceae* grow well under aerobic conditions on routine laboratory media including blood agar, as well as on differential media such as MacConkey agar or selective differential media such as Hektoen enteric (HE) agar or xylose lysine deoxycholate (XLD) agar. In general, the *Enterobacteriaceae* grow abundantly after 18 to 24 h at 35°C.

On blood agar, colonies of the *Enterobacteriaceae* may be beta-hemolytic and are usually medium to large, glistening, and gray; however, some species have a characteristic morphology. For example, *Klebsiella* may have mucoid colonies, *Proteus* colonies swarm, and *Yersinia* colonies are usually tiny and pinpoint. Additionally, some species, e.g., *Serratia marcescens*, *Serratia rubidaea*, *Enterobacter/Cronobacter sakazakii*, and *Pantoea agglomerans*, produce a pigment.

MacConkey and eosin methylene blue agars are used to distinguish rapid lactose fermenters from delayed lactose fermenters or non-lactose fermenters. Other differential media, such as HE and XLD agars, further help to characterize the species and differentiate some of the enteric pathogens from members of the normal intestinal flora. Most genera considered to be members of the normal enteric flora ferment salicin and produce a salmon color on HE agar, whereas the enteric pathogens do not ferment salicin and appear as green colonies. Both HE and XLD agars contain ferric ammonium citrate, which permits the detection of H_2S-producing species such as *Salmonella* and *Proteus*. Selective media can also be used to enhance the isolation of some species. For example, MacConkey agar with sorbitol can be used to distinguish *Escherichia coli* O157:H7 from other *Enterobacteriaceae*. *E. coli* O157:H7 produces colorless colonies on MacConkey agar with sorbitol because it is sorbitol negative, whereas most other serotypes of *E. coli* are sorbitol positive and appear as pink colonies. CHROMagar O157 is also a selective medium for *E. coli* O157:H7. Cefsulodin-irgasan-novobiocin (CIN) agar is a selective medium for *Yersinia*.

The *Enterobacteriaceae* are biochemically active. They ferment glucose and other carbohydrates, often with the production of gas; are oxidase negative and catalase positive; and reduce nitrate to nitrite. Since all members of the *Enterobacteriaceae* are cytochrome oxidase negative, a rapid spot test is usually performed to confirm that the isolate belongs to this family.

Four commonly used tests to identify the *Enterobacteriaceae* are indole, methyl red, Voges-Proskauer, and citrate. These are usually referred to as the IMViC tests, and the various reactions are listed in Table 10-1. Other commonly used biochemical tests that assist in the identification of the *Enterobacteriaceae* are phenylalanine, tryptophan, lysine, ornithine, arginine, urea, *o*-nitrophenyl-β-D-galactopyranoside (ONPG), gelatin, and 4-methylumbelliferyl-β-D-glucuronidase (MUG). Lysine and ornithine decarboxylase and arginine dihydrolase are supplemental tests that are very helpful in identifying the *Enterobacteriaceae*, especially the commonly isolated genera *Klebsiella*, *Enterobacter*, and *Serratia* (Table 10-2). Triple sugar iron (TSI) agar is also very helpful in identifying the *Enterobacteriaceae* (Table 10-3).

Some of the *Enterobacteriaceae* have the ability to utilize sodium malonate as the sole carbon source and ammonium dihydrogen as the sole nitrogen source. The reaction is similar to that described for citrate utilization. Table 10-4 lists the positive reactions for some of the commonly used tests for the *Enterobacteriaceae*.

In general, the approach in the clinical microbiology laboratory is to use one or more screening tests to determine if additional testing with an identification system is necessary.

Table 10-1 IMViC lactose reactions of various *Enterobacteriaceae*

Lactose fermentation	Organism(s) with reaction[a]:				
	++00	00++	0+0+	++0+	0+00
Rapid	*Escherichia*	*Klebsiella* *Klebsiella oxytoca* (+0++) *Raoultella* (V0++) *Enterobacter*	*Citrobacter*		
Late	*Escherichia* *Leclercia*	*Cedecea lapagei* *Hafnia alvei* (00+0) *Klebsiella* *Enterobacter* *Serratia*	*Citrobacter freundii* *Cedecea davisae* *Salmonella*	*Kluyvera* *Citrobacter*	*Shigella sonnei* *Klebsiella pneumoniae* subsp. *ozaenae* *Klebsiella pneumoniae* subsp. *rhinoscleromatis* *Proteus penneri*
Negative	*Edwardsiella* *Proteus vulgaris* *Morganella*		*Salmonella* *Salmonella enterica* serovar Typhi (0+00) *Proteus mirabilis*	*Providencia*	*Shigella* *Yersinia*

[a]Reactions are positive (+), negative (0), or variable (V) for indole, methyl red, Voges-Proskauer, and citrate.

Table 10-2 Decarboxylase-dihydrolase reactions of various *Enterobacteriaceae*

Organism	Reaction[a] for:		
	Lysine	Arginine	Ornithine
Cedecea davisae	0	+	+
Cedecea lapagei	0	+	0
Citrobacter koseri (*diversus*)	+	+	+
Citrobacter freundii	+	0	+
Edwardsiella	+	0	+
Enterobacter aerogenes	+	0	+
Enterobacter agglomerans	0	0	0
Enterobacter cloacae	0	+	+
Enterobacter (*Cronobacter*) *sakazakii*	0	+	+
Enterobacter gergoviae	+	0	+
Escherichia	+	0	+
Hafnia alvei	+	0	+
Klebsiella spp. other than *K. rhinoscleromatis*	+	0	0
Klebsiella rhinoscleromatis	0	0	0
Kluyvera	+	0	+
Leclercia	0	0	0
Morganella morganii	0	0	+
Proteus mirabilis	0	0	+
Proteus vulgaris	0	0	0
Providencia	0	0	0
Salmonella spp. other than *S. enterica* serovar Typhi	+	+	+
Salmonella enterica serovar Typhi	+	0	0
Serratia spp. other than *S. rubidaea*	+	0	+
Serratia rubidaea	+	0	0
Shigella spp. other than *S. sonnei*	0	0	0
Shigella sonnei	0	0	+
Yersinia	0	0	+

[a]+, positive; 0, negative.

Table 10-3 TSI reactions[a] of various *Enterobacteriaceae*

A/AG	A/AG H_2S+	ALK/A	ALK/AG	ALK/AG H_2S+	ALK/A H_2S^w
Citrobacter spp.	*Citrobacter* spp.	*Escherichia coli*	*Escherichia coli*	*Citrobacter* spp.	*Salmonella enterica* serovar Typhi
Escherichia coli	*Proteus vulgaris*	*Klebsiella rhinoscleromatis*	*Citrobacter* spp.	*Edwardsiella tarda*	
Enterobacter spp.		*Morganella*	*Enterobacter* spp.	*Proteus mirabilis*	
Klebsiella spp.		*Proteus penneri*	*Hafnia*	*Salmonella* spp. other than *S. enterica* serovars Typhi and Paratyphi	
Yersinia spp.[b]		*Providencia* spp.	*Klebsiella* spp.		
		Serratia spp.	*Proteus myxofaciens*		
		Shigella spp.	*Providencia alcalifaciens*		
		Yersinia spp.	*Salmonella enterica* serovar Paratyphi		
			Serratia spp.		
			Yersinia kristensenii		

[a]A, acid; ALK, alkaline; G, gas; +, positive; w, weak.
[b]*Yersinia frederiksenii* can produce gas from glucose; *Yersinia enterocolitica* does not produce gas. Both ferment sucrose, resulting in an acid slant.

Table 10-4 Positive reactions of organisms in commonly used tests

Phenylalanine deaminase	Urease	ONPG	Malonate	Gelatin hydrolysis
Morganella	*Citrobacter*[a]	*Cedecea*	*Cedecea*	*Proteus*
Proteus	*Edwardsiella*[a]	*Citrobacter*	*Citrobacter koseri*	*Serratia*
Providencia	*Klebsiella*[a]	*Enterobacter*	*Enterobacter*	
	Morganella[b]	*Escherichia*	*Klebsiella*	
	Proteus[b]	*Hafnia alvei*	*Kluyvera*	
	Providencia rettgeri[b]	*Klebsiella*	*Leclercia*	
	Yersinia[a]	*Kluyvera*	*Serratia rubidaea*	
		Leclercia		
		Pantoea		
		Raoultella		
		Serratia		
		Shigella sonnei		
		Yersinia		

[a]Overnight incubation.
[b]Within 3 h.

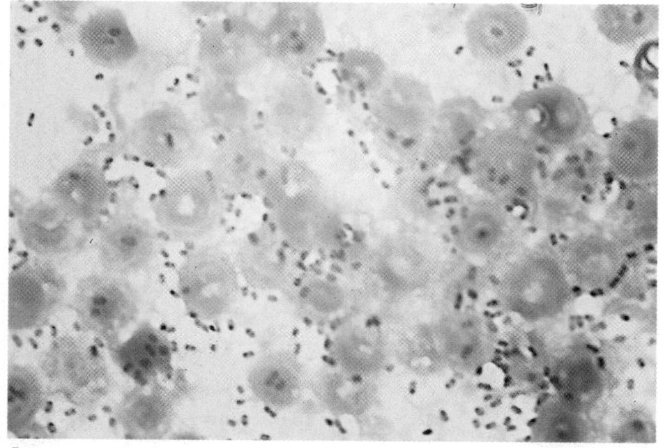

A

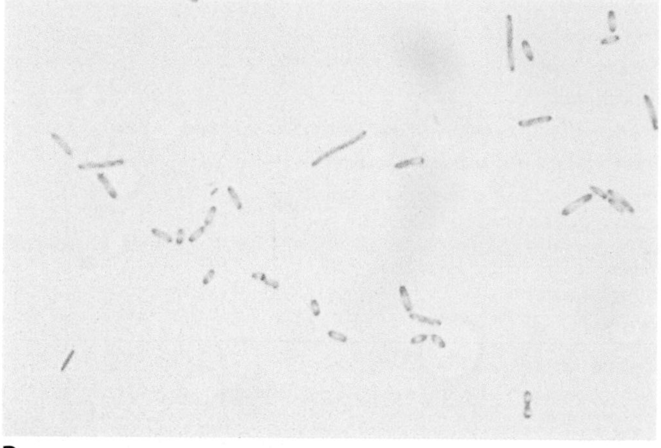

B

Figure 10-1 Gram stain of *Enterobacteriaceae*. Some species, such as *E. coli*, are short (2 to 3 μm long), plump, gram-negative bacilli with bipolar staining (A), while others, such as *Proteus* spp., are long (6 to 7 μm long) with bipolar staining (B).

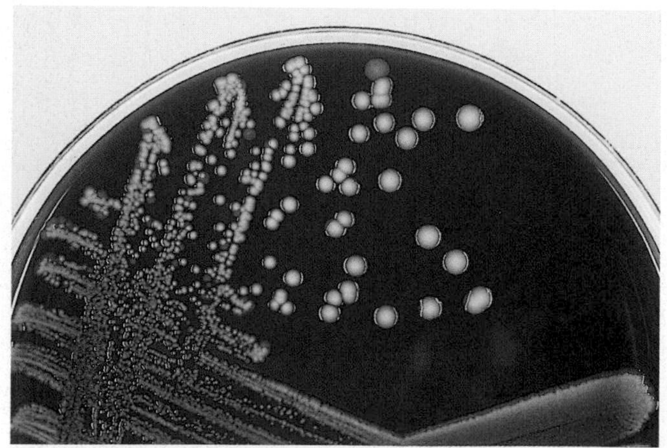

Figure 10-2 *Klebsiella pneumoniae* on blood agar. Colonies of *K. pneumoniae* are large (approximately 4 to 6 mm in diameter), gray, opaque, and somewhat mucoid.

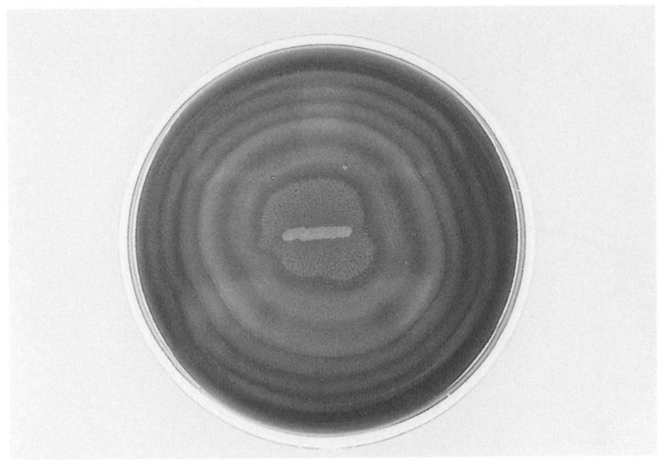

Figure 10-3 ***Proteus* spp. on blood agar.** *Proteus* species exhibit a characteristic swarming on blood agar, causing a wave-like appearance across the agar plate. Individual colonies are not distinguishable due to the swarming effect resulting from this motility.

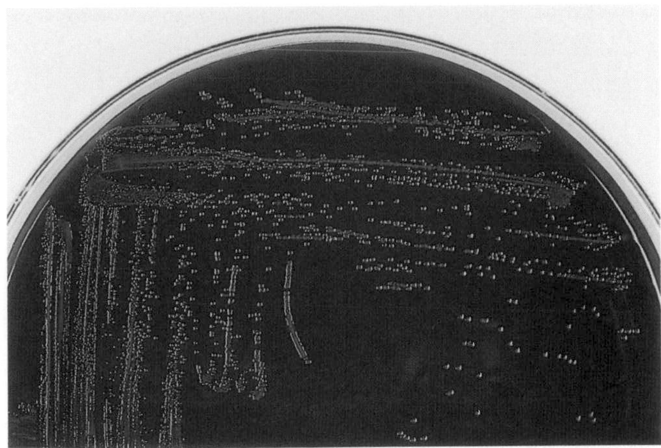

Figure 10-4 ***Yersinia enterocolitica* on blood agar.** Colonies of *Y. enterocolitica* are small (approximately 1 to 2 mm in diameter), gray, opaque, and pinpoint. Because of their small size, colonies of *Y. enterocolitica* do not resemble commonly isolated *Enterobacteriaceae*.

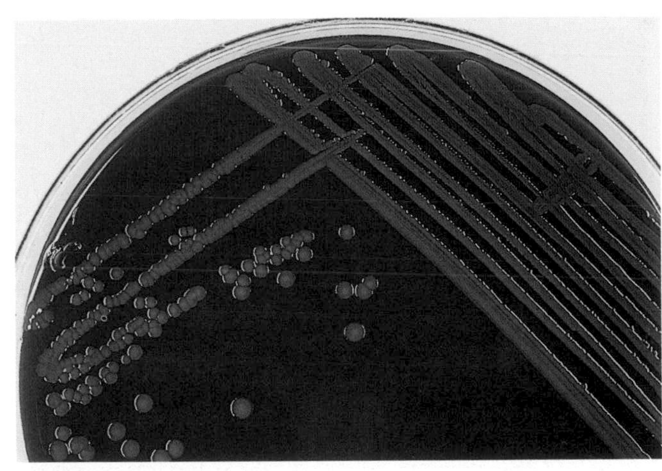

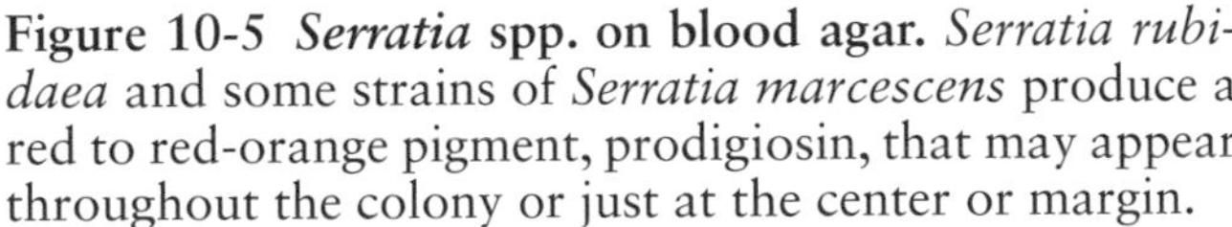

Figure 10-5 ***Serratia* spp. on blood agar.** *Serratia rubidaea* and some strains of *Serratia marcescens* produce a red to red-orange pigment, prodigiosin, that may appear throughout the colony or just at the center or margin.

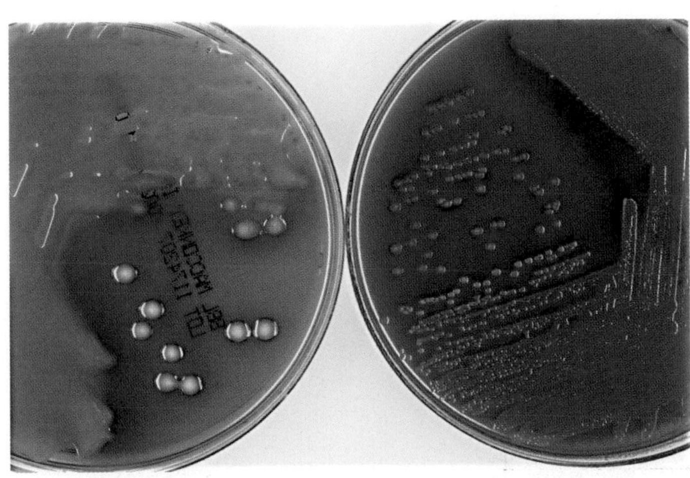

Figure 10-6 ***Escherichia coli* and *Klebsiella* spp.** on MacConkey agar. Presumptive identification of *E. coli* and *Klebsiella* spp. can be made based on their characteristic morphology on MacConkey agar. *E. coli* colonies are dry, donut shaped, and dark pink, approximately 2 to 4 mm in diameter (right), while *Klebsiella* colonies are often mucoid, larger (4 to 6 mm), and dark to faint pink (left).

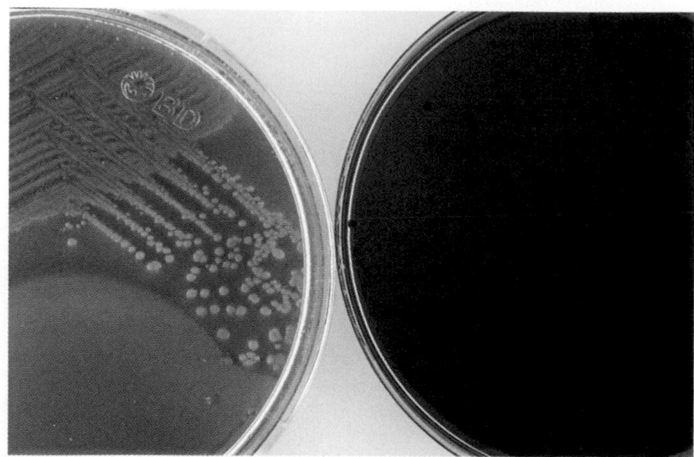

Figure 10-7 *Escherichia coli* and *Shigella* spp. on HE agar. HE agar is a selective and differential medium for the isolation and differentiation of enteric pathogens from members of the normal enteric flora. The medium contains bile salts; carbohydrates including lactose, sucrose, and salicin; indicator dyes (bromthymol blue and acid fuchsin); sodium thiosulfate; and ferric ammonium citrate for the detection of H_2S. The increased carbohydrate and peptone contents counteract the inhibitory effects of the bile salts and indicators. The carbohydrates distinguish the fermenters from the nonfermenters. Rapid fermenters, such as *E. coli*, appear as salmon pink to orange, surrounded by a zone of bile precipitate (left), while *Shigella* colonies are green (right).

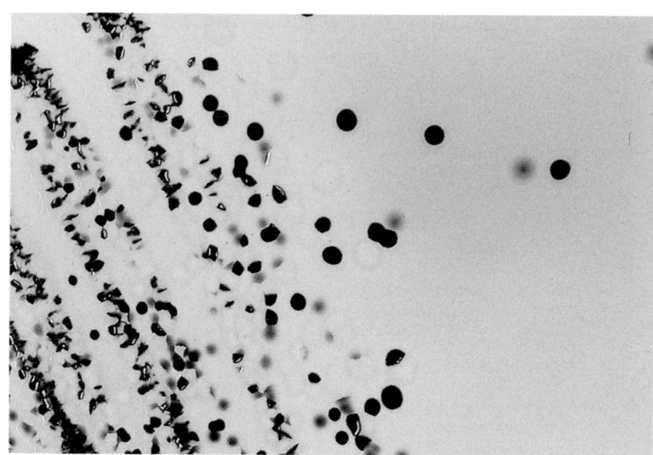

Figure 10-8 H_2S-positive *Salmonella* colonies on HE agar. *Salmonella* and some *Proteus* strains form green to blue-green colonies with black centers when the colonies are H_2S positive.

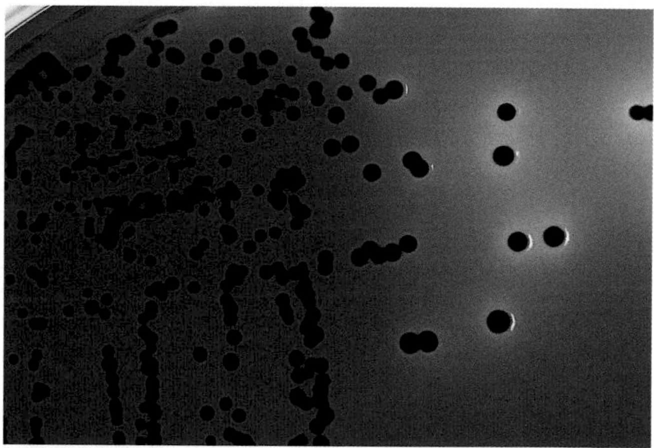

Figure 10-9 H_2S-positive *Salmonella* colonies on XLD agar. On XLD agar, *Salmonella* can be differentiated from members of the normal enteric flora by three reactions: xylose fermentation, lysine decarboxylation, and hydrogen sulfide production. On this medium, the production of hydrogen sulfide under alkaline conditions results in the formation of red colonies with black centers, characteristic of *Salmonella*, whereas under acidic conditions, this black precipitate is not formed.

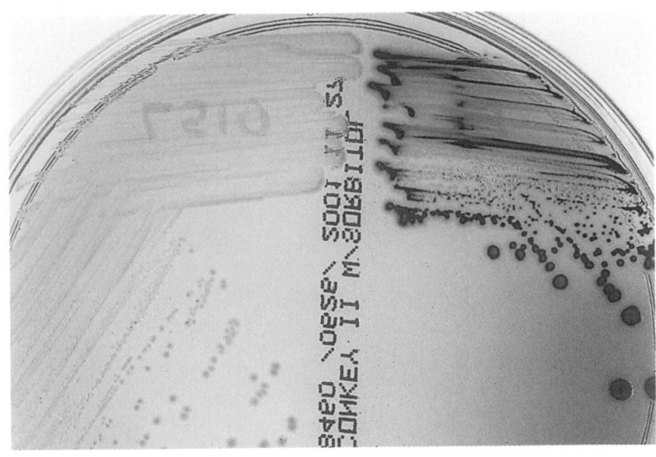

Figure 10-10 ***Escherichia coli*** **and** ***E. coli*** **O157:H7 on MacConkey agar with sorbitol.** *E. coli* O157:H7 is sorbitol negative, and colonies appear colorless (left), whereas other strains of *E. coli* ferment sorbitol and appear as pink colonies (right).

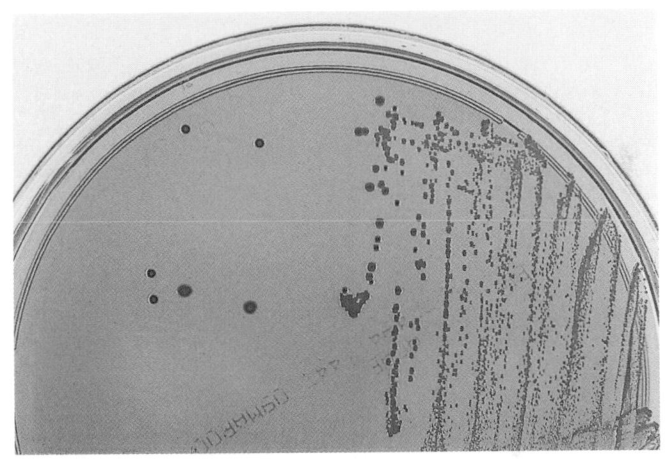

Figure 10-11 ***Yersinia enterocolitica*** **on CIN agar.** CIN agar is a selective medium specifically used for the isolation of *Y. enterocolitica* from fecal specimens. This medium contains yeast extract, mannitol, and bile salts, with neutral red and crystal violet as pH indicators. Colonies are small (1 to 2 mm in diameter). *Y. enterocolitica* ferments mannitol, causing a drop in pH around the colony. The colony absorbs neutral red, which may appear as a red bull's-eye in the center of the colony. Most other bacteria, including other enteric bacteria that ferment mannitol, are inhibited on CIN agar.

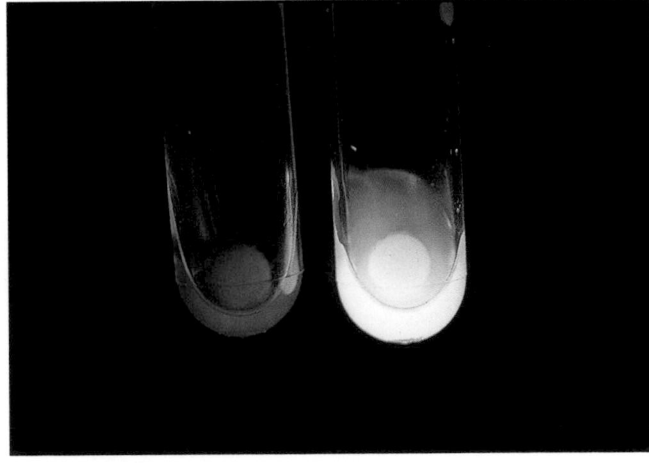

Figure 10-12 **MUG test.** In the presence of the enzyme β-glucuronidase, the substrate MUG releases 4-methylumbelliferone, a fluorescent compound that is easily detected by long-wave (360-nm) UV light (right tube). Since approximately 97% of all *E. coli* strains possess β-glucuronidase, the MUG test provides a rapid (30-min) method for the identification of this species. However, *E. coli* O157:H7 rarely posseses β-glucuronidase.

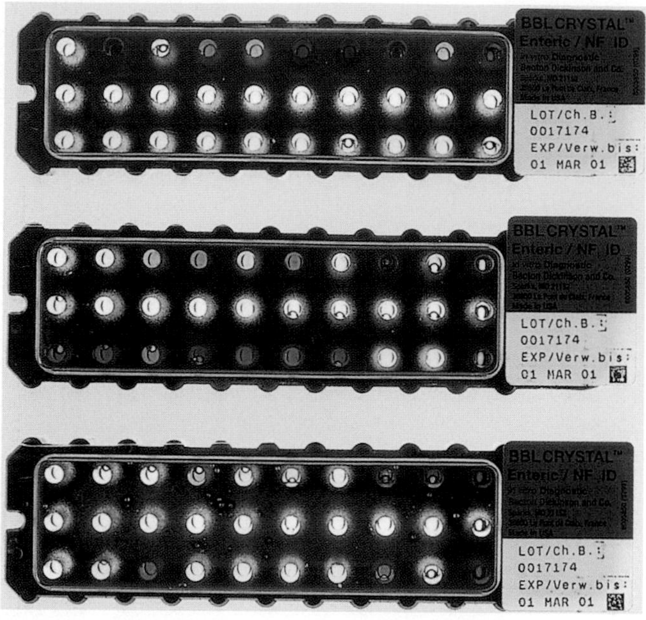

Figure 10-13 BBL CRYSTAL Enteric/Nonfermenter ID Kit. The BBL CRYSTAL Enteric/Nonfermenter ID panel (BD Diagnostic Systems, Franklin Lakes, NJ) is a modified microplate consisting of 30 wells of organic and inorganic substrates for the identification of both the *Enterobacteriaceae* and other gram-negative bacilli. Following an 18- to 20-h incubation period, the wells are examined for color changes. The resulting pattern of reactions is converted into a 10-digit profile number that is used as the basis for identification. Shown here are *K. pneumoniae* (top), *Proteus mirabilis* (middle), and *E. coli* (bottom).

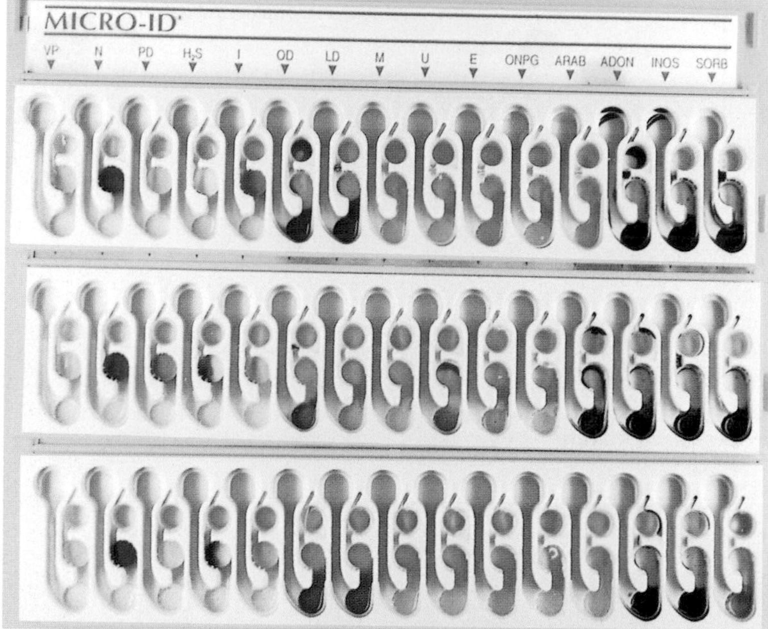

Figure 10-14 Micro-ID system. The Micro-ID system (bioMérieux, Inc., Durham, NC) is a self-contained unit with 15 biochemical tests for the rapid identification of the *Enterobacteriaceae*. The system is based on the principle that bacteria contain preformed enzymes that can be detected in 4 h. Each reaction chamber contains a filter paper disk impregnated with a reagent that detects an enzyme or metabolic product. Following inoculation and incubation for 4 h, the reaction chambers are inspected and the findings are interpreted based on color changes. Shown here are *K. pneumoniae* (top), *P. mirabilis* (middle), and *E. coli* (bottom).

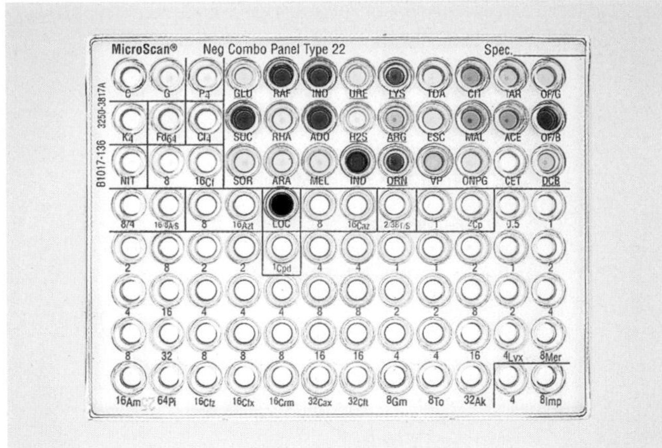

Figure 10-15 MicroScan Combo plate system. The MicroScan Combo plate system (Siemens Healthcare Diagnostics, Inc., West Sacramento, CA) utilizes modified conventional and chromogenic tests for the identification of fermentative and nonfermentative, gram-negative bacilli. Identification is based on detection of pH changes, substrate utilization, and growth in the presence of antimicrobial agents after 16 to 42 h of incubation at 35°C. Shown here is *E. coli.*

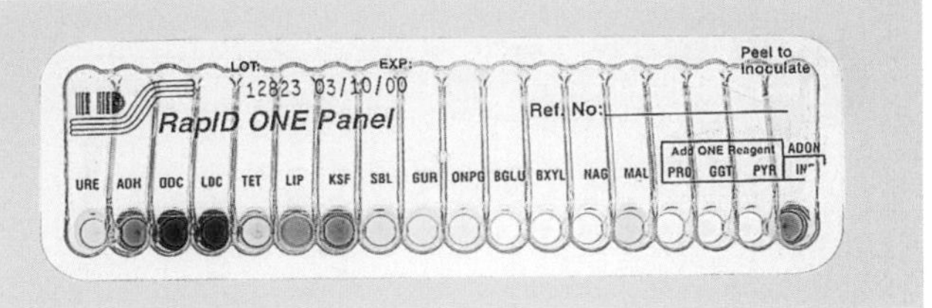

Figure 10-16 RapID onE system. The RapID onE system (Thermo Scientific Remel Products, Lenexa, KS) is a qualitative micromethod in which conventional and chromogenic substrates are used for the identification of medically important *Enterobacteriaceae* and other selected oxidase-negative, gram-negative bacilli. A suspension of test organisms is used to rehydrate and initiate the test reactions. After 4 h at 35°C, each test cavity is examined for reactivity by noting the development of a color. The pattern of positive and negative results is used as the basis for identification of the isolate by comparison of the test results to reactivity patterns in a database. Shown here is *E. coli.*

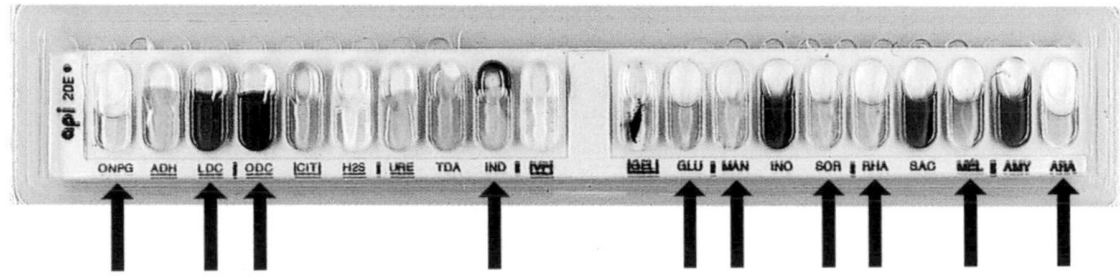

Figure 10-17 API 20E system. The API 20E (bioMérieux, Inc., Durham, NC) is a self-contained system consisting of 20 microtubes of dehydrated substrates designed to measure standard biochemical tests for *Enterobacteriaceae*. Substrates are rehydrated by adding a bacterial suspension of a colony in 0.85% NaCl. For a rapid interpretation (4 h), the inoculum must equal a no. 1 McFarland turbidity standard. The substrates/tests included in the system are ONPG, arginine (ADH), lysine (LDC), ornithine (ODC), citrate (CIT), H_2S, urea (URE), tryptophan (TDA), indole (IND), Voges-Proskauer (VP), gelatin (GEL), glucose (GLU), mannitol (MAN), inositol (INO), sorbitol (SOR), rhamnose (RHA), saccharose (sucrose) (SAC), melibiose (MEL), amygdalin (AMY), and arabinose (ARA). Identification is made by adding the required reagents and visually interpreting the results. A numerical code is derived by dividing the tests into seven groups of three. The test results are converted to a seven-digit profile. The oxidase reaction is the third test in the last set. If any of the tests are positive, a score is assigned to each tube; the first test of each set is given a score of 1, the second test is assigned a score of 2, and the third test is assigned a score of 4. If the test is negative, it is given a 0. The total scores in a set can range from 0 to 7. Shown here is *E. coli* with positive reactions (above the arrows) for ONPG, LDC, ODC, IND, GLU, MAN, SOR, RHA, MEL, and ARA. The oxidase test was negative. Therefore, the profile code number is 5144552.

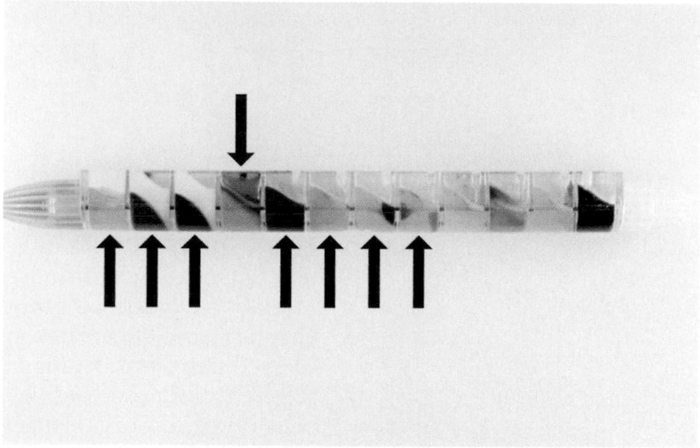

Figure 10-18 Enterotube II Identification System for *Enterobacteriaceae*. The Enterotube II System (BD Diagnostic Systems, Franklin Lakes, NJ) is a compartmented plastic tube containing 12 different conventional media and an enclosed inoculating wire, resulting in the reactions of 15 standard biochemical tests using a single colony. The tests include glucose, gas production from glucose, lysine decarboxylase, ornithine decarboxylase, H_2S production, indole, adonitol, lactose, arabinose, sorbitol, Voges-Proskauer, dulcitol, phenylalanine deaminase, urea, and citrate. Identification is made by adding the required reagents and visually interpreting the results. The resulting combination of color reactions, together with the Computer Coding System, allows identification of *Enterobacteriaceae*. The system should only be used on oxidase-negative bacteria. The organism represented in this image is *E. coli*. The positive reactions, indicated by the arrows, are glucose, gas production from glucose, lysine decarboxylase, ornithine decarboxylase, indole, lactose, arabinose, and sorbitol. The five-digit ID value is 36560.

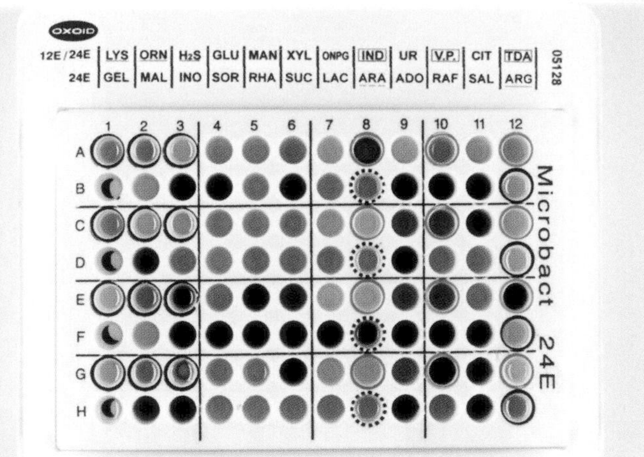

Figure 10-19 Microbact Gram-Negative Identification System. The Microbact 24E Identification System (Oxoid Ltd., Basingstoke, United Kingdom) consists of two separate strips, 12A (also referred to as 12E) and 12B, each containing 12 different biochemical substrates. Use of one strip alone will limit the ability to identify a wide range of gram-negative bacilli. For example, the 12A strip will identify 15 genera within the family *Enterobacteriaceae* that are oxidase negative, nitrate positive, and glucose fermenters. When the 12B strip is added, identification is expanded to include organisms that are oxidase positive, nitrate negative, and glucose nonfermenters. The substrates included in the Microbact 24E (with their abbreviations and expected positive reactions in parentheses), beginning with the top row, left to right, are lysine (LYS, blue-green), ornithine (ORN, blue), H_2S (black), glucose (GLU, yellow), mannitol (MAN, yellow), xylose (XYL, yellow), ONPG (yellow), indole (IND, pink-red), urease (URE, pink-red), Voges-Proskauer (VP, pink-red), citrate (CIT, blue), and tryptophan deaminase (TDA, cherry red). The bottom row includes gelatin (GEL, black), malonate (MAL, blue), inositol (INO, yellow), sorbitol (SOR, yellow), rhamnose (RHA, yellow), sucrose (SUC, yellow), lactose (LAC, yellow), arabinose (ARA, yellow), adonitol (ADO, yellow), raffinose (RAF, yellow), salicin (SAL, yellow), and arginine (ARG, green-blue at 24 h and blue at 48 h). Reagents are added to the following wells: IND, VP, and TDA. Additionally, nitrate reagents are added to the ONPG well once its reaction is read. It should be noted that the gelatin well should be read at 24 and 48 h for the *Enterobacteriaceae* and only at 48 h for the other gram-negative bacilli. The arginine color reaction is different at 24 and 48 h, as noted above. Identification is based on an octal coding system similar to the API system described in Fig. 10-17. The organisms shown in this image, from top to bottom, are *E. coli* (rows A and B), *K. pneumoniae* (rows C and D), *P. mirabilis* (rows E and F), and *Enterobacter cloacae* (rows G and H).

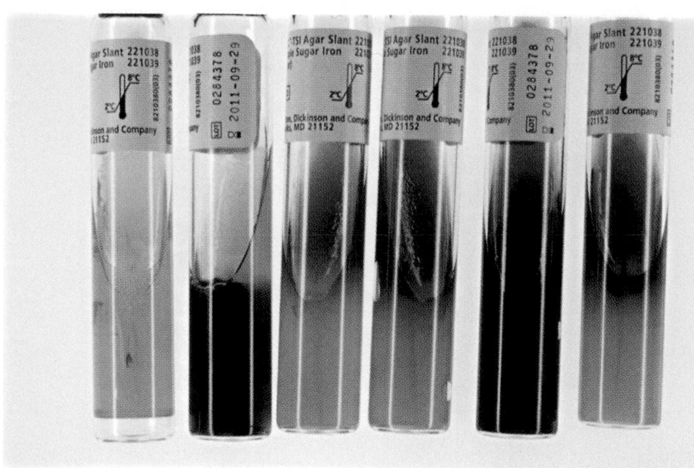

Figure 10-20 TSI agar. A TSI agar slant contains three carbohydrates, sucrose, lactose, and glucose, at a ratio of 10:10:1. For the detection of H_2S, sodium thiosulfate is present in the medium as the source of sulfur atoms. Two iron salts, ferrous sulfate and ferric ammonium citrate, react with the H_2S to form a black precipitate of ferrous sulfide. In the TSI tube, the agar in the top half forms a slant and thus is aerobic due to the exposure to oxygen, while the bottom (butt) is protected from air and, as a result, is considered anaerobic. Production of the gases CO_2 and H_2 is also detected by observing cracks or bubbles in the agar. The tubes should be inoculated with a single, well-isolated colony by using a long, straight wire. No change in the medium, indicated by an alkaline reaction in the slant and butt (Alk/Alk), means that the organism cannot ferment any of the sugars present, thereby excluding the *Enterobacteriaceae*. If glucose alone is fermented, the butt will be yellow due to the acid (A) production by the fermentation of glucose under anaerobic conditions; however, the slant will be alkaline (pink) due to the oxidative degradation of the peptones under aerobic conditions (Alk/A). Fermentation of glucose and lactose or of sucrose results in both an acidic slant and an acidic butt (A/A). As shown in this figure, members of the *Enterobacteriaceae* demonstrate a variety of reactions and these six correspond to those shown in the heading of Table 10-3, beginning with an acid slant and an acid butt and gas in the very bottom of the tube (A/AG). Because they all ferment glucose, the butt will always be acidic (yellow). The last tube on the right shows a characteristic reaction for *Salmonella enterica* serovar Typhi because of the slight H_2S production. An alternative to the TSI system is Kligler iron agar (KIA), which does not contain sucrose. The advantage of the sucrose in TSI is that *Salmonella* and *Shigella* do not metabolize either lactose or sucrose. Thus, any acid-acid reaction on a TSI will exclude *Salmonella* and *Shigella* spp. *Y. enterocolitica* ferments sucrose but not lactose, appearing as an A/A in TSI and Alk/A in KIA.

Escherichia, *Shigella*, and *Salmonella*

11

Escherichia coli is a member of the family *Enterobacteriaceae* and the enteric group *Escherichia-Shigella*. Although the genus *Escherichia* includes six species, *E. coli* is by far the most common, as well as being the bacterial species most frequently isolated in the clinical microbiology laboratory. It is normally found in the gastrointestinal tract of humans and animals.

E. coli can be spread from person to person by the fecal-oral route or by contaminated food, unchlorinated water, raw milk, and improperly cooked beef. The source of contamination is usually bovine manure. *E. coli* causes both gastrointestinal and extraintestinal infections including urinary tract infections, septicemia, nosocomial pneumonia, and wound infections. The strains causing gastroenteritis or enteritis can be grouped into five different clinical presentations: the most common are enterotoxigenic *E. coli* (ETEC), involved in traveler's diarrhea; enteropathogenic *E. coli* (EPEC), the cause of infantile diarrhea worldwide and resulting in fever, vomiting, and watery diarrhea; enteroinvasive *E. coli* (EIEC), involved in a dysentery-like disease; Shiga toxin-producing *E. coli* (STEC) O157 and non-O157, causing hemorrhagic colitis and associated with hemolytic-uremic syndrome (HUS); and enteroaggregative *E. coli* (EAEC), associated with chronic, persistent diarrhea and possibly a common cause of pediatric diarrhea in infants and young toddlers.

Fecal specimens should be collected within 4 days of disease onset, when organisms are usually present in their greatest numbers. Specimens should be processed within 1 to 2 h of collection or stored at 4°C until processed.

Colonies of *E. coli* are gray, smooth, and often beta-hemolytic on blood agar. Hemolytic colonies isolated from urine specimens usually suggest more virulent strains. Most strains ferment lactose rapidly. Aerobic growth appears within 12 to 18 h at 35°C. The colonies are pink on MacConkey agar and yellow to salmon on both Hektoen enteric (HE) and xylose lysine deoxycholate (XLD) agar plates. Sorbitol-containing MacConkey agar medium (SMAC) enhances the identification of *E. coli* O157. Since *E. coli* O157 fails to ferment sorbitol, this aids in differentiating this serogroup from strains normally found in the intestinal tract. In addition to SMAC, other media are available and have been shown to increase the sensitivity of cultures for O157 STEC. These include CHROMagar O157 and cefixime- and tellurite-containing SMAC (CT-SMAC; BD Diagnostic Systems, Franklin Lakes, NJ). There is no selective medium for non-O157; therefore, testing for the presence of Shiga toxin is important.

Presumptive identification of *E. coli* should be based on Gram stain morphology, colony morphology on MacConkey agar, and triple sugar iron (TSI) and IMViC (indole, methyl red, Voges-Proskauer, citrate) reactions (Table 11-1). In addition, *E. coli* can be differentiated from most other members of the *Enterobacteriaceae* because they are methylumbelliferyl-β-D-glucuronide positive. Most strains of *E. coli* are motile, with the exception of the nonmotile enteroinvasive *E. coli*. This strain may also be a non- or late lactose fermenter, and thus may be confused with *Shigella* spp. CDC guidelines recommend that all fecal specimens submitted for testing for routine enteric pathogens and all patients with suspected HUS should be cultured for O157 STEC

Table 11-1 Characteristic reactions of *E. coli* and *Shigella* spp.[a]

Characteristic	*E. coli*	*E. coli* O157	*Shigella*
TSI	A/AG	ALK/AG	ALK/A
Indole	+	+	V
Methyl red	+	+	+
Voges-Proskauer	0	0	0
Citrate	0	0	0
Sorbitol	+	0	V
Lactose	+	+	0/+[b]
Xylose	+	+	0
Lysine	+	+	0
Motility	+	+	0

[a]A, acid; ALK, alkaline; G, gas; +, positive reaction (≥90% positive); V, variable reaction (11 to 89% positive); 0, negative reaction (≤10% positive).

[b]*S. sonnei* is lactose positive.

on selective and differential media and tested for non-O157 STEC using a Shiga toxin assay. These guidelines were proposed to avoid missing STEC infection by testing on selective specimens, such as bloody stools.

Shiga toxins of *E. coli* O157 and non-O157 can be identified by a variety of commercial reagents. If the assay is not available in the laboratory, the specimen should be sent to a reference laboratory for identification. DNA probes, DNA pulsed-field gel electrophoresis, tissue culture, and animal studies may be used to identify other gastrointestinal strains of *E. coli*. *E. coli* O104:H4 carries the gene for a Shiga toxin 2 variant (stx_{2a}). However, STEC genes such as Shiga toxin 1 (stx_1), *eae*, and *ehx* are missing. This is unusual in that most non-O157 strains carry the gene for Shiga toxin 1.

The genus *Shigella* is composed of four species subgroups. These include subgroup A or *Shigella dysenteriae*, subgroup B or *Shigella flexneri*, subgroup C or *Shigella boydii*, and subgroup D or *Shigella sonnei*. Generally they are anaerogenic and nonmotile. They do not ferment lactose, with the exception of *S. sonnei*, which is a late lactose fermenter.

The common clinical symptoms of shigellosis are self-limiting and initially present as fever, abdominal cramps, and watery diarrhea. Within a few days, blood and mucus appear in the feces, suggesting that the organism has penetrated the intestinal mucosa. Large numbers of polymorphonuclear leukocytes can be observed during microscopic examination of feces. Overall, symptoms associated with shigellosis are mild, and some patients are asymptomatic. *S. dysenteriae* causes dysentery, the most severe form of shigellosis, which is related to the production of Shiga toxin. HUS is one of the most serious complications of infection. Reactive arthritis or Reiter's chronic syndrome has been associated with *S. flexneri* infection. Humans are a natural reservoir, and the organism is spread by person-to-person contact or via contaminated water or food. As few as 10 bacteria can cause infection, compared to 10^5 for infection with *Salmonella* and some of the other enteric pathogens. For this reason, shigellosis is the most common infection among laboratory workers. *S. sonnei* is the most common *Shigella* species causing shigellosis in developed countries, followed by *S. flexneri*.

MacConkey agar and either HE or XLD agar are recommended for optimal isolation of *Shigella*. *Shigella* strains appear as colorless colonies on all three media because they do not ferment the carbohydrates contained in the media: lactose, salicin, sucrose, and xylose. *Shigella* spp. produce an alkaline slant and an acid butt (ALK/A) and no gas in TSI agar. IMViC reactions can be similar to those of *E. coli*, i.e., indole positive, methyl red positive, Voges-Proskauer negative, and citrate negative, although *S. sonnei* is indole negative and only 25 to 50% of the other *Shigella* spp. are indole positive (Table 11-1).

Serologic testing is required for the grouping of *Shigella* isolates because *S. flexneri* and *S. boydii* are biochemically indistinguishable. In the diagnostic laboratory, serologic identification is routinely performed by a slide agglutination method with polyvalent somatic antigen antisera. Isolates of *S. dysenteriae* should be sent to a reference laboratory for identification of serotype *S. dysenteriae* 1 for epidemiological follow-up.

The genus *Salmonella* is composed of two species, *Salmonella enterica* and *Salmonella bongori*, and there are more than 2,400 antigenically distinct members of these two species. *S. enterica* is subdivided into six subspecies; however, *S. enterica* subsp. *enterica* (designated subspecies I) is commonly isolated from humans and warm-blooded animals.

Most infections with *Salmonella* are caused by contaminated food or water. Other reservoirs include contact with animals colonized with the organism and human contact. Similar to infections with *Shigella* spp., intestinal infections with *Salmonella* spp. are usually self-limited in the otherwise healthy host; they cause diarrhea that can last as long as 1 week. However, infection with *Salmonella* serotype Typhi causes serious sepsis, known as typhoid fever. The symptoms include fever and headache, often without diarrhea. The infection is more common in developing countries and is usually associated with foreign travel when isolated in the United States. Similar infections are caused by

Salmonella serotypes Paratyphi A, B, and C. Outbreaks of infections caused by *Salmonella* serotype Enteritidis are increasing in the United States and are usually associated with contaminated food, including raw or poorly cooked eggs. Of concern are *Salmonella* infections that are resistant to several antimicrobial agents. These are usually associated with *Salmonella* serotype Typhimurium.

Although MacConkey agar and either HE or XLD agar are recommended for isolation of *Salmonella*, more highly selective media are available. These include xylose lysine Tergitol-4 (XLT4) and Rambach agars. Bismuth sulfite and brilliant green agars are the preferred media for isolation of *Salmonella* serotype Typhi. Suspicious colonies isolated from selective media should be subcultured onto TSI or Kligler iron agar slants. Typically, most *Salmonella* serotypes produce an alkaline reaction on the slant and an acidic reaction in the butt (ALK/A). They also generate gas in the tube, as well as large amounts of H_2S. Although *Salmonella* serotype Typhi produces ALK/A, it produces a very small amount of H_2S and no visible gas in TSI agar. Additional biochemical tests may be used to confirm the identification (Table 11-2).

Testing is required for the serotyping of *Salmonella* spp. These organisms may possess somatic (O), flagellar (H), and capsular (Vi) antigens. In the diagnostic laboratory, serological identification is routinely performed by a slide agglutination method using polyvalent somatic antigen antisera as described for *Shigella*. If *Salmonella* serotype Typhi is suspected, the isolate should be tested with both O group D and Vi antigens. If only Vi is positive, the isolate should be heated in boiling water for 15 min because the capsular antigen is heat labile. On retesting with O antiserum, the group D test should be positive. A laboratory may provide a preliminary report of *Salmonella* spp. based on biochemical reactions and serotyping. The isolate should then be referred to the health department for confirmation.

Table 11-2 Characteristic reactions of *Salmonella* spp.[a]

Characteristic	*Salmonella* spp.[b]	*Salmonella* serotype Typhi
TSI	ALK/AG	ALK/A
H_2S on TSI	+	Slight
Indole	0	0
Methyl red	+	+
Voges-Proskauer	0	0
Citrate	+	0
Ornithine	+	0
Arabinose	+	0
Dulcitol	+	0
Rhamnose	+	0

[a]A, acid; ALK, alkaline; G, gas; +, positive reaction (≥90% positive); V, variable reaction (11 to 89% positive); 0, negative reaction (≤10% positive).
[b]Reactions for most commonly isolated *Salmonella* serotypes.

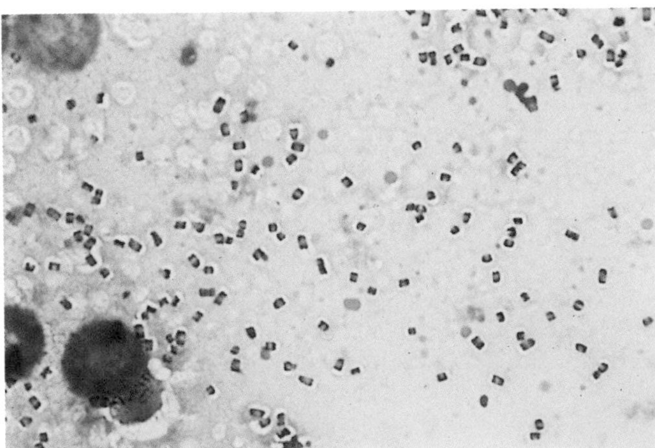

Figure 11-1 Gram stain of *Escherichia coli*. *E. coli* is a gram-negative bacillus appearing as a short, plump, straight rod with bipolar staining, often resembling a safety pin shape. This morphology helps to distinguish *E. coli* from other *Enterobacteriaceae*. Although bipolar staining occurs with the other *Enterobacteriaceae*, they are usually longer bacilli.

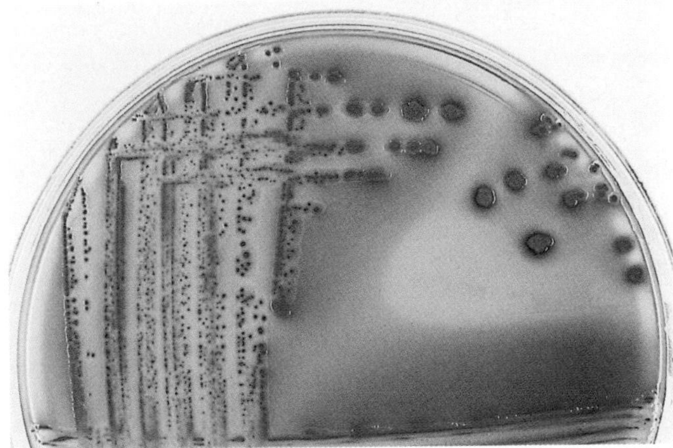

Figure 11-2 Colonies of *Escherichia coli* on MacConkey agar. On MacConkey agar, the colonies are pink, dry, and donut shaped and are surrounded by a dark pink area of precipitated bile salts.

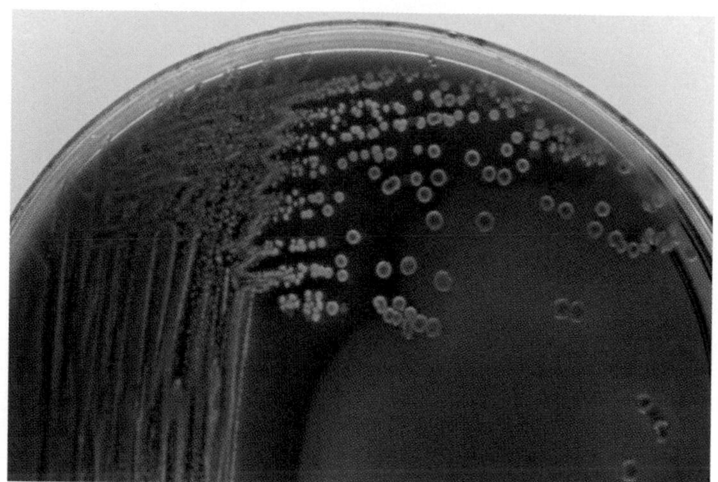

Figure 11-3 Colonies of *Escherichia coli* on HE agar. Colonies of *E. coli* on HE agar appear yellow-orange to salmon pink. This is due to the rapid fermentation of lactose by this organism.

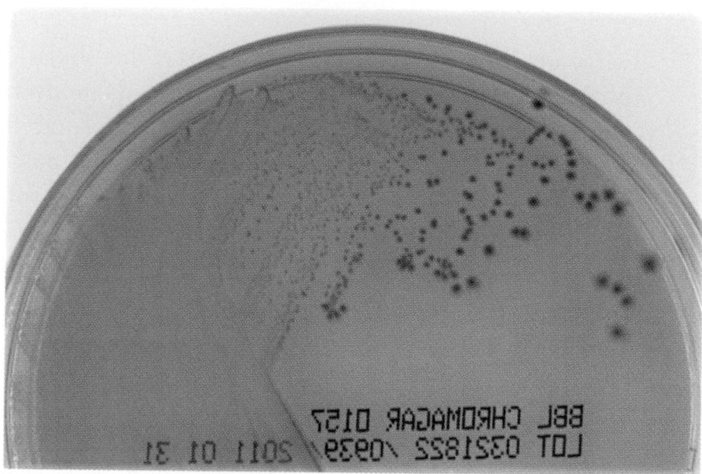

Figure 11-4 Colonies of *Escherichia coli* on CHROMagar O157. BBL CHROMagar O157 medium (BD Diagnostic Systems, Franklin Lakes, NJ) has been shown to increase the sensitivity of culture for O157 STEC. It is intended for the isolation, differentiation, and presumptive identification of *E. coli* O157. Due to the chromogenic substrates in the medium, colonies of *E. coli* O157 produce a mauve color, as shown here, whereas *E. coli* non-O157:H7 produces blue colonies. CHROMagar O157 contains cefixime, cefsulodin, and potassium tellurite, which reduces the number of other bacteria that grow on this medium.

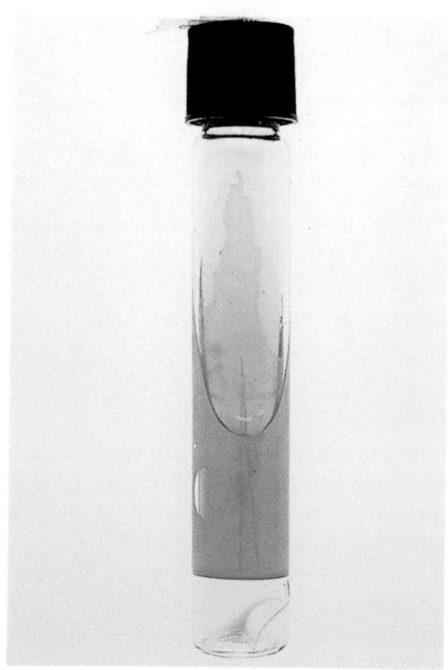

Figure 11-5 *Escherichia coli* on a TSI agar slant. Colonies of *E. coli* on a TSI agar slant produce an acid slant and acid butt due to the rapid fermentation of glucose and lactose. This can result in copious gas production, causing the agar to split or be lifted from the bottom of the tube, as shown in this figure. A description of this test can be found in Fig. 10-20.

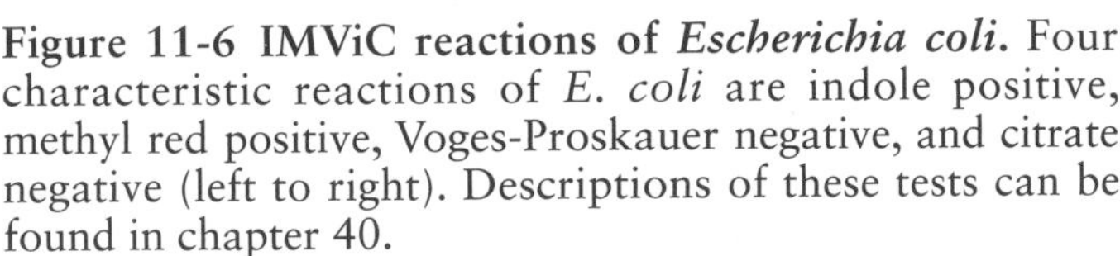

Figure 11-6 IMViC reactions of *Escherichia coli*. Four characteristic reactions of *E. coli* are indole positive, methyl red positive, Voges-Proskauer negative, and citrate negative (left to right). Descriptions of these tests can be found in chapter 40.

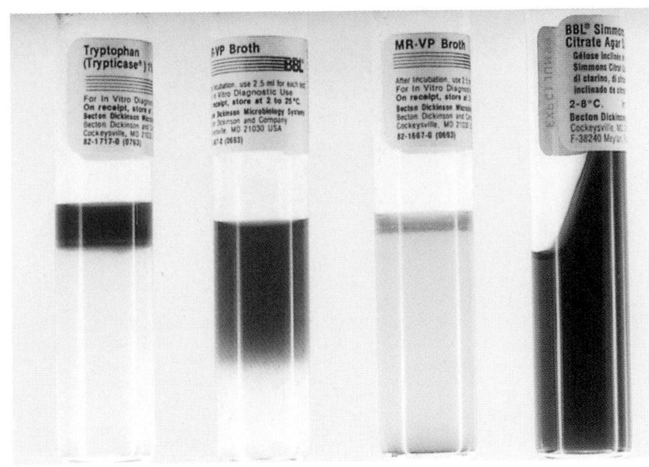

Figure 11-7 Toxin assay for the qualitative detection of Shiga toxins 1 and 2 produced by toxin-producing strains of *E. coli*. The Immuno*Card* STAT! EHEC (Meridian Bioscience, Inc., Cincinnati, OH) is based on the immunochromatographic lateral flow principle. The test device contains immobilized monoclonal anti-Shiga toxin 1 and anti-Shiga toxin 2 antibodies labeled with red-colored gold particles. Each test has an internal control. The toxins in the sample form complexes with the gold-labeled antibody, which migrates through the pad until it encounters the binding zone in the test area. Due to the gold labeling, a distinct red line is formed, as shown here. The test kit on the left is negative for Shiga toxins 1 and 2, the center kit is positive for toxin 2 only, and the test on the right is positive for both toxins 1 and 2.

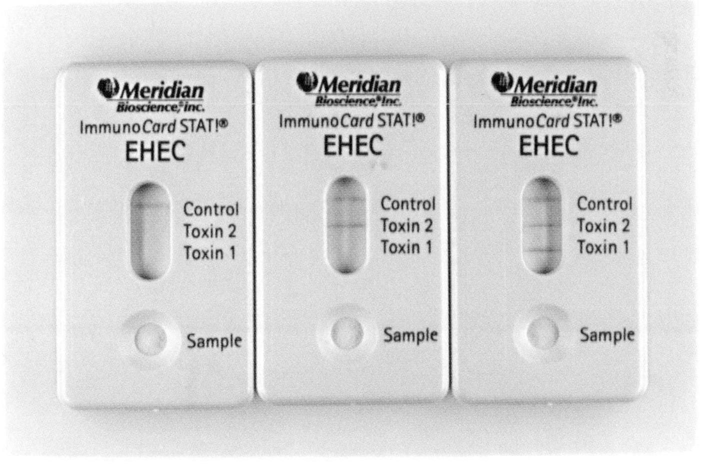

Figure 11-8 Colonies of *Shigella* spp. and *Escherichia coli* on MacConkey agar. *Shigella* spp. are lactose negative and appear as colorless colonies (left), whereas *E. coli* is a rapid lactose fermenter and appears pink (right).

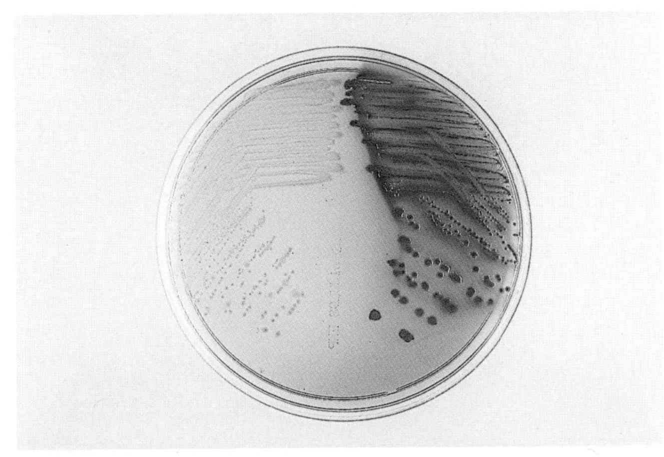

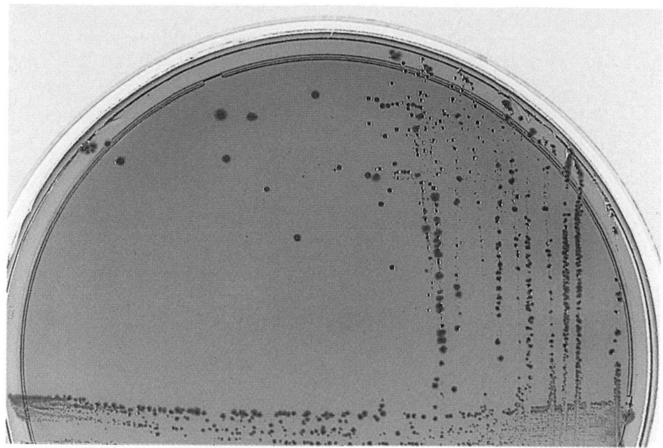

Figure 11-9 ***Shigella*** **spp. on HE agar.** *Shigella* spp. do not ferment lactose, salicin, or sucrose, the carbohydrates contained within HE agar; therefore, they appear as colorless colonies, as shown here.

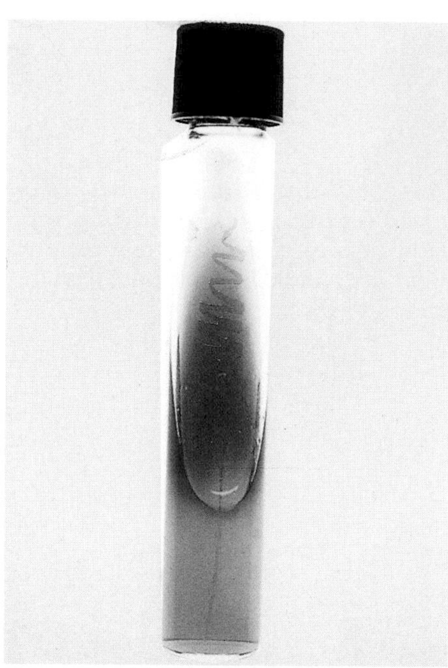

Figure 11-10 ***Shigella*** **spp. on a TSI agar slant.** *Shigella* spp. ferment glucose but not lactose or sucrose present in the TSI slant; therefore, they produce ALK/A. They also do not produce H_2S or gas.

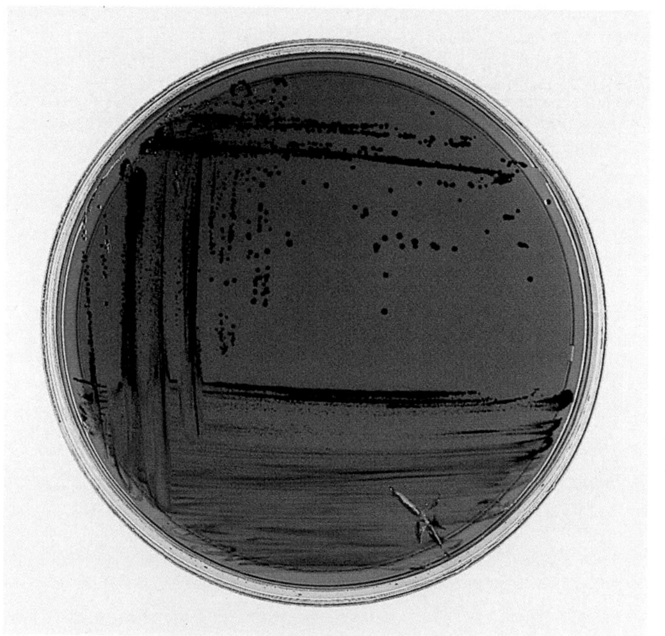

Figure 11-11 ***Salmonella*** **spp. on HE agar.** Although *Salmonella* spp. do not ferment the carbohydrates in HE agar, they do produce H_2S. The presence of ferric ammonium citrate in HE agar causes the colonies of *Salmonella* to appear black.

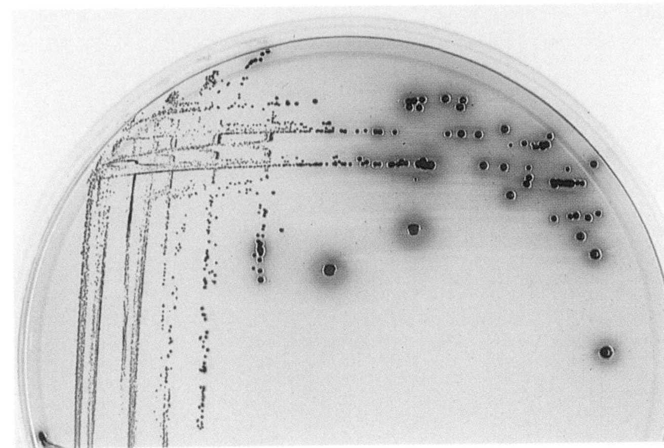

Figure 11-12 *Salmonella* serotype Typhi on bismuth sulfite agar. Bismuth sulfite agar contains ferrous sulfate, bismuth sulfite indicator, and brilliant green. Well-isolated subsurface colonies of *Salmonella* serotype Typhi are circular, jet black, and well defined. The black colony may vary from 1 to 4 mm in diameter, depending on the particular strain, length of incubation, and position of the colony in the agar. The typical discrete surface of a *Salmonella* serotype Typhi colony is black and is surrounded by a black or brownish black zone that appears several times the size of the colony, as shown in this figure. By reflected light, this zone exhibits a distinctly characteristic metallic sheen.

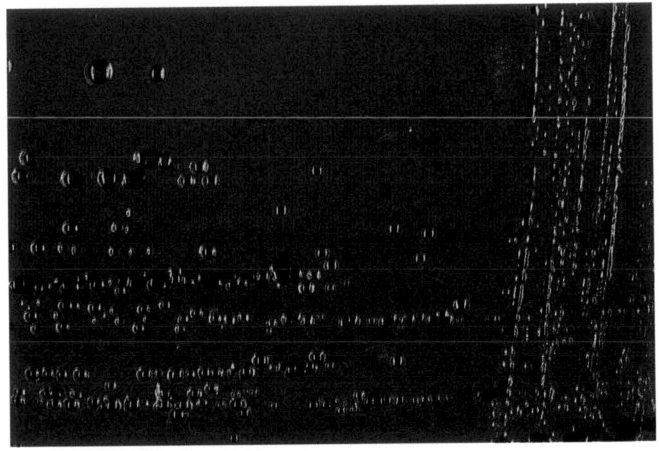

Figure 11-13 *Salmonella* on XLT4 agar. XLT4 agar was introduced in 1990 for the purpose of inhibiting bacterial overgrowth commonly associated with screening of fecal specimens for *Salmonella* spp. contaminated with enteric organisms. This medium is similar to XLD agar; however, the sodium deoxycholate is replaced with a 27% solution of Tergitol-4. This supplement inhibits the growth of non-*Salmonella* organisms. Typical H_2S-positive *Salmonella* colonies, other than *Salmonella* serotype Typhi, appear black after 18 to 24 h of incubation. Colonies of H_2S-negative *Salmonella* strains appear pinkish yellow. Other enterics may appear red or yellow but should appear markedly inhibited, as shown in this figure.

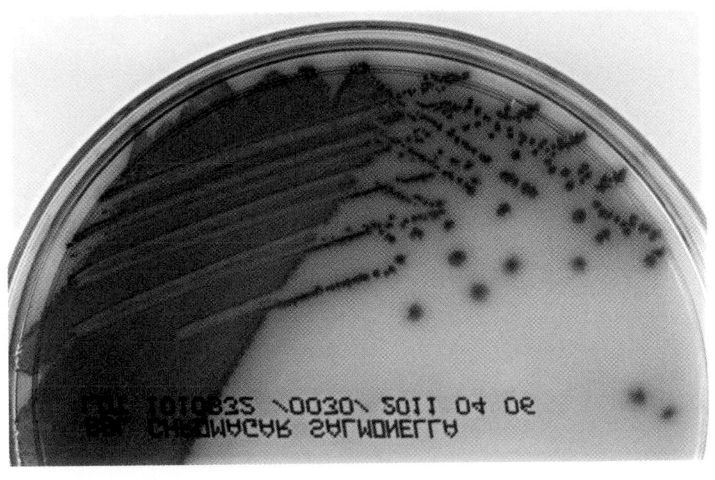

Figure 11-14 *Salmonella* on CHROMagar. BBL CHROMagar Salmonella (BD Diagnostic Systems) is a selective and differential medium for the isolation and presumptive identification of *Salmonella* spp. based on chromogenic substrates in the medium. *Salmonella* spp. appear as mauve-colored (rose to purple) colonies, shown here, whereas other enterics appear blue or colorless.

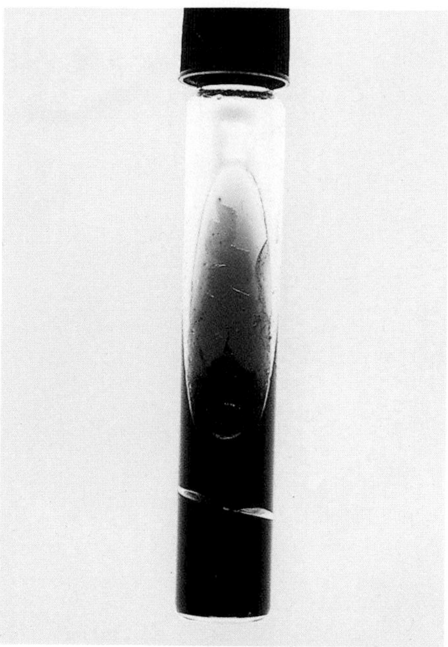

Figure 11-15 *Salmonella* on a TSI agar slant. Most *Salmonella* spp. ferment glucose and produce gas and large amounts of H_2S. Therefore they cause the ALK/AG H_2S^+ reaction on a TSI agar slant.

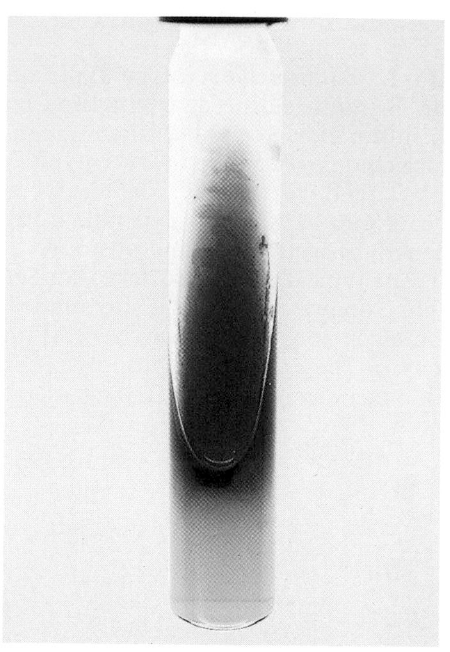

Figure 11-16 *Salmonella* serotype Typhi on a TSI agar slant. Although *Salmonella* serotype Typhi ferments glucose like other *Salmonella* spp., it does not produce gas and produces only a small amount of H_2S. The resulting reaction on a TSI agar slant is ALK/A slight H_2S.

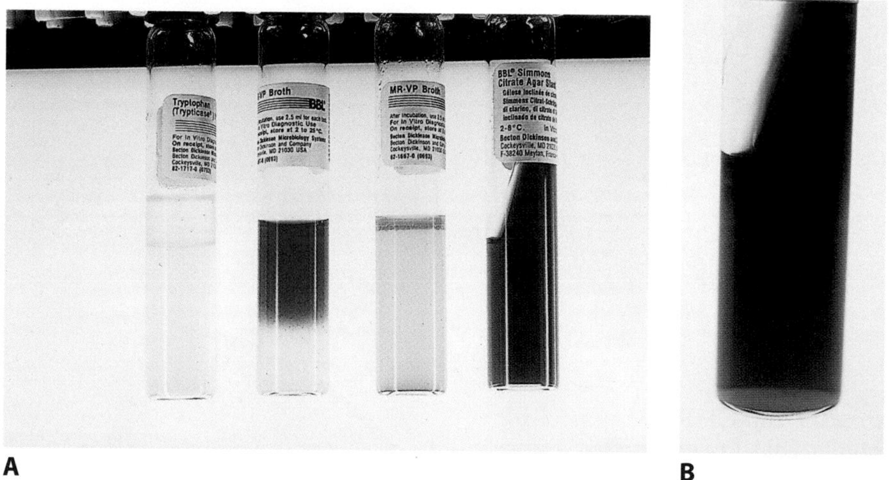

A B

Figure 11-17 IMViC reactions of *Salmonella* serotype Typhi. Four characteristic reactions of *Salmonella* serotype Typhi are indole negative, methyl red positive, Voges-Proskauer negative, and citrate negative (panel A, left to right). Descriptions of these tests can be found in chapter 40. In comparison, most other commonly isolated *Salmonella* species have similar reactions for indole, methyl red, and Voges-Proskauer; however, they are citrate positive (B).

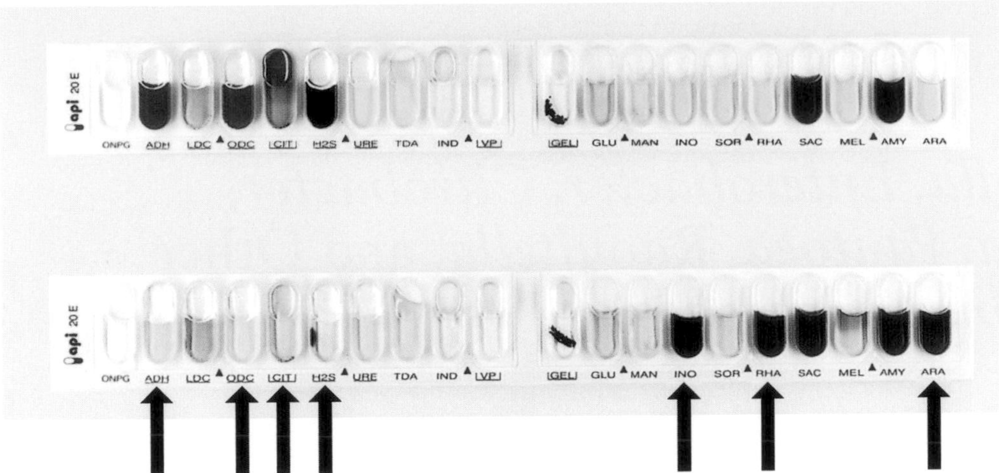

Figure 11-18 ***Salmonella enterica*** **and** ***Salmonella*** **serotype Typhi in the API 20E system.** Shown here are the reactions of *Salmonella enterica* and *Salmonella* serotype Typhi on API 20E (bioMérieux, Inc., Durham, NC). *S. enterica* is in the top strip. The differentiating characteristics, indicated by the arrows, are arginine dihydrolase (ADH), ornithine decarboxylase (ODC), citrate (CIT), and H_2S. *Salmonella* spp. are strongly positive for these reactions, whereas *Salmonella* serotype Typhi is negative ADH, ODC, and CIT and weakly positive for H_2S. The carbohydrate reaction differences are shown in Table 11-2 and in this figure.

Klebsiella, *Enterobacter*, *Citrobacter*, *Serratia*, *Pantoea*, *Raoultella*, and Other *Enterobacteriaceae*

12

Klebsiella, *Enterobacter*, *Citrobacter*, *Pantoea*, *Raoultella*, and *Serratia* are all members of the family *Enterobacteriaceae*. The genus *Klebsiella* is composed of five species: *Klebsiella pneumoniae*, *Klebsiella oxytoca*, *Klebsiella granulomatis*, *Klebsiella singaporensis*, and *Klebsiella varicola*. Additionally, there are three subspecies of *K. pneumoniae*: *K. pneumoniae* subsp. *pneumoniae*, *K. pneumoniae* subsp. *ozaenae*, and *K. pneumoniae* subsp. *rhinoscleromatis*. *K. singaporensis* is not known to cause disease in humans.

There are 14 species within the genus *Enterobacter*. Of these, 10 have been found in clinical specimens. The two most common clinical isolates are *Enterobacter aerogenes* and *Enterobacter cloacae*. *Enterobacter sakazakii* has now been transferred to the genus *Cronobacter*; however, it is acceptable to continue to refer to this organism as *E. sakazakii*. The reason is that because of the lack of discriminatory tests it is difficult to identify the species of *Cronobacter* in the diagnostic laboratory. *Enterobacter agglomerans*, previously a member of the *Enterobacter* spp., is now in the genus *Pantoea*.

The genus *Citrobacter* is composed of 11 species. All have been isolated from clinical specimens with the exception of *Citrobacter rodentium*, a mouse pathogen. The three most common clinical isolates are *Citrobacter freundii*, *Citrobacter braakii*, and *Citrobacter youngae*.

There are nine *Serratia* species, with *Serratia marcescens* and *Serratia odorifera* containing biogroups and *S. marcescens* also containing subspecies. The *Serratia liquefaciens* group actually contains three species, but for the purposes of this discussion, this group is referred to as a species. Seven *Serratia* species have been isolated from clinical specimens.

The genus *Raoultella* contains three species: *Raoultella ornithinolytica*, *Raoultella planticola*, and *Raoultella terrigena*. The latter two species share pathogenicity characteristics with *K. pneumoniae* and therefore are difficult to differentiate biochemically. However, *K. pneumoniae* grows at 44°C but not at 10°C, whereas *R. planticola* and *R. terrigena* grow at 10°C but not at 44°C.

Klebsiella, *Enterobacter*, *Citrobacter*, and *Serratia* cause a wide variety of infections, most frequently in hospitalized patients. These organisms are known to cause sepsis, infections of the respiratory tract and urinary tract, wound infections, and meningitis, although rarely. They are normally found in the gastrointestinal tract, and this is usually the source of the infection; however, they may be spread by person-to-person transmission, intravenous fluids, and medical devices. Multiple-antibiotic-resistant strains have caused outbreaks in hospitals, usually in locations with seriously ill patients, such as intensive care units.

Klebsiella, *Enterobacter*, *Pantoea*, *Raoultella*, *Citrobacter*, and *Serratia* are gram-negative bacilli that range from approximately 3 to 6 μm in length and up to 1 μm in width. In general, these genera grow well on blood and MacConkey agars when incubated aerobically at 35°C for 18 to 24 h. Although encapsulated strains of *Klebsiella* are known to produce mucoid colonies, strains from the other genera can also have the same appearance. Some of the *Serratia* spp. are pigmented, including *Serratia rubidaea*, *Serratia plymuthica*, and some strains of *S. marcescens*. They produce a red pigment known as prodigiosin. Another characteristic that aids in the identification is the potato-like odor produced by *S. odorifera*. *E. sakazakii* and *P. agglomerans* also produce a pigment that ranges from bright to pale yellow.

Overall, these genera provide a challenge for the commercial identification systems. Therefore, if identification by these systems is <90% for any species, the identification should be confirmed using conventional methods. Most *Klebsiella*, *Enterobacter*, *Pantoea*, *Raoultella*, *Citrobacter*, and *Serratia* spp. are identified using commercial kits, along with triple sugar iron (TSI) agar slants. These organisms, in the absence of pigment, may have similar colony morphologies. They may also be indistinguishable on TSI agar slants. Lysine, arginine, and ornithine tests are very helpful in the identification of *Klebsiella*, *Enterobacter*, *Citrobacter*, and *Serratia* (Tables 12-1 through 12-4). The IMViC (indole, methyl red, Voges-Proskauer, citrate) reactions of *Klebsiella* and *Enterobacter* are similar: negative for indole and methyl red and positive for Voges-Proskauer and citrate. However, *K. oxytoca* and *R. ornithinolytica* are indole positive (Table 12-1). Four species of *Citrobacter*, including *C. freundii*, may produce H_2S; however, some of the more common clinical isolates are H_2S negative (Table 12-4). The late lactose-fermenting, H_2S-producing *Citrobacter* spp. resemble *Salmonella* on TSI agar slants and in IMViC reactions.

Table 12-1 Key characteristics of some *Klebsiella* and *Raoultella* species and subspecies[a]

Species	Indole	Ornithine	VP	Malonate	ONPG	Growth at 10°C	Growth at 44°C
K. pneumoniae subsp. *pneumoniae*	0	0	+	+	+	0	+
K. pneumoniae subsp. *ozaenae*	0	0	0	0	V	NA	NA
K. pneumoniae subsp. *rhinoscleromatis*	0	0	0	+	0	NA	NA
K. oxytoca	+	0	+	+	+	0	+
R. ornithinolytica	+	+	V	+	+	+	NA
R. planticola	V	0	+	+	+	+	0
R. terrigena	0	0	+	+	+	+	0

[a]VP, Voges-Proskauer; ONPG, *o*-nitrophenyl-D-galactopyranoside; +, positive reaction (≥90% positive); V, variable reaction (11 to 89% positive); 0, negative reaction (≤10% positive); NA, not available.

Table 12-2 Key characteristics of *Enterobacter* and *Pantoea* spp.[a]

Species	LDC	ADH	ODC	Malonate	Sorbitol	Yellow pigment
E. aerogenes	+	0	+	+	+	0
E. cloacae subsp. *cloacae*	0	+	+	V	+	0
E. gergoviae	+	0	+	+	0	0
E. sakazakii	0	+	+	0	0	+
E. cancerogenus	0	+	+	+	0	0
E. amnigenus biogroup 1	0	0	V	+	0	0
E. asburiae	0	V	+	0	+	0
E. hormaechei subsp. *hormaechei*	0	V	+	+	0	0
E. intermedius	0	0	V	+	+	0
E. cowanii	0	0	0	NA	+	V
E. kobei	0	+	+	NA	+	0
P. agglomerans	0	0	0	V	V	V

[a]LDC, lysine decarboxylase; ADH, arginine dihydrolase; ODC, ornithine decarboxylase; +, positive reaction (≥90% positive); V, variable reaction (11 to 89% positive); 0, negative reaction (≤10% positive); NA, not available.

Table 12-3 Differentiating characteristics of *Serratia* spp. isolated from clinical specimens[a]

Species	Indole	LDC	ODC	Malonate	Sorbitol	Arabinose	Red pigment
S. ficara	0	0	0	0	+	+	0
S. fonticola	0	+	+	+	+	+	0
S. liquefaciens group	0	+	+	0	+	+	0
S. marcescens subsp. *marcescens*	0	+	+	0	+	0	V
S. marcescens biogroup 1	0	V	V	0	+	0	0
S. odorifera biogroup 1	V	+	+	0	+	+	0
S. odorifera biogroup 2	V	+	0	0	+	+	0
S. plymuthica	0	0	0	0	V	+	+
S. rubidaea	0	V	0	+	0	+	+

[a]LDC, lysine decarboxylase; ODC, ornithine decarboxylase; +, positive reaction (≥90% positive); V, variable reaction (11 to 89% positive); 0, negative reaction (≤10% positive).

Table 12-4 Key characteristics of *Citrobacter* spp.[a]

Species	Indole	Citrate	H_2S on TSI	LDC	ODC	Malonate
C. amalonaticus	+	+	0	0	+	0
C. braakii	0	V	V	0	+	0
C. farmeri	+	0	0	0	+	0
C. freundii sensu stricto	V	V	V	0	0	0
C. gillenii	0	V	V	0	0	+
C. koseri (diversus)	+	+	0	0	+	+
C. murliniae	+	+	V	0	0	0
C. sedlakii	V	V	0	0	+	+
C. werkmanii	0	+	+	0	0	+
C. youngae	V	V	V	0	0	0

[a]LDC, lysine decarboxylase; ODC, ornithine decarboxylase; +, positive reaction (≥90% positive); V, variable reaction (11 to 89% positive); 0, negative reaction (≤10% positive).

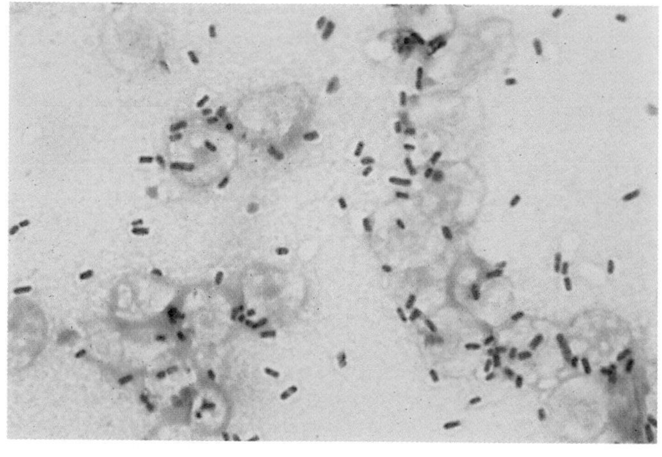

Figure 12-1 Gram stain of a sputum specimen with *Klebsiella*. This Gram stain from a sputum specimen containing *Klebsiella* demonstrates gram-negative bacilli with bipolar staining, approximately 6 μm long and up to 1 μm wide. These bacilli are longer than the characteristic *E. coli* cells shown in Fig. 11-1.

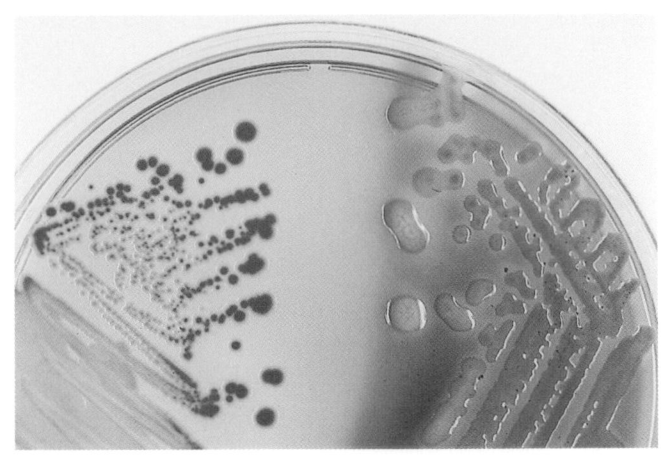

Figure 12-2 *Enterobacter* and *Klebsiella* on MacConkey agar. *Enterobacter* colonies are shown on the left of the MacConkey agar plate, and *Klebsiella* colonies are on the right. *Enterobacter* colonies are smaller (approximately 2 to 3 mm in diameter) than *Klebsiella* colonies (approximately 4 to 5 mm). Two distinguishing characteristics are lactose fermentation on the medium and the viscosity of the colonies. *Enterobacter* spp. are often late lactose fermenters, and thus the colonies can appear colorless to light pink, as shown here, whereas *Klebsiella* colonies are darker pink. Encapsulated strains of *Klebsiella* are also mucoid in appearance, a characteristic of some strains of this genus.

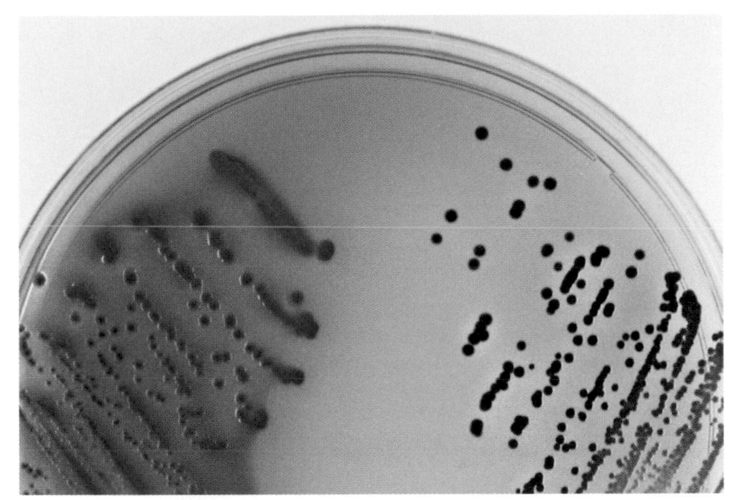

Figure 12-3 *Serratia marcescens* and *Citrobacter freundii* on MacConkey agar. Colonies of *S. marcescens* are shown on the right of this MacConkey agar plate, and *C. freundii* colonies are on the left. Comparing the two colony types, the *Serratia* colonies appear red whereas the *Citrobacter* colonies are dark pink. The red color of the *Serratia* colonies is due to the pigment prodigiosin. *Citrobacter* closely resembles *E. coli* (Fig. 11-2) in colony morphology (both size and color).

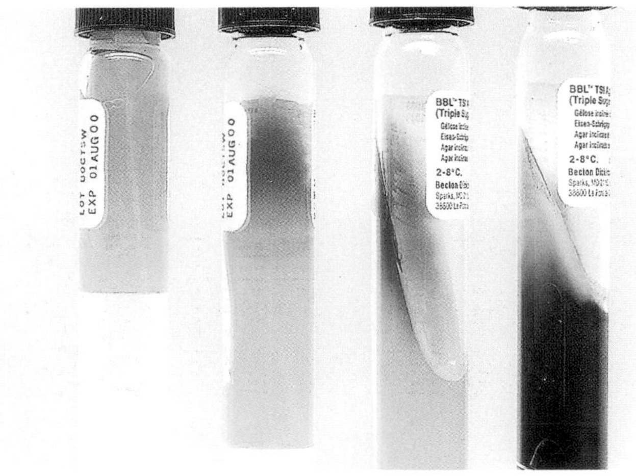

Figure 12-4 *Klebsiella*, *Enterobacter*, *Serratia*, and *Citrobacter* on a TSI agar slant. Shown from left to right are the TSI reactions of *Klebsiella*, *Enterobacter*, *Serratia*, and *Citrobacter*. Large amounts of gas are produced by both *Klebsiella* and *Enterobacter*, causing the agar medium to be lifted from the bottom of the tubes. *Serratia* can be a slow lactose fermenter, resulting in an alkaline reaction in the slant, as seen in the figure. Some species of *Citrobacter* produce H_2S, which can easily be detected in the TSI slant.

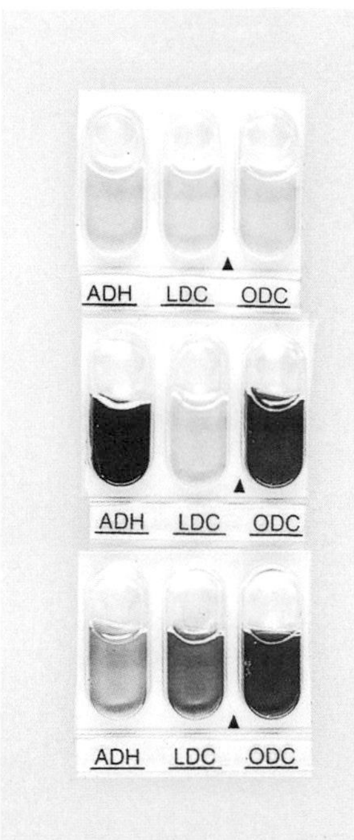

Figure 12-5 Arginine, lysine, and ornithine decarboxylase reactions of *Enterobacter*. Shown here are three sets of reactions for arginine dihydrolase (ADH), lysine decarboxylase (LDC), and ornithine decarboxylase (ODC). The top three reactions are negative, suggestive of *P. agglomerans*. In the center set, both ADH and ODC are positive and LDC is negative. These are characteristic reactions for *E. cloacae* and *E. sakazakii*. In the bottom set, both LDC and ODC are positive, suggesting either *E. aerogenes* or *Enterobacter gergoviae*.

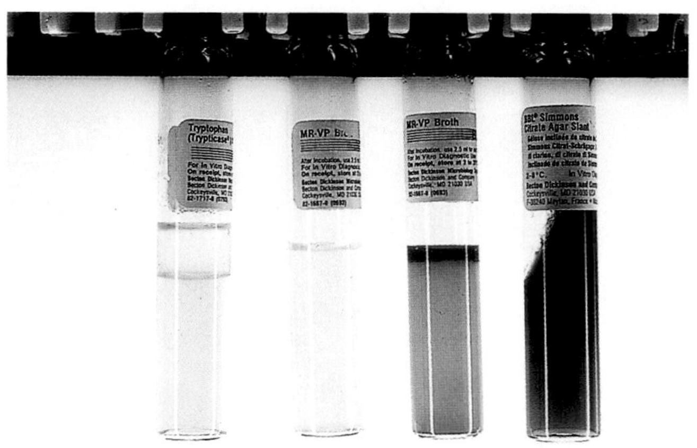

Figure 12-6 IMViC reactions of *Klebsiella*, *Enterobacter*, and *Serratia*. *Klebsiella*, *Enterobacter*, and *Serratia* have similar IMViC reactions; the indole and methyl red reactions (the two tubes on the left) are negative, and the Voges-Proskauer and citrate reactions (the two tubes on the right) are positive, as shown in the figure.

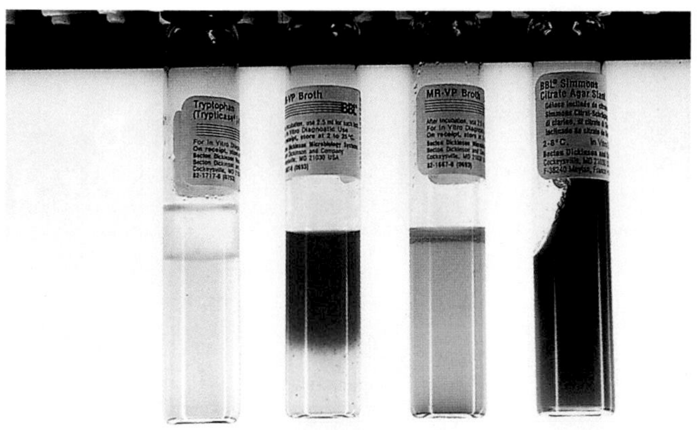

Figure 12-7 IMViC reactions of *Citrobacter*. The IMViC reactions of *Citrobacter* differ from those of *Klebsiella*, *Enterobacter*, and *Serratia* (Fig. 12-6). As shown here, the indole and Voges-Proskauer reactions (tubes 1 and 3 from the left) are negative and the methyl red and citrate reactions (tubes 2 and 4 from the left) are positive, characteristic findings of *Citrobacter*.

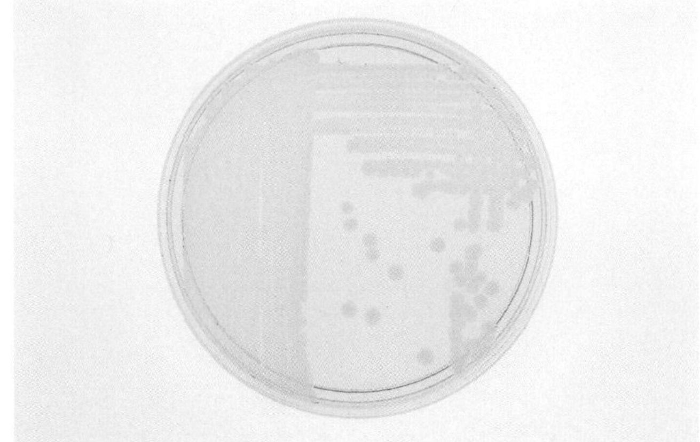

Figure 12-8 Colonies of *Enterobacter sakazakii* grown on nutrient agar. *E. sakazakii* is easily distinguished from most other *Enterobacter* spp. by its characteristic bright yellow pigment, as shown here.

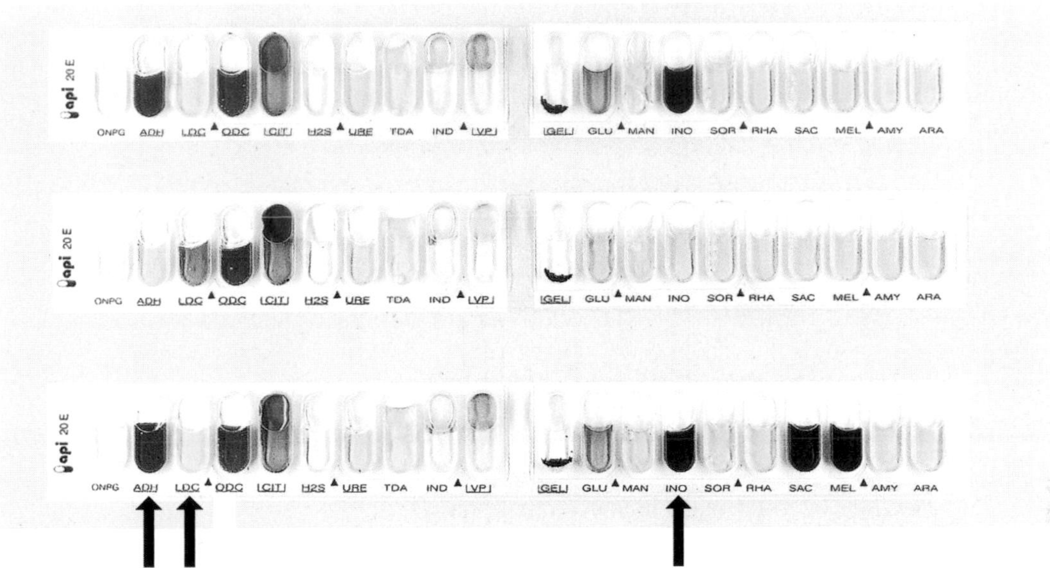

Figure 12-9 *Enterobacter aerogenes*, *Enterobacter cloacae*, and *Enterobacter cancerogenus* (formerly *Enterobacter taylorae*) in the API 20E system. The API 20E strips (bioMérieux, Inc., Durham, NC) were inoculated with *E. cloacae* (top strip), *E. aerogenes* (middle strip), and *E. cancerogenus* (bottom strip). *E. aerogenes* and *E. cloacae* are the most common *Enterobacter* spp. isolated in the diagnostic laboratory. Although the reactions of these two species are similar, the distinguishing biochemicals, indicated by the arrows, are arginine dihydrolase (ADH), lysine decarboxylase (LDC), and inositol (INO). *E. cloacae* (top) is ADH positive, LDC negative, and INO negative, whereas *E. aerogenes* (middle) is ADH negative, LDC positive, and INO positive, as shown in this figure. *E. cloacae* and *E. cancerogenus* are also very similar, with the exception of the sucrose (SAC) and melibiose (MEL) reactions, both of which are positive for *E. cloacae* and negative for *E. cancerogenus*.

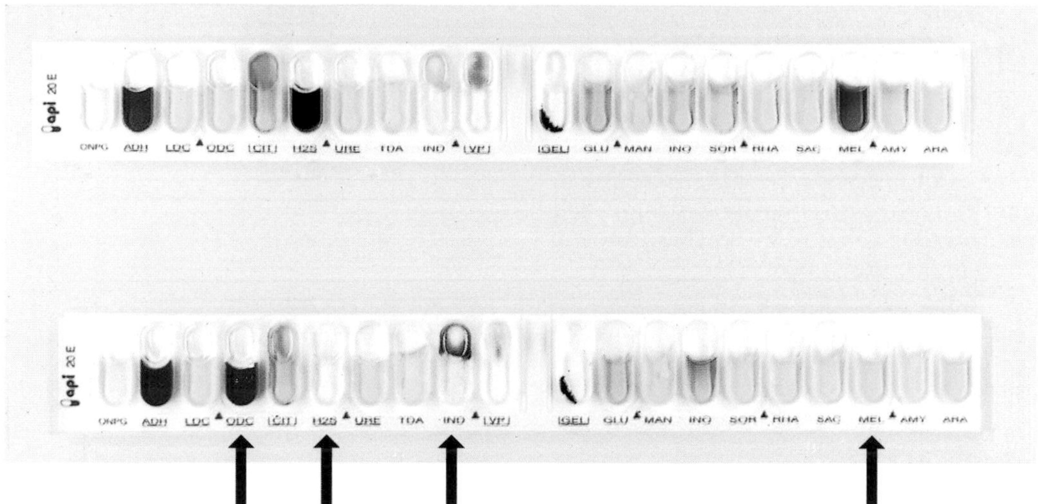

Figure 12-10 ***Citrobacter freundii*** **and** ***Citrobacter amalonaticus*** **in the API 20E system.** *C. freundii* was inoculated in the top strip and *C. amalonaticus* was inoculated in the bottom strip. The differences between the two species, indicated by the arrows, are the reactions for ornithine decarboxylase (ODC), H_2S, indole (IND), and melibiose (MEL). *C. freundii* produces H_2S and is negative for the other three tests, whereas *C. amalonaticus* is negative for H_2S and positive for the other three.

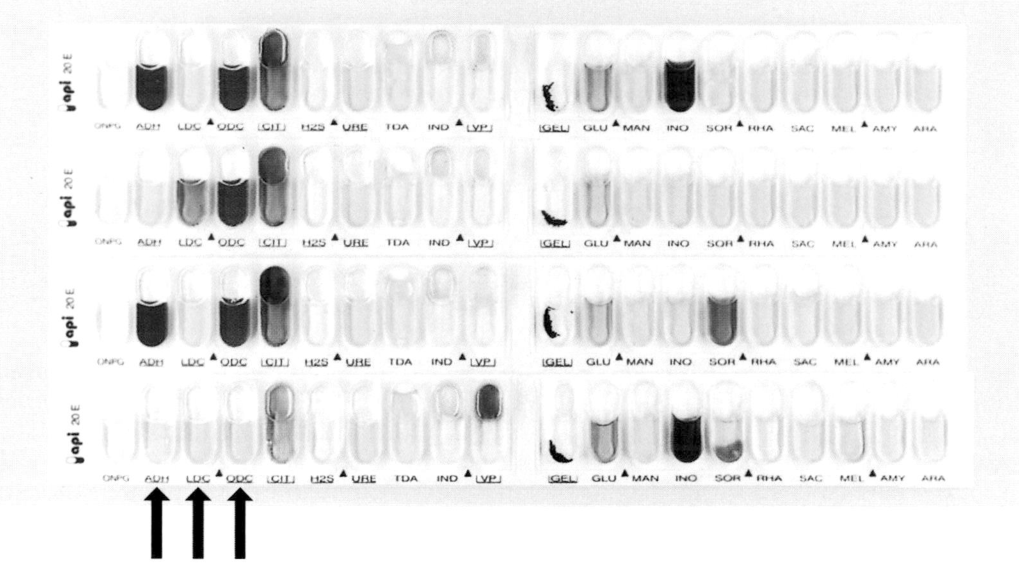

Figure 12-11 ***Enterobacter cloacae*****,** ***Enterobacter aerogenes*****,** ***Enterobacter sakazakii*****, and** ***Pantoea agglomerans*** **in the API 20E system.** From top to bottom, the organisms are *E. cloacae*, *E. aerogenes*, *E. sakazakii*, and *P. agglomerans*. The major differentiating reactions among these four organisms, indicated by the arrows, are arginine dihydrolase (ADH), lysine decarboxylase (LDC), and ornithine decarboxylase (ODC). These reactions are listed in Table 12-2.

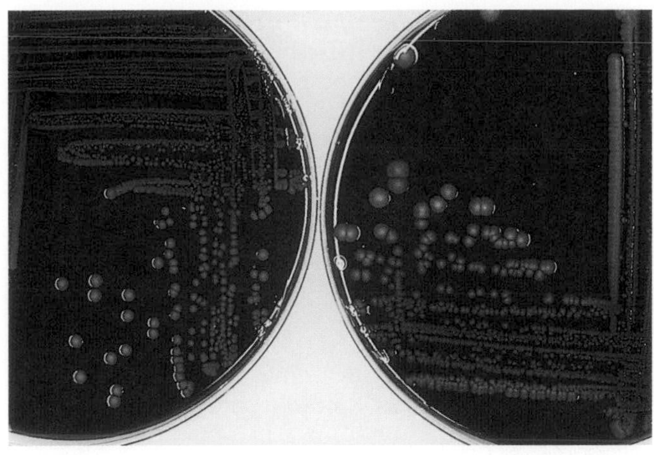

Figure 12-12 Colonies of *Enterobacter sakazakii* and *Enterobacter cloacae* on blood agar. Yellow colonies produced by *E. sakazakii* are shown on the blood agar plate on the left, in comparison to the gray colonies of *E. cloacae* on the right.

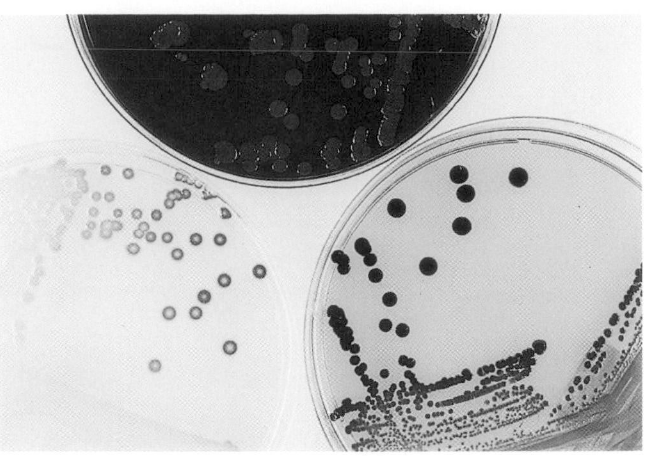

Figure 12-13 Colonies of *Serratia rubidaea* on blood, MacConkey, and nutrient agars. The red pigment produced by *S. rubidaea* is easily detected when the organism is grown on nutrient agar (bottom right) or Mueller-Hinton agar, in contrast to growth on blood agar (top) and MacConkey agar (bottom left).

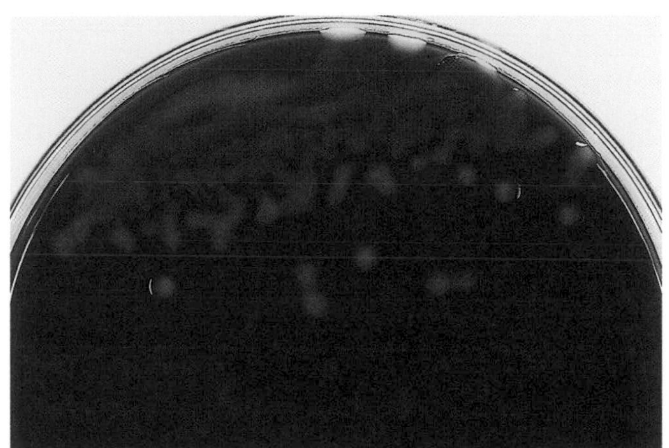

Figure 12-14 Colonies of *Klebsiella ozaenae* on blood agar. Colonies of *K. ozaenae* on blood agar after a 24-h incubation at 35°C are 2 to 4 mm in diameter, gray, and mucoid. The organism contains a large polysaccharide capsule, which gives rise to mucoid colonies. *K. ozaenae* is a subspecies of *K. pneumoniae*, but most laboratories still treat and report it as a separate species.

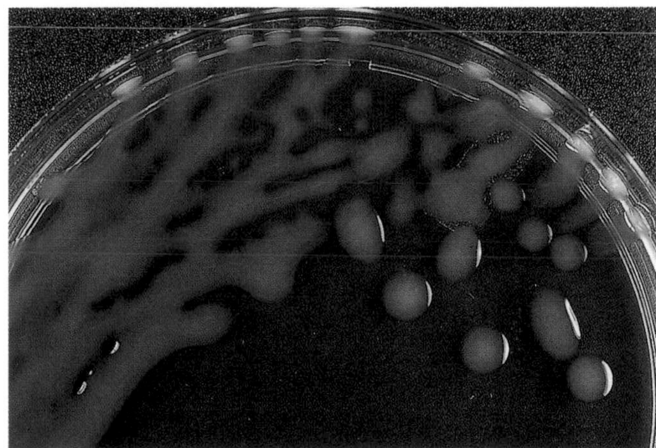

Figure 12-15 Colonies of *Klebsiella ozaenae* on MacConkey agar. Colonies of *K. ozaenae* on MacConkey agar after a 48-h incubation at 35°C are 5 to 6 mm in diameter, pink, and mucoid, as shown here.

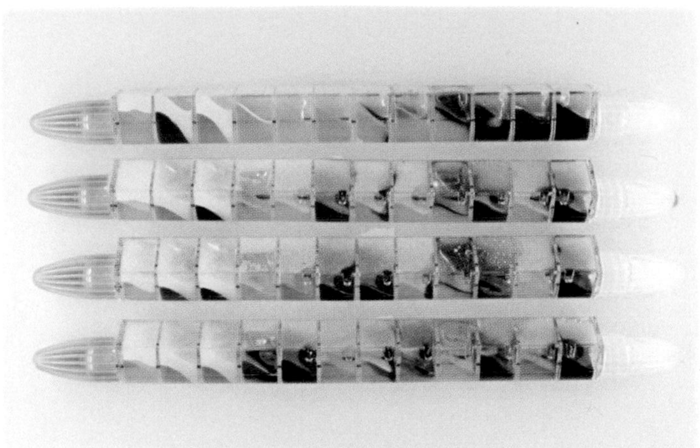

Figure 12-16 *Klebsiella*, *Enterobacter*, *Serratia*, and *Citrobacter* identified by the Enterotube II Identification System. The Enterotube II System (BD Diagnostic Systems, Franklin Lakes, NJ) is described in Fig. 10-18. The organisms in this figure, from top to bottom, are *Klebsiella*, *Enterobacter*, *Serratia*, and *Citrobacter*. As shown, the reactions for lysine decarboxylase (LDC), ornithine decarboxylase (ODC), H_2S, adonitol (ADON), lactose (LAC), arabinose (ARAB), Voges-Proskauer (VP), and urease (URE) will help to differentiate the four genera, whereas the reactions for glucose (GLU), indole (IND), sorbitol (SOR), dulcitol (DUL), phenylalanine deaminase (PAD), and citrate (CIT) are the same, as indicated below.

Organism	GLU	Gas	LDC	ODC	H_2S	IND	ADON	LAC	ARAB	SOR	VP	DUL	PAD	URE	CIT
Klebsiella	+	+	+	0	0	0	+	+	+	+	+	0	0	+	+
Enterobacter	+	+	0	+	0	0	0	0	+	+	+	0	0	0	+
Serratia	+	0	+	+	0	0	0	+	0	+	+	0	0	0	+
Citrobacter	+	+	0	0	+	0	0	+	+	+	0	0	0	0	+

Yersinia, the *Proteeae*, *Edwardsiella*, and *Hafnia*

13

The genus *Yersinia* includes three pathogenic species: *Yersinia pestis*, *Yersinia enterocolitica*, and *Yersinia pseudotuberculosis*. Other members of the *Enterobacteriaceae* that have been isolated from clinical specimens, and are discussed in this chapter, include *Proteus*, *Providencia*, and *Morganella* (members of the tribe *Proteeae*); *Edwardsiella tarda*; and *Hafnia alvei*.

Y. pestis is known as the plague bacillus; its natural reservoir is rodents, and it is transmitted to humans by rodent fleas. In recent years, outbreaks have occurred in Africa, South America, and India. The organism can be isolated from blood, bubo aspirates, respiratory secretions, and cerebrospinal fluid.

Y. enterocolitica and *Y. pseudotuberculosis* are distributed worldwide, and infections due to these organisms are usually acquired by ingestion of contaminated food or water. *Y. enterocolitica* can cause enterocolitis in humans and may mimic acute appendicitis because it can result in mesenteric lymphadenitis, which is associated with severe abdominal pain. This organism is found in the gastrointestinal tracts of many animal species, mostly dogs, rodents, and swine. Its growth is enhanced by cold temperatures, and therefore it is likely to be found in temperate and subtropical regions. The species is divided into six biogroups that can be differentiated biochemically: 1A, 1B, 2, 3, 4, and 5. Biotype 1B appears to be the most pathogenic. The production of urease allows *Y. enterocolitica* to survive in the stomach and colonize the small intestine. It can multiply at 4°C; therefore, blood contaminated from an asymptomatic donor can transmit infection through a transfusion. *Y. pseudotuberculosis* is primarily a pathogen of rodents, rabbits, and wild birds and rarely causes infections in humans. Other *Yersinia* spp. have been isolated from clinical specimens, but their pathogenicity has not been established. If they are isolated from fecal specimens, they should be reported as nonpathogenic yersiniae. The biochemical differentiation of the pathogenic *Yersinia* spp. is shown in Table 13-1.

Yersinia spp. are small, gram-negative bacilli, approximately 0.5 to 0.8 μm wide and 1 to 3 μm long. All species except *Y. pestis* are motile. They grow both aerobically and anaerobically at temperatures ranging between 4 and 40°C, with optimal growth at 25 to 28°C; growth at ≥35°C is not consistent. Growth above 28°C may be delayed (>24 h), or inconsistent biochemical reactions may occur. However, commercial identification systems are based on results obtained at 35°C. Preferred media include blood agar, as well as MacConkey agar and cefsulodin-irgasan-novobiocin (CIN) agar, which is the recommended medium if *Yersinia* is suspected. On CIN agar, colonies of *Y. enterocolitica* are approximately 2 mm in diameter and usually have red centers surrounded by a translucent zone. *Aeromonas* spp. can have a similar appearance; however, they are oxidase positive. *Yersinia* spp. ferment glucose, reduce nitrate to nitrite, and are catalase positive. All species except *Y. pestis* are also urea positive at 25 to 28°C; however, the reaction may be negative at 35°C. Ornithine is decarboxylated by most *Yersinia* spp.; the exceptions are *Y. pestis* and *Y. pseudotuberculosis*. For identification, the API 20E system (bioMérieux, Inc., Durham, NC) seems to have the greatest sensitivity and specificity for *Y. enterocolitica* and *Y. pseudotuberculosis*.

Table 13-1 Biochemical reactions of *Yersinia* spp. after incubation at 35°C[a]

Species	Indole	Motility at 25°C	Urea	Ornithine	Sucrose	Rhamnose	Melibiose
Y. pestis	0	0	0	0	0	0	V
Y. enterocolitica	V	+	+	+	+	0	0
Y. pseudotuberculosis	0	+	+	0	0	+	+

[a]+, positive reaction (≥90% positive); V, variable reaction (11 to 89% positive); −, negative reaction (≤10% positive).

Y. pestis is best seen when stained with Giemsa, Wright's, Wayson, or methylene blue stain rather than the Gram stain. The organisms are small (1 to 2 μm by 0.5 μm), gram-negative bacilli and may appear bipolar, resembling safety pins, when isolated from clinical material; however, this bipolar morphology is not seen in Gram stains or from colonies growing on culture media. On solid media, *Y. pestis* appears as pinpoint colonies after a 24-h incubation at 35°C. Colonies are usually nonhemolytic on blood agar and mucoid on brain heart infusion agar and look like fried eggs after prolonged incubation. In a broth medium, organisms tend to clump along the side of the tube and then fall to the bottom after a 24-h incubation. The metabolic activity of this organism is best demonstrated at 13 to 25°C. Prolonged incubation (2 to 5 days) may be necessary to determine the biochemical reactions. Automated systems may misidentify *Y. pestis* as *Y. pseudotuberculosis* or as *Salmonella*, *Shigella*, or *Acinetobacter*. It is recommended that suspicious isolates of *Y. pestis* be sent to a reference laboratory, especially if the identification does not agree with the clinical picture.

Proteus, *Providencia*, and *Morganella* are normally found in the human gastrointestinal tract and can cause urinary tract infections, although they have been isolated from other specimen types. Of the *Proteeae* isolated from clinical specimens, there are four species of *Proteus* (*Proteus mirabilis*, *Proteus vulgaris*, *Proteus penneri*, and *Proteus hauseri*), five species of *Providencia* (*Providencia rettgeri*, *Providencia stuartii*, *Providencia alcalifaciens*, *Providencia rustigianii*, and *Providencia heimbachae*), and one species that includes two subspecies of *Morganella* (*Morganella morganii* subsp. *morganii* and *M. morganii* subsp. *sibonii*). A majority of *Proteeae* infections appear to be community acquired, although *Providencia* spp. usually cause nosocomial infections. *P. mirabilis* is a common cause of urinary tract infections, whereas *P. vulgaris* is isolated more often from wounds than from urine.

The *Proteeae* grow well on routine laboratory media. Characteristic reactions of the *Proteeae* are shown in Table 13-2. All species are lactose negative. *P. mirabilis* and *P. vulgaris* are easily recognized by their swarming growth on blood or chocolate agar media and their distinct odor, often resembling chocolate cake. They can be differentiated by an indole spot test and ampicillin susceptibility. *P. mirabilis* is indole negative and ampicillin susceptible, and *P. vulgaris* is indole positive and ampicillin resistant. All *Proteeae* produce phenylalanine deaminase. *Proteus*, *Morganella*, and *P. rettgeri* produce urease. Commercially available systems accurately identify *Proteus*; however, *Providencia* can be misidentified.

Table 13-2 Biochemical differentiation between members of the *Proteeae*[a]

Species	Indole	H_2S	Urea	Ornithine	Maltose	Trehalose	Inositol
Proteus							
P. hauseri	+	V	+	0	+	0	0
P. mirabilis	0	+	+	+	0	+	0
P. penneri	0	V	+	0	0	V	0
P. vulgaris	+	+	+	0	+	V	0
Providencia							
P. alcalifaciens	+	0	0	0	+	0	0
P. heimbachae	0	0	0	0	V	0	V
P. rettgeri	+	0	+	0	0	0	+
P. rustigianii	+	0	0	0	0	0	0
P. stuartii	+	0	V	0	0	+	+
Morganella morganii	+	0	+	+	0	0	0

[a]+, positive reaction (≥90% positive); V, variable reaction (11 to 89% positive); −, negative reaction (≤10% positive).

Also, rapid 2-h identification systems can misidentify *M. morganii* subsp. *morganii.*

There are three species of *Edwardsiella*, but *E. tarda* is the only one associated with human disease. The organism, an infrequent cause of gastroenteritis and infections, has been linked to contact with fish and turtles. Serious wound infections have been reported in immunocompetent individuals with aquatic exposure, whereas patients with liver disease may acquire serious systemic infections. *E. tarda* resembles *Salmonella* on many media, including MacConkey agar, xylose lysine desoxycholate agar (XLD), and triple sugar iron (TSI) agar slant, but is indole positive and citrate negative.

The genus *Hafnia* has a single species, *H. alvei*, which is found in the intestinal tracts of humans and is responsible for a wide variety of opportunistic infections. It may also produce abscesses in the biliary tree. Like other members of the family *Enterobacteriaceae*, *H. alvei* grows well on routine laboratory media. It produces lysine and ornithine decarboxylases. Like the *Enterobacter* spp., it is positive for the Voges-Proskauer test and for citrate at 22°C, but it is not consistently positive at 35°C.

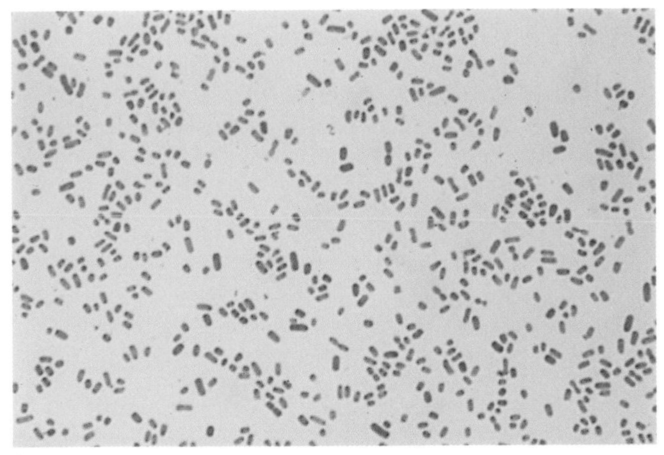

A

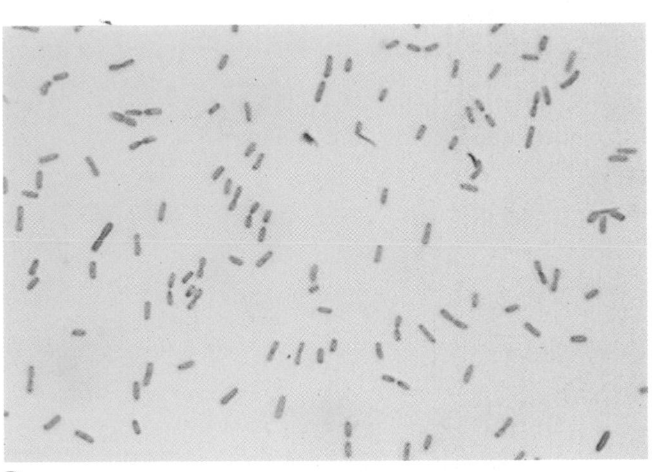

B

Figure 13-1 Gram stain of *Yersinia enterocolitica* and *Yersinia pestis.* (A) *Yersinia* spp. are small, plump, gram-negative bacilli, measuring approximately 0.8 μm in width and 2 μm in length. These cells appear coccoid with bipolar staining. (B) *Y. pestis* is coccoid or rod shaped. The appearance of *Yersinia* spp. in the Gram stain is similar to other members of the family *Enterobacteriaceae.*

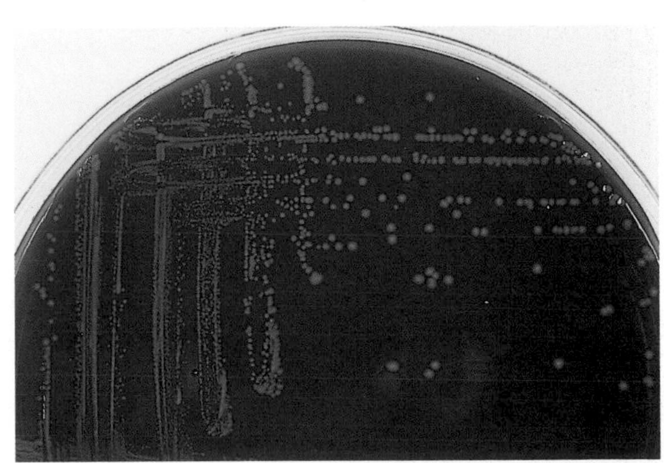

Figure 13-2 *Yersinia enterocolitica* on blood agar. Colonies of *Y. enterocolitica* are small and gray to grayish white, measuring 1 to 2 mm in diameter after overnight incubation at 35°C under 5% CO_2.

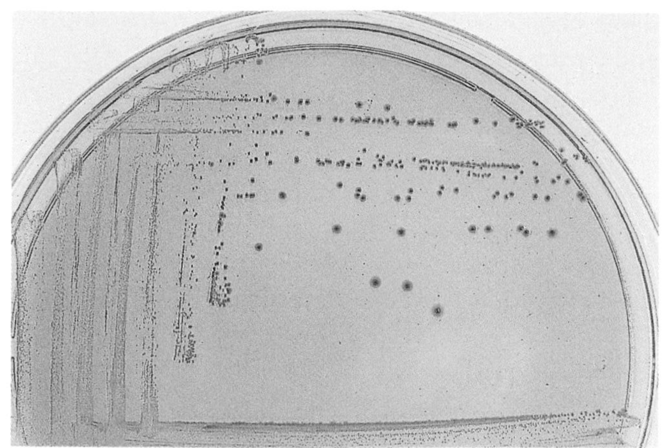

Figure 13-3 *Yersinia enterocolitica* on MacConkey agar. *Y. enterocolitica* is a lactose nonfermenter; therefore, colonies appear colorless or transparent on MacConkey agar. Colonies are small compared to other members of the *Enterobacteriaceae*, ranging in size from 1 to 3 mm after overnight incubation at 35°C. Incubation at 25°C for 48 h enhances their growth.

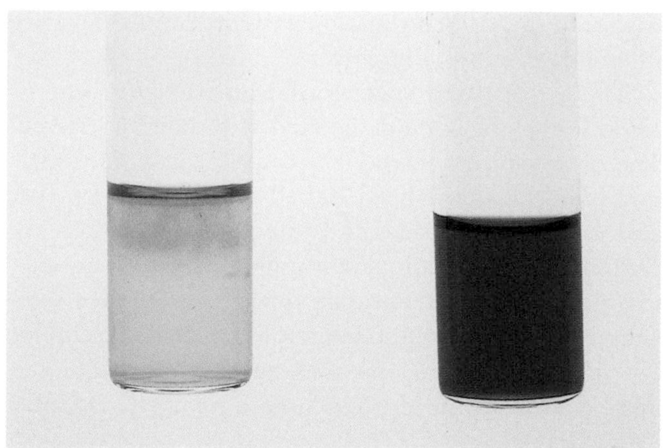

Figure 13-4 *Yersinia enterocolitica* in methyl red and Voges-Proskauer broth. The methyl red reaction is positive, as shown by the presence of a red color (right tube), and the Voges-Proskauer reaction is negative (left tube). These reactions alone do not differentiate *Yersinia* spp. from other members of the *Enterobacteriaceae*. For example, *Y. enterocolitica* can be confused with *Shigella* spp., and therefore it is important to do further biochemical tests, as shown in Fig. 13-5 and 13-6.

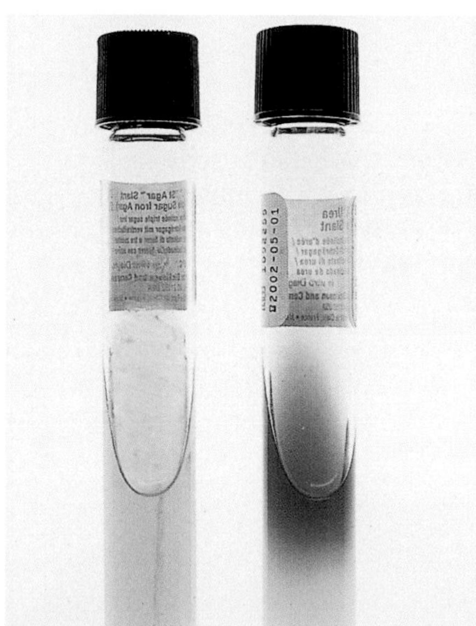

Figure 13-5 *Yersinia enterocolitica* on TSI and urea agar slants. *Y. enterocolitica* ferments glucose and sucrose; therefore, the expected TSI reaction is an acid slant and an acid butt with no gas production. Urea is hydrolyzed by *Y. enterocolitica*, as shown by the tube on the right. Optimal reactions for *Y. enterocolitica* occur at 25°C, rather than at 35°C as for other members of the *Enterobacteriaceae*. Therefore, if *Yersinia* spp. are suspected but the biochemical reactions are questionable, the tests should be repeated with incubation at 25°C for 48 h.

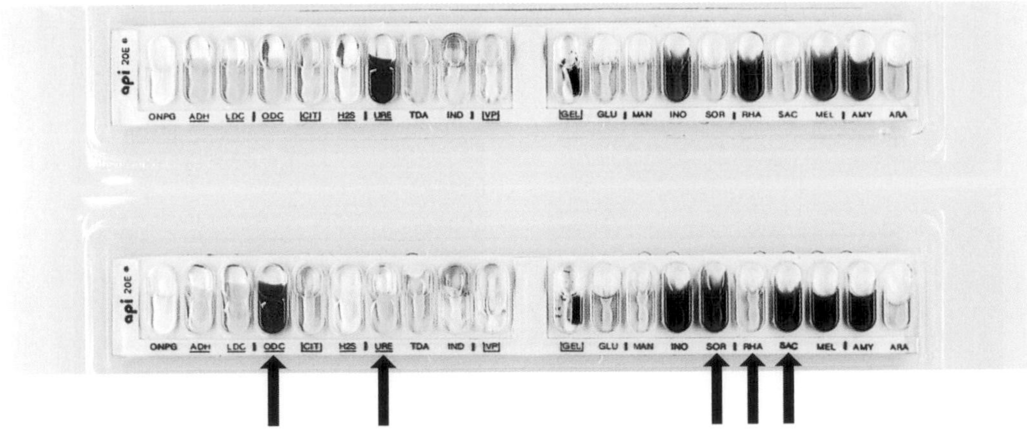

Figure 13-6 *Yersinia enterocolitica* and *Shigella sonnei* in the API 20E system. Because *Y. enterocolitica* sometimes resembles *Shigella* spp., the following example of the API 20E reactions for both organisms is shown in this figure. *Y. enterocolitica* is shown at the top. The differentiating characteristics in the first 10 reactions, indicated by the arrows in the figure and the table below, are urea (URE) and ornithine decarboxylase (ODC). *Y. enterocolitica* is URE positive and ODC negative, and *S. sonnei* is URE negative and ODC positive. However, *Shigella* A, B, and C are ODC negative. Regarding the carbohydrates, sorbitol (SOR) and sucrose (SAC) are metabolized by *Y. enterocolitica* but not by *Shigella* spp., whereas S. sonnei metabolizes rhamnose (RHA), as indicated by the arrows. The reactions of *Y. enterocolitica* and *S. sonnei* are as follows. It should be noted that a commercial system may give reactions that are different from those on conventional media because the databases of commercial systems are derived from a 4- to 24-h incubation time and an organism's delayed reactions may not be detected. As an example, in this figure *S. sonnei* is o-nitrophenyl-β-D-galactopyranoside (ONPG) negative, but it can have a delayed lactose action and is usually ONPG positive when a conventional method is used.

Organism	ONPG	ADC	LDC	ODC	CIT	H_2S	URE	TDA	IND	VP	GEL	GLU	MAN	INO	SOR	RHA	SAC	MEL	AMY	ARA
Y. enterocolitica	0	0	0	0	0	0	+	0	0	0	0	+	+	0	+	0	+	0	0	+
S. sonnei	0	0	0	+	0	0	0	0	0	0	0	+	+	0	0	+	0	0	0	+
				↑			↑								↑	↑	↑			

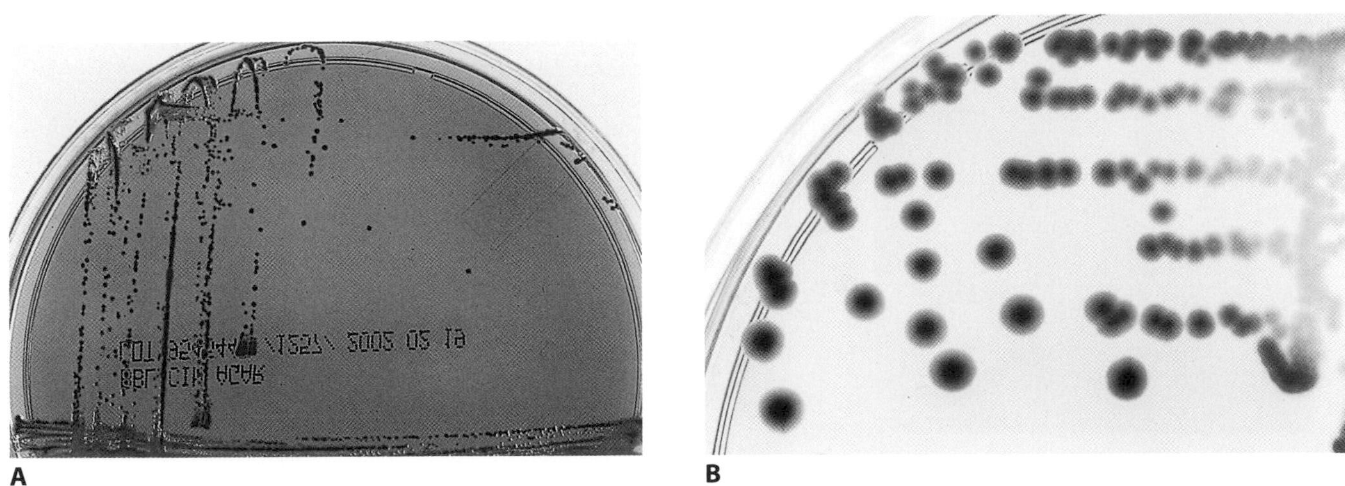

A B

Figure 13-7 *Yersinia enterocolitica* on CIN agar incubated at 25°C for 24 and 48 h. CIN agar is an excellent medium for the isolation of *Y. enterocolitica*, especially from fecal specimens. For optimal growth, the specimen should be inoculated onto the medium and incubated at 25°C for 48 h. Colonies of *Y. enterocolitica* appear bright pink with a red center surrounded by a translucent zone, giving the typical appearance of a bull's-eye. Very few other organisms grow on this medium, the exception being *Aeromonas* spp. (A) Colonies incubated for 24 h at 25°C. They measure approximately 1 mm in diameter. (B) Colonies incubated for 48 h at 25°C. These colonies measure approximately 3 to 4 mm in diameter.

Figure 13-8 *Yersinia pestis* on blood agar. Colonies of *Y. pestis* on blood agar are pinpoint at 24 h, as shown here. On prolonged incubation, they can exhibit a rough, cauliflower-like appearance. When grown in a broth medium, the colonies form clumps of cells that adhere to one side of the tube, resembling a stalactite pattern or hammered copper.

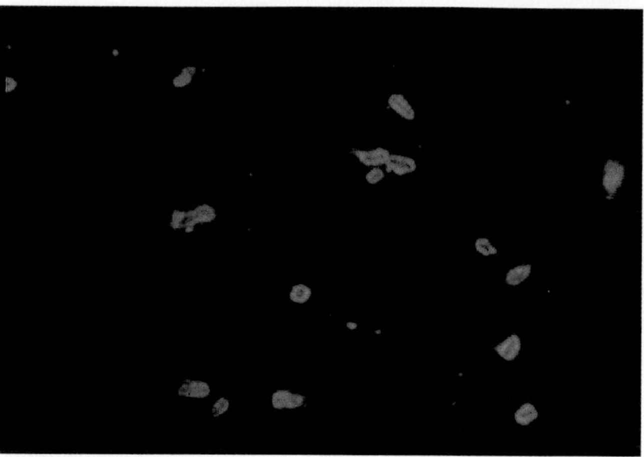

Figure 13-9 Direct fluorescent-antibody stain of *Yersinia pestis*. Direct microscopic detection of the *Y. pestis* capsular F1 antigen is performed using a fluorescent-antibody stain, as shown here. A positive immunofluorescence stain is a presumptive diagnosis of the plague bacillus.

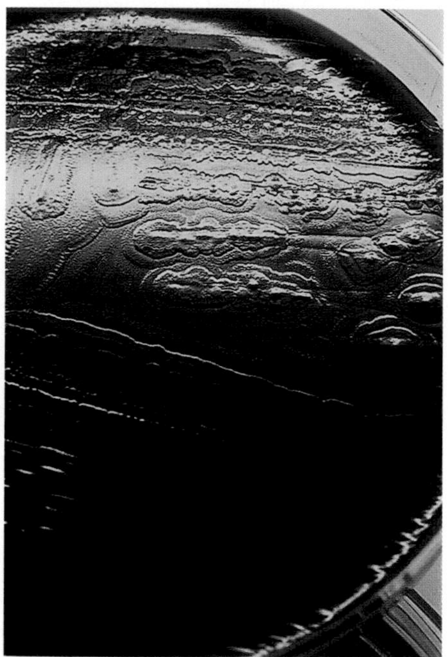

Figure 13-10 *Proteus mirabilis* on blood agar. As a result of motility, *Proteus* spp. swarm on blood and chocolate agars. Swarming results in the production of a thin film of growth on the agar surface. The organism was inoculated across the center of the blood agar, causing the growth to occur in waves, spreading across the entire plate. Colonies can produce a chocolate cake-like odor.

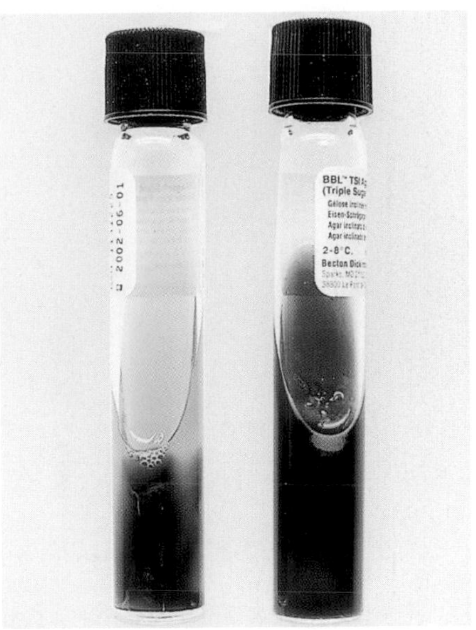

Figure 13-11 *Proteus vulgaris* and *Proteus mirabilis* on a TSI agar slant. The TSI agar slant on the left, acid/acid and H_2S positive, is the expected reaction for *P. vulgaris*, and the alkaline/acid and H_2S positive (right) is the expected reaction for *P. mirabilis*. *P. vulgaris* ferments glucose and sucrose, resulting in an acid slant and acid butt because TSI agar contains both carbohydrates. However, *P. mirabilis* ferments glucose but not sucrose, resulting in an alkaline slant and an acid butt. TSI alone cannot be used to identify these two species or any of the *Enterobacteriaceae*, since many of these organisms have the same reactions as those in this figure. For example, some *Citrobacter* spp. have the same TSI reactions as *P. vulgaris*. Also, the TSI reactions for *P. mirabilis*, *Salmonella* spp., and *E. tarda* are the same. Refer to Fig. 10-20 for a complete description of TSI agar slant.

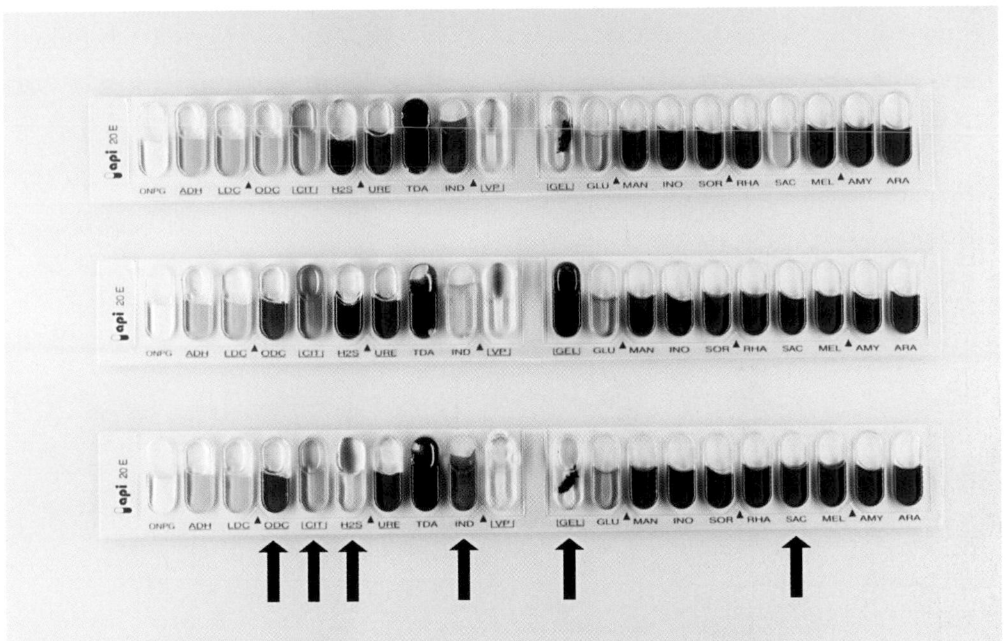

Figure 13-12 *Proteus vulgaris, Proteus mirabilis,* and *Morganella morganii* in the API 20E system. *Proteus* spp. and *M. morganii* are closely related and have many similar biochemical reactions. The similarities and differences of *P. vulgaris*, *P. mirabilis*, and *M. morganii* are shown in this figure. All three species are urea (URE) and tryptophan deaminase (TDA) positive, characteristic reactions of these organisms. *M. morganii* is H_2S negative, while the *Proteus* spp. are positive. *P. mirabilis* is citrate (CIT) positive and indole (IND) negative, differentiating it from the other two species. The differentiating reactions are indicated by the arrows. The reactions of *P. vulgaris*, *P. mirabilis*, and *M. morganii* are as follows.

Organism	ONPG	ADC	LDC	ODC	CIT	H_2S	URE	TDA	IND	VP	GEL	GLU	MAN	INO	SOR	RHA	SAC	MEL	AMY	ARA
P. vulgaris	0	0	0	0	0	+	+	+	+	0	+	+	0	0	0	0	+	0	0	0
P. mirabilis	0	0	0	+	+	+	+	+	0	0	0	+	0	0	0	0	0	0	0	0
M. morganii subsp. *morganii*	0	0	0	+	0	0	+	+	+	0	0	+	0	0	0	0	0	0	0	0
				↑	↑	↑			↑		↑						↑			

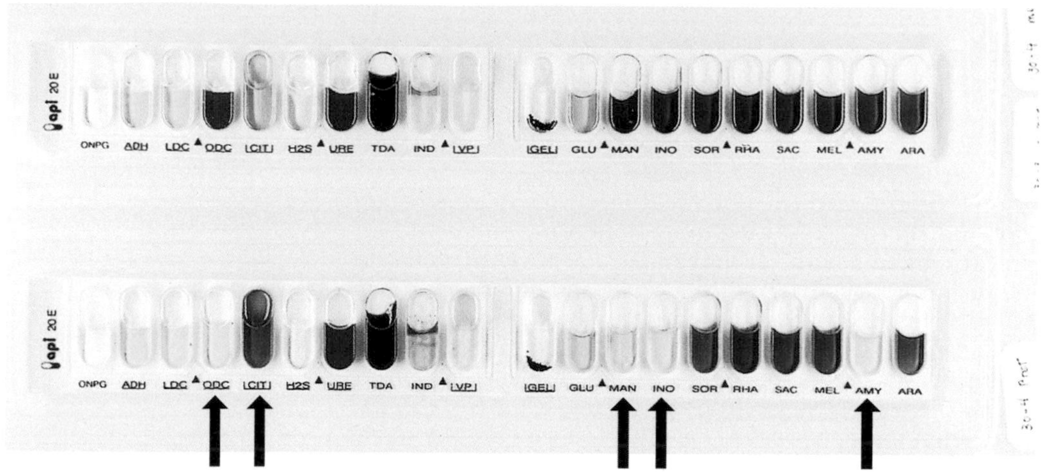

Figure 13-13 ***Morganella morganii*** **and** ***Providencia rettgeri*** **in the API 20E system.** *M. morganii* and *P. rettgeri* are urea (URE) and tryptophan deaminase (TDA) positive and H_2S negative. They also have similar TSI reactions. By observing the reactions in this figure, one can easily see that the ornithine (ODC), citrate (CIT), mannitol (MAN), inositol (INO), and amygdalin (AMY) reactions, indicated by the arrows in the figure and the table below, readily distinguish the two species. The reactions of *M. morganii* and *P. rettgeri* are as follows.

Organism	ONPG	ADC	LDC	ODC	CIT	H_2S	URE	TDA	IND	VP	GEL	GLU	MAN	INO	SOR	RHA	SAC	MEL	AMY	ARA
M. morganii subsp. *morganii*	0	0	0	+	0	0	+	+	+	0	0	+	0	0	0	0	0	0	0	0
P. rettgeri	0	0	0	0	+	0	+	+	+	0	0	+	+	+	0	0	0	0	+	0
				↑	↑										↑	↑			↑	

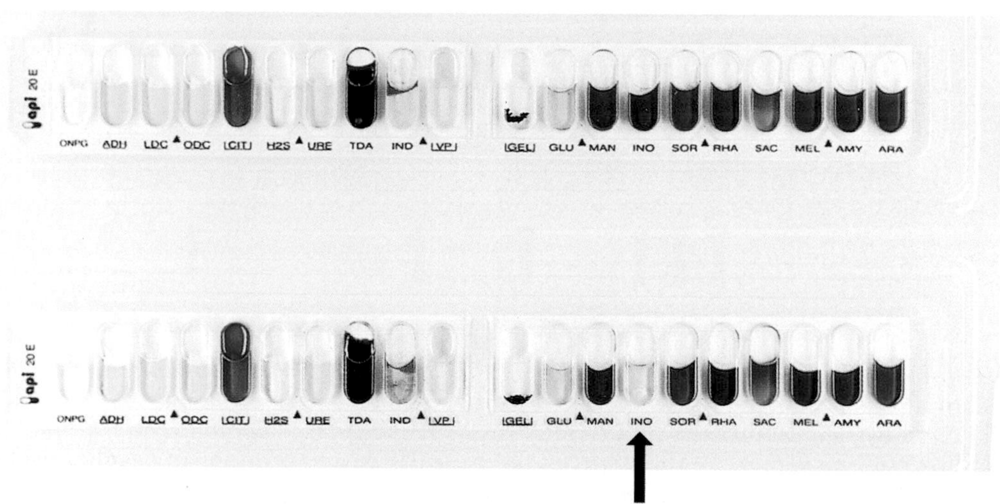

Figure 13-14 ***Providencia alcalifaciens*** **and** ***Providencia stuartii*** **in the API 20E system.** This figure shows the API 20E reactions of *P. alcalifaciens* and *P. stuartii*. The only difference between these two species is the inositol (INO) reaction indicated by the arrow.

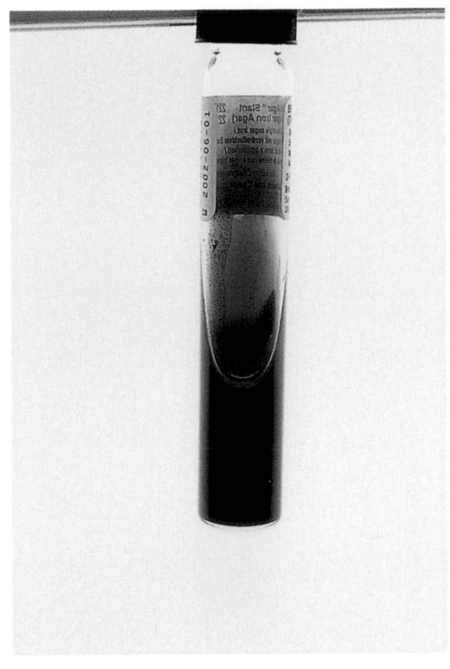

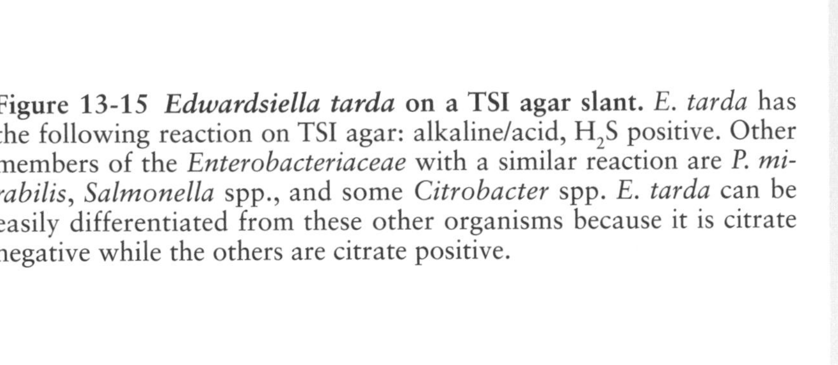

Figure 13-15 ***Edwardsiella tarda*** **on a TSI agar slant.** *E. tarda* has the following reaction on TSI agar: alkaline/acid, H_2S positive. Other members of the *Enterobacteriaceae* with a similar reaction are *P. mirabilis*, *Salmonella* spp., and some *Citrobacter* spp. *E. tarda* can be easily differentiated from these other organisms because it is citrate negative while the others are citrate positive.

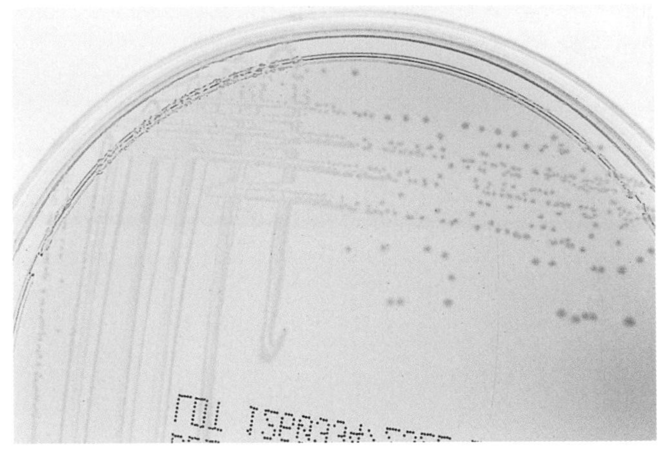

Figure 13-16 ***Hafnia alvei*** **on MacConkey agar.** Colonies of *H. alvei* are small (1 to 3 mm in diameter) and appear colorless on MacConkey agar. This organism was previously classified as an *Enterobacter* sp.; however, it is lactose negative while the *Enterobacter* spp. are all lactose fermenters.

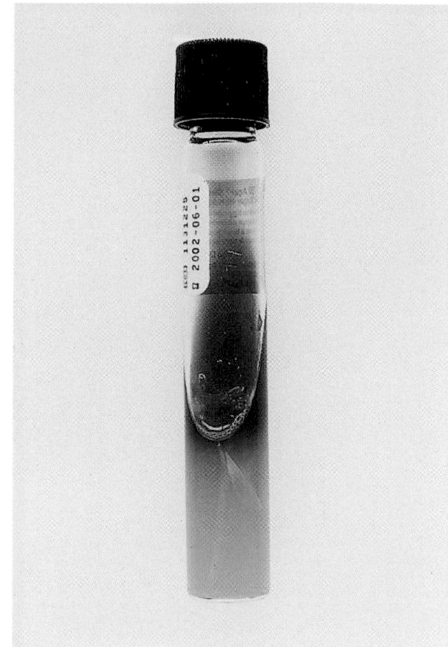

Figure 13-17 ***Hafnia alvei*** **on a TSI agar slant.** *H. alvei* has the following reaction on TSI agar slant: alkaline/acid. This organism was previously classified as an *Enterobacter* sp., and its reactions, including TSI, are very similar to those for organisms within this genus.

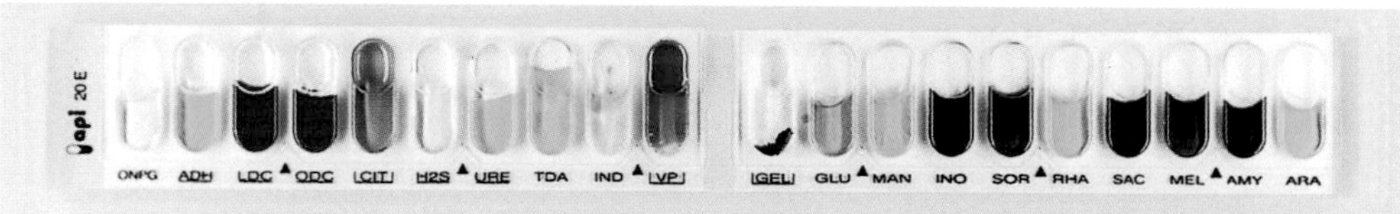

Figure 13-18 ***Hafnia alvei*** **in the API 20E system.** *H. alvei* is o-nitrophenyl-β-D-galactopyranoside (ONPG) and citrate (CIT) negative, while the *Enterobacter* spp. are positive for both reactions. Also, many of the *Enterobacter* spp. are sucrose (SAC) positive, but *H. alvei* is SAC negative.

Vibrionaceae

14

Vibrio spp. are classified in the family *Vibrionaceae* along with five other genera: *Aliivibrio*, *Enterovibrio*, *Grimontia*, *Photobacterium*, and *Salinivibrio*. Pathogenic species are found in the genera *Vibrio* (10 species), *Grimontia* (1 species), and *Photobacterium* (1 species). Of these, *Vibrio cholerae*, *Vibrio parahaemolyticus*, and *Vibrio vulnificus* are the most frequently isolated, followed by *Vibrio alginolyticus*, *Vibrio mimicus*, and *Vibrio fluvialis*. *Vibrio damsela* has now been classified as *Photobacterium damselae* based on gene sequencing. *Vibrio hollisae* has also been reclassified as *Grimontia hollisae*. The remaining *Vibrio* spp. are rarely encountered.

The *Vibrionaceae* are isolated mainly in marine environments. They cause both intestinal and extraintestinal infections that occur more frequently during the warmer months and usually occur following consumption of raw fish or as a result of wounds associated with contact with contaminated fish. *V. cholerae* is the only species that causes endemic, epidemic, and pandemic cholera. It is divided into three major subgroups: *V. cholerae* O1, *V. cholerae* O139, and *V. cholerae* non-O1. The most important pathogens in this group are *V. cholerae* serogroups O1 and O139. There are two biotypes of *V. cholerae* O1: classical and El Tor. The classical biotype was responsible for six of the seven historical pandemics, while the El Tor biotype was responsible for the seventh pandemic, which began in 1961. The El Tor biotype is Voges-Proskauer positive, hemolyzes erythrocytes, and is inhibited by polymyxin B, whereas the classical biogroup has the opposite reactions. In 2007, the World Health Organization (WHO) reported more than 177,000 cases of cholera worldwide. More than 70,000 infections were reported in Zimbabwe alone within a 3-month period.

In 1992, an epidemic of cholera occurred in India, Bangladesh, and elsewhere in Asia. The new subgroup of *V. cholerae* was designated O139 to distinguish it from the other somatic antigen groups of *V. cholerae* known prior to 1998. Thus, there are now two serogroups of *V. cholerae*, O1 and O139, that have the heat-labile cholera toxin (CT) and produce cholera. O139 and O1 strains carry similar virulence factors. As of 1998, 11 countries had reported cases of *V. cholerae* O139 cholera. In 2002, O139 reemerged in Bangladesh, and it has been speculated that its emergence may be the beginning of an eighth pandemic. According to a recent WHO report, most of the *V. cholerae* O139 cases in Asia were reported from China. In contrast, $<0.5\%$ of cholera cases reported from Thailand were O139 and no cases of O139 have been reported from Africa.

The epidemiological characteristics of serogroup O139 are similar to those of serogroup O1. The isolation and identification characteristics of serogroup O139 are identical to those of serogroup O1; therefore, antiserum to serogroup O139 is needed for definitive identification. The severe symptoms caused by these serogroups are the result of CT. The clinical presentation of cholera ranges from an asymptomatic infection to a severe form, resulting in watery diarrhea known as "rice water" stools, with a fluid loss of 500 to 1,000 ml/h. Fluid and electrolyte replacement is the recommended treatment.

V. cholerae non-O1 (non-O1, non-O139), the non-epidemic-associated cholera organisms, are the third most commonly isolated vibrios following *V. parahemolyticus* and *V. vulnificus*. *V. cholerae* non-O1 usually does not produce CT, although it may produce other toxins. The non-O1 *V. cholerae* causes self-limiting gastroenteritis, sepsis, and wound infections. *V. mimicus* is very similar to *V. cholerae* non-O1 with respect to clinical presentation and the characteristics of the organism. For these reasons, it was previously classified as sucrose-negative *V. cholerae*.

V. parahaemolyticus is frequently associated with gastroenteritis following the consumption of raw, contaminated fish or shellfish. In Japan, a majority of foodborne diarrhea is due to *V. parahaemolyticus*. In the United States, it is the *Vibrio* species most frequently isolated from clinical specimens. The infection is usually self-limited, with watery, sometimes bloody, diarrhea lasting 2 to 3 days. Urease-positive strains are thought to be more virulent than urease-negative ones, and this has been linked to the production of thermostable direct hemolysin, a hemolysin that lyses human erythrocytes.

V. vulnificus is associated with very severe disease and a high mortality rate. It causes septicemia and wound infections, usually following the consumption or handling of raw oysters. The disease is known to occur mainly in individuals with preexisting liver disease. It appears that the increased availability of iron resulting from the liver disease puts these individuals at increased risk of acquiring the infection. *V. alginolyticus* is also associated with wound and ear infections following exposure to seawater. The organism can grow in salt concentrations as high as 10%. The remaining members of the pathogenic *Vibrionaceae* are less commonly isolated.

Vibrio spp. are curved or straight, gram-negative bacilli measuring approximately 0.5 to 0.8 μm wide and 1.5 to 2.5 μm long. Most species are motile by a polar flagellum, whereas those that swarm on agar media have peritrichous flagella. All but *Vibrio metschnikovii* are oxidase positive, and all ferment glucose. *Vibrio* spp. grow best on nutrient agar or in broth in the presence of NaCl. Apart from the nonhalophilic species, *V. cholerae* and *V. mimicus*, they do not grow without at least 0.5% NaCl. Most primary culture media contain at least 0.5% NaCl; therefore, *Vibrio* spp. grow well on blood and MacConkey agars. However, in a suspected outbreak, the use of a selective medium such as thiosulfate citrate bile salts sucrose (TCBS) agar may be helpful, especially when the specimen source is feces. On this medium, *V. cholerae* produces yellow colonies because it ferments sucrose whereas most of the other *Vibrio* spp. causing gastroenteritis are sucrose negative and appear as green colonies.

The string test is very helpful in differentiating *Vibrio* spp. from closely related organisms such as *Aeromonas* and *Plesiomonas* spp. In this test, *Vibrio* spp. are lysed in the presence of 0.5% sodium deoxycholate, resulting in a positive string test, whereas *Aeromonas* and *Plesiomonas* give negative tests. Other key tests that assist in the identification of *Vibrio* spp. are the oxidase test, reactions on a triple sugar iron (TSI) agar slant, *o*-nitrophenyl-β-D-galactopyranoside, lysine decarboxylase, ornithine decarboxylase, and arginine dihydrolase. Key differentiating characteristics of the more commonly isolated *Vibrio* spp. are shown in Table 14-1. Isolates with a presumptive identification of *V. cholerae* should be reported and submitted immediately to a public health laboratory.

Molecular detection of *Vibrio* spp. is also available. PCR-based assays have the advantage over culture methods in that fecal specimens can be frozen and tested at a later time. Current PCR assays allow for the differentiation of serotypes O1 and O139, as well as the El Tor and classical biotypes.

Table 14-1 *Vibrionaceae* isolated from clinical specimens[a]

Species	Oxidase	Motility	ONPG	ADH	LDC	ODC	0% NaCl	6% NaCl	Salicin	Sucrose
Vibrio										
V. alginolyticus	+	+	0	0	+	V	0	+	0	+
V. cincinnatiensis	+	V	V	0	V	0	0	+	+	+
V. cholerae	+	+	+	0	+	+	+	V	0	+
V. fluvialis	+	V	V	+	0	0	0	+	0	+
V. furnissii	+	V	V	+	0	0	0	+	0	+
V. harveyi	+	0	0	0	+	0	0	+	0	V
V. metschnikovii	0	V	V	V	V	0	0	V	0	+
V. mimicus	+	+	+	0	+	+	+	V	0	0
V. parahaemolyticus	+	+	0	0	+	+	0	+	0	0
V. vulnificus	+	+	V	0	+	V	0	V	+	V
Grimontia hollisae	+	0	0	0	0	+	0	V	0	0
Photobacterium damselae	+	V	0	+	V	0	0	+	0	0

[a]ONPG, *o*-nitrophenyl-β-D-galactopyranoside; ADH, arginine dihydrolase; LDC, lysine decarboxylase; ODC, ornithine decarboxylase; +, positive reaction (≥90% positive); V, variable reaction (11 to 89% positive); 0, negative reaction (≤10% positive).

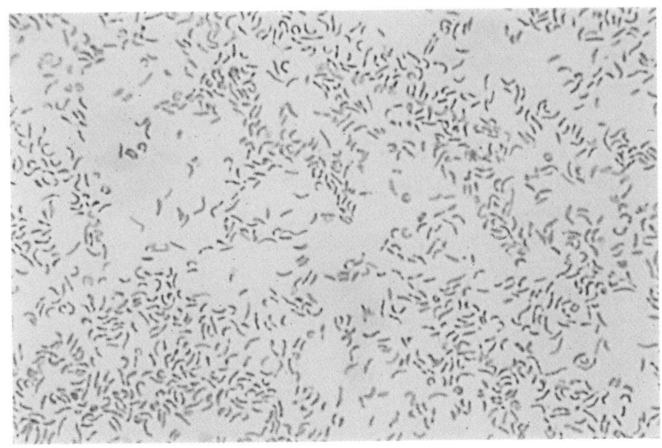

Figure 14-1 Gram stain of *Vibrio* spp. A Gram stain of *Vibrio* spp. shows typical curved and straight, gram-negative bacilli measuring approximately 0.5 to 0.8 μm wide and 1.5 to 2.5 μm long.

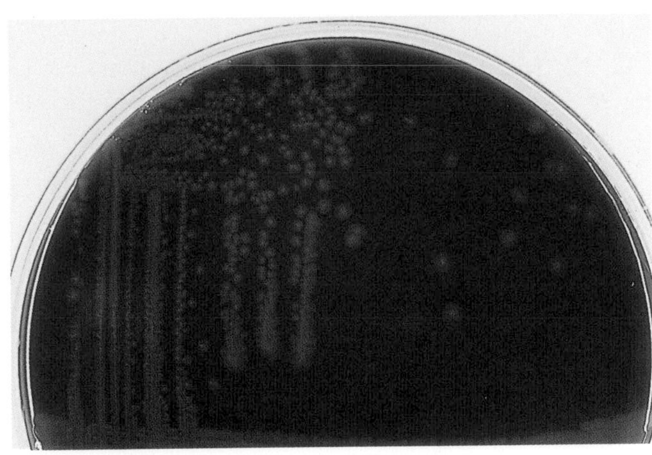

Figure 14-2 *Vibrio cholerae* on blood agar. Colonies of *V. cholerae* on blood agar are small to medium, measuring approximately 1 to 3 mm in diameter; nonhemolytic; smooth; and opaque, with a greenish hue.

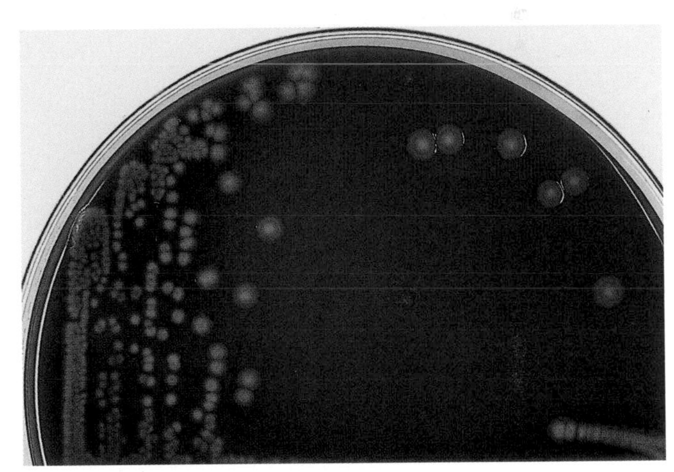

Figure 14-3 *Vibrio alginolyticus* on blood agar. Colonies of *V. alginolyticus* on blood agar are medium to large, measuring approximately 3 to 5 mm in diameter; nonhemolytic; smooth; and opaque, with a slight greenish hue. Most *Vibrio* spp. are nonhemolytic, with the exception of *V. fluvialis* and *V. mimicus*.

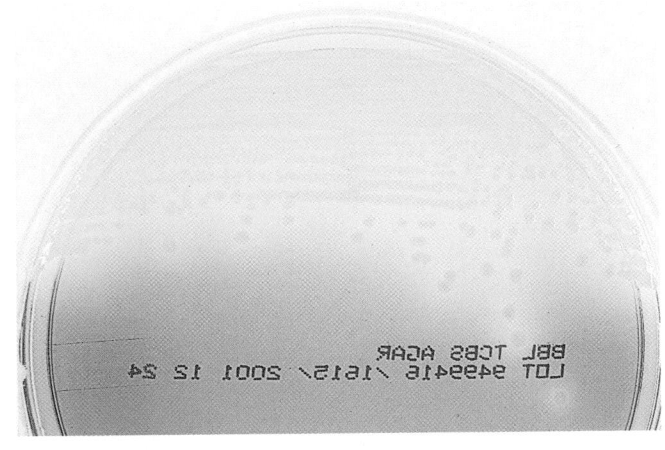

Figure 14-4 *Vibrio cholerae* on TCBS agar. TCBS agar is a selective medium developed for the isolation of *Vibrio* spp., especially *V. cholerae*, from fecal specimens. Some *Vibrio* spp. grow poorly on this medium, while others grow well and produce yellow or green colonies, depending on whether they ferment sucrose. *V. cholerae* is a sucrose fermenter; as shown in this figure, the colonies are yellow. TCBS agar should be incubated at 35°C in ambient air rather than under 5 to 10% CO_2.

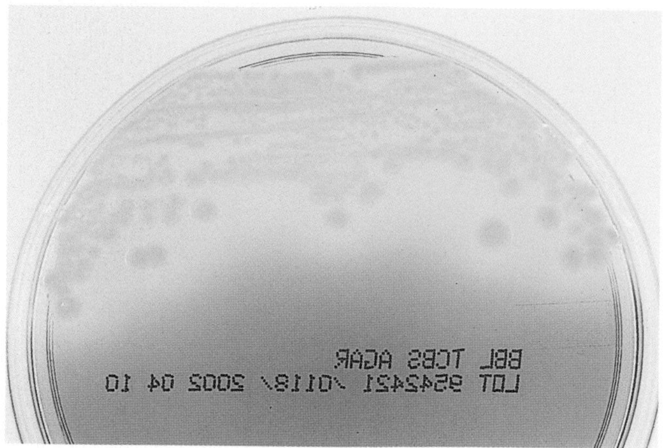

Figure 14-5 ***Vibrio alginolyticus*** **on TCBS agar.** TCBS agar is not selective for *V. cholerae* alone. Other species also ferment sucrose, including *V. metschnikovii*, *V. fluvialis*, *V. alginolyticus* (shown here), and some strains of *V. vulnificus*. Colonies of *V. alginolyticus* on TCBS are larger than those of *V. cholerae* (Fig. 14-4).

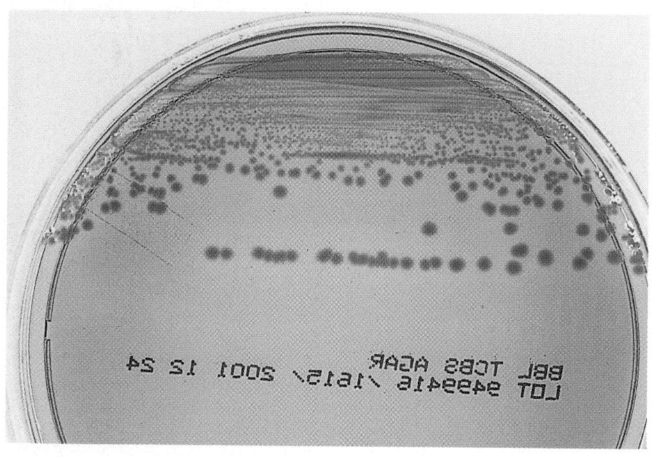

Figure 14-6 ***Vibrio parahaemolyticus*** **on TCBS agar.** Unlike the *Vibrio* spp. described in Fig. 14-4 and 14-5, *V. parahaemolyticus* does not ferment sucrose, and therefore the colonies are green on TCBS agar.

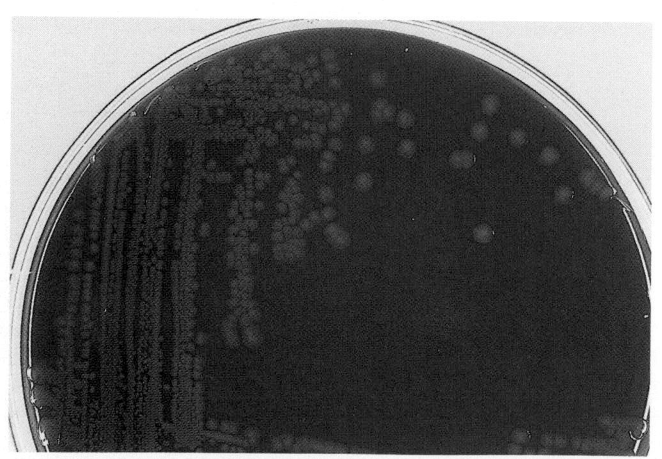

Figure 14-7 ***Vibrio parahaemolyticus*** **on blood agar.** Colonies of *V. parahaemolyticus* on blood agar are very similar to those of *V. cholerae* (Fig. 14-2), although they are slightly larger, measuring 2 to 4 mm in diameter, with a darker greenish coloration.

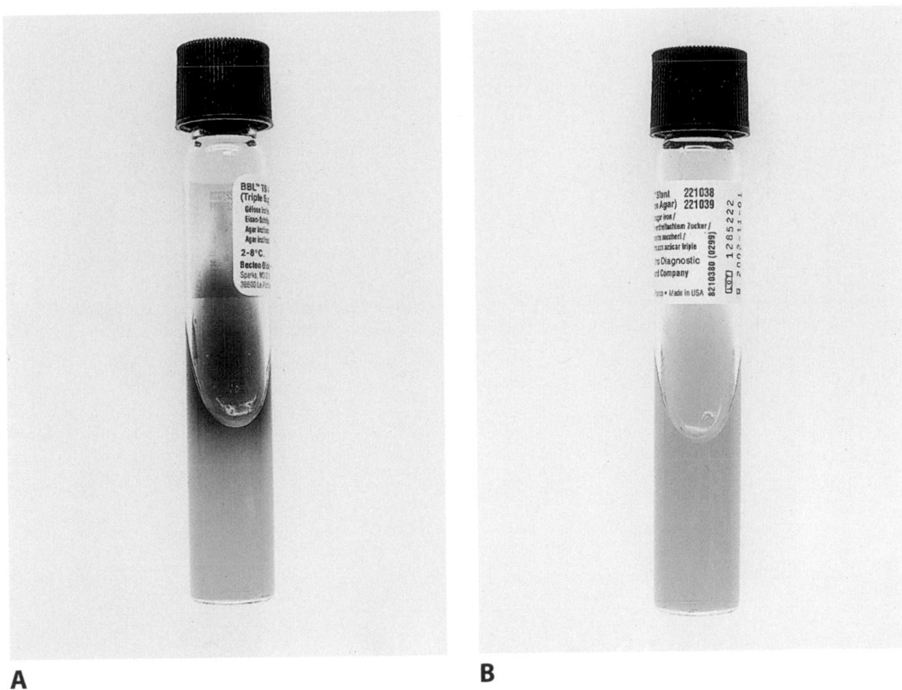

Figure 14-8 ***Vibrio* spp.** on a TSI agar slant. *Vibrio* spp. grow well on a TSI agar slant. Since they ferment glucose without gas production, the reaction in the butt of the tube is acid (yellow). The reaction in the slant depends on whether the organism ferments lactose and/or sucrose. (A) *V. parahaemolyticus* does not ferment lactose or sucrose, and therefore the slant is alkaline (pink). (B) *V. alginolyticus* ferments sucrose and therefore gives an acid (yellow) reaction in the TSI agar slant.

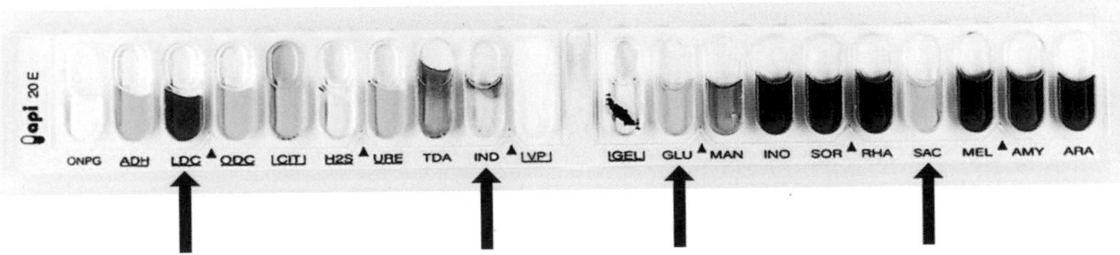

Figure 14-9 ***Vibrio alginolyticus* identified by the API 20E system.** Identification of *Vibrio* spp. by commercial systems is unreliable. However, more commonly isolated species, such as *V. alginolyticus*, are included in the databases. The positive reactions in this API 20E test (bioMérieux, Inc., Durham, NC), shown above the arrows, are characteristic for *V. alginolyticus*, including lysine decarboxylase (LDC), indole (IND), glucose (GLU), and sucrose (SAC). The identification is based on the combination of these reactions, along with a positive oxidase test.

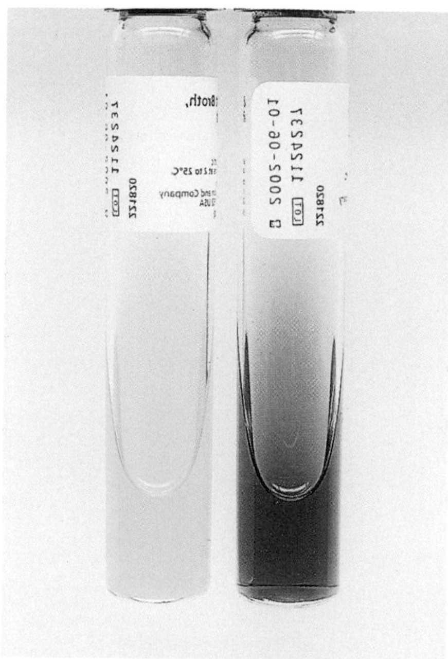

Figure 14-10 *Vibrio alginolyticus* and *Aeromonas hydrophila* inoculated into 6.5% NaCl broth. The growth of *Vibrio* spp. on primary culture media is very similar to that of *Aeromonas* and *Plesiomonas* spp., all three of which are oxidase positive. One of the distinguishing characteristics of the *Vibrio* spp. is their ability to grow in the presence of high concentrations of NaCl. In this figure, *V. alginolyticus* is growing in 6.5% NaCl (left) but *A. hydrophila* shows no growth (right). The 6.5% NaCl broth also contains glucose and an indicator; the medium becomes acid (yellow) due to the fermentation of glucose.

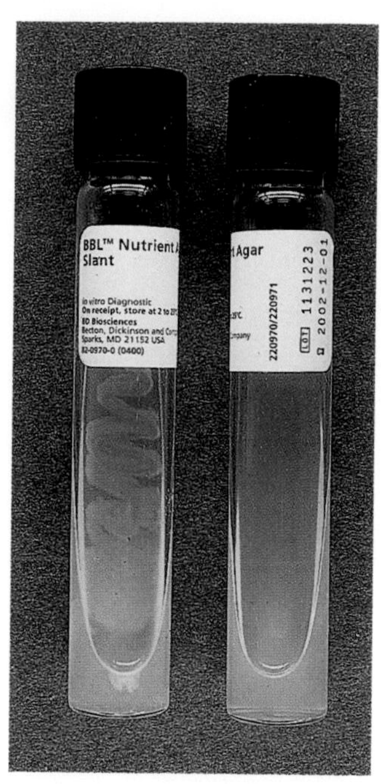

Figure 14-11 *Vibrio alginolyticus* and *Aeromonas hydrophila* inoculated on nutrient agar. Most *Vibrio* spp. require NaCl for growth. Here, one nutrient agar slant was inoculated with *A. hydrophila* (left) and the other was inoculated with *V. alginolyticus* (right). Since the nutrient agar does not contain sufficient NaCl to support the growth of *V. alginolyticus*, growth appears only in the tube inoculated with *A. hydrophila*.

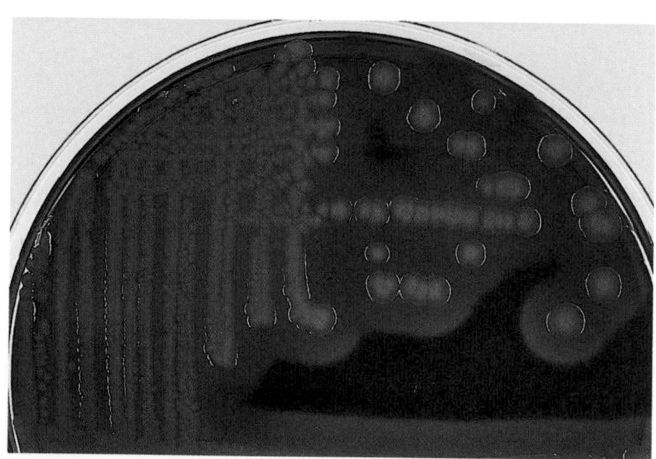

Figure 14-12 *Vibrio mimicus* on blood agar. Most *Vibrio* spp. are nonhemolytic; however, two species can be beta-hemolytic: *V. fluvialis* and *V. mimicus*. In this figure, colonies of *V. mimicus* on blood agar are medium to large, measuring 4 to 5 mm in diameter, and are surrounded by wide zones of beta-hemolysis. *Photobacterium damselae* (formerly *V. damsela*) is also beta-hemolytic.

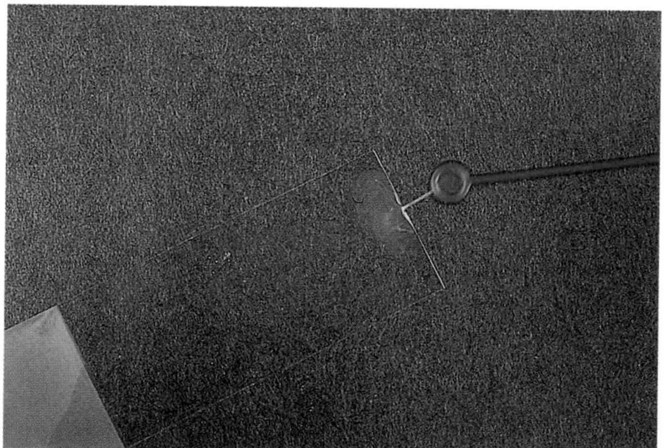

Figure 14-13 Presumptive identification of *Vibrio* spp. by the string test. The string test is used to differentiate *Vibrio* from other related organisms, such as *Aeromonas* and *Plesiomonas*. Suspected colonies are suspended in 0.5% sodium deoxycholate on a glass slide. *Vibrio* spp. lyse when mixed with this reagent, forming a viscous suspension. A string of viscous material appears when the suspension is pulled away from the test surface with a loop, as shown here.

Aeromonas and *Plesiomonas* 15

Aeromonas spp. belong to the family *Aeromonadaceae* along with the genera *Oceanimonas* and *Tolumonas*; however, *Aeromonas* is the only genus pathogenic for humans. Of the 27 species and subspecies classified in the genus *Aeromonas*, only 12 have been isolated from clinical specimens; *Aeromonas hydrophila* subsp. *hydrophila* sensu stricto, *Aeromonas caviae*, and *Aeromonas veronii* biovar *sobria* are the most commonly isolated and account for >95% of all *Aeromonas* blood-borne infections. The other *Aeromonas* species encountered in clinical specimens, although infrequently, include *A. veronii* biovar *veronii*, *Aeromonas jandaei*, *Aeromonas media*, *Aeromonas schubertii*, *Aeromonas popoffii*, *Aeromonas bestiarum*, *Aeromonas salmonicida*, *Aeromonas trota*, and *Aeromonas eucrenophila*.

The genus *Aeromonas* is widely distributed in aquatic and marine environments. The aeromonads not only produce disease in fish and cold-blooded animal species, but they also cause infections in both immunocompetent and immunocompromised individuals. Humans become infected during the warmer months through a variety of pathways. Although water is often the source for infection acquired through the environment and recreational activities, consumable products, pets, and zoonoses have been implicated. *Aeromonas* spp. cause a wide variety of intestinal and extraintestinal disease ranging from a self-limiting gastroenteritis to life-threatening infections including septicemia and necrotizing fasciitis. Although rare, other infections have been reported, including genitourinary, ocular, respiratory, and surgical infections. Previously, *Aeromonas* appeared to represent a low risk to human health. However, following natural disasters early in the 21st century, including flooding in New Orleans and the tsunami in Thailand, *Aeromonas* was a significant cause of infection. In Thailand, *Aeromonas* was the single most common pathogen in skin and soft tissue, accounting for 20% of infections. There is also an increased risk of *Aeromonas* infection following medicinal leech therapy since leeches harbor aeromonads.

Aeromonas spp. are small, gram-negative bacilli and coccobacilli, measuring 1.0 to 4.0 μm long and 0.3 to 1.0 μm wide. Most species are motile by polar flagella; however, lateral flagella may be observed in cultures that are <8 h old. *Aeromonas* spp. grow well on routine laboratory media, including blood and MacConkey agars, and approximately 90% of isolates are beta-hemolytic on blood agar, with the exception of *A. popoffii*, which is nonhemolytic (Table 15-1). The use of modified cefsulodin-irgasan-novobiocin (CIN) agar containing 4 μg/ml of cefsulodin may be helpful when attempting to isolate the organism from feces. Other media, such as ampicillin blood agar with 20 μg/ml of ampicillin, have been used to enhance the recovery of aeromonads from feces. However, ampicillin-susceptible species, e.g., *A. trota*, will be inhibited. *Aeromonas* agar is another selective medium for the isolation of aeromonads. It is a highly selective medium containing D-xylose, which *Aeromonas* spp. do not ferment. This reaction differentiates *Aeromonas* spp. from *Yersinia* spp. and *Citrobacter* spp., the two genera with similar colony morphology to *Aeromonas* on CIN agar. Another advantage is that an oxidase test can be performed directly from colonies on *Aeromonas* agar but not from colonies on CIN agar.

Table 15-1 Differentiation of *Aeromonas* spp. and *Plesiomonas shigelloides* encountered in clinical specimens[a]

Species	Esculin hydrolase	Voges-Proskauer	Gas from glucose	LDC	ADH	ODC
A. caviae complex						
A. caviae sensu stricto	+	0	0	0	+	0
A. eucrenophila	V	0	V	0	+	0
A. media	+	0	0	0	+	0
A. hydrophila complex						
A. bestiarum	+	V	V	V	+	0
A. hydrophila sensu stricto	+	+	+	+	+	0
A. salmonicida	+	V	V	V	+	0
Other *Aeromonas* spp.						
A. jandaei	0	+	+	+	+	0
A. popoffii	0	+	+	0	+	0
A. schubertii	0	V	0	+	+	0
A. trota	0	0	V	+	+	0
A. veronii biovar *sorbia*	0	+	+	+	+	0
A. veronii biovar *veronii*	+	+	+	+	0	+
Plesiomonas shigelloides	0	0	0	+	+	+

[a]LDC, lysine decarboxylase; ADH, arginine dihydrolase; ODC, ornithine decarboxylase; +, positive reaction (>85% positive); V, variable reaction (15 to 85% positive); 0, negative reaction (<15% positive).

Aeromonas spp. are oxidase and catalase positive, reduce nitrate to nitrite, and ferment glucose along with other carbohydrates. However, not all aeromonads produce gas from glucose. Other than *A. schubertii* and an occasional strain of *A. caviae*, most species are indole positive. The aeromonads grow over a wide range of temperatures (10 to 42°C). Use of commercial systems to identify these organisms may present a problem since not all of the species appear in the databases, although the more common clinical isolates are usually included. These systems tend to identify the genus correctly but not the species, and in some instances strains are completely misidentified. Fortunately, it is not necessary to definitively identify members of the *A. hydrophila* complex or *A. caviae* complex isolated from feces. On the other hand, it is important to distinguish *A. hydrophila* and *A. veronii* biovar *sobria* from other *Aeromonas* spp. because they can cause serious, aggressive extraintestinal infections. Fermentation of L-arabinose and esculin hydrolysis are the two most helpful tests in differentiating these two species (Table 15-1).

The genus *Plesiomonas* has only a single species, *Plesiomonas shigelloides*. It is a member of the family *Vibrionaceae*. However, because *Plesiomonas* is closer to the family *Enterobacteriaceae* than *Vibrionaceae* and because it contains the enterobacterial common antigen, it has been included in the family *Enterobacteriaceae*. Since *Plesiomonas* is oxidase positive and the *Enterobacteriaceae* are oxidase negative, its classification in the family *Enterobacteriaceae* may be tentative.

Plesiomonas is found in surface waters and in soil. Its minimum growth temperature of 8°C and its inability to grow in a salty environment limits its distribution to freshwater and estuarine water. It infects cold-blooded animals. Humans are infected as a result of ingesting contaminated foods, especially raw fish, and handling infected cold-blooded animals. *P. shigelloides* is known to cause gastroenteritis, septicemia, and meningitis, although the last two infections are rare. Infections have been associated with travel to areas where the organism is endemic, mostly tropical and subtropical countries, or with residence in areas of endemic infection, such as Thailand, where the organism is found in approximately 25% of the population. As with *Aeromonas* spp., infections occur in the warmer months. Symptoms can range from short episodes of watery diarrhea to several days of dysentery-like diarrhea.

P. shigelloides is a straight, short, gram-negative bacillus, measuring approximately 3.0 μm long by 1.0 μm wide. It is usually motile by two to five lophotrichous flagella, although nonmotile strains do occur. The organism grows well on blood agar and most enteric media but not on ampicillin-containing selective medium, which is recommended for the enhanced recovery of *Aeromonas* spp. Colonies are nonhemolytic, gray, shiny, and smooth, measuring approximately 1.5 mm in diameter after overnight incubation at 30 to 35°C, with optimal growth at 30°C. A selective medium, inositol-bile salts-brilliant green agar, can be used if

P. shigelloides is suspected; however, because of the low incidence of infection, it is not recommended for routine use. *P. shigelloides* is oxidase, indole, and catalase positive; reduces nitrate to nitrite; and ferments glucose along with other carbohydrates. It is positive for arginine, lysine, and ornithine and is DNase negative, a differentiating characteristic that separates it from *Aeromonas* spp. Additional biochemical characteristics of *P. shigelloides* and some of the *Aeromonas* spp. are presented in Table 15-1.

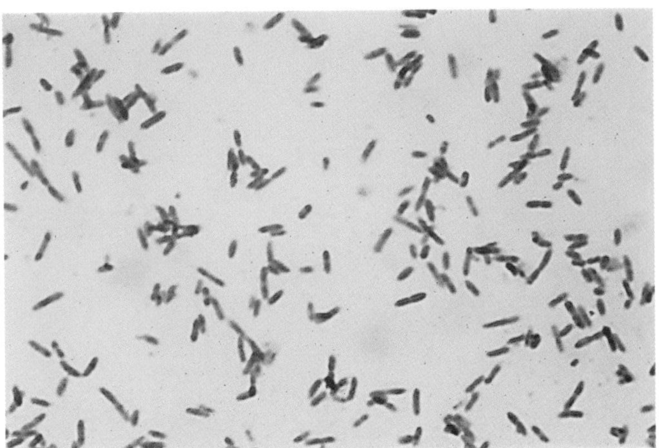

Figure 15-1 Gram stain of *Aeromonas hydrophila*. *A. hydrophila* appears as small, straight, gram-negative bacilli and coccobacilli, measuring 1.0 to 4.0 μm long and 0.3 to 1.0 μm wide.

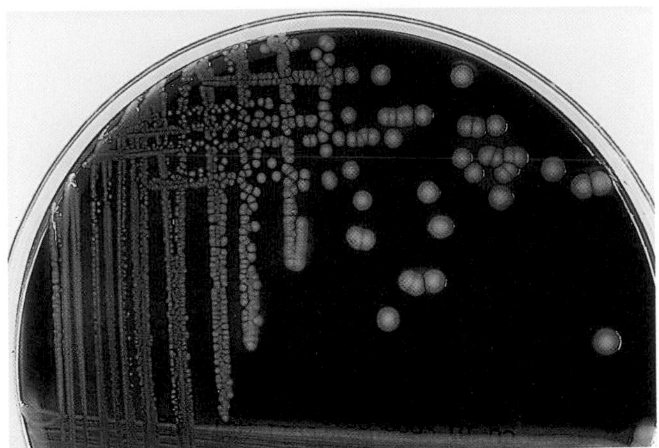

Figure 15-2 *Aeromonas hydrophila* on blood agar. Colonies of *A. hydrophila* on blood agar are approximately 4 mm in diameter, round, raised, opaque, and beta-hemolytic. This is characteristic of most species of *Aeromonas*, except *A. caviae*, which is usually nonhemolytic. Colonies of *Aeromonas* spp. can be confused with enteric gram-negative bacilli, although they are usually more opaque.

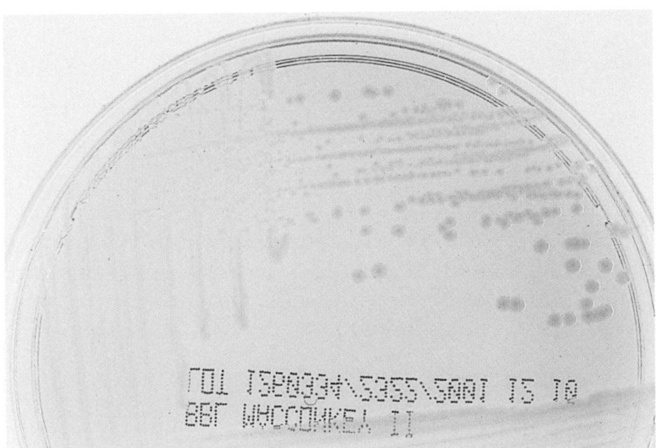

Figure 15-3 *Aeromonas hydrophila* on MacConkey agar. Colonies of *A. hydrophila* on MacConkey agar are lactose nonfermenting, appearing as colorless or pinkish beige. This is characteristic of most species of *Aeromonas*, except *A. caviae*, which ferments lactose, resulting in pink colonies on this medium.

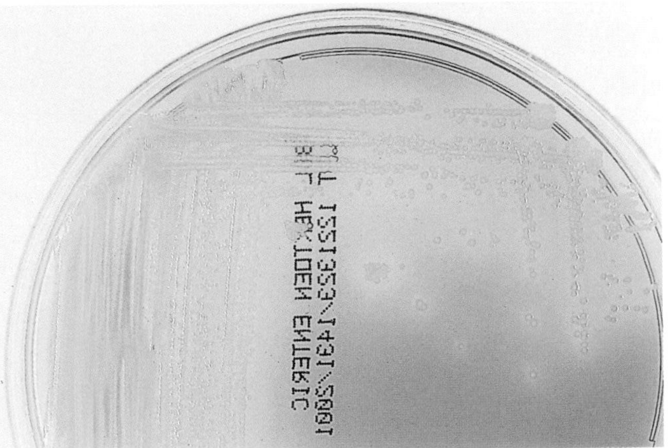

Figure 15-4 *Aeromonas hydrophila* on Hektoen agar. *A. hydrophila* grows well on Hektoen agar, producing yellow colonies because it ferments sucrose. These colonies are similar in appearance to colonies of many of the nonpathogenic enteric organisms; therefore, it is difficult to differentiate them from members of the normal intestinal flora in fecal specimens.

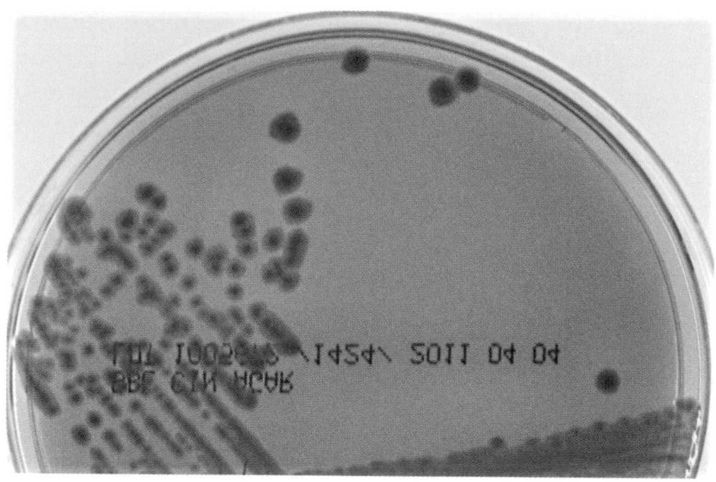

Figure 15-5 ***Aeromonas caviae*** **on CIN agar.** CIN agar is an excellent isolation medium for aeromonads. On this medium, *Aeromonas* spp. colonies have a pink center with an uneven, clear area. *Yersinia enterocolitica* has a similar appearance on this medium.

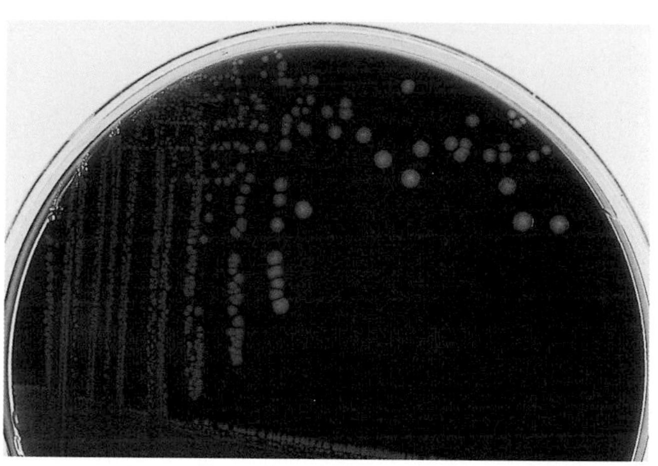

Figure 15-6 ***Plesiomonas shigelloides*** **on blood agar.** Colonies of *P. shigelloides* on blood agar are approximately 2 to 3 mm in diameter, shiny, opaque, smooth, and nonhemolytic. Like *Aeromonas* spp., colonies of *P. shigelloides* can be confused with other enteric gram-negative bacilli.

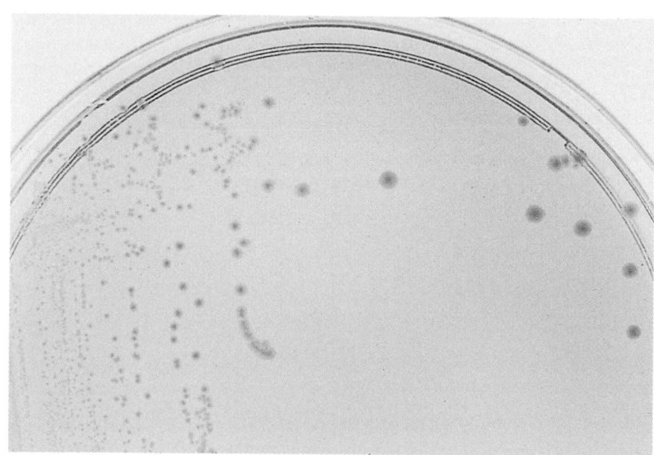

Figure 15-7 ***Plesiomonas shigelloides*** **on MacConkey agar.** Colonies of *P. shigelloides* on MacConkey agar are usually colorless or pinkish beige, measuring 1 to 2 mm in diameter. The colonies look very similar to those of *Shigella* spp.

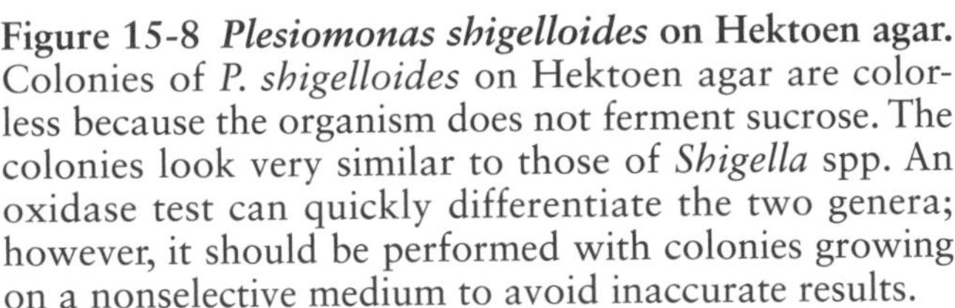

Figure 15-8 ***Plesiomonas shigelloides*** **on Hektoen agar.** Colonies of *P. shigelloides* on Hektoen agar are colorless because the organism does not ferment sucrose. The colonies look very similar to those of *Shigella* spp. An oxidase test can quickly differentiate the two genera; however, it should be performed with colonies growing on a nonselective medium to avoid inaccurate results.

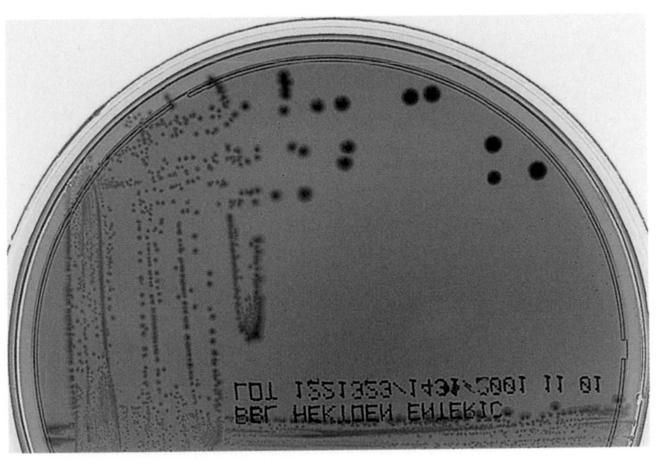

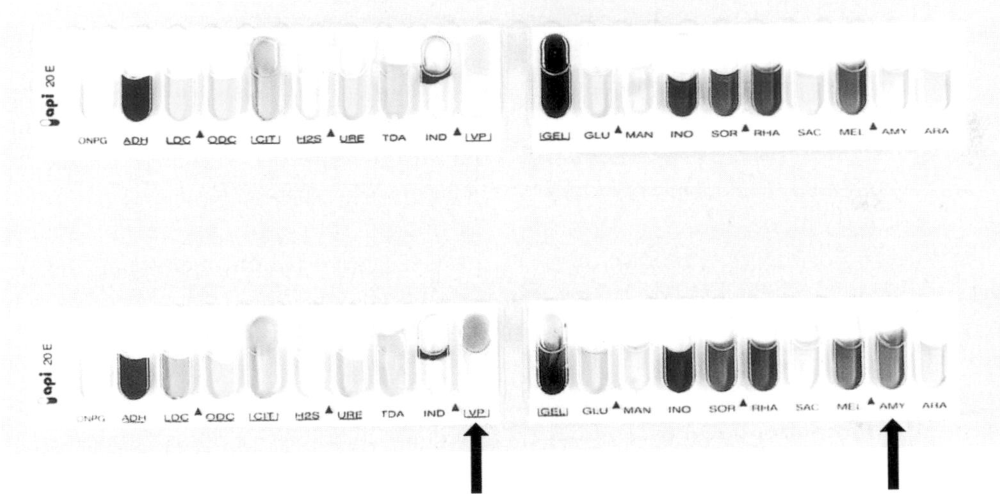

Figure 15-9 ***Aeromonas hydrophila*** **and** ***Aeromonas caviae*** **identified by the API 20E system.** Both *A. hydrophila* and *A. caviae* are included in the API 20E (bioMérieux, Inc., Durham, NC) database; therefore, this system can be used to identify these two *Aeromonas* spp. In this example, *A. caviae* appears in the top strip and *A. hydrophila* is in the bottom strip. The reactions that differentiate them, shown above the arrows, are Voges-Proskauer (VP) and amygdalin (AMY). *A. hydrophila* is VP positive (red), while *A. caviae* is negative (no color). *A. caviae* is AMY positive (yellow), while *A. hydrophila* is negative (blue). The combination of the reactions in each of the strips, as well as the positive oxidase reactions, confirms the identification of these two isolates.

Pseudomonas

16

Twelve *Pseudomonas* spp. have been found in clinical specimens: *Pseudomonas aeruginosa*, *Pseudomonas alcaligenes*, *Pseudomonas fluorescens*, *Pseudomonas luteola*, *Pseudomonas mendocina*, *Pseudomonas monteilii*, *Pseudomonas mosseilii*, *Pseudomonas oryzihabitans*, *Pseudomonas pseudoalcaligenes*, *Pseudomonas putida*, *Pseudomonas stutzeri*, and *Pseudomonas veronii*. There are several other *Pseudomonas* spp.; however, they are saprophytes or plant pathogens.

Pseudomonas spp. are widely distributed in the environment and are often found in moist areas. This has caused problems in hospitals because they have been isolated from a variety of aqueous solutions including dialysis and irrigation fluids and the instruments and equipment associated with them.

P. aeruginosa is a member of the normal flora of the intestinal tract. It has been associated with a variety of infections, including nosocomial infections especially in burn patients. The common source of these infections is usually the water used in hydrotherapy baths. The source of nosocomial respiratory infections due to *P. aeruginosa* is usually respiratory therapy equipment. *P. aeruginosa* is by far the most frequent cause of nosocomial infections and the most important pathogen in this genus. Other types of infections caused by *P. aeruginosa* are folliculitis acquired in swimming pools and hot tubs, "swimmer's ear" associated with aquatic sports, eye infections due to trauma to the cornea, osteomyelitis due to puncture wound of the foot, and endocarditis in intravenous drug users. Mucoid strains of *P. aeruginosa* cause chronic infections in a high percentage of cystic fibrosis (CF) patients. Immunocompetent individuals are resistant to serious *Pseudomonas* infections. However, immunocompromised hosts are occasionally infected with *Pseudomonas* spp. other than *P. aeruginosa*, especially CF patients.

Pseudomonas spp. are aerobic, non-spore-forming, gram-negative bacilli, measuring 0.5 to 1 μm by 2 to 7 μm. The bacilli are longer and thinner than the *Enterobacteriaceae* but have a similar appearance to other nonfermenters. Microscopically mucoid strains, frequently found in CF patients, tend to cluster or produce filaments of short, gram-negative bacilli surrounded by darker pink material known as alginate. Observation of these morphologies intracellularly in polymorphonuclear leukocytes is clinically significant and should be documented.

Pseudomonas spp. grow well on blood and MacConkey agars and are catalase positive, motile by one or more polar flagella, and oxidase positive. However, exceptions to the oxidase-positive species are *P. luteola* and *P. oryzihabitans*, which are oxidase negative. Most species oxidize glucose and reduce nitrate to either nitrite or nitrogen gas. Six species—*P. aeruginosa*, *P. fluorescens*, *P. monteilii*, *P. mosseilii*, *P. putida*, and *P. veronii*—produce a water-soluble, yellow-green or yellow-brown pigment known as pyoverdin. As a result of this pigment, these six species are classified as members of the fluorescent pseudomonad group. Additionally, *P. aeruginosa* also produces a blue-green pigment, pyocyanin, which combines with pyoverdin, resulting in a bright green color. Occasional strains of *P. aeruginosa* produce only pyoverdin, making it difficult to differentiate those strains from the other five fluorescent pseudomonads. However, *P. aeruginosa* grows at 42°C, whereas the other fluorescent pseudomonads do not. *P. luteola*, *P. mendocina*, and *P. pseudoalcaligenes* also grow at 42°C. *P. stutzeri*, a frequent isolate but an unusual cause of infection, is easily recognized by its characteristic growth on blood and chocolate agars. *P. stutzeri* colonies are dry and wrinkled and can pit the agar. The differentiating characteristics of the *Pseudomonas* spp. encountered in clinical specimens are presented in Table 16-1. A number of identification systems accurately identify glucose-nonfermenting, gram-negative bacilli, including the *Pseudomonas* spp.

Although *Pseudomonas* spp. grow on routine culture media, more rapid, nucleic acid detection methods have been used for certain situations, e.g., evaluating sputum from CF patients and screening environmental niches. The reason is that commercial identification systems perform poorly, especially with mucoid *P. aeruginosa* isolates. Also, isolates from sites of chronic infection, e.g., CF respiratory sites, exhibit multiple morphotypes that can make identification difficult. PCR amplification has been valuable in the identification of *Pseudomonas* spp. other than *P. aeruginosa* as well as biochemically inactive *Pseudomonas* spp. Recently, peptide nucleic acid fluorescent in situ hybridization (PNA FISH) has been described as a highly sensitive and specific assay for the identification of *P. aeruginosa*.

Table 16-1 Differentiating characteristics of *Pseudomonas* spp. encountered in clinical specimens[a]

Species	Oxidase	Growth at 42°C	Nitrate		Gelatin hydrolysis at 7 days	ADH	Glucose	Xylose	Maltose
			NO_2[b]	N_2[c]					
P. aeruginosa	+	+		+	V	+	+	+	0
P. alcaligenes	+	V at 41°C	V		0	V	0	0	0
P. fluorescens	+	0	V		+	+	+	+	0
P. luteola	0	+	V		V	+	+	+	+
P. mendocina	+	+		+	0	+	+	V	0
P. monteilii	+	0	0		0	0	+	0	0
P. mosseilii	+	0	0		+	+	+	0	V
P. oryzihabitans	0	V	0		V	V	+	+	+
P. pseudoalcaligenes	+	+	+		0	V	0	V	0
P. putida	+	0	0		0	+	+	+	V
P. stutzeri	+	V		+	0	0	+	+	+
P. veronii	+	0		+	V	+	+	+	ND

[a]ADH, arginine dihydrolase; +, positive reaction (≥90% positive); V, variable reaction (11 to 89% positive); 0, negative reaction (≤10% positive); ND, no data.

[b]Reduces nitrate to nitrite.

[c]Reduces nitrate to nitrogen gas.

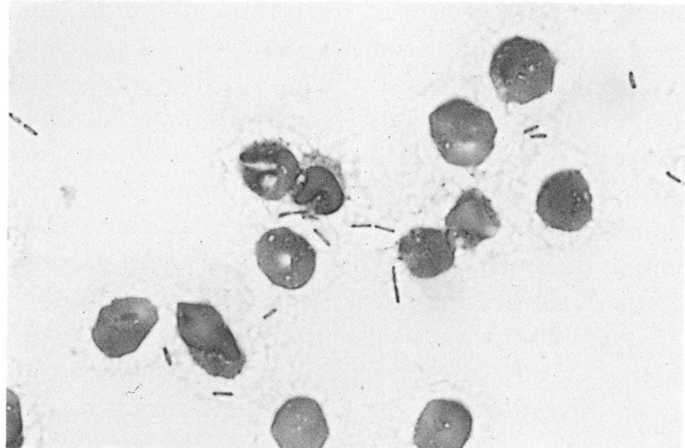

Figure 16-1 Gram stain of *Pseudomonas aeruginosa* in blood culture broth. A Gram stain of a blood culture shows slender, gram-negative bacilli, measuring approximately 1 μm by 5 to 7 μm, with rounded ends. *P. aeruginosa* was isolated from this blood culture.

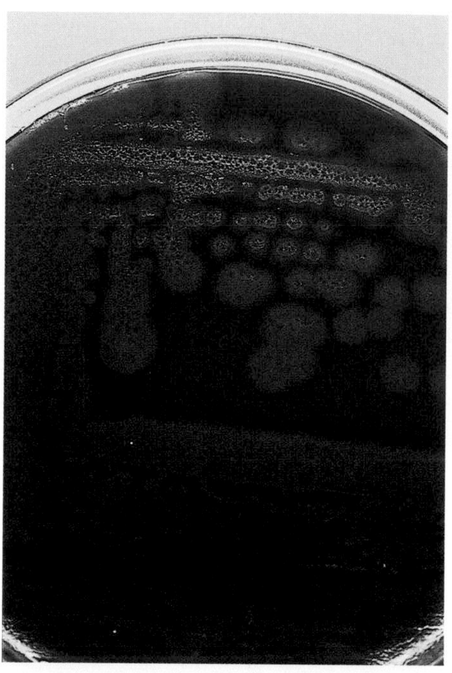

Figure 16-2 *Pseudomonas aeruginosa* on blood agar. Colonies of *P. aeruginosa* are approximately 4 mm in diameter with a blue-green color produced by pyoverdin and pyocyanin pigments. The colonies are beta-hemolytic, flat, and spreading, with serrated edges and confluent growth. Most isolates have a grape-like odor due to aminoacetophenone.

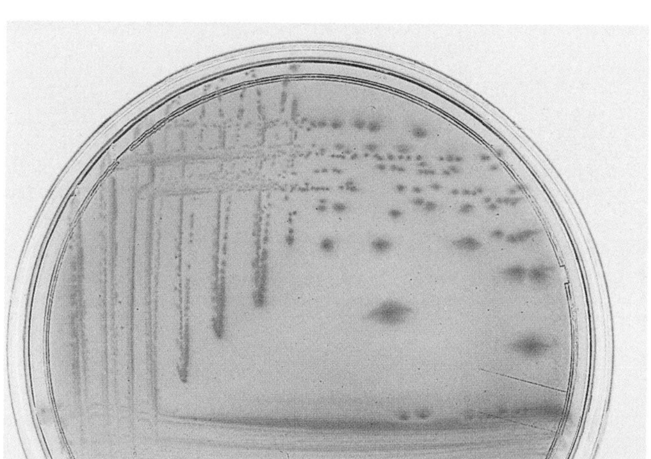

Figure 16-3 *Pseudomonas aeruginosa* on MacConkey agar. Colonies of *P. aeruginosa* on MacConkey agar are approximately 2 mm in diameter and lactose nonfermenting, with a brownish green coloration and irregular, feathered edges.

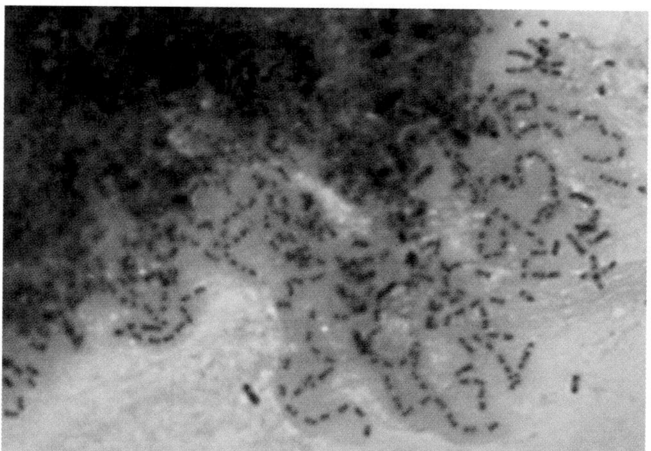

Figure 16-4 Gram stain of mucoid *Pseudomonas aeruginosa*. This figure shows a Gram stain of *P. aeruginosa* from a sputum specimen of a CF patient. The gram-negative bacilli are surrounded by a distinctive orange alginate material, a characteristic finding, since mucoid strains synthesize a large quantity of alginate exopolysaccharide. This alginate material causes the organism to resist phagocytosis and destruction by antimicrobials. (Gram stain courtesy of Barbara McKee, Long Beach Memorial/Healthtech Laboratories, Long Beach, CA.)

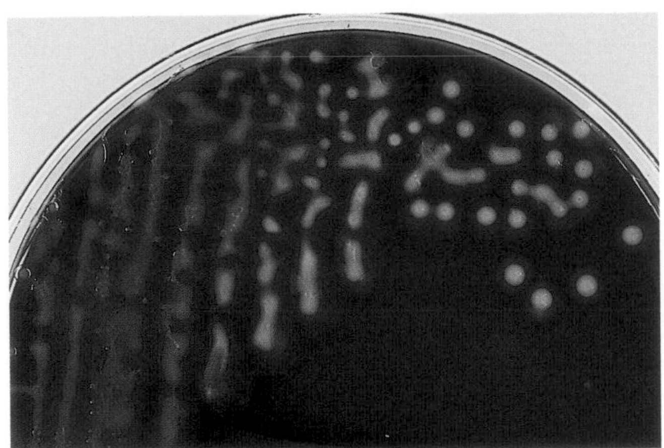

Figure 16-5 Mucoid colonies of *Pseudomonas aeruginosa* on blood agar. This figure shows a highly mucoid, nonpigmented strain of *P. aeruginosa*. This is the typical appearance of isolates recovered from respiratory secretions of patients with CF. The colonies are approximately 2 to 3 mm in diameter and are usually smaller than those of the typical pigmented strains shown in Fig. 16-2.

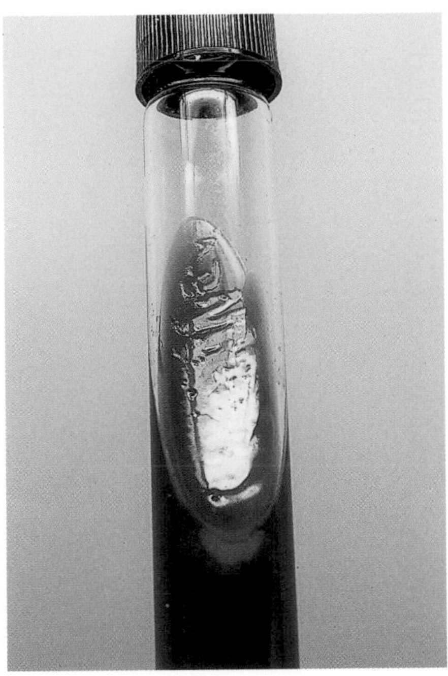

Figure 16-6 *Pseudomonas aeruginosa* on a triple sugar iron agar slant. On a triple sugar iron agar slant, *P. aeruginosa* appears as a blue-green, somewhat metallic greenish fluorescent layer of growth.

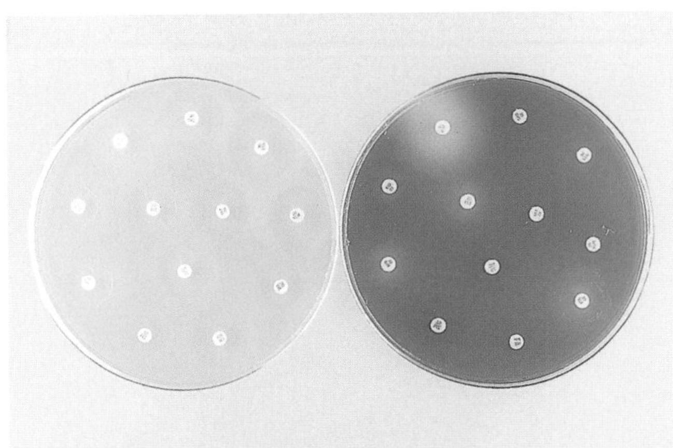

Figure 16-7 *Pseudomonas aeruginosa* on Mueller-Hinton agar. The very distinct green pigment of *P. aeruginosa* colonies is clearly demonstrated when the isolate is grown on a medium without blood, dyes, or other indicators.

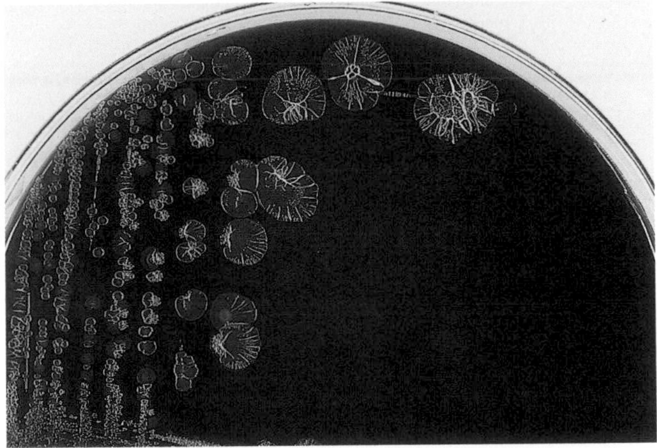

Figure 16-8 *Pseudomonas stutzeri* on blood agar. Colonies of *P. stutzeri* on blood agar have a characteristic dry, wrinkled appearance. They vary in size from approximately 1 to 6 mm in diameter. In areas where there are fewer colonies, the colonies are larger than in areas where there are many.

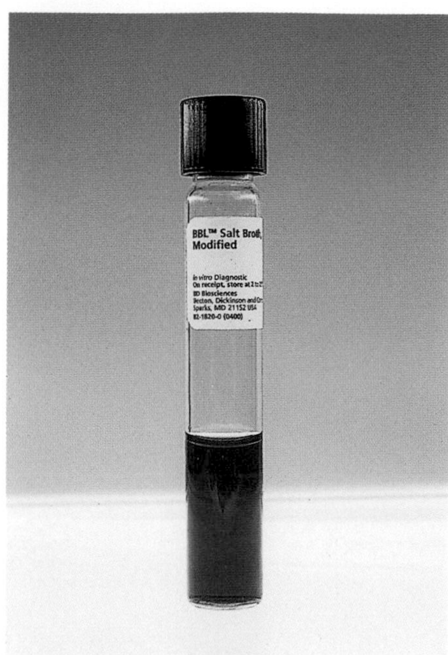

Figure 16-9 ***Pseudomonas stutzeri*** **in 6.5% NaCl broth.** *P. stutzeri*, along with *P. mendocina* and CDC group Vb-3 (*P. stutzeri* biovar), can grow in the presence of 6.5% NaCl. This biochemical characteristic, along with the ability to reduce nitrates to nitrogen gas and oxidize glucose but not lactose, distinguishes the *P. stutzeri* group from the other *Pseudomonas* spp.

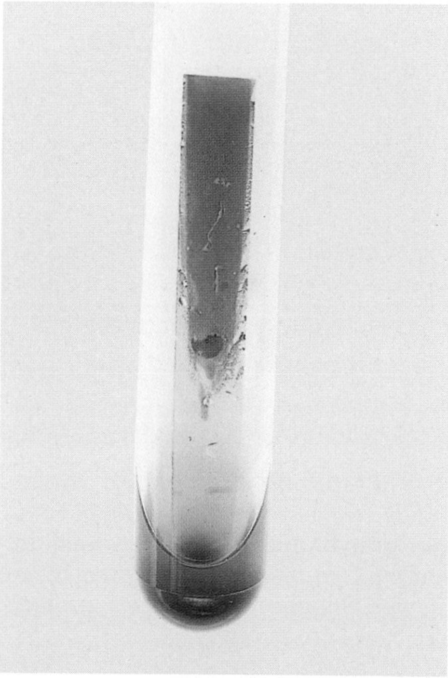

Figure 16-11 ***Pseudomonas fluorescens*** **incubated with gelatin strips.** *P. fluorescens* can be differentiated from most of the other *Pseudomonas* spp. because it hydrolyzes gelatin. Although some strains of *P. aeruginosa* can also hydrolyze gelatin, they grow at 42°C and reduce nitrate to N_2, whereas *P. fluorescens* does not.

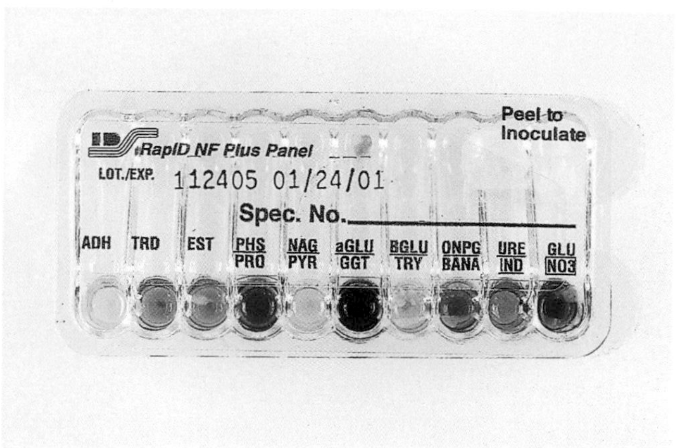

Figure 16-10 ***Pseudomonas stutzeri*** **identified by the RapID NF Plus system.** The RapID NF Plus system (Thermo Scientific Remel Products, Lenexa, KS) is a 4-h test system for the identification of glucose-nonfermenting, gram-negative bacilli. It contains 10 reaction wells that, along with the oxidase reaction, provide 18 test scores. Wells 4 through 10 are bifunctional, with two separate tests in the same well. The results from the 10 wells are interpreted before the addition of reagents. Reagents are added, and the additional tests are interpreted. In this example, the positive reactions are proline-β-naphthylamide (PRO), γ-glutamyl-β-naphthylamide (GGT), *N*-benzoylarginine-β-naphthylamide (BANA), and nitrate (NO_3). The oxidase test was also positive. The combination of these test reactions confirms the identification of *P. stutzeri.*

Figure 16-12 ***Pseudomonas aeruginosa*** **identified by PNA FISH.** PNA FISH (AdvanDx, Woburn, MA) is a rapid and highly sensitive and specific fluorescent assay for the detection of gram-negative pathogens including *P. aeruginosa*. The specimen is placed on a slide and fixed. After fixation, a drop of the probe solution is added and hybridized. The slide is washed and read using a fluorescent microscope. The red color signifies hybridization with *P. aeruginosa*. (Image courtesy of AdvanDx.)

Burkholderia, Stenotrophomonas, Ralstonia, Cupriavidus, Pandoraea, Brevundimonas, Comamonas, Delftia, and *Acidovorax*

17

Several species previously in the genus *Pseudomonas* have been reclassified into several new genera as a result of DNA-rRNA hybridization experiments. These genera include *Burkholderia*, *Stenotrophomonas*, *Ralstonia*, *Cupriavidus*, *Pandoraea*, *Brevundimonas*, *Comamonas*, *Delftia*, and *Acidovorax*.

The genus *Burkholderia* comprises 59 species. The species known to cause a majority of human infections are *Burkholderia cepacia* complex (17 species), *Burkholderia gladioli*, *Burkholderia mallei*, and *Burkholderia pseudomallei*, while *Burkholderia fungorum*, *Burkholderia glumae*, and *Burkholderia thailandensis* are uncommon causes of infection. The human pathogens within the genus *Ralstonia* include *Ralstonia pickettii*, *Ralstonia mannitolilytica*, and *Ralstonia insidiosa*. The genus *Pandoraea* was created for species previously classified in the genera *Burkholderia* and *Ralstonia*. There are five distinct species and four unnamed, most occurring in clinical specimens. The named species include *Pandoraea apista*, *Pandoraea pulmonicola*, *Pandoraea pnomenusa*, *Pandoraea sputorum*, and *Pandoraea norimbergensis*.

Organisms previously classified in the *Pseudomonas* rRNA homology group III have been reclassified into the family *Comamonadaceae*, which includes the genera *Comamonas*, *Delftia*, and *Acidovorax*. The human clinical isolates in the genus *Comamonas* are *Comamonas terrigena*, *Comamonas aquatica*, and *Comamonas kerstersii*. *Comamonas acidovorans* now has been reclassified as *Delftia acidovorans*. The genus *Acidovorax* comprises *Acidovorax facilis*, *Acidovorax delafieldii*, and *Acidovorax temperans*, along with five other plant and environmental species.

The genus *Brevundimonas* was previously classified as *Pseudomonas* rRNA homology group IV. There are 14 species, most of which are environmental, with the exception of *Brevundimonas diminuta* and *Brevundimonas vesicularis*. *Pseudomonas maltophilia* was originally represented in the *Pseudomonas* rRNA homology group V. It was transferred to the genus *Xanthomonas* and finally to the genus *Stenotrophomonas*. There are eight species of *Stenotrophomonas*, and all but *Stenotrophomonas maltophilia* are environmental species.

By Gram stain, these genera appear as straight or slightly curved, gram-negative bacilli, measuring 0.5 to 1.0 μm by 1.8 to 5 μm, with the exception of *Stenotrophomonas* spp., which appear as straight bacilli and may be slightly smaller than the other genera. They are motile by polar flagella, with the exception of *B. mallei*, which is nonmotile. Additionally, *B. pseudomallei* may appear as small, gram-negative bacilli with bipolar staining. Most of these organisms grow on routine laboratory media, are nonfermenters, oxidize glucose, and reduce nitrate. They are catalase positive, and most are weakly or strongly oxidase positive, with the exception of *Stenotrophomonas* spp. and *B. gladioli*.

The nine genera discussed in this chapter are opportunistic pathogens isolated primarily from patients in health care settings. Many of these organisms cause infections in cystic fibrosis (CF) patients. For example, of the 17 species of *B. cepacia* complex, 16 have been isolated from CF patients. *Burkholderia multivorans* and *Burkholderia cenocepacia* account for a majority of these infections. The source of infection can usually be traced to contaminated equipment or aqueous solutions, which is due to the organisms' ability to survive in those environments.

The organisms in *B. cepacia* complex, previously designated *Pseudomonas aeruginosa*, *Pseudomonas multivorans*, *Pseudomonas kingae*, and CDC EO-1, cause infection with low virulence. Patients with chronic granulomatous disease and with CF are more susceptible to infection. *B. mallei*, which causes glanders disease in horses, mules, and donkeys, can also be transmitted to humans. *B. pseudomallei* is the cause of melioidosis, a disease prevalent in Southeast Asia and northern Australia, especially during the monsoon seasons. Melioidosis is becoming more common in Europe and the United States due to travel to these locations, especially for individuals with CF. The organism infects humans by inhalation or through contact with broken skin, and there is a very high mortality rate in patients with sepsis. Chronic infections can mimic *Mycobacterium tuberculosis* infection because *B. pseudomallei* can produce granulomatous lesions in tissue. The sources of infection are usually contaminated respiratory therapy equipment and disinfectants. *B. gladioli*, previously considered a plant pathogen, has also been isolated from the sputa of patients with CF as well as those with chronic granulomatous disease.

S. maltophilia, a nosocomial pathogen, can cause a wide variety of serious disseminated infections in immunocompromised patients whose respiratory tracts are colonized with this organism. *R. pickettii*, formerly designated *Burkholderia pickettii*, *Pseudomonas pickettii*, and CDC Va1, Va2, has been isolated from a variety of clinical specimens and can cause bacteremia, meningitis, endocarditis, and osteomyelitis. Although it has been isolated from the respiratory tract of CF patients, it does not appear to cause pulmonary disease. It has also been identified in pseudobacteremia and nosocomial outbreaks due to contaminated intravenous medications, "sterile" solutions, and intravenous catheters. *R. mannitolilytica* accounts for a majority of *Ralstonia* infections in CF patients and twice as many as *R. pickettii*. *Cupriavidus* spp. have also been implicated in human infection; however, their role in lung disease needs further study.

The two species of *Brevundimonas*, *B. diminuta* and *B. vesicularis*, are occasionally isolated from clinical specimens and can produce bacteremia in patients with various underlying diseases, including cancer. *D. acidovorans* and *Comamonas testosteroni* have been associated with infections in humans and have been recovered from the sputa of patients with CF. *D. acidovorans* can cause bacteremia, endocarditis, and infections of the eye and ear. *C. testosteroni* has been isolated from the peritoneal cavity. *Acidovorax*, *D. acidovorans*, and *C. testosteroni* have been recovered from sputa of CF patients; however, the roles of these organisms in contributing to lung disease in CF also need to be established. *Pandoraea* spp. also cause infections in CF patients and have been recovered from blood and from patients with chronic obstructive pulmonary disease.

The nine genera discussed in this chapter grow well on enriched primary isolation media, including blood and chocolate agars. With the exception of *B. vesicularis*, these organisms also grow on MacConkey agar. Selective media, such as PC (*Pseudomonas cepacia*) and OFPBL (oxidative-fermentative base, polymyxin B, bacitracin, lactose) agars, can be used to isolate *B. cepacia* complex and *B. pseudomallei*. Both media contain antibiotics that inhibit the growth of *P. aeruginosa*, which may be helpful when culturing sputa from CF patients. Ashdown agar, which contains crystal violet and gentamicin, is a selective medium for the isolation of *B. pseudomallei* from clinical specimens. However, Ashdown broth medium, supplemented with 50 mg of colistin per liter, increases organism recovery by 25% compared with direct plating of clinical specimens on Ashdown agar. *B. cepacia* medium is a good alternative when Ashdown medium is not available. A selective medium containing vancomycin, imipenem, and amphotericin B (VIA medium) increases the recovery of *S. maltophilia*.

Colony morphology and pigment production can be helpful in the differentiation of these organisms. For example, *B. vesicularis* produces dark yellow to orange colonies on blood agar after 48 h of incubation at 35°C. Some strains of *B. cepacia* complex produce a yellow pigment on some media and a dark pink or red color on MacConkey agar after 4 days of incubation at 35°C. This is due to lactose oxidation after prolonged incubation. *B. gladioli* produces a bright yellow pigment on OFPBL agar and can therefore be confused with *B. cepacia*. *B. cepacia* may also be slow growing when isolated from the sputa of CF patients, with at least 3 days of incubation required before colonies appear on isolation media; the colonies appear wet, runny, and mucoid. Colonies of *B. pseudomallei* can appear as either smooth and mucoid or dry and wrinkled and resemble *Pseudomonas stutzeri*. Because of the clinical importance of *B. pseudomallei*, it is necessary to distinguish between these two organisms. *Acidovorans* spp. may also produce a yellow pigment, while *B. diminuta*,

C. testosteroni, and *S. maltophilia* can produce a tan to brown pigment. Colonies of *R. pickettii* are slow growing and pinpoint after 24 h of incubation on blood agar incubated at 35°C.

Several key biochemical tests, including oxidase, nitrate reduction, arginine dihydrolase, gelatinase activity, DNase reaction, and oxidation of carbohydrates, can be used to differentiate these organisms. Conventional biochemicals or identification kits are available. However, the identification kits should be used with caution because of their low level of accuracy with some of these organisms, especially those isolated from CF patients. On Gram stains prepared from specimens from CF patients infected with *B. cepacia*, the gram-negative bacilli are surrounded by large capsules. Key characteristics of *Burkholderia*, *Stenotrophomonas*, *Ralstonia*, *Cupriavidus*, *Pandoraea*, *Acidovorax*, *Brevundimonas*, and *Comamonas* are shown in Table 17-1.

Rapid direct detection methods have been developed for *B. pseudomallei* because of its high mortality rate. These include urine antigen detection by latex agglutination and enzyme immunoassay. Enzyme immunoassay is more sensitive than latex agglutination; however, results should be interpreted with caution because of cross-reactivity with other urinary tract pathogens. Several molecular assays are available for the organisms discussed in this chapter. However, they are not sufficiently sensitive to replace conventional culture.

Table 17-1 Key characteristics of *Acidovorax*, *Brevundimonas*, *Burkholderia*, *Comamonas*, *Cupriavidus*, *Delftia*, *Pandoraea*, *Ralstonia*, and *Stenotrophomonas* isolates from clinical specimens[a]

Organism	Oxidase	Nitrate	LYS	Growth at 42°C	Glucose	Xylose	Lactose	Sucrose	Maltose	Mannitol
Acidovorax spp.	+	+	0	V	+	V	0	0	0	V
Brevundimonas										
B. diminuta	+	0	0	V	V	0	0	0	0	0
B. vesicularis	+	0	0	V	V	V	0	0	+	0
Burkholderia										
B. cepacia	+	0	+	V	+	+	+	V	V	+
B. gladioli	V	V	0	V	+	+	0	0	0	+
B. mallei	V	+	0	0	+	V	V	0	0	0
B. pseudomallei	+	+, gas[b]	+	V	+	V	+	V	+	+
Comamonas testosteroni	+	+[c]	0	V	0	0	0	0	0	0
Cupriavidus spp.	+	0	0	V	0	0	0	0	ND	ND
Delftia acidovorans	+	+[c]	0	+	0	0	0	0	0	+
Pandoraea spp.	V	V	0	V		0	0	0	0	ND
Ralstonia										
R. picketti	+	+, gas[b]	0	V	+	+	V	0	V	0
R. insidiosa	+	+	0	ND	0	+	V	0	ND	ND
R. mannitolilytica	+	0	0	+	+	+	+	0	+	+
Stenotrophomonas maltophilia	V	V	+	V	V	V	V	V	+	0

[a]LYS, lysine decarboxylase; +, positive reaction (≥90% positive); V, variable reaction (11 to 89% positive); 0, negative reaction (≤10% positive); ND, no data.

[b]Organism reduces nitrate to nitrogen gas.

[c]Organism reduces nitrate to nitrite.

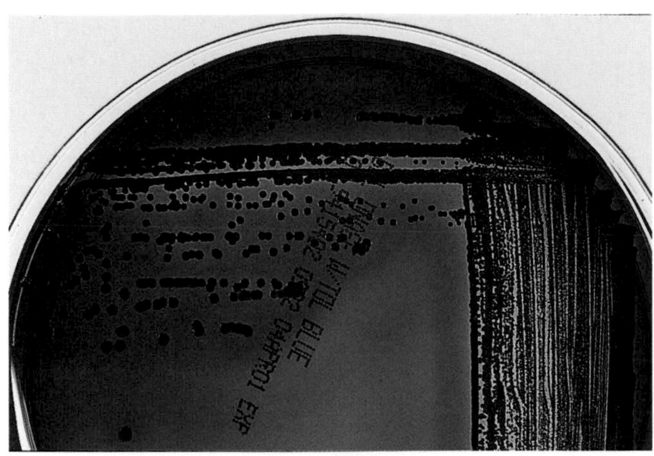

Figure 17-6 ***Stenotrophomonas maltophilia*** **on DNase agar.** Colonies of *S. maltophilia* have a positive DNase reaction. Detection of extracellular DNase activity by *S. maltophilia* is key in differentiating this species from most glucose-oxidizing, gram-negative bacilli. As shown here, DNase-positive organisms produce a zone of clearing around the colonies on this medium.

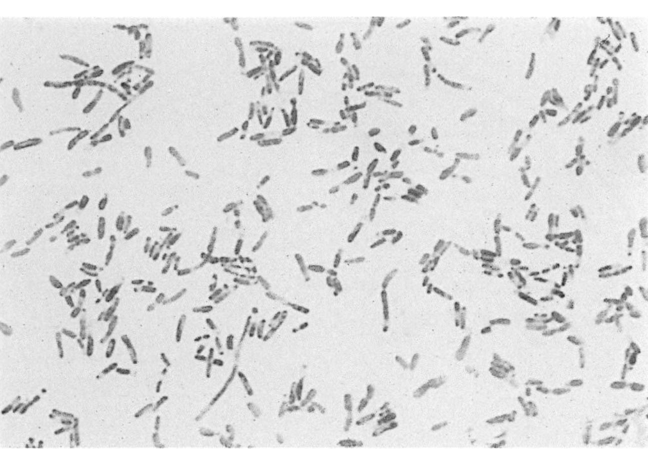

Figure 17-7 Gram stain of ***Comamonas*** **spp.** *Comamonas* spp. are straight to slightly curved, gram-negative bacilli, measuring 0.5 to 1.0 μm by 1 to 4 μm and occurring singly and in pairs. Lipid inclusions of poly-β-hydroxybutyrate accumulate in the cells, giving them a moth-eaten appearance.

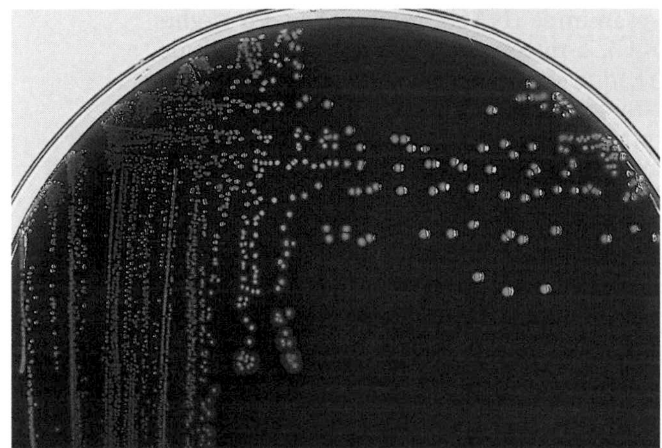

Figure 17-8 ***Comamonas*** **spp.** on blood agar. Colonies of *Comamonas* spp. on blood agar are round and tan, measuring approximately 2 mm in diameter.

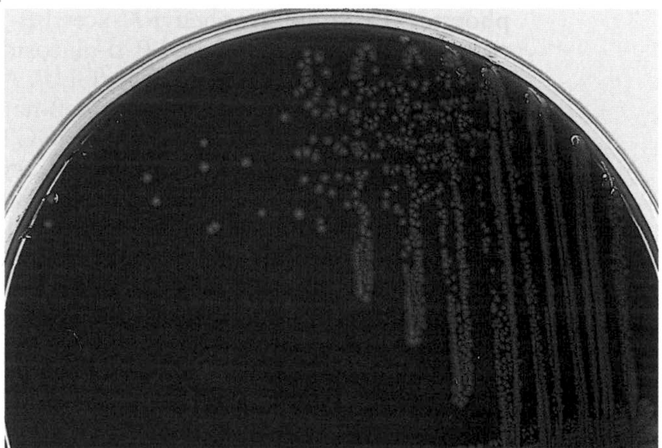

Figure 17-9 ***Ralstonia pickettii*** **on blood agar.** Colonies of *R. pickettii* after a 48-h incubation at 35°C on blood agar are pinpoint, measuring approximately 1 mm in diameter. This organism is slow growing and may require 72 h to produce visible colonies.

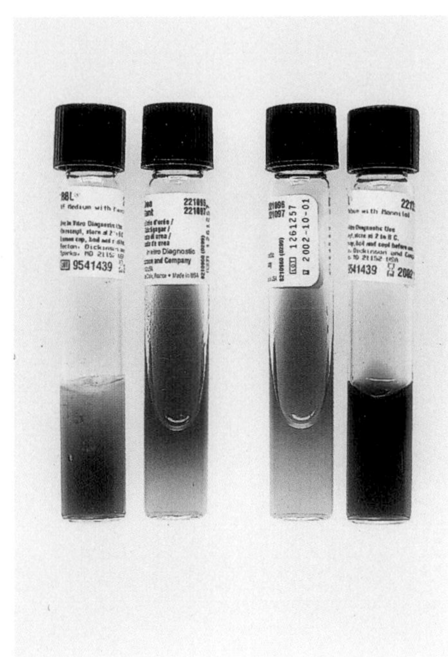

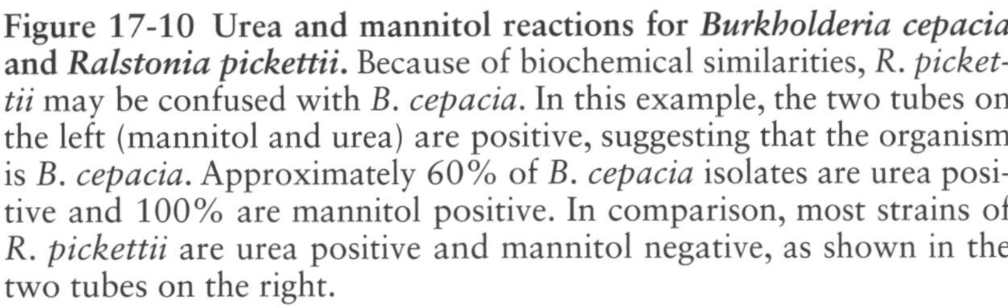

Figure 17-10 Urea and mannitol reactions for *Burkholderia cepacia* and *Ralstonia pickettii*. Because of biochemical similarities, *R. pickettii* may be confused with *B. cepacia*. In this example, the two tubes on the left (mannitol and urea) are positive, suggesting that the organism is *B. cepacia*. Approximately 60% of *B. cepacia* isolates are urea positive and 100% are mannitol positive. In comparison, most strains of *R. pickettii* are urea positive and mannitol negative, as shown in the two tubes on the right.

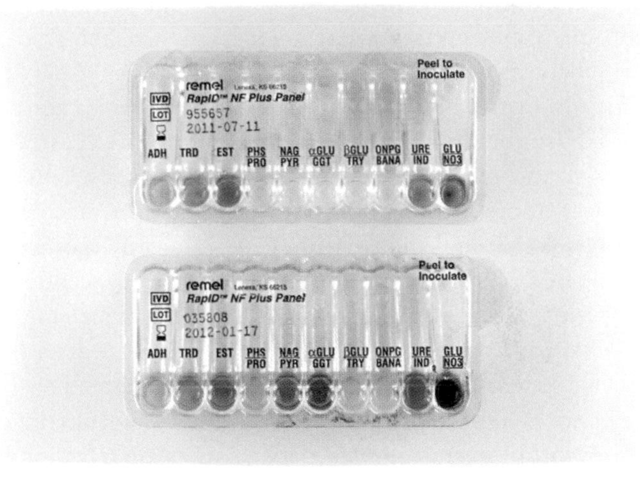

Figure 17-11 Identification of *Delftia acidovorans* by the RapID NF Plus system. The RapID NF Plus system is described in Fig. 17-4. Shown here are positive reactions for triglyceride (EST; yellow-orange) in the top panel and pyrrolidine-β-naphthylamide (PYR; dark pink), γ-glutamyl-β-naphthylamide (GGT; dark pink), and sodium nitrate (NO_3; red) in the bottom panel. These reactions confirm the identification of *D. acidovorans*. Although the indole (IND) may be interpreted as positive due to the reddish orange color, an indole-positive reaction in this system is indicated by a brown or black color.

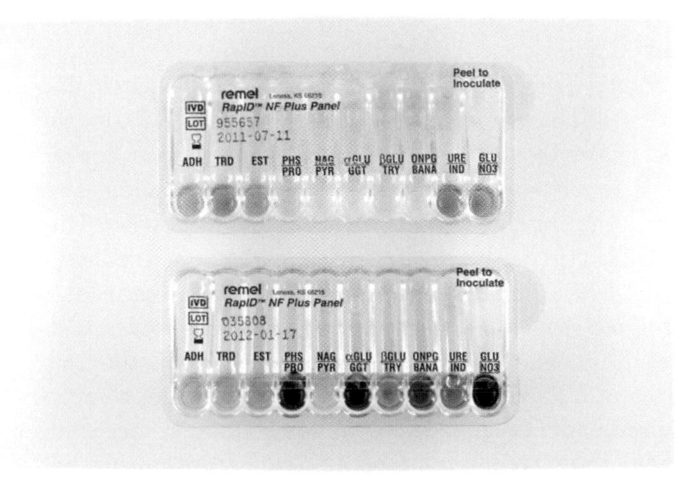

Figure 17-12 Identification of *Stenotrophomonas maltophilia* by the RapID NF Plus system. In this figure, *p*-nitrophenyl-phosphoester (PHS) and *p*-nitrophenyl-β-D-glucoside (βGLU) are positive in the top panel and proline-β-naphthylamide (PRO), γ-glutamyl-β-naphthylamide (GGT), *N*-benzoylarginine-β-naphthylamide (BANA), and sodium nitrate (NO_3) in the bottom panel, confirming the identification of *S. maltophilia*.

Acinetobacter, *Chryseobacterium*, *Moraxella*, *Methylobacterium*, and Other Nonfermentative Gram-Negative Bacilli

18

The organisms described in this chapter form a diverse group of nonfermentative, catalase-positive, gram-negative bacilli and coccobacilli. They can be divided into five groups based upon oxidase, indole, and trypsin reactions and pigment production (Table 18-1). A majority of these organisms grow at 35°C in an aerobic environment, although some species grow best at <30°C and some will not grow anaerobically. Most of these nonfermenters are found in soil; water, including tap water; and the environment. Clinically they are considered opportunistic pathogens, with the exception of *Elizabethkingia meningoseptica*, *Moraxella lacunata*, and *Moraxella catarrhalis*.

The genus *Acinetobacter* consists of 21 named species and 11 unnamed species. Of these, 14 are of clinical importance. *Acinetobacter* spp. can cause infections involving wounds, including catheter sites, and the respiratory and urinary tracts. Risk factors for infection include the use of respiratory care equipment, antimicrobial therapy, extended stay in an intensive care unit, and surgery. These organisms are small, gram-negative coccobacilli, measuring 1 to 1.5 μm by 1.5 to 2.5 μm, and occur singly and in pairs. On Gram stain, their appearance is very similar to that of *Neisseria* spp. Colonies are smooth, opaque, and grayish white to yellowish. They are oxidase-negative, nitrate-negative, nonmotile organisms. They are the second-most-common nonfermenters isolated from clinical specimens, after *Pseudomonas aeruginosa*. *Acinetobacter* spp. are usually nonpathogenic; however, they can cause infections in immunocompromised patients. The most commonly isolated species are *Acinetobacter baumannii*, *Acinetobacter lwoffii*, and *Acinetobacter haemolyticus*. *A. baumannii* strains are the glucose-oxidizing, nonhemolytic strains; *A. lwoffii* strains are the glucose-nonoxidizing, nonhemolytic strains; and *A. haemolyticus* strains are the glucose-nonoxidizing, hemolytic strains. Over time, *Acinetobacter* spp. have developed resistance to multiple antimicrobial agents.

Moraxella spp. are small, plump, gram-negative coccobacilli that occur in pairs and short chains. On Gram stain, they also resemble *Neisseria* spp. *Moraxella* spp. are oxidase positive, nonmotile, indole negative, and asaccharolytic. The species isolated from clinical specimens are *Moraxella nonliquifaciens*, *M. lacunata*, *M. catarrhalis*, *Moraxella osloensis*, and *Moraxella lincolnii*. Most species do not grow on MacConkey agar. Colonies on primary isolation media are small, measuring approximately 0.5 mm in diameter after a 24-h incubation and up to 1.0 mm in diameter after a 48-h incubation. Colonies of *M. catarrhalis* are slightly larger than other *Moraxella* spp. and can easily be pushed around the plate with a loop. Colonies of *M. lacunata* and *M. nonliquifaciens* tend to pit the agar, and *M. nonliquifaciens* may also spread. *M. lacunata* is the only proteolytic species with gelatin activity. Tween 80 esterase activity is a rapid test to differentiate it from other *Moraxella* spp.

The genus *Oligella* consists of two species, *Oligella urealytica* (formerly CDC group IVe) and *Oligella urethralis* (formerly *Moraxella urethralis* and CDC group M-4). Both species have been isolated from the urinary tract and cause urosepsis. *O. urealytica* grows slowly on blood agar, resulting in pinpoint colonies after 24 h;

Table 18-1 Nonfermentative, gram-negative bacilli

Oxidase-negative	Oxidase-positive, indole-negative, trypsin-negative	Oxidase-positive, indole-negative, trypsin-positive	Oxidase-positive, indole-positive	Pink-pigmented
Acinetobacter	*Haematobacter*	*Alishewanella*	*Balneatrix*	*Asaia*
Granulibacter	*Moraxella*	*Inquilinus*	*Bergeyella*	*Azospirillum*
	Oligella	*Myroides*	*Chryseobacterium*	*Methylobacterium*
	Paracoccus	*Ochrobactrum*	*Elizabethkingia*	*Roseomonas*
	Psychrobacter	*Pannonibacter*	*Empedobacter*	
		Rhizobium	*Flavobacterium*	
		Shewanella	*Wautersiella*	
		Sphingobacterium	*Weeksella*	
		Sphingomonas		

however, large colonies develop after 3 days of incubation. A key characteristic of this organism is that it hydrolyzes urea within a few minutes after inoculation onto a urea-containing medium. *O. urethralis* is similar to *M. osloensis* both in colonial morphology and biochemically. They can be differentiated based on nitrate reduction and phenylalanine deaminase. *O. urethralis* reduces nitrate and has a weakly positive phenylalanine deaminase reaction, while *M. osloensis* is negative for both.

The genus *Psychrobacter* includes more than 30 species; however, only a few are of clinical importance. A majority of clinical isolates belong to *Psychrobacter phenylpyruvicus* (formerly *Moraxella phenylpyruvica*), *Psychrobacter faecalis*, and *Psychrobacter pulmonis*. The latter two species were previously classified as *Psychrobacter immobilis* and are uncommon causes of infection. *P. phenylpyruvicus* is similar to the moraxellae both microscopically and on culture, except that it is urease and phenylalanine deaminase positive. Colonies on Trypticase soy agar with 1% Tween 80 are at least double in size compared with those grown on sheep blood agar.

Infections due to *Myroides* spp. are rare, although the organisms have been isolated from a variety of clinical specimens. *Myroides* spp., formerly classified as *Flavobacterium* spp., are small, gram-negative bacilli, measuring 0.5 μm by 1.0 to 2.0 μm. Colonies on blood agar have a yellow pigment and tend to spread on the surface of the agar, similar to *Bacillus* spp. They also produce a fruity odor, similar to *Alcaligenes faecalis*. *Myroides* spp. grow on MacConkey agar and are oxidase, urease, and gelatinase positive and indole negative. Nitrate is negative, but nitrite is reduced to nitrogen gas. There are two species in this genus, *Myroides odoratus* and *Myroides odoratimimus*. Both species were previously classified as *Flavobacterium odoratum*.

Rhizobium radiobacter (formerly *Agrobacterium radiobacter*) is a small to medium-size, gram-negative bacillus, measuring 0.6 to 1.0 μm by 1.5 to 3.0 μm. It grows on routine laboratory media at 35°C aerobically, but optimal growth occurs at 25 to 28°C. After a 48-h incubation, colonies on blood agar are approximately 2 mm in diameter, round, smooth, and nonpigmented to buff colored. Colonies are pink on MacConkey agar and can become mucoid after prolonged incubation. *R. radiobacter* is motile, and the reactions for urease, phenylalanine deaminase, and esculin are positive. It also oxidizes glucose, maltose, sucrose, mannitol, and xylose. These reactions distinguish it from other, closely related organisms. *R. radiobacter* has been isolated most frequently from blood, and the source is usually contaminated indwelling catheters or implanted prostheses.

Sphingomonas paucimobilis (formerly *Pseudomonas paucimobilis*) and *Sphingomonas parapaucimobilis* are the only clinically significant species in the genus *Sphingomonas*. They are widely distributed in nature, including the hospital environment, and have been isolated from a variety of clinical specimens. Microscopically, by Gram stain, the organisms are long, slender, gram-negative bacilli, resembling *Pseudomonas* spp. They are motile by polar flagella at 18 to 22°C but nonmotile at 37°C. Colonies on blood agar are approximately 2 mm in diameter and produce a strong yellow pigment when incubated at 30°C. They are oxidase, O-nitrophenyl-β-D-galactopyranoside, and esculin positive. They also oxidize glucose, maltose, sucrose, and xylose. Since the two species are difficult to distinguish biochemically, it is recommended that they be reported as *Sphingomonas* spp.

The genus *Sphingobacterium* consists of two species that have been isolated from clinical specimens: *Sphingobacterium multivorum* and *Sphingobacterium spiritivorum*. They are nonmotile bacilli that produce yellowish colonies. Both species are indole negative and urease positive and oxidize glucose and xylose; however, only *S. spiritivorum* oxidizes mannitol. Of the two species, *S. multivorum* is more frequently isolated and from a variety of clinical specimens. *S. spiritivorum* is usually recovered from blood and urine.

The genus *Shewanella* consists of two species, *Shewanella putrefaciens* (formerly *Pseudomonas putrefaciens*, *Alteromonas putrefaciens*, *Achromobacter putrefaciens*, and CDC group Ib) and *Shewanella algae*. They have been isolated from a wide variety of clinical specimens and are associated with many types of infections. *Shewanella* spp. are oxidase-positive, indole-negative, gram-negative bacilli that are motile by a single polar flagellum. Colonies on blood agar are round and smooth, measuring approximately 2 to 3 mm in diameter, with a brown to tan-colored pigment and greenish discoloration of the medium. *Shewanella* spp. are nitrate, alkaline phosphatase, trypsin, and ornithine decarboxylase positive. A distinguishing characteristic is the production of H_2S in either Kligler iron or triple sugar iron (TSI) agar slants. *S. algae* is very similar to *S. putrefaciens*, except that it is halophilic, requires NaCl for growth, and does not oxidize maltose or sucrose.

Four named *Chryseobacterium* spp. have been isolated from clinical specimens: *Chryseobacterium indologenes* and *Chryseobacterium gleum* (both formerly CDC group IIb), *Chryseobacterium anthropi* (formerly CDC group IIe), and *Chryseobacterium hominis* (formerly CDC group IIc). Microscopically, they are gram-negative bacilli that are thinner in the center than at the ends and can also appear as filamentous forms. *Chryseobacterium* spp. are nonmotile and catalase-, oxidase-, and indole-positive organisms. Most strains of *C. indologenes* and *C. gleum* produce flexirubin, a water-soluble pigment, and are esculin and gelatin hydrolysis positive. Colonies of *C. indologenes* are beta-hemolytic after 3 days of incubation, and they will not grow at 42°C. In contrast, *C. gleum* is alpha-hemolytic and grows at 42°C. Colonies of *C. anthropi* are very sticky and are usually nonpigmented but may develop a salmon pinkish color after a few days. Colonies of *C. hominis* are usually mucoid, and some strains produce a pale yellow pigment. Although *C. indologenes* is the most common species isolated from clinical specimens, its clinical significance is rare.

E. meningoseptica, formerly *Chryseobacterium meningosepticum*, has been associated with neonatal meningitis, endocarditis, and a variety of other infections including nosocomial infections associated with dialysis. Colonies are large and either nonpigmented or produce a pale yellow or salmon pinkish pigment after 2 to 3 days of incubation. *E. meningoseptica* is mannitol, *o*-nitrophenyl-β-D-galactopyranoside, gelatin, and esculin positive.

Methylobacterium spp. are pink nonfermenters, whose name is derived from their ability to utilize methanol as the sole carbon source. *Methylobacterium mesophilicum* and *Methylobacterium zatmanii* are the species found in clinical specimens and are nosocomial organisms that have been associated with a wide variety of infections, including septicemia and peritoneal dialysis-associated peritonitis. On Gram stain, the organisms appear as large, vacuolated, pleomorphic, gram-negative bacilli that stain poorly and may not be easily decolorized. These organisms are very slow growing, requiring 4 to 5 days before colonies can be visualized. The colonies are dry and appear pink or coral, measuring approximately 1 mm in diameter, on agar media. *Methylobacterium* spp. do not grow on MacConkey agar. Optimal growth occurs between 25 and 30°C. These organisms are oxidase positive and hydrolyze urea and starch.

Roseomonas is also a pink-pigmented nonfermenter. The following have been isolated from clinical specimens: *Roseomonas gilardi* subsp. *gilardi*, *R. gilardi* subsp. *rosea*, *Roseomonas mucosa*, *Roseomonas cervicalis*, *Roseomonas* genomospecies 4, and *Roseomonas* genomospecies 5. *Roseomonas* spp. have been associated with infections in immunocompromised individuals. A majority of infections are from blood; however, these organisms have also been isolated from wounds, abscesses, and urogenital sites. Microscopically, isolates are plump, nonvacuolated, gram-negative bacilli, occurring in pairs and short chains. Although they grow on a variety of laboratory media including MacConkey agar, optimal growth occurs on Sabouraud agar. Colonies are large, pink, mucoid, and runny, measuring up to 6 mm in diameter. *R. cervicalis* is strongly oxidase positive, whereas the other species are weakly oxidase positive or oxidase negative. They all hydrolyze starch and urea.

Key characteristics of the genera discussed in this chapter are listed in Table 18-2.

Table 18-2 Differentiating characteristics of miscellaneous nonfermentative, gram-negative bacilli[a]

Genus	Oxidase	Nitrate	Pigment	Motility	Growth on MacConkey agar	Indole
Acinetobacter	0	0	0	0	+	0
Chryseobacterium	+	V	Yellow	0	V	+
Elizabethkingia	+	+	V	0	+	+
Methylobacterium[b]	0	0	Coral pink	+	0	0
Moraxella	+	V	0	0	Scant, 0	0
Myroides	+	+, gas	Yellow	0	V	0
Oligella	+	+	0	V	V	0
Psychrobacter	+	V	0	0	+	0
Rhizobium	+	V	V, pale yellow	+	+	0
Roseomonas[b]	Weak, 0	0[c]	Pink	+	+	
Shewanella	+	+	Brown-tan	+	+	0
Sphingobacterium	+	0	Yellowish	0	V	0
Sphingomonas	+	0	Yellow	+	0	0

[a]+, positive reaction (≥90% positive); V, variable reaction (11 to 89% positive); 0, negative reaction (≤10% positive).
[b]Grows best on Sabouraud agar.
[c]*Roseomonas* genomospecies 4 is nitrate positive.

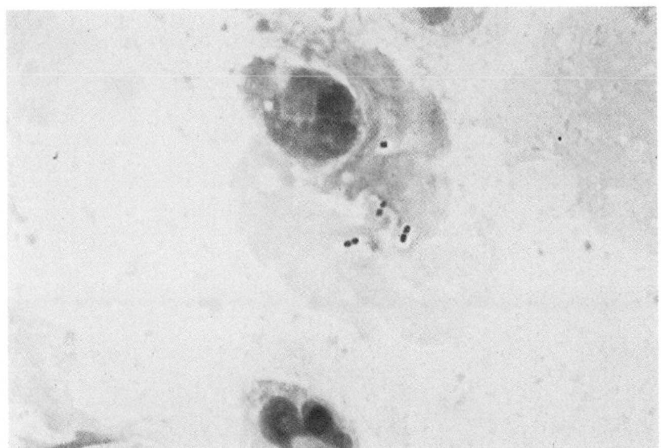

Figure 18-1 Gram stain of *Acinetobacter* spp. Shown is a Gram stain of a sputum specimen containing intracellular, small, gram-negative coccobacilli, measuring 1.0 by 1.5 μm, occurring singly and in pairs, and resembling *Neisseria* spp. This organism was identified as *Acinetobacter baumannii.*

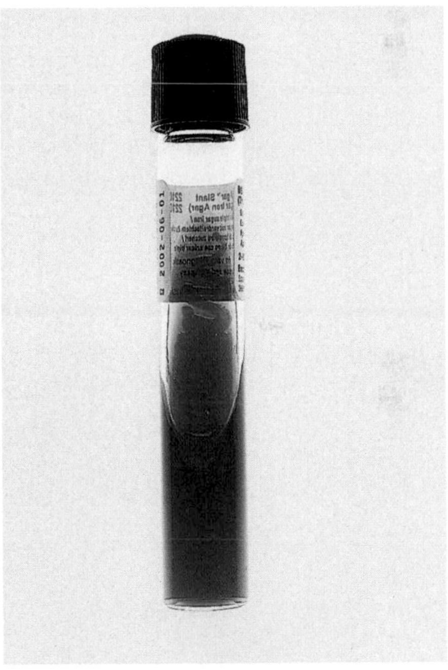

Figure 18-2 TSI agar slant inoculated with a nonfermenter. Most nonfermenters grow on the surface of a TSI agar slant, resulting in an alkaline reaction, as shown here. There is no color change in the butt of the medium because these organisms do not ferment carbohydrates. This is a typical reaction of most nonfermenters on a TSI agar slant.

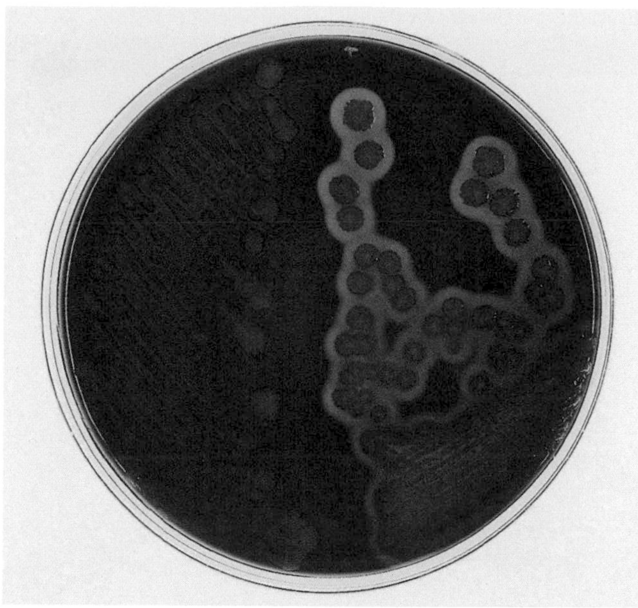

Figure 18-3 ***Acinetobacter baumannii*** **and** ***Acinetobacter haemolyticus*** **on blood agar.** After 48 h of growth on blood agar, colonies of *A. baumannii* (left) measure approximately 1.5 mm in diameter and are translucent to opaque, convex, entire, nonhemolytic, and nonpigmented. Colonies of *A. haemolyticus* (right) appear very similar to those of *A. baumannii*; however, they are surrounded by a wide zone of beta-hemolysis.

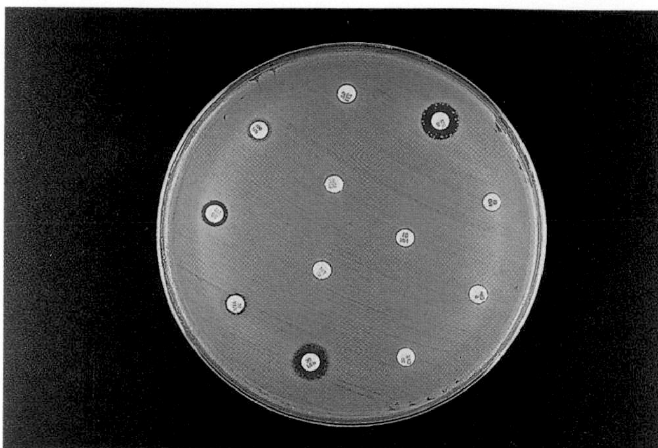

Figure 18-4 Antimicrobial susceptibility testing of ***Acinetobacter*** **spp. by the disk diffusion method.** *Acinetobacter* spp. are resistant to multiple antimicrobial agents. In this example, antimicrobial susceptibility testing of *Acinetobacter* spp. was performed on a Mueller-Hinton agar plate by the disk diffusion method. As expected, this *Acinetobacter* isolate was resistant to the antimicrobials tested.

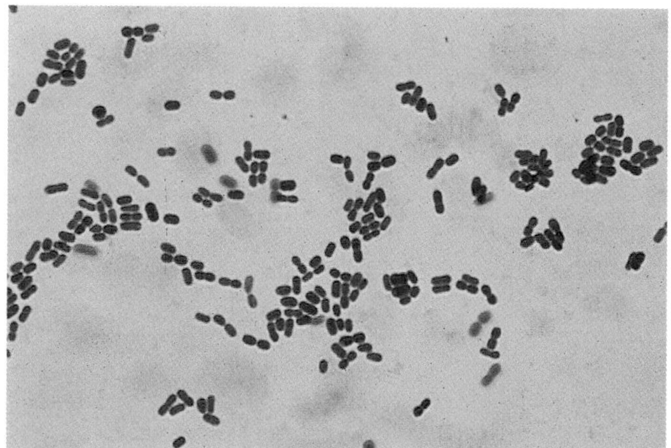

Figure 18-5 Gram stain of ***Moraxella*** **spp.** *Moraxella* spp. appear as gram-negative coccobacilli that occur in pairs and short chains, measuring 1.0 to 1.5 μm by 1.5 to 2.5 μm. Although the organisms in this figure are clearly gram negative, some strains resist decoloration and appear gram variable. Cells may be capsulated and pleomorphic when deprived of oxygen.

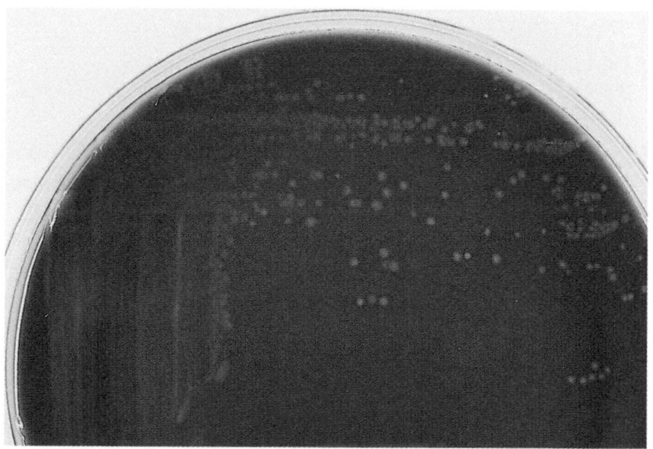

Figure 18-6 ***Moraxella lacunata*** **on chocolate agar incubated for 48 h.** Colonies of *M. lacunata* on chocolate agar are small, measuring 0.5 to 1 mm in diameter, and have a greenish hue. Occasionally these colonies spread and pit the agar after prolonged incubation.

Figure 18-7 *Psychrobacter phenylpyruvicus* on blood agar. Colonies of *P. phenylpyruvicus* on blood agar are small, pinpoint, smooth, translucent, and tan, measuring 0.5 mm in diameter.

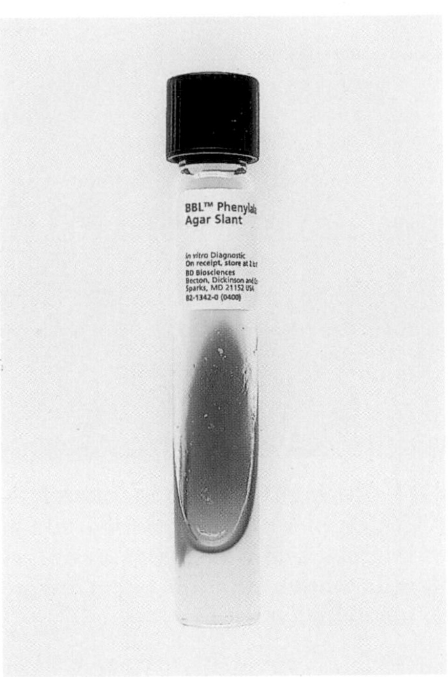

Figure 18-8 *Psychrobacter phenylpyruvicus* on a phenylalanine agar slant. The phenylalanine deaminase test is used to determine the ability of an organism to oxidatively deaminate phenylalanine to phenyl pyruvic acid. On addition of a few drops of 10% ferric chloride, a green color is formed between the two compounds. *P. phenylpyruvicus* produces the enzyme phenylalanine deaminase, resulting in a positive test, as shown here. This reaction differentiates *P. phenylpyruvicus* from most other oxidase-positive, indole-negative coccobacillary nonfermenters.

Figure 18-9 *Myroides* spp. (formerly *Flavobacterium odoratum*) on blood agar. Colonies of *Myroides* spp. grown on blood agar are small, translucent, smooth, shiny, convex, and circular, measuring 0.5 to 1.0 mm in diameter. The colonies have a slight yellow pigment and tend to spread, as shown in this figure; however, nonpigmented strains do occur. Colonies produce a characteristic fruity odor.

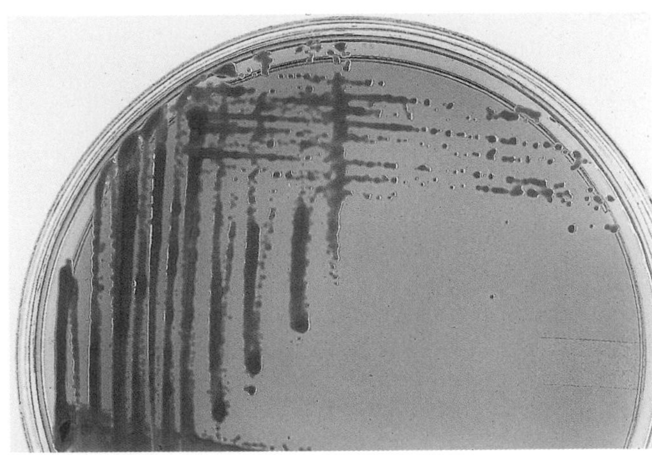

Figure 18-10 *Rhizobium radiobacter* on MacConkey agar. Colonies of *R. radiobacter* on MacConkey agar are small (0.5 to 1.0 mm), convex, circular, smooth, pink, wet, and mucoid after a 48-h incubation at 35°C.

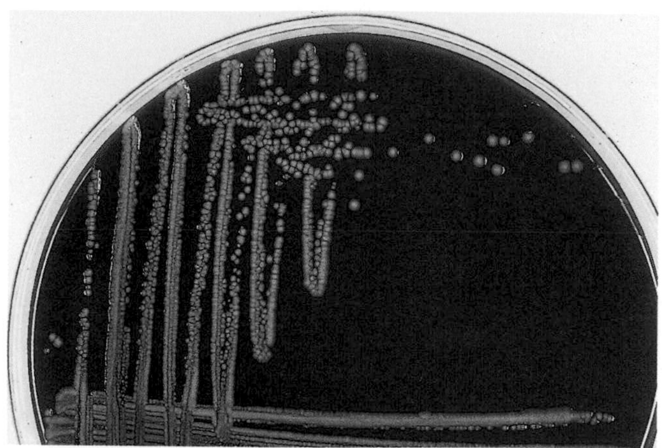

Figure 18-11 ***Sphingomonas paucimobilis*** **on blood agar at 30°C.** Colonies of *S. paucimobilis* on blood agar are approximately 2 mm in diameter and produce a strong yellow, insoluble, nonfluorescent, carotenoid pigment when incubated at 30°C.

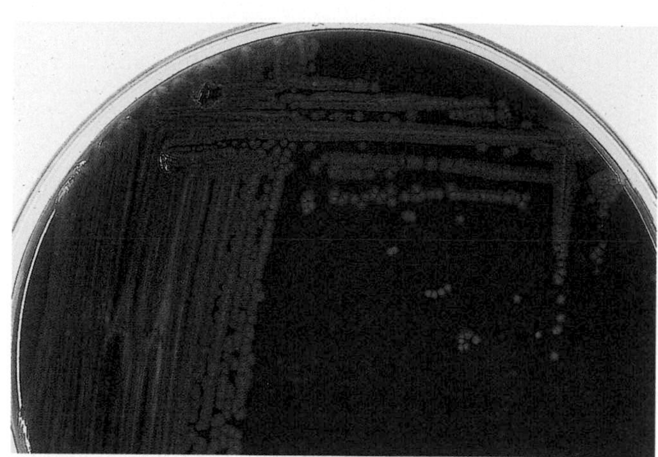

Figure 18-12 ***Shewanella putrefaciens*** **on blood agar.** Colonies of *S. putrefaciens* on blood agar are round and smooth, measuring approximately 2 to 3 mm in diameter, with a tan pigment and a greenish discoloration of the medium.

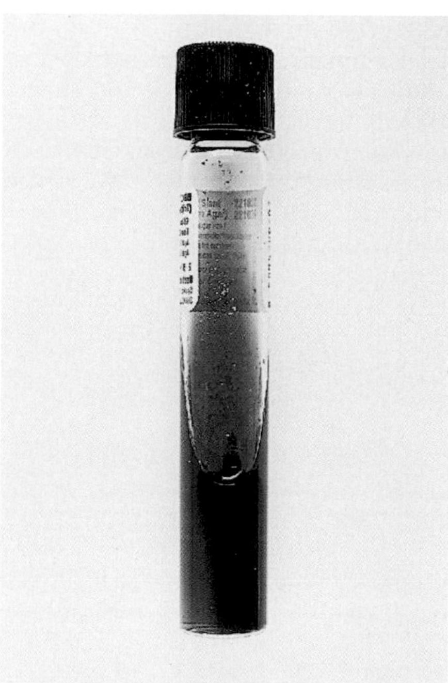

Figure 18-13 ***Shewanella putrefaciens*** **on a TSI agar slant.** A distinguishing characteristic of *Shewanella* spp. is the production of H_2S. *S. putrefaciens* is the only nonfermenter that produces large amounts of H_2S on a TSI agar slant (shown here) or a Kligler iron agar slant.

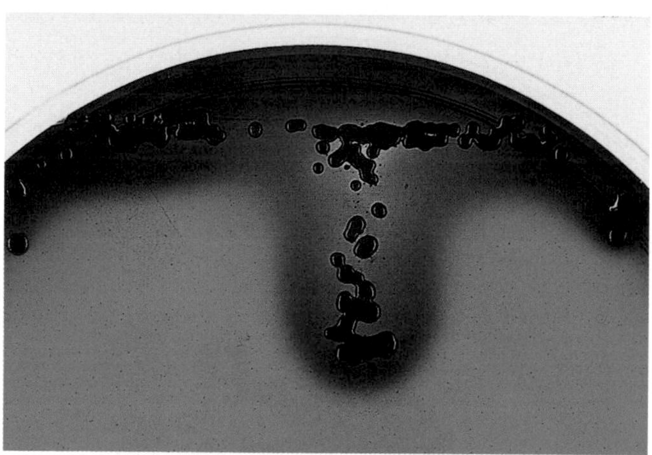

Figure 18-14 ***Shewanella putrefaciens*** **on DNase agar.** *S. putrefaciens* produces the enzyme DNase, which hydrolyzes DNA. The DNase test medium contains toluidine blue complexed with DNA. Hydrolysis of DNA causes changes in the structure of the dye to yield a pink color surrounding the colonies.

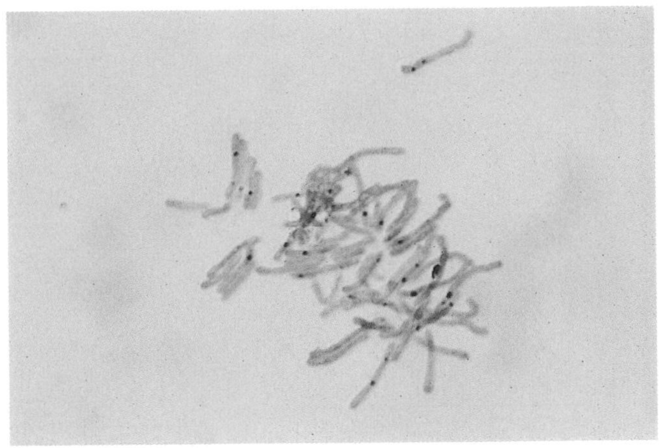

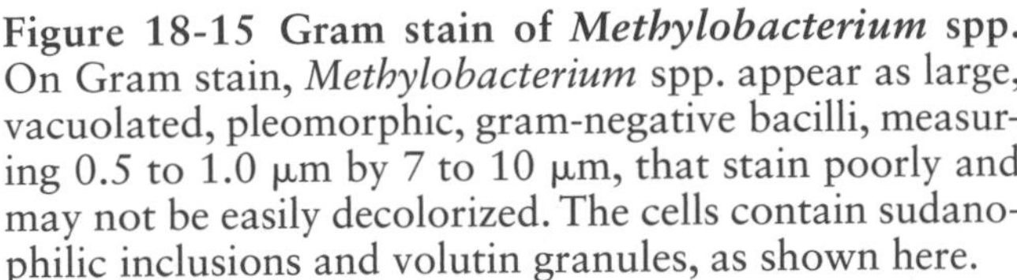

Figure 18-15 Gram stain of *Methylobacterium* spp. On Gram stain, *Methylobacterium* spp. appear as large, vacuolated, pleomorphic, gram-negative bacilli, measuring 0.5 to 1.0 μm by 7 to 10 μm, that stain poorly and may not be easily decolorized. The cells contain sudanophilic inclusions and volutin granules, as shown here.

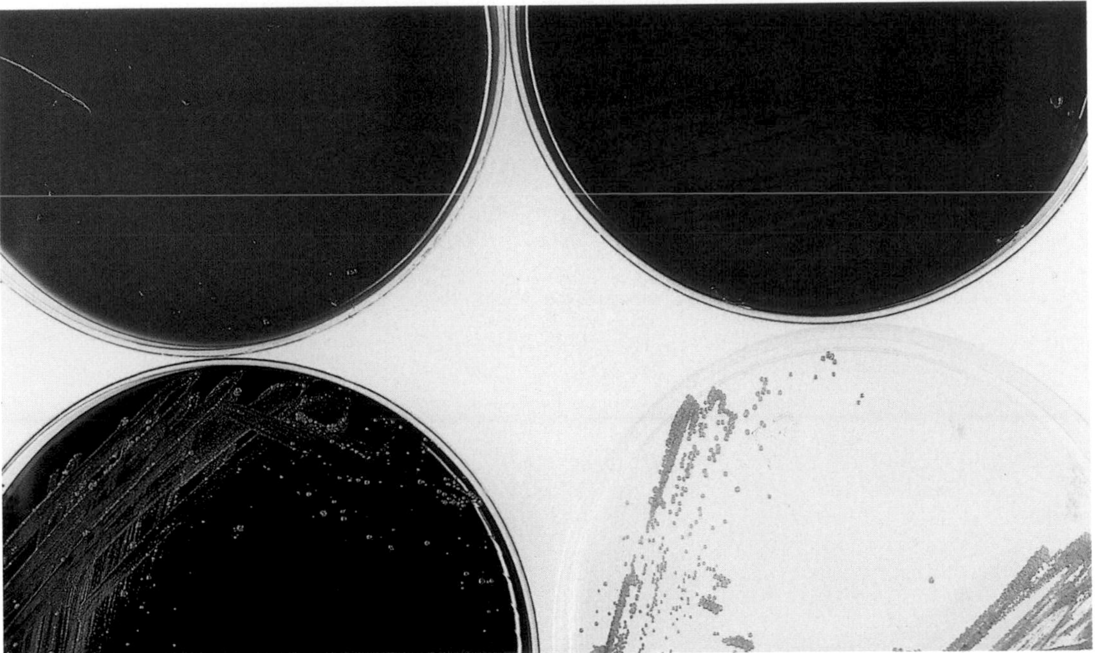

Figure 18-16 *Methylobacterium* spp. on blood agar, modified Thayer-Martin agar, Sabouraud agar, and buffered charcoal-yeast extract. Isolates of *Methylobacterium* spp. are slow growing on routine laboratory media, producing 1-mm-diameter pink colonies after incubation for 4 to 5 days. Some strains do not grow on nutrient agar. Here, the organism was inoculated onto modified Thayer-Martin agar (top left), blood agar (top right), Sabouraud agar (bottom right), and buffered charcoal-yeast extract agar (bottom left). The best growth occurred on Sabouraud agar. The optimal temperature for growth of *Methylobacterium* spp. is between 25 and 30°C.

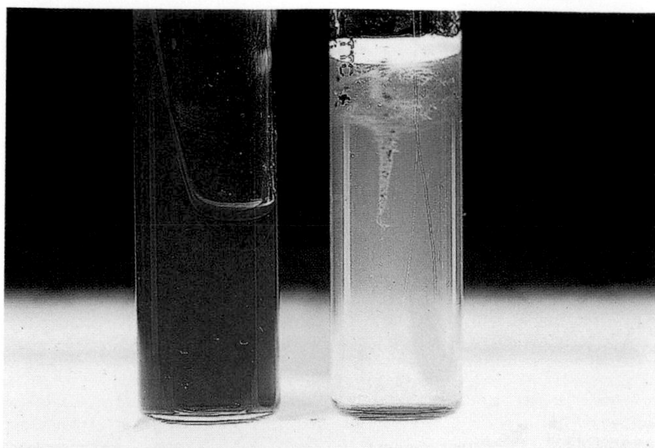

Figure 18-17 *Methylobacterium* spp. on a urea agar slant and in motility medium. *Methylobacterium* spp. are urease positive, causing the urea agar to become bright pink (left tube). They are also motile by a single polar or lateral flagellum, although motility is difficult to demonstrate. Here (right tube), the organism appears to be growing away from the stab line in the motility medium, confirming that it is a motile organism.

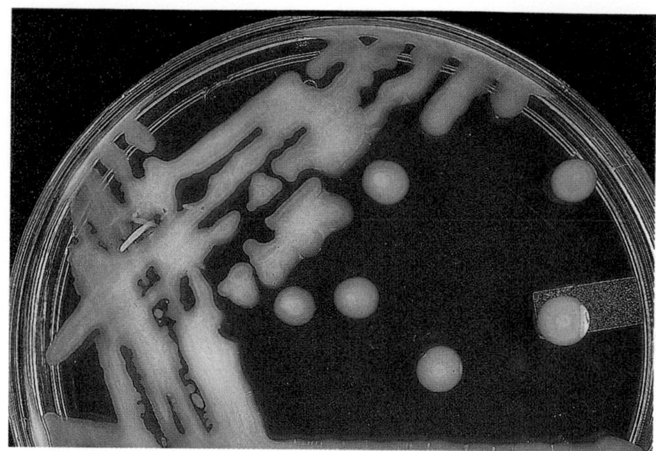

Figure 18-18 *Roseomonas* spp. on Sabouraud agar incubated at 35°C. Colonies of *Roseomonas* spp. on Sabouraud agar are large, pink, mucoid, and runny and measure approximately 6 mm in diameter. Although they are pink nonfermenters like *Methylobacterium* spp. (Fig. 18-16), their colony morphologies are very different. *Roseomonas* spp. grow on a variety of laboratory media including MacConkey agar, whereas *Methylobacterium* spp. do not grow on MacConkey agar.

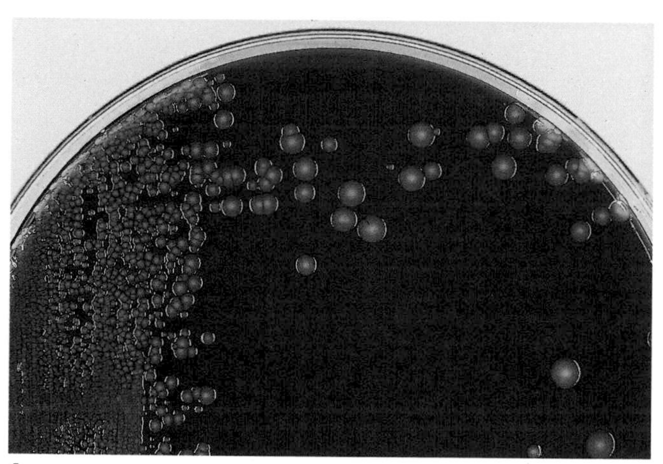

A

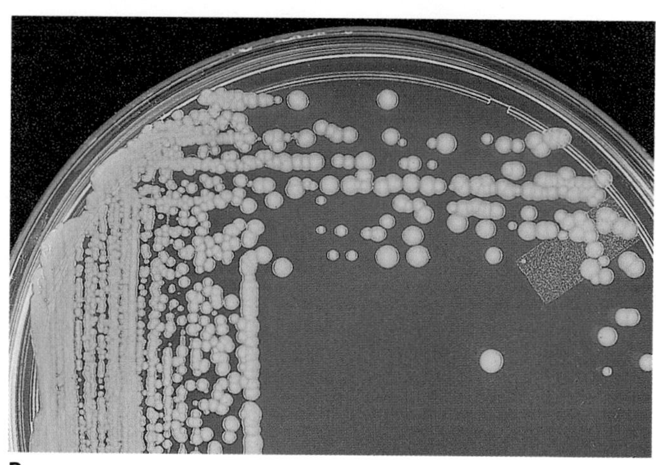

B

Figure 18-19 Colonies of *Chryseobacterium indologenes* on blood agar (A) and Mueller-Hinton agar (B). Colonies of *C. indologenes* are deep yellow due to the production of flexirubin.

Actinobacillus, Aggregatibacter, Capnocytophaga, Eikenella, Kingella, and Other Fastidious or Rarely Encountered Gram-Negative Bacilli

19

The organisms described in this chapter are termed fastidious because most do not grow well on routine laboratory media; they require special atmospheric conditions and prolonged incubation for growth. They include *Actinobacillus*, *Aggregatibacter*, *Capnocytophaga*, *Cardiobacterium*, *Dysgonomonas*, *Eikenella*, *Kingella*, *Suttonella*, *Chromobacterium*, and *Streptobacillus*. With a few exceptions, these organisms are members of the normal flora of the oral cavity. This group can cause endocarditis, particularly in immunocompromised patients. Five of these genera—*Actinobacillus*, *Aggregatibacter*, *Cardiobacterium*, *Eikenella*, and *Kingella*—belong to the HACEK group of bacteria, whose other member is *Haemophilus*. Microscopically, these gram-negative bacilli vary in size and shape from coccoid forms to long fusiform rods that can be straight or curved. The colony morphology varies on agar media from tiny to large to colonies that pit the agar or spread across the agar surface. Most of the HACEK bacteria require 2 to 4 days for growth at 35 to 37°C under either 5 to 10% CO_2 or a microaerophilic atmosphere (candle jar), with increased moisture.

The genus *Actinobacillus* is classified in the family *Pasteurellaceae*. The most common species of this genus associated with disease in humans was *Actinobacillus actinomycetemcomitans*; however, this organism is now classified in the genus *Aggregatibacter*. Other *Actinobacillus* spp. also cause infections in humans; however, they are usually associated with animal bites or contact with animals. These include *Actinobacillus hominis*, *Actinobacillus lignieresii*, *Actinobacillus equuli*, *Actinobacillus minor*, *Actinobacillus muris*, *Actinobacillus pleuropneumoniae*, *Actinobacillus suis*, and *Actinobacillus ureae*. These organisms usually cause disease following trauma or localized injury to otherwise healthy tissue. The most susceptible hosts are immunocompromised and elderly individuals and those with recent viral infections. On Gram stain, *Actinobacillus* spp. appear as small, oval coccobacilli. Most *Actinobacillus* spp. grow on chocolate and blood agars as pinpoint to small colonies, measuring 0.5 to 2 mm in diameter, and are grayish white, adherent, and nonhemolytic, requiring 48 h before visible growth is detected. *A. ureae* may show light growth on MacConkey agar, whereas the other species do not grow on this medium. *Actinobacillus* spp. are oxidase positive and reduce nitrate, and some strains produce acid from glucose and maltose and hydrolyze urea. Acid production from carbohydrates is used along with other distinguishing characteristics to differentiate the species. For example, *A. equuli* produces H_2S when a lead acetate strip is used and is o-nitrophenyl-β-D-galactopyranoside (ONPG) positive. *A. suis* hydrolyzes esculin and is also ONPG positive.

The genus *Aggregatibacter* is in the family *Pasteurellaceae* and was recently reclassified to include the bacteria previously named *Haemophilus aphrophilus* and *Haemophilus paraphrophilus* along with *Actinobacillus actinomycetemcomitans*. Currently *Aggregatibacter* includes three species: *Aggregatibacter actinomycetemcomitans*, *Aggregatibacter aphrophilus*, and *Aggregatibacter segnis*. *A. aphrophilus* includes the organisms formerly named *H. aphrophilus* and *H. paraphrophilus*. The habitat of *Aggregatibacter* spp. is the human oral cavity, including dental plaque. *A. actinomycetemcomitans* is the most common cause of periodontal disease, a predisposing factor for infective endocarditis following dental manipulations. It can also occur with *Actinomyces* spp. in sulfur granules. *A. aphrophilus* may cause systemic disease as well as bone and joint infections. *A. segnis* may also cause endocarditis. *Aggregatibacter* spp. are gram-negative, coccoid or rod-shaped bacilli and can exhibit filamentous forms. *A. aphrophilus* and *A. segnis* require V factor for growth but not hemin (X factor). *A. actinomycetemcomitans* produces small colonies (0.5 to 3 mm in diameter) after 48 to 72 h of incubation on blood agar and, on further incubation, develops a star-like structure and pitting of the agar medium. In liquid media the colonies form granules that adhere to the sides of the tube. Colonies of *A. aphrophilus* and *A. segnis* are granular to smooth and may be grayish to yellowish. Testing for X and V factors helps to distinguish them from *Haemophilus* spp. They are not dependent on the X factor and are indole, ornithine, and urea negative.

Capnocytophaga spp. are thin, gram-negative bacilli with pointed ends, resembling *Fusobacterium* spp. They have a characteristic movement described as "gliding" motility. On blood and chocolate agars, the organism produces tiny pinpoint, yellow-orange colonies in 24 h when grown under 5 to 10% CO_2 or anaerobically, but it does not grow aerobically. The colonies pit the agar and spread or swarm due to the gliding motility. Five species are members of the normal oral flora of humans: *Capnocytophaga gingivalis*, *Capnocytophaga granulosa*, *Capnocytophaga haemolytica*, *Capnocytophaga ochracea*, and *Capnocytophaga sputigena*. The organisms have been isolated from the oral cavity, including dental pockets and subgingival plaque; respiratory secretions; wounds; and blood, particularly in patients with granulocytopenia. *Capnocytophaga* spp. isolated from humans are indole, oxidase, and catalase negative. *C. haemolytica* and *C. sputigena* reduce nitrate, and all species except *C. granulosa* hydrolyze esculin.

The genus *Dysgonomonas* belongs to a group of facultative anaerobic, nonmotile, gram-negative coccobacilli. There are four species: *Dysgonomonas capnocytophagoides*, *Dysgonomonas gadei*, *Dysgonomonas mossii*, and "Dysgonomonas hofstadii." These species have been isolated from feces, blood and other body fluids, gall bladder, and wounds. Isolates are primarily from immunocompromised hosts. Colonies are 1 to 2 mm in diameter and have a strawberry-like odor. They are catalase, nitrate, and oxidase negative and ONPG positive. *D. capnocytophagoides*, *D. gadei*, and *D. mossii* produce acid from lactose, sucrose, and xylose. If *Dysgonomonas* spp. are suspected as a cause of diarrhea, a selective medium containing cefoperazone, vancomycin, and amphotericin B is recommended for fecal cultures.

The genus *Eikenella*, in the family *Neisseriaceae*, has one species, *Eikenella corrodens*. It has been isolated from the oral cavity, including dental pockets and subgingival plaque; respiratory secretions; wounds; and blood. *E. corrodens* is frequently associated with trauma, in particular with trauma due to human bites. The organism is a thin, gram-negative bacillus, measuring 0.5 μm by 2 to 4 μm. Growth on agar media occurs after 2 to 4 days of incubation under 5% CO_2 at 35 to 37°C. The organism requires heme and therefore does not grow on MacConkey agar. Colonies are 0.2 to 0.5 mm in diameter at 24 h and 0.5 to 1.0 mm at 48 h. They appear gray when young but may become pale yellow after prolonged incubation. Most strains form small pits or corrode the surface of the agar and produce a bleach-like odor. In broth medium, the organism adheres to the side of the tube and produces granules. *E. corrodens* is oxidase and ornithine decarboxylase positive and reduces nitrate, but it is catalase negative.

The genus *Kingella* belongs to the family *Neisseriaceae*. These organisms are small, gram-negative coccobacilli, measuring 0.5 to 1.0 μm by 2 to 3 μm. *Kingella* spp. occur in pairs and short chains resembling *Neisseria* spp. There are four species of *Kingella*: *Kingella kingae*, *Kingella oralis*, *Kingella potus*, and *Kingella denitrificans*. *Kingella* spp. are part of the normal flora of the respiratory tract of humans. As mentioned above, *Kingella* spp. are members of the HACEK group and two species, *K. kingae* and *K. denitrificans*, cause endocarditis. *K. kingae* has also been associated with osteomyelitis, septic arthritis, and septicemia, and *K. oralis* has been isolated from dental plaque, but its role in disease is unknown. *K. kingae* osteomyelitis and arthritis are most often found in infants and young children (younger than 6 years). *Kingella* spp. grow on blood and chocolate agars after 2 to 4 days of incubation under 5% CO_2. Colonies of *K. kingae* are beta-hemolytic, while the others are not. They are oxidase positive and catalase negative. *K. denitrificans* reduces nitrate, but the other *Kingella* spp. do not. *K. kingae* produces acid in both glucose and maltose after prolonged incubation, while the other *Kingella* spp. produce acid in glucose alone. *K. denitrificans* may grow on Thayer-Martin medium and may be misidentified as *Neisseria gonorrhoeae*. They differ based on their catalase reaction: *K. denitrificans* is catalase negative and *N. gonorrhoeae* is catalase positive. CDC group EF-4a is closely related to *Kingella* spp.; however, it is now classified in the genus *Neisseria*.

The genus *Cardiobacterium* has two species: *Cardiobacterium hominis* and *Cardiobacterium valvarum*. *C. hominis* is pathogenic, causing endocarditis. It is a gram-negative bacillus, measuring 1.0 μm by 2.0 to 4.0 μm. The cells of *C. hominis* have a characteristic appearance on Gram stain; they are pleomorphic bacilli with swollen ends arranged in rosette clusters. Colonies of *C. hominis* grow on blood and chocolate agars as pale yellow to white colonies, measuring 1 mm, after 2 to 4 days of incubation at 36°C in a microaerophilic atmosphere. Like other fastidious gram-negative bacilli, they do not grow on MacConkey agar.

The genus *Suttonella* is a member of the family *Cardiobacteriaceae*, and *Suttonella indologenes* is the only species. It is a plump, gram-negative bacillus measuring 3 μm in length, which may appear in pairs, chains, and rosette formations. These organisms can appear gram variable because they tend to resist decolorization, similar to *Kingella* and *Cardiobacterium*. The colonies grow slowly on blood agar and may spread or pit the agar, similar to those of *C. hominis*, except that *S. indologenes* colonies are gray and translucent. Both organisms are oxidase and indole positive and produce acid from glucose and sucrose. *S. indologenes* can be differentiated from *C. hominis* by its positive alkaline phosphatase reaction.

Chromobacterium violaceum is the only species in this genus that has been isolated from clinical specimens; it is associated with disease in humans mainly in tropical and subtropical climates. The infection site is usually a cutaneous lesion that becomes contaminated with soil and water. Diarrhea, urinary tract infection, and disseminated infection have also been reported, with a high mortality rate reported for disseminated infections. *C. violaceum* is a curved or straight, gram-negative bacillus, measuring 1.5 to 3.5 μm in length and occurring singly and in pairs and short chains. Colonies are smooth and round, measuring 3 mm in diameter, with a deep violet pigment called violacin. This pigment may interfere with the oxidase reaction. Nonpigmented colonies may appear on the same medium with the pigmented ones. This organism also grows on MacConkey agar. Its characteristic violet pigment aids in its identification, along with positive urea, indole, and arginine dihydrolase tests. Most strains are oxidase positive and produce acid from glucose.

The genus *Streptobacillus* consists of one species, *Streptobacillus moniliformis*. *S. moniliformis* is normally found in the upper respiratory tract of rats and is the cause of streptobacillary rat bite fever. When the organism is acquired by ingestion of water or milk, it is called Haverhill fever or epidemic arthritic erythema. Complications can result in more serious infections such as endocarditis, septic arthritis, pneumonia, pancreatitis, and prostatitis. An interesting feature of the organism is that it can spontaneously develop L forms in culture. Organisms have been isolated from blood and from aspirates from various sites, including lymph nodes. *S. moniliformis* is inhibited by sodium polyanethol sulfonate at concentrations present in commercially available blood culture media. Specimens should be mixed with equal volumes of 2.5% sodium citrate to prevent clotting, inoculated into media without sodium polyanethol sulfonate, and stained with either Gram or Giemsa stain. Cells of *S. moniliformis* are pleomorphic, gram-negative bacilli with areas of swelling, usually measuring 0.3 to 0.5 μm by 1.0 to 5.0 μm, although extremely long filaments can be observed. *S. moniliformis* requires the presence of blood, serum, or ascitic fluid for growth. It grows on blood agar incubated in a very moist environment with 5 to 10% CO_2. In broth medium, the organism grows toward the bottom of the tube and can have a bread crumb or cotton ball appearance. Colonies on supplemented agar medium are 1 to 2 mm in diameter, smooth, glistening, and colorless to gray with irregular edges, and they may exhibit a fried-egg appearance like *Mycoplasma*. *S. moniliformis* is oxidase, catalase, and indole negative and does not reduce nitrate; however, it hydrolyzes arginine and produces weak acid from glucose and maltose.

Key characteristics of the genera discussed in this chapter are listed in Table 19-1.

Table 19-1 Differentiating characteristics of *Actinobacillus*, *Aggregatibacter*, *Capnocytophaga*, *Cardiobacterium*, *Chromobacterium*, *Dysgonomonas*, *Eikenella*, *Kingella*, *Streptobacillus*, and *Suttonella*[a]

Organism	Indole	Oxidase	Catalase	Nitrate	Growth on MacConkey agar	Urea	Esculin hydrolysis	Glucose	Sucrose
Actinobacillus	0	+	V	+	V	+	V	+	+
Aggregatibacter	0	V	V	+	0[b]	0	0	V	V[c]
Capnocytophaga	0	V	V	0	0	0	V	+	+
Cardiobacterium	+	+	0	0	0	0	0	+	+
Chromobacterium	V	V	+	+	+	V	0	+	V
Dysgonomonas	V	0	0	0	0	0	V	+	+
Eikenella	0	+	0	+	0	0	0	0	0
Kingella	0	+	0	V	0	0	0	+	0
Streptobacillus	0	0	0	0	0	0	V	+	0
Suttonella	+	+	V	0	V	0	0	+	+

[a]+, positive reaction (≥90% positive); V, variable reaction (11 to 89% positive); 0, negative reaction (≤10% positive).
[b]*A. aphrophilus* may grow on MacConkey with a weak reaction.
[c]*A. actinomycetemcomitans* is sucrose negative.

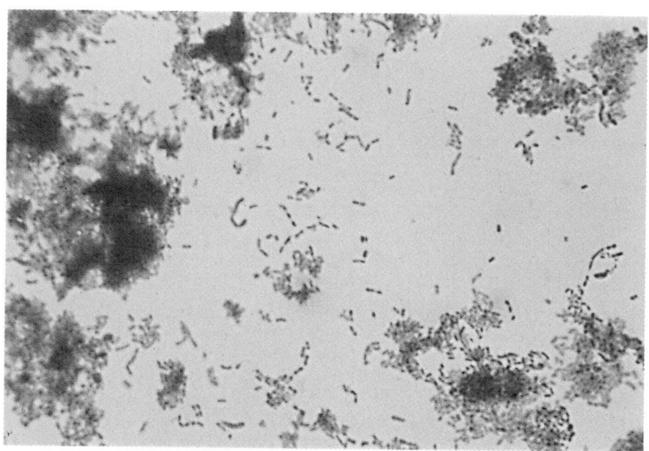

Figure 19-1 Gram stain of *Aggregatibacter actinomycetemcomitans*. *A. actinomycetemcomitans* organisms appear as small, gram-negative coccobacilli, measuring 0.5 by 1.0 μm. They can become elongated (up to 6 μm) after repeated subcultures on media containing glucose or maltose.

Figure 19-2 *Aggregatibacter actinomycetemcomitans* on blood agar. *A. actinomycetemcomitans* produces pinpoint to small colonies 0.5 mm in diameter after a 24-h incubation on blood agar, as shown. The colonies are smooth or rough, sticky, adherent, and surrounded by a slight greenish tinge after 48 h, as shown here. Sticky colonies may be difficult to remove from the surface of the agar. A characteristic morphology is the development of a star-like configuration in the center of a 4- to 5-day-old colony when grown on a clear medium such as brain heart infusion agar. This morphology can be visualized under low-power magnification (×100).

Figure 19-3 *Actinobacillus ureae* on blood agar. Colonies of *A. ureae* on blood agar are small, wet, slightly mucoid, and gray, measuring 1 to 2 mm in diameter. Growth on agar media resembles that of the *Pasteurella.*

Figure 19-4 *Actinobacillus hominis* on blood agar. Colonies of *A. hominis* on blood agar after a 72-h incubation in a microaerophilic atmosphere are small, slightly alpha-hemolytic, smooth, round, glistening, and opaque, measuring 1 mm in diameter. As the colonies mature, they tend to pit the agar.

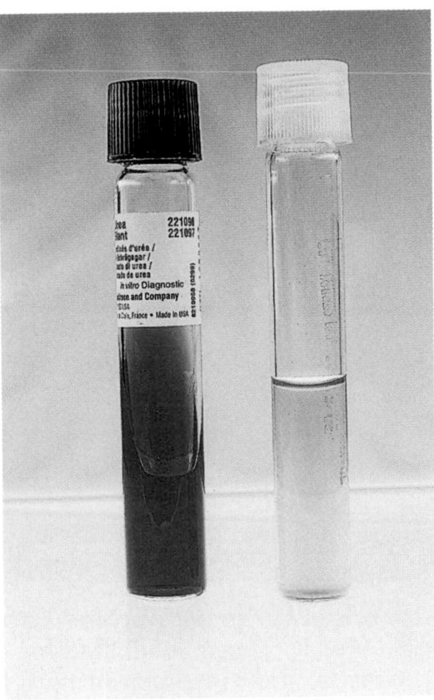

Figure 19-5 Reaction of *Actinobacillus* spp. on urea agar and in mannitol broth. The urea agar slant is positive (left tube) and the mannitol broth is weakly positive (right tube) after a 48-h incubation. All *Actinobacillus* spp. are urease positive, and they all produce acid from mannitol; however, only *A. ureae* has a delayed reaction. The positive urea reaction and delayed reaction from mannitol, shown in this figure, are suggestive of *A. ureae.*

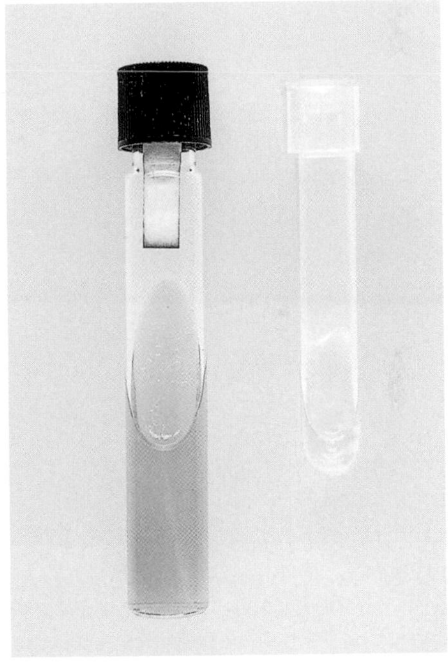

Figure 19-6 *Actinobacillus equuli* on a triple sugar iron (TSI) agar slant. *A. equuli* was inoculated onto a TSI agar slant with a lead acetate strip placed above the slant (left tube) and into a tube containing an ONPG tablet (right tube). *A. equuli* produces acid from glucose, lactose, and sucrose, the three carbohydrates in TSI medium, causing an acid reaction in the slant and butt. It produces a small amount of H_2S, which is not detected by the ferrous sulfate in the TSI medium. Therefore, a more sensitive reagent, lead acetate, is used to detect H_2S production. As shown here, the presence of a black color at the bottom of the strip is a positive reaction. *A. equuli* is also one of the *Actinobacillus* spp. that is ONPG positive within 2 to 4 h, resulting in a yellow color.

Figure 19-7 *Capnocytophaga* spp. on chocolate agar. Colonies of *Capnocytophaga* spp. incubated on chocolate agar for 48 h are small to medium sized, measuring 1 to 3 mm in diameter, and nonhemolytic. There is a haze or swarming on the surface of the agar, similar to *Proteus* spp. This is due to the gliding motility of the organism, a characteristic of *Capnocytophaga* spp.

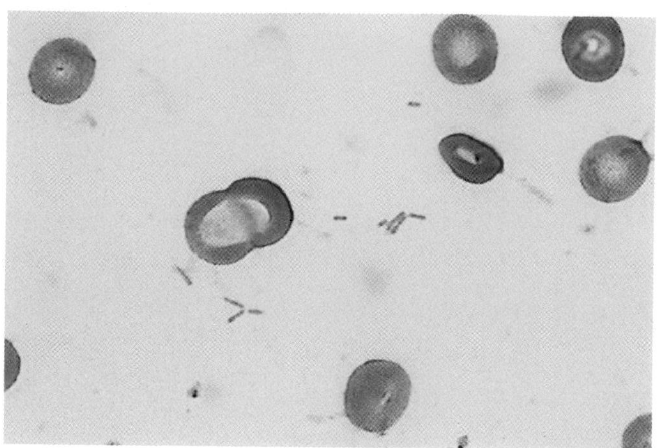

Figure 19-8 Gram stain of *Eikenella corrodens* isolated from a blood culture. This Gram stain of *E. corrodens* isolated from a blood culture shows slender, gram-negative bacilli, measuring 0.5 μm by 1.5 to 4 μm, with rounded ends.

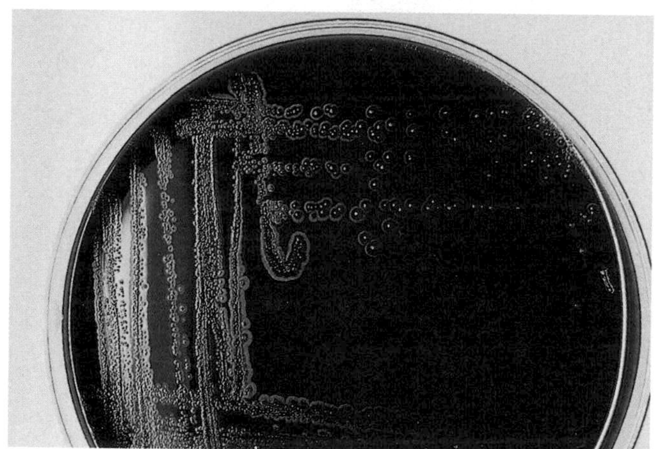

Figure 19-9 *Eikenella corrodens* on blood agar. Shown here are colonies of *E. corrodens* grown on blood agar and incubated for 48 h. The colonies are clear, pinpoint to small, and surrounded by flat, spreading growth. The center of the colony is pitting the agar surface, a characteristic of this organism. The colonies also produce a characteristic bleach-like odor.

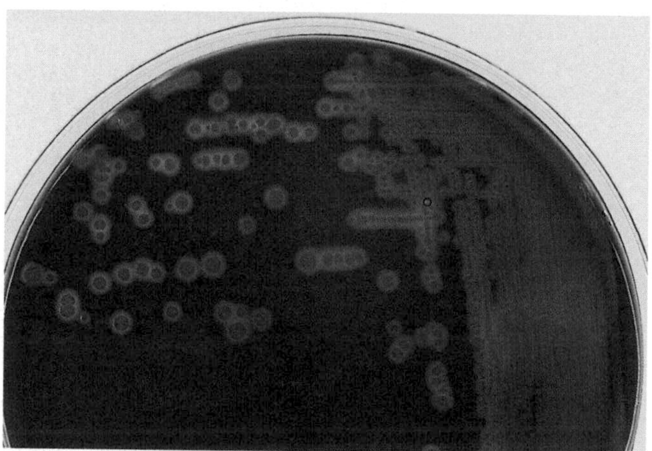

Figure 19-10 *Kingella kingae* on blood agar. Shown here are colonies of *K. kingae* incubated for 48 h. They are smooth, convex, and gray, measuring 0.5 to 1 mm in diameter, and are surrounded by a zone of beta-hemolysis. In contrast, colonies of *K. denitrificans* are small, spreading, and nonhemolytic, and they frequently pit the agar.

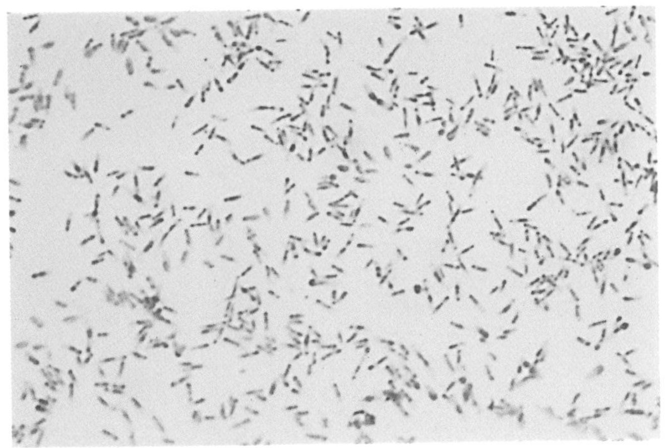

Figure 19-11 Gram stain of *Cardiobacterium hominis*. This Gram-stained smear of *C. hominis* from an agar plate shows pleomorphic, gram-negative bacilli with pointed and swollen ends in palisade formation, measuring 0.5 to 0.75 µm by 1.0 to 3.0 µm. Some strains retain the crystal violet in the swollen ends or central portion of the cells. They also can appear in rosette clusters.

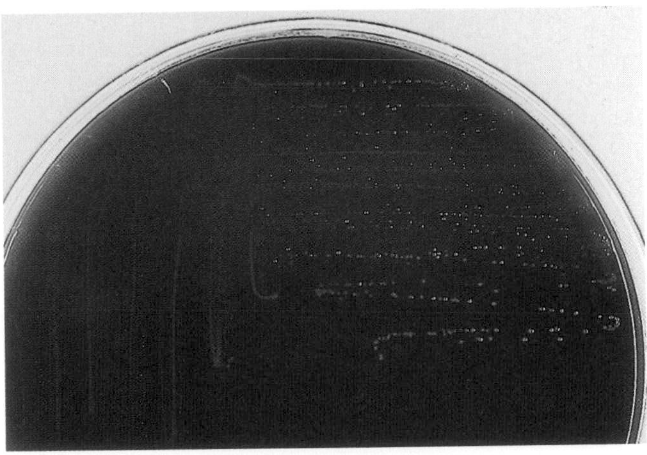

Figure 19-12 *Cardiobacterium hominis* on blood agar. Colonies of *C. hominis* on chocolate or blood agar are small (0.5 to 1.0 mm in diameter), slightly alpha-hemolytic, smooth, round, glistening, and opaque after a 48-h incubation. If they are incubated aerobically, growth is scant unless the humidity is increased or they are incubated under a microaerophilic atmosphere (candle jar). Mature colonies tend to pit the agar.

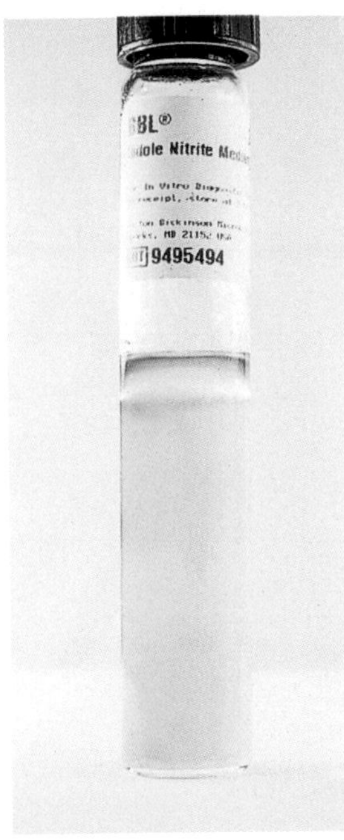

Figure 19-13 Indole reaction of *Cardiobacterium hominis*. Indole formation is an important characteristic of *C. hominis*. Indole production may be weak and may not be detected by procedures that do not concentrate the indole by xylene extraction.

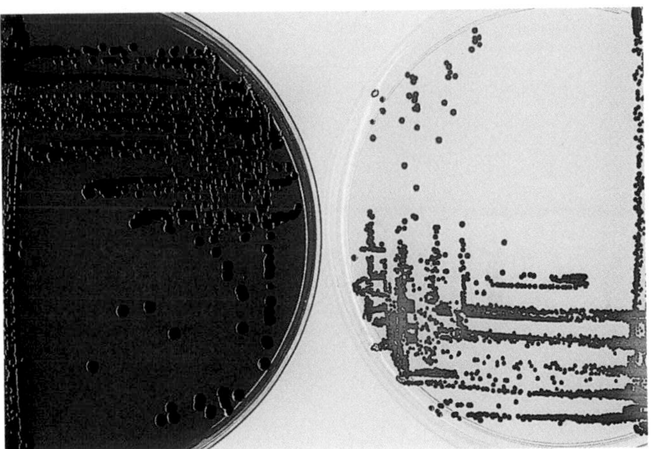

Figure 19-14 *Chromobacterium violaceum* on blood agar and Mueller-Hinton agar. Colonies of *C. violaceum* are 2 to 4 mm in diameter, round, smooth, and convex, with a very dark purple (violet) pigment. Shown here are colonies of *C. violaceum* growing on blood agar (left) and Mueller-Hinton agar (right). It is difficult to determine the pigment color on blood agar because of the presence of erythrocytes in the medium, while the color on Mueller-Hinton agar is clearly violet. These colonies produce an odor of ammonium cyanide.

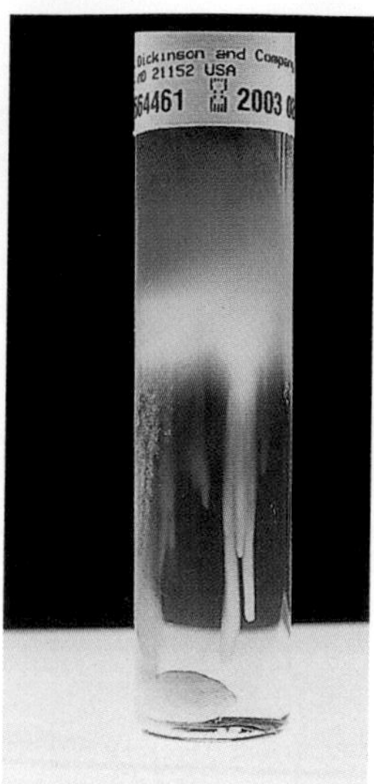

Figure 19-15 ***Streptobacillus moniliformis*** **in broth medium.** *S. moniliformis* is a fastidious organism that requires supplementation with blood or horse serum for growth. Growth on agar media may require a 7-day incubation before it is visualized. As shown here, the organism is growing toward the bottom of the tube with bread crumb-like morphology on the left side of the tube, a characteristic of *S. moniliformis*.

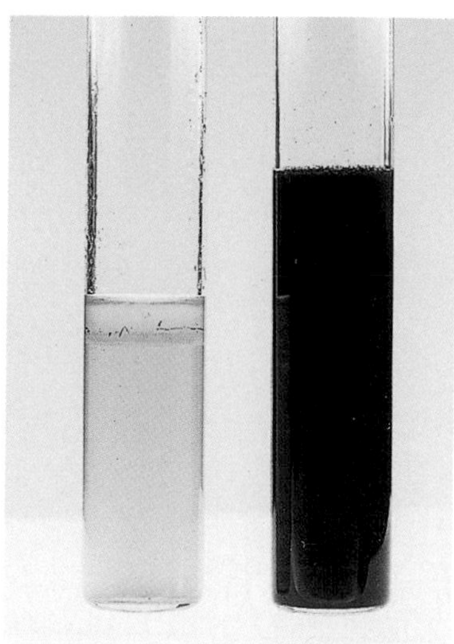

Figure 19-16 Indole and nitrate reactions of ***Chromobacterium violaceum*****.** The indole test is shown on the left, and the nitrate test is shown on the right. In contrast to *C. hominis*, the indole test is negative and nitrate is reduced to nitrite.

Legionella

20

Legionella spp. are thin, faint-staining, non-spore-forming, pleomorphic, gram-negative bacilli that are found in the environment, particularly in bodies of water and in domestic sources of stagnant or warm water, e.g., cooling systems and hot tubs. They are known to survive low levels of chlorine and thus can colonize water supplies. There are currently 52 species. The majority of human infections are are caused by *Legionella pneumophila*, *Legionella micdadei*, *Legionella longbeachae*, and *Legionella dumoffii*. These organisms are thought to be transmitted to humans mainly by aerosols, and thus *Legionella* infections primarily affect the respiratory tract; however, dissemination and extrapulmonary involvement have been documented (e.g., pericarditis, pyelonephritis, and peritonitis). The two main forms of *Legionella* infections are pneumonia (Legionnaires' disease) and Pontiac fever. *L. pneumophila* serogroup 1 is responsible for >90% of the pneumonia cases, even though there are more than 50 serogroups of *L. pneumophila*. Legionnaires' disease has been reported to have a mortality rate of 12%. Once inhaled, *Legionella* infects human macrophages, in particular alveolar macrophages. The organisms possess several genes that enable them to evade host defenses and are capable of multiplying and surviving in an intracellular host environment. Unlike Legionnaires' disease, Pontiac fever, an acute, self-limiting flu-like illness, is thought to be due to an inhaled toxin or allergic reaction.

Legionella spp. are difficult to see on a routine Gram stain and therefore can be better visualized with a carbol fuchsin counterstain or the Gimenez stain. Organisms visualized from direct smears are coccobacillary, in contrast to the long, slender, gram-negative bacilli seen in cultures. A direct fluorescent-antibody test is commercially available but is limited to the detection of *L. pneumophila*. In general, direct staining of specimens, due to the small number of organisms present, yields a low sensitivity. Culture is the recommended laboratory test because it detects all species and serogroups. Specimens for culture can be from all sites; however, lower respiratory tract specimens are the most common. Often there is a paucity of polymorphonuclear leukocytes in the respiratory specimens, and therefore cellular evaluation of the specimen should not be an exclusion criterion for culture. In cases of pneumonia, transtracheal aspirates may give better recovery than sputum or bronchoscopy specimens.

Legionella spp. are aerobic organisms that require L-cysteine for growth, exhibit enhanced growth with iron and under 5% CO_2, and are relatively inert biochemically. Enriched media, such as buffered charcoal-yeast extract (BCYE) containing α-ketoglutaric acid, with and without antibiotics, should be included among the primary culture media. Growth can be detected on plates that have been incubated in 5% CO_2 for 3 to 5 days at 35°C. Microscopically, colonies resemble cut glass and some species have a brown pigment or fluorescence. While biochemicals have not been particularly helpful in identifying *Legionella* spp., hippurate hydrolysis has been used to differentiate *L. pneumophila*, which is hippurate positive, from the majority of the other *Legionella* spp. *Francisella tularensis*, mainly due to its delayed growth and dependence on cysteine, has the potential to be misidentified as *Legionella*. Colonies, however, of the two genera differ greatly. Monoclonal or polyclonal antibodies can be used to presumptively identify the organism, but definitive identification usually requires genetic analysis. Antimicrobial susceptibility testing is not routinely performed due to a lack of standardized methods.

Testing for *L. pneumophila* urinary antigen is a rapid test with a specificity of ≥99% but is limited to the detection of *L. pneumophila* serogroup 1. The sensitivity of the assay depends on the severity and stage of the pneumonia, but a general figure of 80% has been established in at least one large study.

Molecular assays are available mainly in reference laboratories but are still being developed so as to be more useful in the routine diagnosis of pneumonia due to *Legionella*. While commercial assays are available, they have not been extensively evaluated. Serological testing of single serum specimens may be helpful in establishing a diagnosis when a high titer (>128) to *Legionella* is present, especially if the patient is from a geographical area where background titers are known to be relatively low. Paired serum specimens that show seroconversion or a fourfold rise in titer are highly suggestive of active infection.

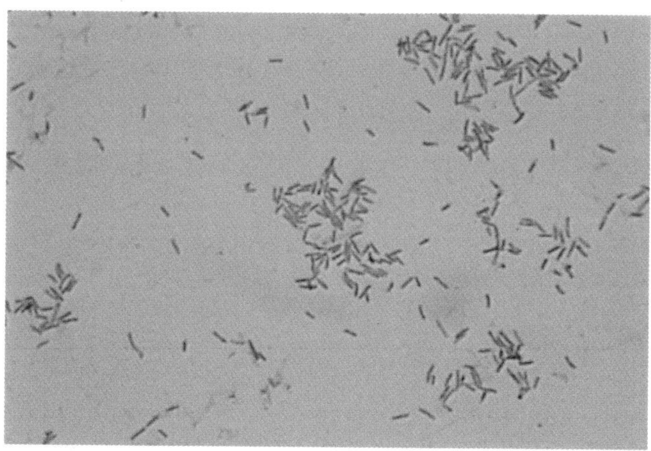

Figure 20-1 Gram stain of *Legionella*. *Legionella* spp. are thin, gram-negative bacilli that stain faintly with a safranin counterstain. They measure 1 to 2 μm by 0.5 μm but can show variation, with bacilli up to 20 μm in length.

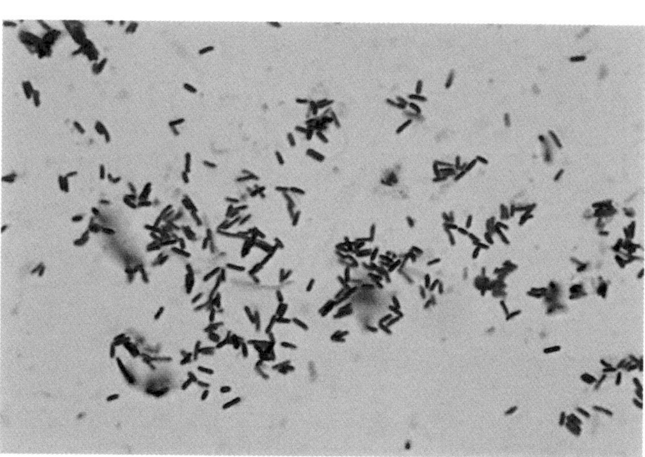

Figure 20-2 Gram stain of *Legionella* using carbol fuchsin as the counterstain. A Gram stain of the same *Legionella* isolate as that shown in Fig. 20-1 was performed using carbol fuchsin as the counterstain. Here the organisms are easier to see because they stain much darker.

Figure 20-3 Direct fluorescent-antibody stain of *Legionella pneumophila*. A direct fluorescent-antibody stain of an expectorated sputum specimen was positive for *L. pneumophila*. This organism was identified as *L. pneumophila* serogroup 1. The fluorescent-antibody stain is more sensitive for detecting this organism directly from sputum than is the Gram stain because there are often few organisms and the specimen may be mixed with members of the oropharyngeal flora.

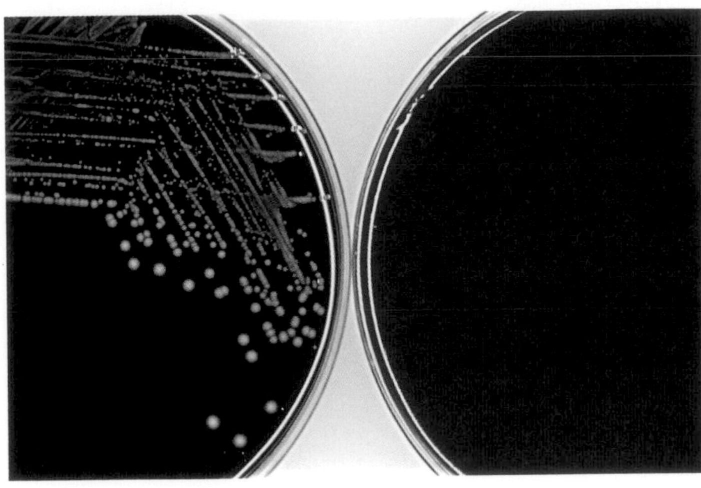

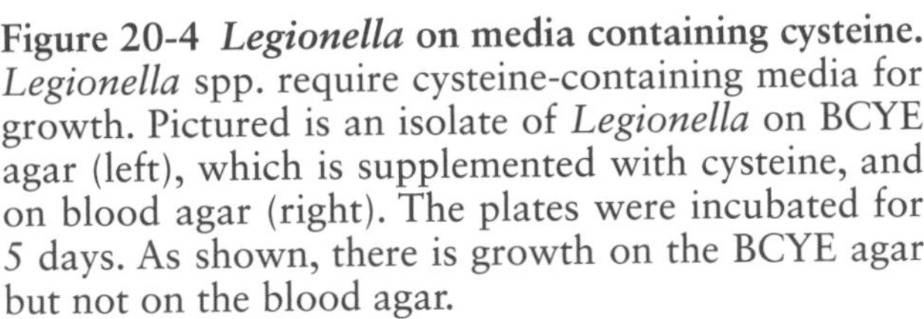

Figure 20-4 *Legionella* on media containing cysteine. *Legionella* spp. require cysteine-containing media for growth. Pictured is an isolate of *Legionella* on BCYE agar (left), which is supplemented with cysteine, and on blood agar (right). The plates were incubated for 5 days. As shown, there is growth on the BCYE agar but not on the blood agar.

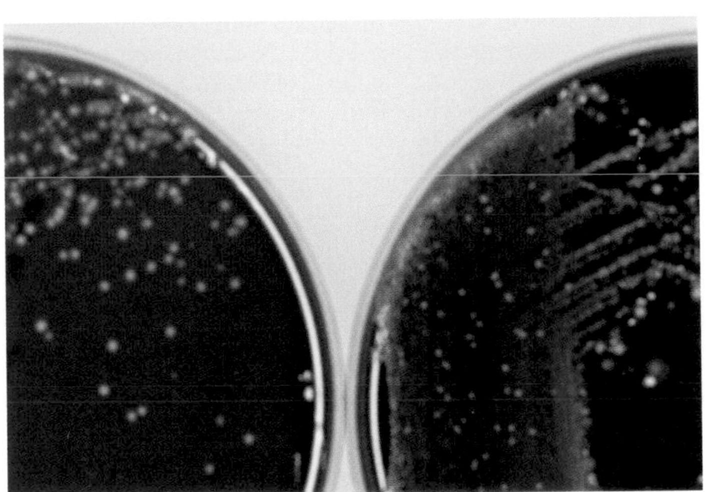

Figure 20-5 Sputum specimen cultured on BCYE agar with and without antibiotics. Pictured is a sputum specimen that was plated onto BCYE agar with (left) and without (right) antibiotics. Since the normal respiratory flora can grow on BCYE agar, specimens from nonsterile sites from patients who are suspected to have a *Legionella* infection should be plated onto BCYE agar, or its equivalent, with and without antibiotics. To improve the recovery of *Legionella* from sites contaminated with normal flora, specimens can be treated with acid prior to culture.

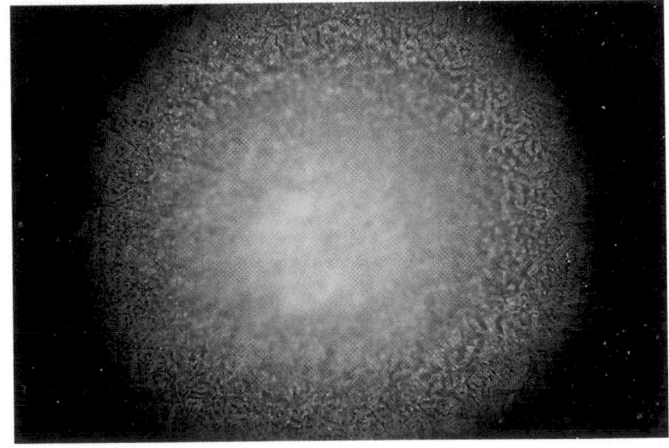

Figure 20-6 *Legionella pneumophila* on BCYE agar. Colonies of *L. pneumophila* viewed microscopically under low-power magnification have a cut-glass appearance, as shown for this 5-day-old colony grown on BCYE agar.

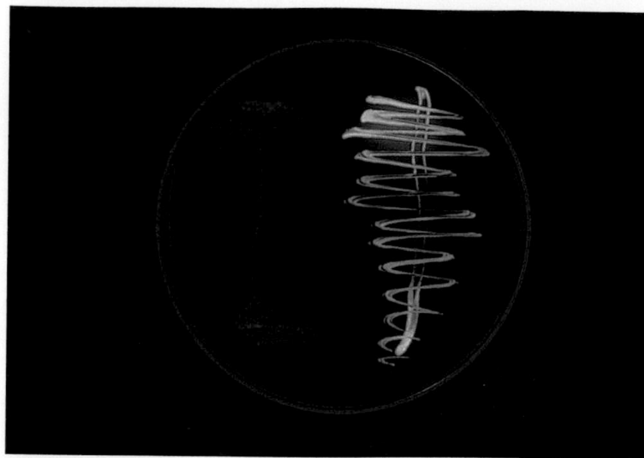

Figure 20-7 *Legionella* viewed under long-wavelength UV light. Some species of *Legionella* fluoresce when exposed to long-wave UV light. Depending on the species, the color resulting from autofluorescence can vary from that seen here to red or yellow-green. The isolates shown here were grown on BCYE agar. *L. pneumophila* (left) does not fluoresce, while *Legionella bozemanae* (right) exhibits blue-white fluorescence.

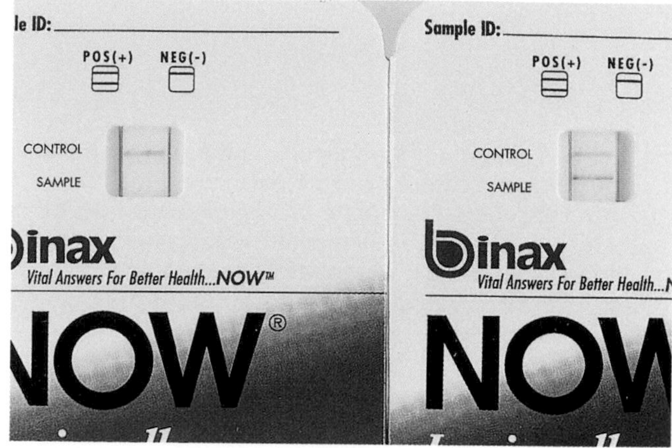

Figure 20-8 Rapid test for *Legionella* antigen in urine. Testing for the presence of *Legionella* antigen in urine is a rapid and sensitive way to aid in the diagnosis of a *Legionella* infection. While this test can been performed in an enzyme immunoassay and radioimmunoassay format, a commercially available rapid immunochromatographic assay, BinaxNOW Legionella Urinary Antigen Test (Alere, Waltham, MA), is shown here. The advantages of this test are its simplicity and rapidity. A limitation of the urinary antigen tests is that they detect antigen of only *L. pneumophila* serogroup 1.

Neisseria

21

Neisseria spp. are gram-negative diplococci. They are described as kidney bean shaped owing to the flattened side where the two cocci appear to touch. With the exception of *Neisseria gonorrhoeae*, *Neisseria* spp. are part of the human endogenous flora and typically inhabit the mucosal membranes of the oral cavity and occasionally the genital tract. Most *Neisseria* spp. are commensal organisms, including *Neisseria cinerea*, *Neisseria elongata*, *Neisseria flavescens*, *Neisseria lactamica*, *Neisseria mucosa*, *Neisseria sicca*, and *Neisseria subflava*. However, *N. gonorrhoeae* and *Neisseria meningitidis* are commonly associated with human disease.

N. gonorrhoeae is restricted to humans and is always considered a pathogen when isolated or detected. It is sexually transmitted, causing gonorrhea, and is found most frequently from genital, rectal, and throat specimens. It is capable of dissemination and has been isolated from blood and joint fluid. Transmission of the organism at birth can occur and typically manifests as an ocular infection in the newborn. Isolation of this organism is often attempted from a specimen that has an abundance of normal flora; therefore, selective media must be used to optimize recovery. Modified Thayer-Martin agar is one of the most widely used media for isolation of *N. gonorrhoeae*. It contains colistin (to inhibit gram-negative organisms), vancomycin (to inhibit gram-positive organisms), nystatin (to inhibit yeast), and trimethoprim (to inhibit the swarming of *Proteus* spp.). *N. gonorrhoeae* is fastidious and susceptible to cold and requires a capnophilic atmosphere. To optimize recovery, medium is incorporated into devices that provide a CO_2 atmosphere so that the organisms can be transported under the appropriate environmental conditions. Some transport systems are flushed with CO_2 and the medium simply has to be inoculated, while with others a CO_2 environment is chemically generated after inoculation. Alternatively, the candle jar is the traditional method of generating a CO_2 environment for holding inoculated media.

While *N. meningitidis* colonizes oral mucosal membranes of about 10% of the population, it can cause a variety of clinical presentations, the most common and serious being meningitis and septicemia. This organism is known for its potential to take a fulminant course, with rapid progression leading to considerable morbidity or mortality. Patients with disseminated infection may have extensive vascular involvement manifested by a petechial or purpuric skin rash or even disseminated intravascular coagulation. Vaccines to prevent meningococcemia are available but do not cover all the possible serogroups of this organism.

Neisseria spp. differ in their nutritional requirements. Species such as *N. gonorrhoeae* require enriched media, e.g., chocolate agar; however, many species, including *N. meningitidis*, grow well on blood agar. As stated above, selective media are commonly used to facilitate the isolation of these organisms from other members of the normal flora of mucosal surfaces. Growth of *Neisseria* spp. is enhanced by humidity and a CO_2-enriched atmosphere and should be evident after 24 h of incubation at 35 to 37°C. Depending on the species and strain, colonies can appear moist to mucoid (e.g., strains of *N. meningitidis*) or even dry and tenacious, being described as a "hockey puck" in that they stay intact when

Table 21-1 Selected biochemical reactions used to distinguish between the more commonly isolated *Neisseria* spp. and *Moraxella catarrhalis*[a]

Species	Glucose	Maltose	Lactose	Sucrose	DNase	Butyrate esterase
N. gonorrhoeae	+	0	0	0	0	0
N. meningitidis	+	+	0	0	0	0
N. lactamica	+	+	+	0	0	0
N. sicca	+	+	0	+	0	0
N. flavescens	0	0	0	0	0	0
M. catarrhalis	0	0	0	0	+	+

[a]+, positive reaction; 0, negative reaction.

removed from a plate or suspended in liquid. Most strains produce gray-brown colonies, but some species appear yellow (e.g., *N. subflava*).

A key characteristic of *Neisseria* spp. is their distinctive microscopic morphology. They are gram-negative diplococci, referred to as being coffee bean or kidney bean shaped, that are commonly intracellular, predominantly in polymorphonuclear leukocytes. When direct smears from clinical specimens are stained, it is not unusal for these organisms to avoid decolorization, thus appearing gram positive. *Moraxella catarrhalis*, a cause of a variety of upper respiratory tract infections, can appear microscopically similar to *Neisseria* spp., as it also is a gram-negative diplococcus that is frequently seen in polymorphonuclear leukocytes. For this reason identification kits for the speciation of *Neisseria* usually include *M. catarrhalis* in their identification scheme.

Neisseria spp. are oxidase and catalase positive. *N. gonorrhoeae* can be differentiated from the other *Neisseria* spp. by the superoxal test, which is similar to the catalase test except that it is performed with 30% hydrogen peroxide rather than the standard 3%. *Neisseria* spp. utilize carbohydrates oxidatively and, as such, produce small amounts of acid, thus making carbohydrate utilization tests, such as those involving cystine Trypticase agar (CTA) sugars, difficult to interpret. However, rapid sugar utilization tests based on acid production from glucose, maltose, lactose, and sucrose are more commonly used. With the patterns generated from these carbohydrates, along with additional tests such as nitrate and tributyrin hydrolysis, most isolates can be identified (Table 21-1). Alternative identification methods include detection of preformed enzymes by using chromogenic substrates and monoclonal antibody-based tests, as well as nucleic acid hybridization and amplification assays. Some identification kits combine both carbohydrate utilization and enzymatic substrate tests.

Direct detection of *N. gonorrhoeae* from urine or genital specimens based on nucleic acid amplification methods has, for the most part, replaced traditional culture methods. This is in part due to the ease of obtaining urine from males and the ability to test for *Chlamydia trachomatis* from the same specimen.

Figure 21-1 Gram stain of *Neisseria gonorrhoeae*. A Gram stain of a urethral smear from a symptomatic male shows intracellular gram-negative diplococci with kidney bean-shaped organisms. *N. gonorrhoeae* was isolated from this specimen.

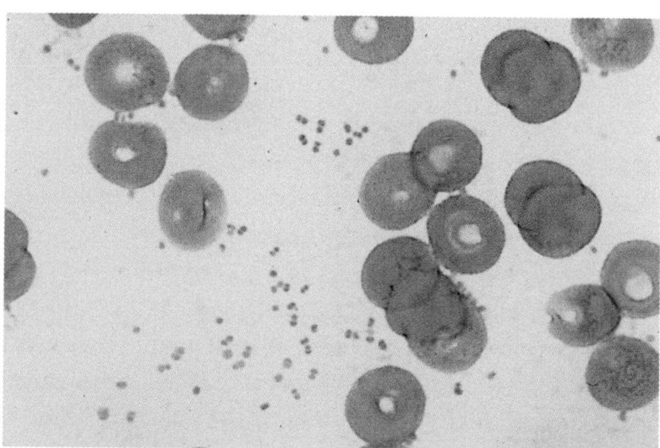

Figure 21-2 Gram stain of *Neisseria meningitidis*. A Gram stain of a positive blood culture bottle shows typical kidney bean-shaped, gram-negative diplococci. *N. meningitidis* was isolated from this blood culture.

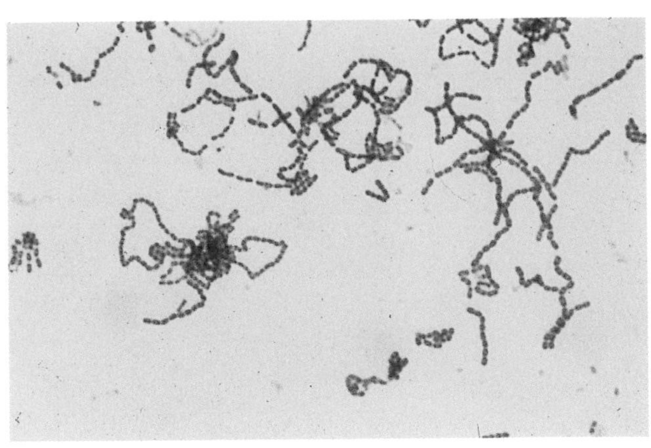

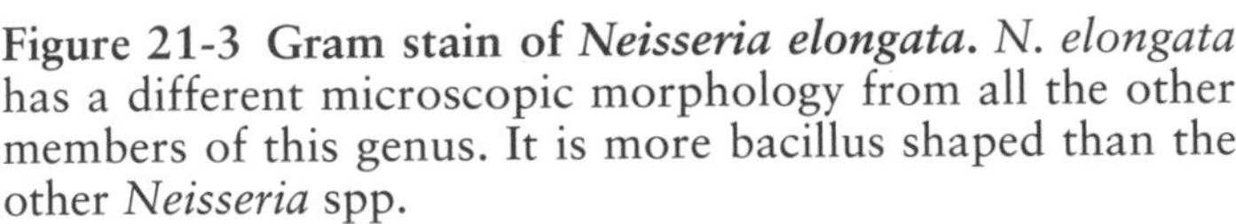

Figure 21-3 Gram stain of *Neisseria elongata*. *N. elongata* has a different microscopic morphology from all the other members of this genus. It is more bacillus shaped than the other *Neisseria* spp.

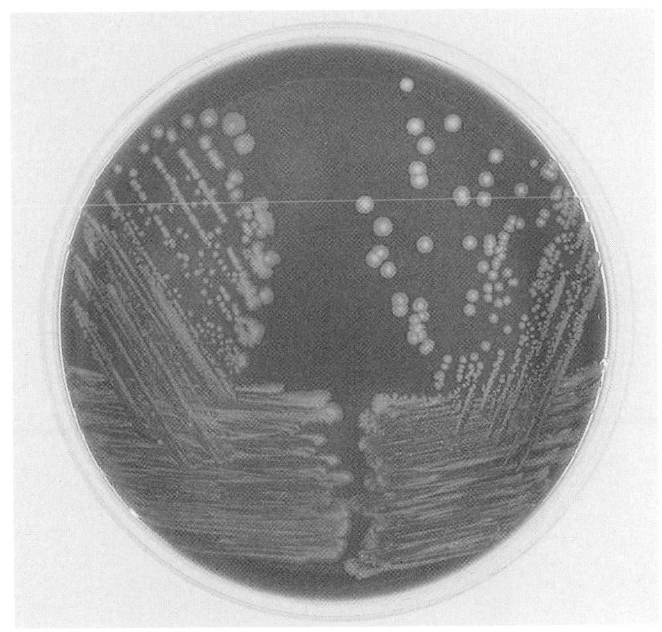

Figure 21-4 Comparison of colonies of *Neisseria meningitidis* and *Neisseria gonorrhoeae*. Colonies of *N. meningitidis* and *N. gonorrhoeae* can be differentiated when grown on chocolate agar. *N. gonorrhoeae* (right) produces an off-white colony with no discoloration of the agar. In contrast, *N. meningitidis* (left) grows as a gray colony and imparts a green color to the agar immediately surrounding the colony.

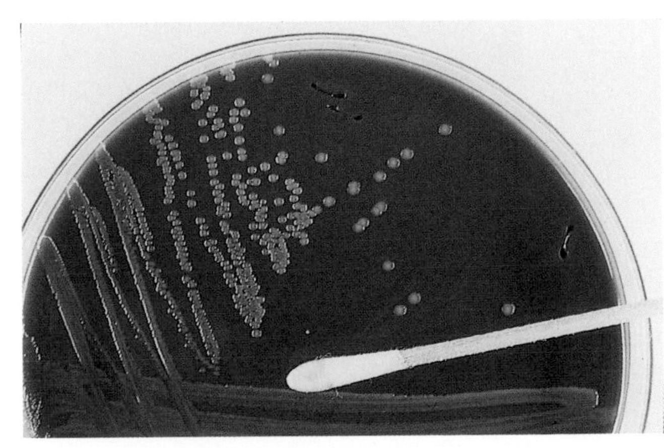

Figure 21-5 *Neisseria flavescens* on chocolate agar. Colonies of *N. flavescens*, considered part of the normal oral pharyngeal flora, are smooth with a defined edge and often have a yellow cast. The pigment is obvious when the colonies are picked up with a cotton swab.

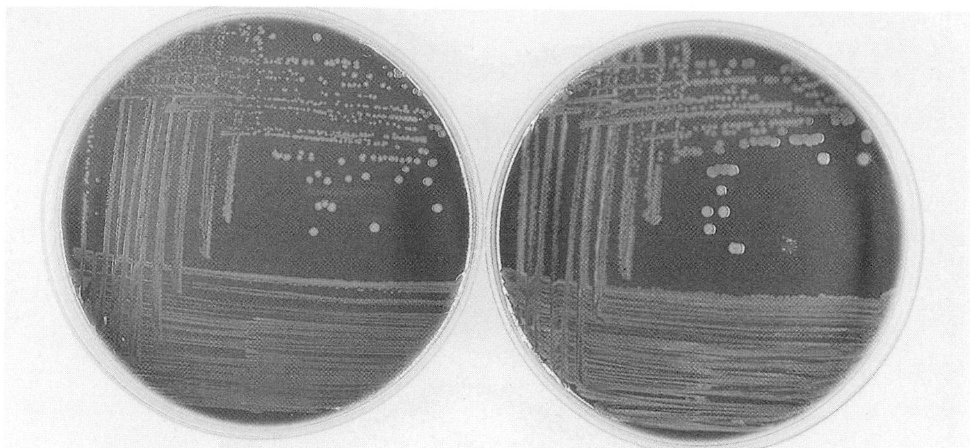

Figure 21-6 ***Neisseria meningitidis*** **and** ***Neisseria lactamica*** **on chocolate agar.** Growth of *N. meningitidis* (right) and *N. lactamica* (left) on chocolate agar illustrates that differentiation between colonies of these two species is difficult. Both produce gray colonies that have a green haze in the agar immediately under and adjacent to the colonies.

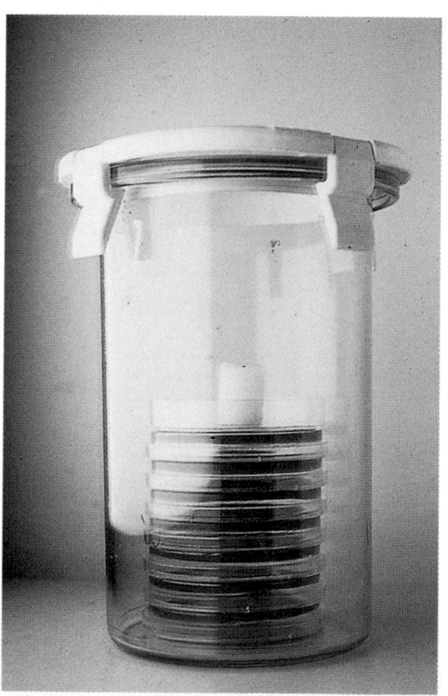

Figure 21-7 Candle jar. Agar plates are placed in a jar, a candle is lit, and the jar is sealed. When the O_2 has been consumed, the candle extinguishes, leaving an atmosphere of 3% CO_2. Inoculated agar is then transported and/or incubated at 35 to 37°C in this CO_2 environment. Candle jars are an alternative method to the commercially available systems for the transport and recovery of *N. gonorrhoeae*.

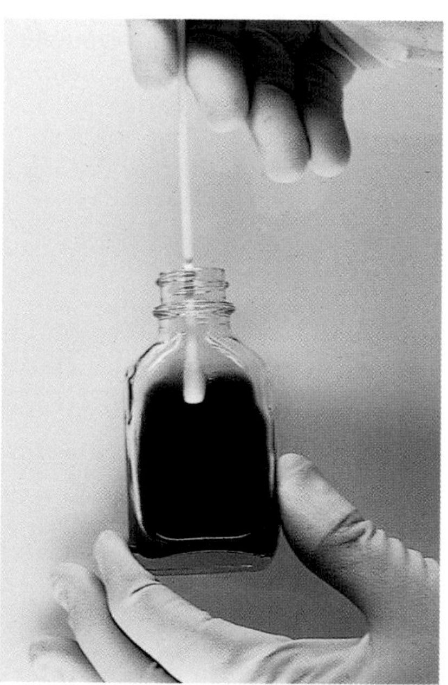

Figure 21-8 Transgrow bottle inoculation. Transgrow bottles contain Thayer-Martin medium and a CO_2 atmosphere (5 to 30% CO_2). They should be brought to room temperature before inoculation. The bottle should be held in an upright position so as to retain the CO_2. Once inoculated, it is transported to the laboratory at room temperature, where it is incubated at 35 to 37°C for up to 72 h.

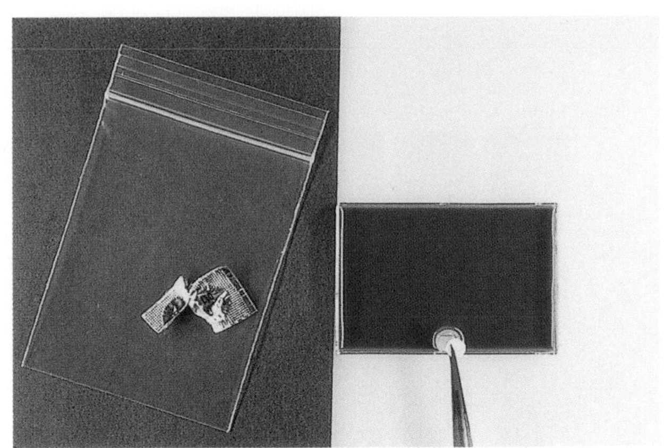

Figure 21-9 JEMBEC plates. The JEMBEC plate shown here contains selective agar, GC-Lect agar (BD Diagnostic Systems, Franklin Lakes, NJ), designed for the enhanced recovery of *N. gonorrhoeae*. Upon inoculation of the medium with the specimen, a CO_2-generating tablet consisting of citric acid and sodium bicarbonate is placed in the JEMBEC plate, as shown. The plate is covered, sealed in the plastic bag provided, and transported to the laboratory.

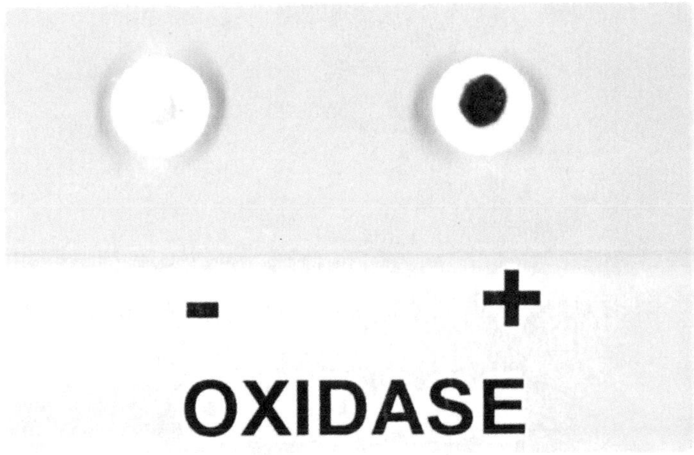

Figure 21-10 Oxidase test. For the identification of *Neisseria* spp., oxidase is a key test. All members of this species are oxidase positive. In this test, filter paper is saturated with an aqueous solution of *N*′,*N*′,*N*′,*N*′-tetramethyl-*p*-phenylenediamine dihydrochloride and then the colony is rubbed onto the paper. The presence of a purple color within 2 min indicates a positive test.

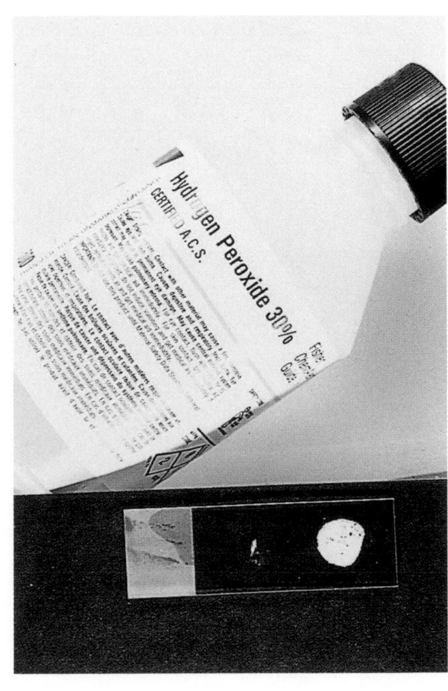

Figure 21-11 Superoxal test. The superoxal test is performed the same way as a catalase test, except that 30% hydrogen peroxide, rather than the usual 3%, is used. The test can be used to differentiate *N. gonorrhoeae* (right) from other, related *Neisseria* spp. (left). If the test is positive, bubbles will appear on the slide when mixed with H_2O_2 (right); if no or few bubbles appear (left), the test is negative. However, while most other *Neisseria* spp. give weak reactions, a few species may react as strongly as *N. gonorrhoeae*.

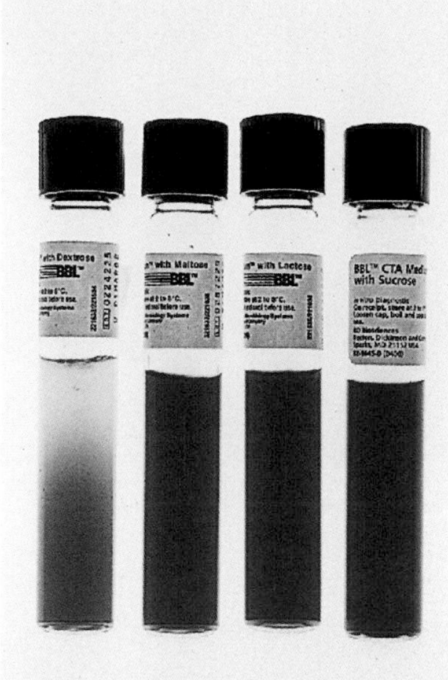

Figure 21-12 CTA sugars for the identification of *Neisseria* species. A conventional method used for the identification and differentiation of *Neisseria* spp. involves the use of CTA sugars. Tubes of semisolid medium containing 1% of the indicated carbohydrate and phenol red as the indicator are inoculated with the unknown organism. The sugars used to differentiate the *Neisseria* spp. are glucose, maltose, sucrose, and lactose. In addition, basal medium with no added carbohydrate is used as a control. The top portion of the agar is inoculated, and the sugars are incubated at 35°C in an aerobic incubator with tight caps for 24 to 72 h. Some *Neisseria* spp. produce a slight amount of acid, and therefore the reactions can be easily missed. In general, CTA sugars have been replaced by other rapid commercial systems for identification. Shown is an isolate of *N. gonorrhoeae* that is positive for glucose (dextrose), as shown by the yellow reaction, and negative for the other three sugars.

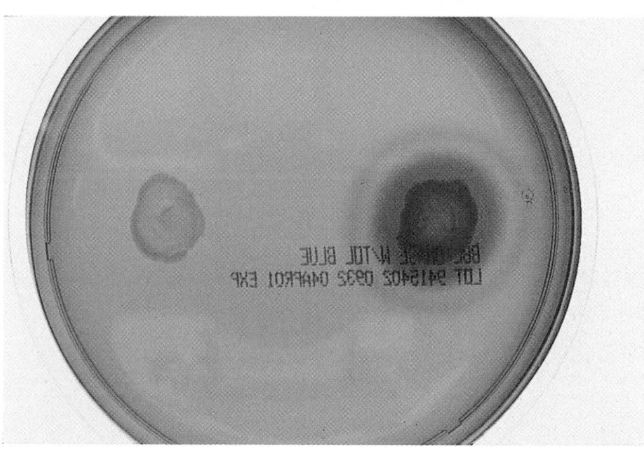

Figure 21-13 DNase plate for the differentiation of *Moraxella catarrhalis* and *Neisseria* spp. *M. catarrhalis* can be distinguished from *Neisseria* spp. by its positive reaction on DNase agar containing toluidine blue. *M. catarrhalis*, which has been used to inoculate the right side of the plate in this figure, is DNase positive, which is apparent from the rose color surrounding the inoculum, whereas the *Neisseria* sp. on the left is DNase negative, since there is no change in the color of the agar around the inoculum.

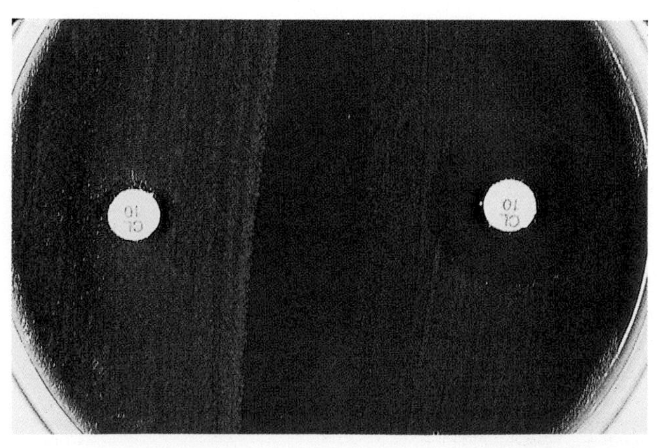

Figure 21-14 Colistin disk differentiation test. In general, commensal *Neisseria* strains are susceptible to colistin. As shown here, *N. gonorrhoeae* (left) is resistant to colistin yet *N. sicca* (right) is susceptible, as illustrated by the large zone of growth inhibition surrounding the colistin disk. However, not all commensal strains are susceptible to colistin, as evidenced by their isolation from selective media such as colistin-containing Thayer-Martin medium.

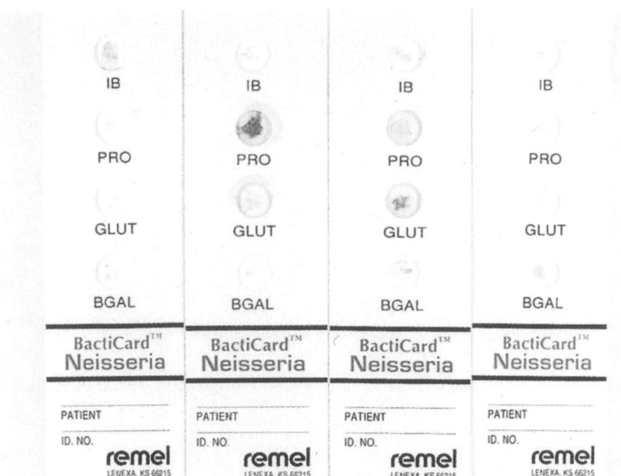

Figure 21-15 BactiCard Neisseria. The BactiCard Neisseria test (Thermo Scientific Remel Products, Lenexa, KS) is an identification system consisting of four substrates that are used for the rapid presumptive identification of *Neisseria* spp. isolated from selective media. The enzymes detected and the substrates used (in parentheses) are β-galactosidase (5-bromo-4-chloro-3-indolyl-D-galactoside), butyrate esterase (5-bromo-4-chloro-3-indolyl-butyrate), γ-glutamyl-aminopeptidase (γ-glutamyl-naphthylamide), and prolyl-aminopeptidase (L-proline-naphthylamide). Shown from left to right are *M. catarrhalis*, *N. gonorrhoeae*, *N. meningitidis*, and *N. lactamica*.

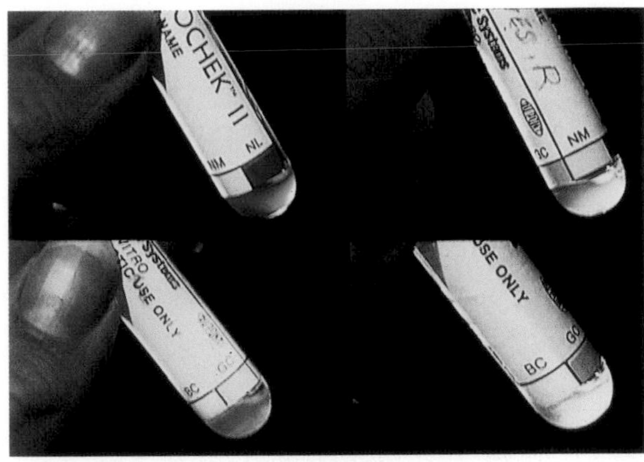

Figure 21-16 The Gonochek-II system. The Gonochek-II system (EY Laboratories Inc., San Mateo, CA) is used for the presumptive identification of *N. gonorrhoeae*, *N. meningitidis*, *N. lactamica*, and *M. catarrhalis*. Identification is based on the detection of the three preformed enzymes prolyl-aminopeptidase, γ-glutamyl-aminopeptidase, and β-galactosidase. Each enzyme breaks down a different substrate, resulting in one of three colors. *M. catarrhalis* should be negative for all three enzyme tests. As shown here, these colors represent identification of the following species: *N. lactamica*, blue (top left); *N. gonorrhoeae*, red/pink (bottom left); *N. meningitidis*, yellow (top right); *M. catarrhalis*, white/no color (bottom right).

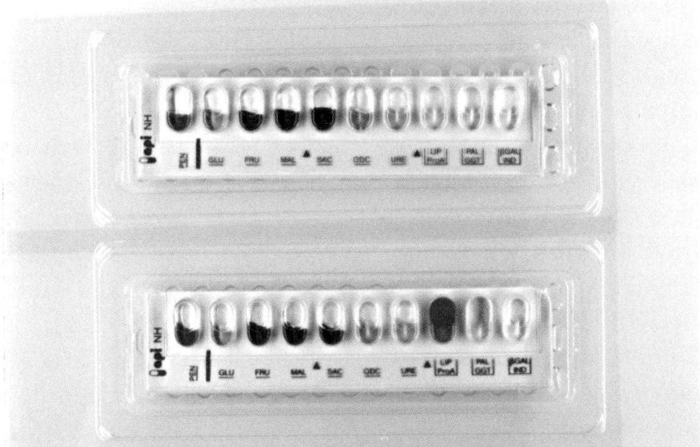

Figure 21-17 API NH identification system. The API NH system (bioMérieux, Inc., Durham, NC) is composed of 13 tests: penicillinase detection and 12 identification tests including 4 fermentation tests (glucose, fructose, maltose, and sucrose) and 8 enzymatic reactions (ornithine decarboxylase, urease, lipase, alkaline phosphatase, β-galactosidase, proline arylamidase, γ-glutamyl-transferase, and indole production). This system requires a heavy inoculum and is read after 2 h of incubation at 35 to 37°C. After the last three wells are read for lipase, alkaline phosphatase, and β-galactosidase, additional reagents are added to determine proline arylamidase, γ-glutamyl-transferase, and indole production. This system can be used for the identification of *Neisseria* spp., *M. catarrhalis*, and *Haemophilus* spp. Shown is a test strip inoculated with *N. gonorrhoeae* and read before (top) and after (bottom) the reagents are added to the last three wells.

Haemophilus 22

Haemophilus spp. are small, gram-negative bacilli that can be found as members of the normal flora of the upper respiratory, gastrointestinal, and genital tracts of humans and animals. Human infections range from uncomplicated upper respiratory infections including conjunctivitis, sinusitis, and otitis media to serious and life-threatening infections such as epiglottitis, endocarditis, and meningitis. Within this genus, the majority of infections are caused by *Haemophilus influenzae*. However, with the advent of a vaccine against *H. influenzae* type b, there has been a dramatic reduction of childhood infections with this organism. *Haemophilus aegyptius*, also known as the Kocks-Weeks bacillus, is a cause of acute purulent conjunctivitis, or pinkeye, seen most frequently in young children. *Haemophilus ducreyi*, unlike most members of this genus, is a sexually transmitted organism characterized by a painful genital soft chancre that can progress to inguinal lymphadenopathy. While less frequently reported, *Haemophilus parainfuenzae*, *Haemophilus haemolyticus*, and *Haemophilus parahaemolyticus* are also capable of causing human disease. *Haemophilus aphrophilus* and *Haemophilus paraphrophilus* have recently been transferred to a new genus, *Aggregatibacter*, and are discussed in chapter 19. *Aggregatibacter* spp. are better known for their association with the HACEK group of organisms, which is made up of gram-negative bacilli that are associated with endocarditis.

Visualization of *Haemophilus* in direct patient material may be difficult because of its small size and faint staining. Members of this genus often exhibit pleomorphic properties, taking on filamentous forms in addition to a gram-negative coccobacillary morphology. *H. ducreyi* tends to arrange in what is referred to as "schools of fish" or "railroad tracks." When this morphology is seen in a smear prepared from a specimen obtained from a soft chancre, it serves as a presumptive identification of this organism.

Haemophilus spp. are facultatively anaerobic, with maximal growth attained in an atmosphere of 5% CO_2 at 35°C. The majority of *Haemophilus* spp. grow on solid media within 24 to 48 h of inoculation. However, *H. aegyptius* and *H. ducreyi* can require up to 5 days to grow, and lower temperatures, 30 to 33°C, may favor the growth of *H. ducreyi*. These organisms are fastidious since most members have special nutritional requirements. All members require either X factor (provided by hemin) or V factor (NAD) or both. Both of these factors are found in chocolate agar, and therefore this is a reliable medium on which to isolate *Haemophilus* spp. The exception to this is *H. ducreyi*, which can be difficult to recover even on chocolate agar. It is not unusual for *Haemophilus* spp. that require both X and V factors to be found growing on blood agar as tiny colonies in proximity to a beta-hemolytic, NAD-producing organism such as *Staphylococcus aureus*. This is referred to as "satellite phenomenon" or "satellitism," with the growth of *Haemophilus* being supported by the release of X factor from the red blood cells and production of V factor from *Staphylococcus*. A key test in differentiating among *Haemophilus* spp. is the X and V factor requirement (Table 22-1). This can be accomplished by

Table 22-1 Key reactions for the differentiation of the more common *Haemophilus* spp.[a]

Organism	Factor required		Hemolysis of horse blood	Fermentation of:			
	X	V		Glucose	Sucrose	Lactose	Mannose
H. influenzae	+	+	0	+	0	0	0
H. parainfluenzae	0	+	0	+	+	0	+
H. haemolyticus	+	+	+	+	0	0	0
H. ducreyi	+	0	0	0	0	0	0

[a]+, positive reaction; 0, negative reaction.

preparing a lawn of *Haemophilus* on Mueller-Hinton agar that contains no X or V factor. Strips impregnated with these factors alone and in combination are then placed on the freshly inoculated plate and incubated overnight, and growth of the organism around the strips reveals the X and V factor requirement(s) for this organism. The porphyrin test is another common method to determine an X factor requirement. Here, if the organism requires X factor, owing to an enzymatic deficiency in the hemin biosynthetic pathway, it should not be able to break down the substrate δ-aminolevulinic acid. On the other hand, if an organism can break down this substrate, the by-product, a porphyrin, is detected due to its red fluorescence at 360 nm.

In addition to the X and V factor requirements, carbohydrate fermentation patterns and hemolysis on horse blood can be used to differentiate the species. For the fermentation reactions, phenol red broth supplemented with X and V factors is generally employed. Biotypes within *H. influenzae* and *H. parainfluenzae* can also be differentiated by using indole, urea, and ornithine decarboxylase tests (Table 22-2). Identification and biotyping can also be accomplished using commercially available kits.

Molecular techniques have been employed to identify *H. influenzae* directly in clinical specimens, in particular cerebrospinal fluid, as well as *H. ducreyi* in suspected cases of chancroid. Identification of other species of *Haemophilus* has not commonly been performed because of problems of sensitivity and specificity due to low numbers of organisms in clinical specimens and the inability to discriminate between pathogenic and commensal *Haemophilus* spp.

Table 22-2 Biochemical reactions for determining *Haemophilus influenzae* biotypes[a]

Biotype	Indole	Urease	Ornithine decarboxylase
I	+	+	+
II	+	+	0
III	0	+	0
IV	0	+	+
V	+	0	+
VI	0	0	+
VII	+	0	0
VIII	0	0	0

[a]+, positive reaction; 0, negative reaction.

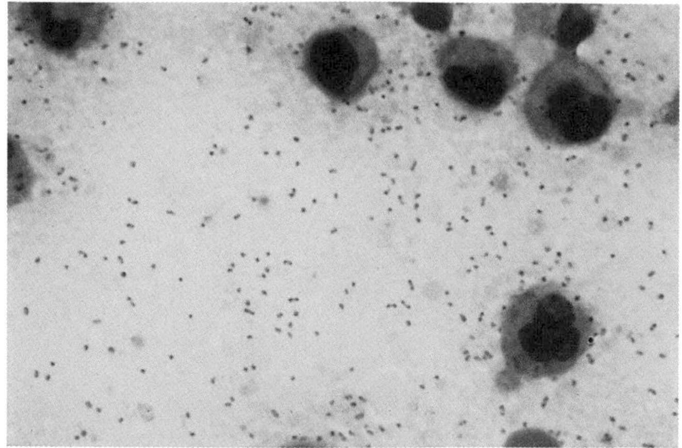

Figure 22-1 Gram stain of *Haemophilus influenzae*. Shown here is a direct smear from a sputum specimen that grew a predominance of a nontypeable *H. influenzae*. The organisms are small, gram-negative coccobacilli and are fairly uniform in morphology. However, it is not unusual for this organism in a direct smear to be pleomorphic, displaying long, filamentous forms.

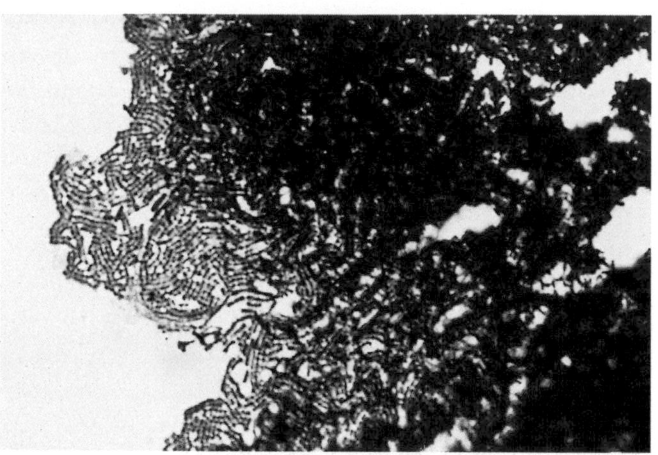

Figure 22-2 Gram stain of *Haemophilus ducreyi*. A characteristic of *H. ducreyi* is a tendency to arrange itself in what resembles schools of fish. The organisms shown here were grown in thioglycolate broth; however, if this morphology is seen in a direct Gram stain of a soft genital chancre, it is presumptive evidence of *H. ducreyi*. In the Gram stain shown, carbol fuchsin was used as the counterstain to enhance the visibility of the small bacilli.

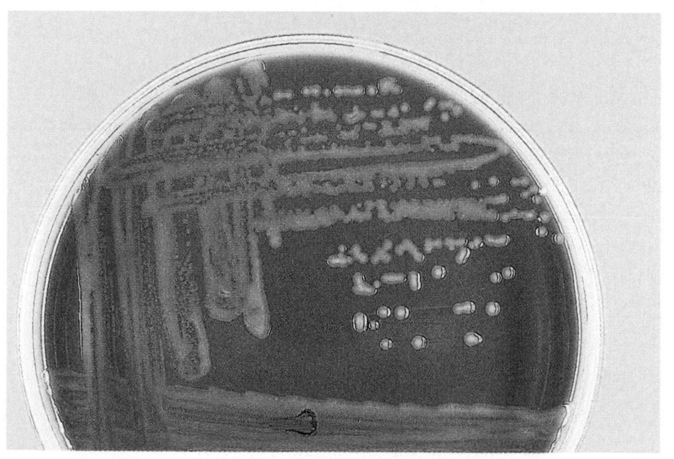

Figure 22-3 *Haemophilus influenzae* on chocolate agar. *H. influenzae* grows well on chocolate agar because, along with other essential nutrients, this medium supplies the X and V factors required for the growth of this species. The plate shown here was inoculated and incubated under 5% CO_2 at 35°C for 24 h. The colonies are gray, mucoid, and glistening.

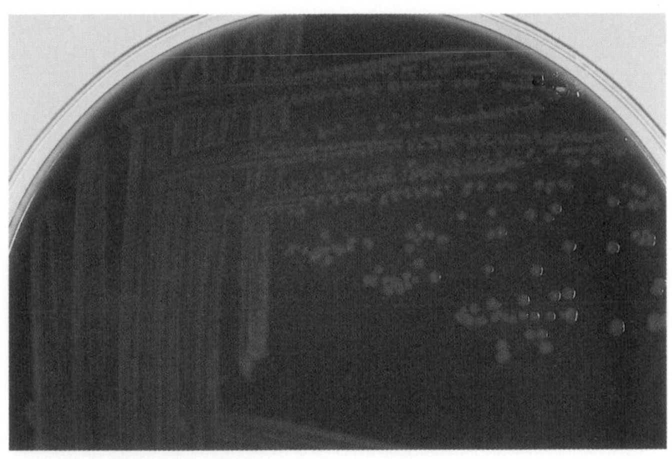

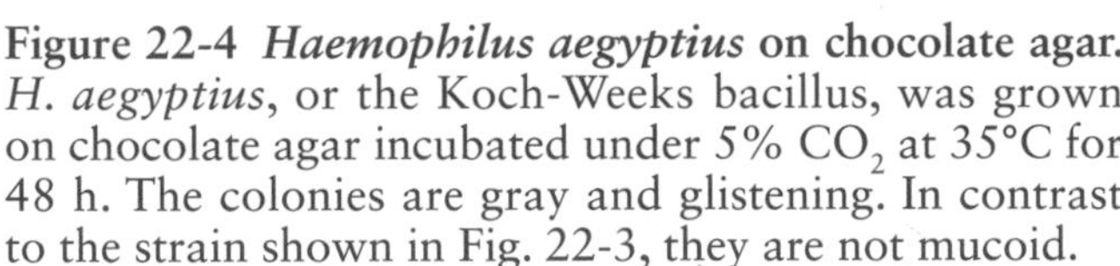

Figure 22-4 ***Haemophilus aegyptius* on chocolate agar.** *H. aegyptius*, or the Koch-Weeks bacillus, was grown on chocolate agar incubated under 5% CO_2 at 35°C for 48 h. The colonies are gray and glistening. In contrast to the strain shown in Fig. 22-3, they are not mucoid.

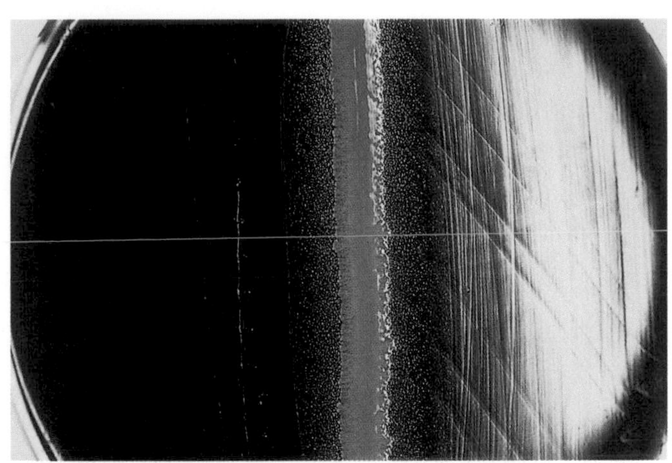

Figure 22-5 Satellite colonies of *Haemophilus influenzae*. On blood agar, *H. influenzae* can be seen growing around beta-hemolytic colonies of *S. aureus*. This phenomenon is called "satellite growth." *H. influenzae* requires both X and V factors, and these are provided by hemolysis of red blood cells (X factor) and by *S. aureus* (V factor). Shown here: a suspension of *H. influenzae* was used to inoculate the surface of blood agar to which a streak of *S. aureus* was applied. Upon incubation, growth of *H. influenzae* can be seen restricted to the area adjacent to *S. aureus*.

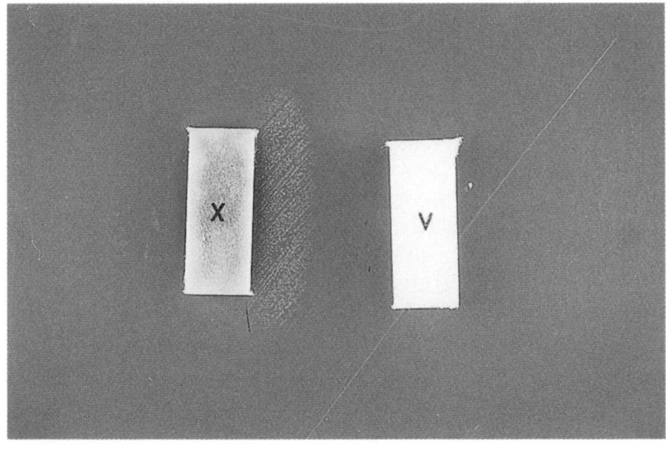

Figure 22-6 Requirement of *Haemophilus influenzae* for X and V factors. *H. influenzae* requires both X and V factors for growth. When grown on Mueller-Hinton agar, which does not contain X or V factor, *H. influenzae* grows only between the strips impregnated with X and V factors. The factors diffuse into the medium, and colonies are seen in the areas where the concentration of each factor is conducive to growth.

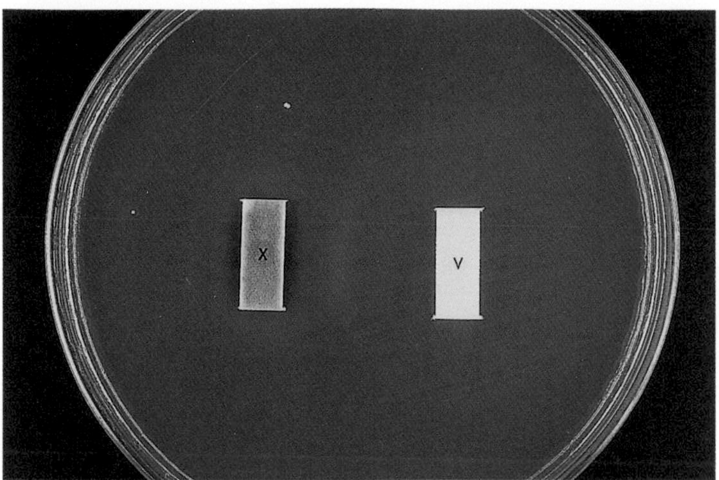

Figure 22-7 Requirement of *Haemophilus parainfluenzae* for V factor. *H. parainfluenzae* requires only V factor for growth. This is demonstrated by its ability to grow around the entire V strip on Mueller-Hinton agar, in contrast to the X strip, which has no V factor; therefore, there is no growth in the areas of the strip not adjacent to the V strip.

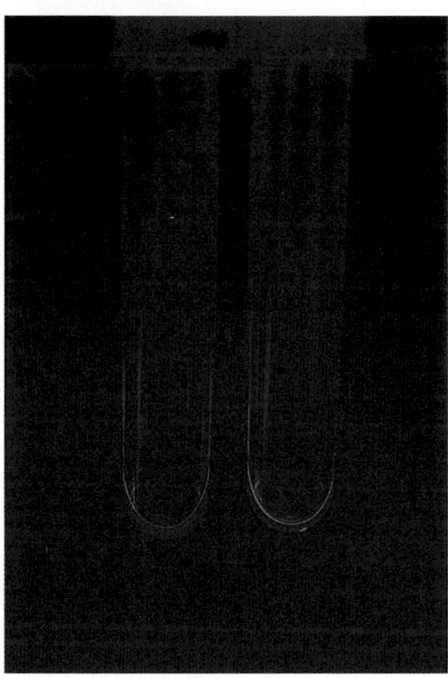

Figure 22-8 Porphyrin production test. The porphyrin production test is an alternative to the use of X strips to determine if an organism requires X factor for growth. In this test, an organism is inoculated into a solution of δ-aminolevulinic acid and incubated for 4 h at 35°C. If the organism can synthesize protoporphyrin compounds in the pathway to hemin production, then it does not require X factor. Since protoporphyrins are fluorescent when exposed to a UV light source such as a Wood's lamp, their presence can be readily detected, as illustrated by the tube on the left, which exhibits fluorescence. As shown here, the organism, *H. parainfluenzae*, used to inoculate the tube on the left does not require X factor. In contrast, *H. influenzae*, used to inoculate the tube on the right, which does not show fluorescence, cannot synthesize protoporphyrins due to a lack of X factor.

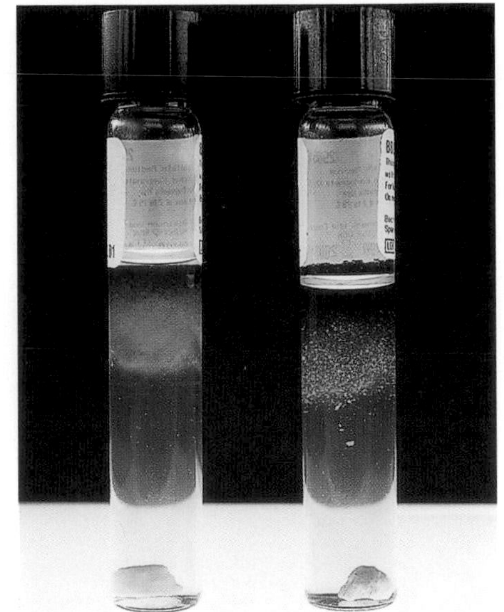

Figure 22-9 *Haemophilus influenzae* and *Haemophilus ducreyi* in thioglycolate broth. *H. influenzae* (left) and *H. ducreyi* (right) were grown for 72 h in thioglycolate broth. *Haemophilus* spp. are facultative anaerobes and grow below the surface of the broth. As shown here, *H. ducreyi* grows in tight, small clumps, in contrast to *H. influenzae*, which forms a homogeneous layer.

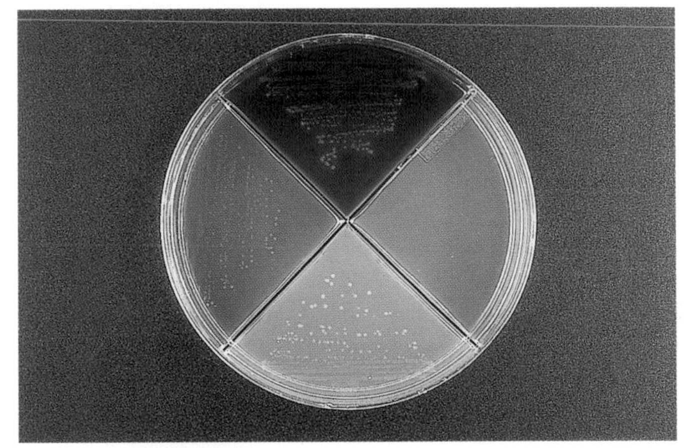

Figure 22-10 Identification of *Haemophilus* spp. using a Hemo-ID Quad plate. As shown here, the Quad plate (BD Diagnostic Systems, Franklin Lakes, NJ) is made of sections that, in clockwise order, contain horse blood agar (top), X factor, V factor, and both X and V factors. The *H. parahaemolyticus* strain used here hemolyzes horse blood and requires only V factor, as evidenced by its growth on the quadrants supplemented with V factor only and with X and V factors but not on the quadrant supplied with X factor alone.

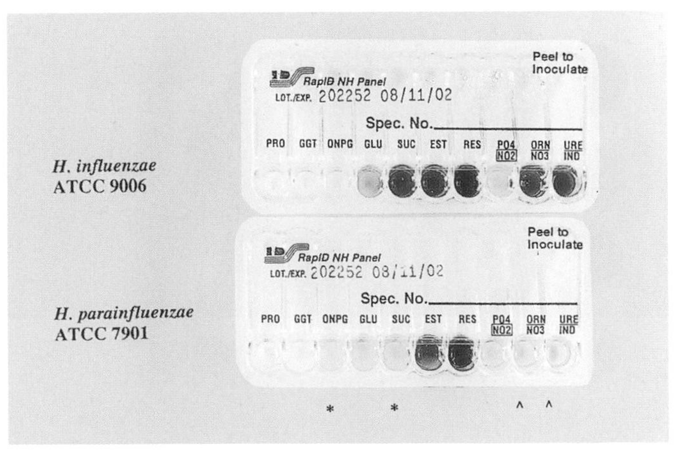

Figure 22-11 Identification of *Haemophilus* spp. by using the RapID NH system. Commercial systems such as the RapID NH system (Thermo Scientific Remel Products, Lenexa, KS) can determine the species and biotype of members of the *Haemophilus* genus. The strip at the top was inoculated with *H. influenzae* and the one at the bottom was inoculated with *H. parainfluenzae*. Key reactions (*) in the differentiation of these two species are *o*-nitrophenyl-β-D-galactopyranoside (ONPG) and sucrose (SUC). In addition, the key biochemicals (^) that are used to biotype *H. influenzae* and *H. parainfluenzae* are included in this rapid panel. In the example shown here, both urea (URE) and indole (IND) reactions can be determined by using the last well.

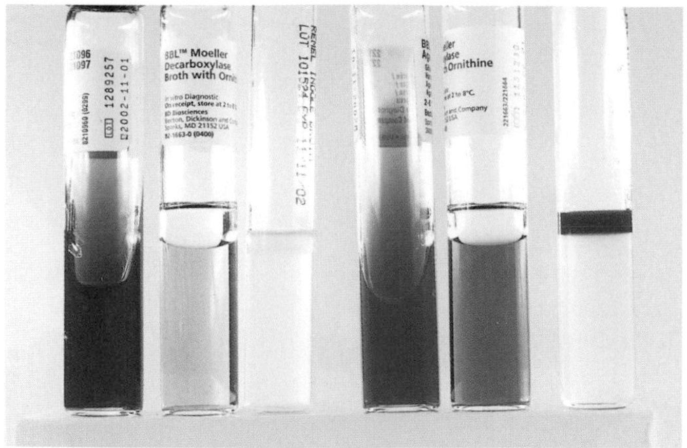

Figure 22-12 Biotyping of *Haemophilus influenzae*. *H. influenzae* and *H. parainfluenzae* strains can be biotyped using urea, ornithine decarboxylase, and indole. As shown here, *H. influenzae* biotype I (right) is positive for all three biochemical reactions, whereas *H. influenzae* biotype III (left), which includes *H. aegyptius*, is positive only for urea.

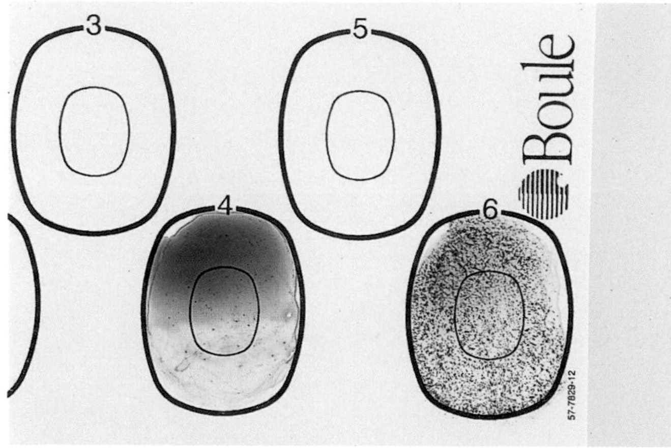

Figure 22-13 Serotyping of *Haemophilus influenzae*. Strains of *H. influenzae* can be serotyped by latex agglutination. Here, antiserum to *H. influenzae* type b (well 6) and types a and c to f (well 4) is coupled to latex particles that coagglutinate when mixed with the corresponding *H. influenzae* type. The Phadebact Haemophilus test (Boule Diagnostics AB, Huddinge, Sweden) shows that the organism is *H. influenzae* type b.

Figure 22-14 Comparison of hemolysis between *Haemophilus influenzae* and *Haemophilus haemolyticus*. Of the more common clinical isolates of *Haemophilus* spp., *H. haemolyticus* (right) is the only one that exhibits beta-hemolysis on horse blood agar. This characteristic can be used to differentiate it from *H. influenzae* (left).

Bordetella and Related Genera

23

Genera of clinical importance that belong to the family *Alcaligenaceae* include *Bordetella*, *Achromobacter*, and *Alcaligenes*. The genus *Bordetella* includes eight species, with *Bordetella pertussis* and *Bordetella parapertussis* the most commonly found in human infections. In general, *Bordetella* spp. inhabit the respiratory tracts of humans and animals by attaching to ciliated epithelial cells. Much of their pathogenesis is due to the elaboration of toxins that act as virulence factors. The pertussis toxin is the best known, being actively expressed by *B. pertussis*.

B. pertussis, the causative agent of whooping cough (pertussis), has only been reported to infect humans. While this infection is commonly thought of as a childhood disease, the protective immunity afforded by the vaccine that is administered in childhood is short-lived. Therefore, adults can serve as an important reservoir for this agent. However, the presentation in symptomatic adults may not be that of typical whooping cough. *B. parapertussis* can mimic the disease caused by *B. pertussis*, but, in general, the course of the infection is milder. It has been estimated that only a small percentage of children with a pertussis-like presentation are infected with *B. parapertussis*. *Bordetella bronchiseptica* is mainly an animal pathogen and is known to cause kennel cough in dogs; however, it can also produce pertussis-like symptoms in immunocompromised humans. *Bordetella holmesii*, which was formerly a member of the CDC nonoxidizer group 2 (NO-2), has only rarely been isolated from blood cultures. *Bordetella trematum* has occasionally been recovered from ears and wounds. Other *Bordetella* species have rarely been isolated from clinical infections.

Bordetella spp. are small, gram-negative coccobacilli. In general, they appear very faint by Gram stain when safranin is used as the counterstain but can be more easily seen when carbol fuchsin is used instead. A direct fluorescent-antibody (DFA) test is commercially available and offers the advantage of rapidity over culture; however, there are sensitivity and specificity problems with the DFA test, and until a more specific antibody can be developed, this test should be used with caution. Nucleic acid amplification methods to directly detect this organism are promising and, with further standardization and expansion of more specific target sequences, may be the preferred approach for detection and identification. However, until that time, culture should be performed in parallel with any direct test.

These organisms are considered fastidious since they require special media and prolonged incubation before colonies can be seen. Timely transportation and plating of specimens are essential for the recovery of *B. pertussis*. Nasopharyngeal specimens, in particular aspirates from young children, are preferred; ideally, they should be plated directly onto solid media. If they must be transported to the laboratory for culture, a transport swab that is known to preserve the viability of this organism should be used, such as one in Casamino Acids broth or a culturette containing charcoal to absorb some of the toxic compounds associated with swabs. The classic medium used for the isolation of *B. pertussis* is Bordet-Gengou agar (BGA), which incorporates potato infusion. Medium that contains horse blood and charcoal, such as Regan-Lowe agar, to which the antibiotic cephalexin has been added, not only supports

Table 23-1 Characteristics of the *Bordetella* spp. isolated from humans[a]

Organism	Growth on: Blood agar	Growth on: MacConkey agar	Oxidase	Urease	Brown pigment[b]
B. pertussis	0	0	+	0	0
B. parapertussis	+	V (delayed)	0	+ (24 h)	+
B. bronchiseptica	+	+	+	+ (4 h)	0
B. trematum	+	+	0	0	0
B. holmesii	+	+ (delayed)	0	0	+

[a]+, positive reaction; V, variable reaction; 0, negative reaction.
[b]On heart infusion agar supplemented with tyrosine.

the growth of most strains of *B. pertussis* but also suppresses normal flora over the prolonged incubation required, thereby increasing the recovery of *Bordetella*. Colonies of *B. pertussis* on BGA have been described as having a "mercury drop-like" appearance. In addition, with prolonged incubation on BGA, a zone of beta-hemolysis may develop around the colonies.

The time required before colonies are visible varies for the different *Bordetella* spp. In general, *B. pertussis* is the slowest growing, taking up to 4 days at 35°C under 5 to 7% CO_2 for visible growth to appear. Colonies of *B. parapertussis* can be seen within 2 to 3 days, and those of *B. bronchiseptica* can be seen within 24 h. The oxidase test can be used to separate *B. parapertussis*, which is negative, from *B. pertussis* and *B. bronchiseptica*, which are both positive. Antisera or nucleic acid amplification can be used to separate the last two species from one another. In addition, *B. parapertussis* and *B. bronchiseptica* are able to grow on blood agar while *B. pertussis* is not. A key characteristic that is useful in distinguishing *B. bronchiseptica* from the other two species is its ability to rapidly hydrolyze urea. This reaction can become positive within 4 h, in contrast to *B. parapertussis*, which is also urease positive but which takes 24 h to give a positive result. On heart infusion medium enriched with tyrosine, *B. parapertussis* and *B. holmesii* can produce a soluble brown pigment. Characteristics that can aid in the differentiation of Bordetella spp. are listed in Table 23-1.

The genus *Achromobacter* is composed of six species, with *Achromobacter xylosoxidans*, the type species, more frequently isolated from clinical material than other members, namely *Achromobacter denitrificans* and *Achromobacter piechaudii*. These organisms have been involved in nosocomial infections related to contaminated solutions or have been recovered from immunocompromised patients and patients with cystic fibrosis. The other three species either have not been recovered or are rarely encountered in clinical infections.

Achromobacter species are motile, aerobic, catalase- and oxidase-positive, gram-negative bacilli. They grow well on standard laboratory media including MacConkey, sheep blood, and chocolate agars. Colonies can range in color from white to tan. *Achromobacter* can be identified by several commercial systems, but the accuracy of these vary over a wide range.

Alcaligenes species, represented by *Alcaligenes faecalis*, have been isolated from a variety of clinical specimens including respiratory specimens obtained from patients with cystic fibrosis. Similar to *Achromobacter* spp., *Alcaligenes* spp. are motile, aerobic, catalase- and oxidase-positive, gram-negative bacilli that grow on standard laboratory media. *A. faecalis* is distinctive for reducing nitrite but not nitrate, and some strains have a fruity odor resembling apples and have a green hue on blood agar.

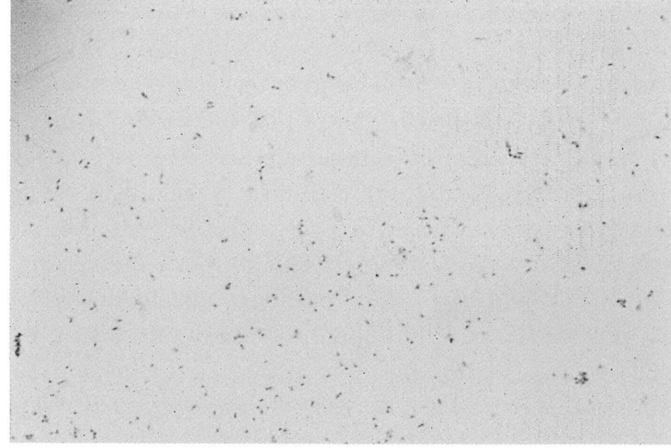

Figure 23-1 Gram stain of *Bordetella pertussis*. A routine Gram stain was performed using safranin as the counterstain. As shown, *B. pertussis* is a short, thin, faint-staining, gram-negative bacillus.

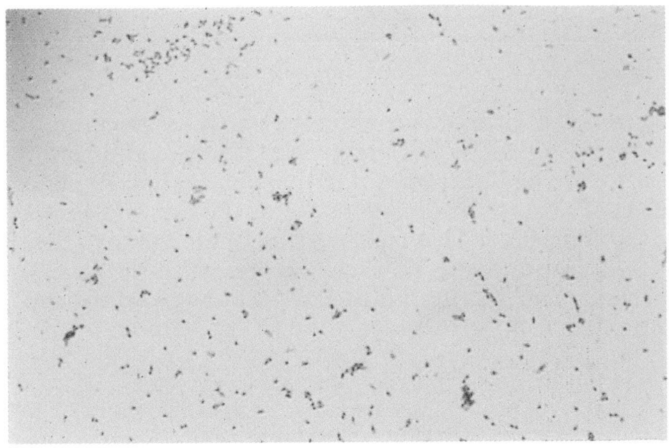

Figure 23-2 Gram stain of *Bordetella pertussis* with carbol fuchsin as the counterstain. In contrast to the Gram stain shown in Fig. 23-1, *B. pertussis* is easier to see in this figure due to the use of carbol fuchsin as the counterstain.

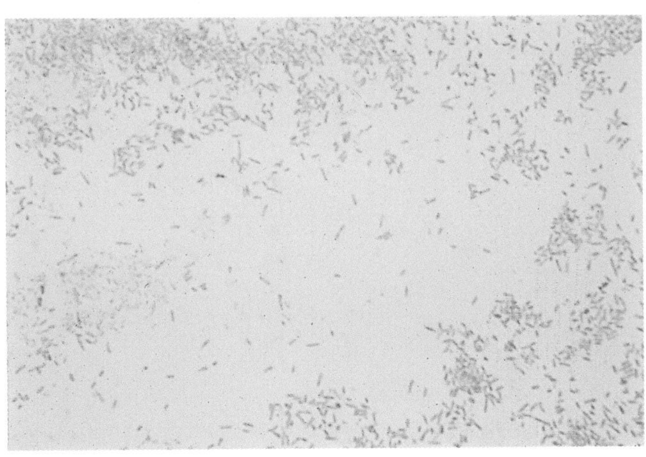

Figure 23-3 Gram stain of *Bordetella parapertussis* with carbol fuchsin as the counterstain. *B. parapertussis* is a larger, longer bacillus than *B. pertussis*. In the Gram stain shown here, carbol fuchsin was used as the counterstain to make the organisms easier to visualize.

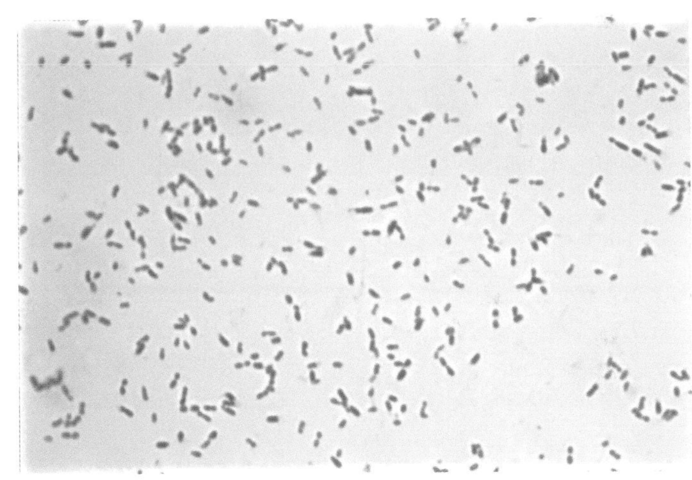

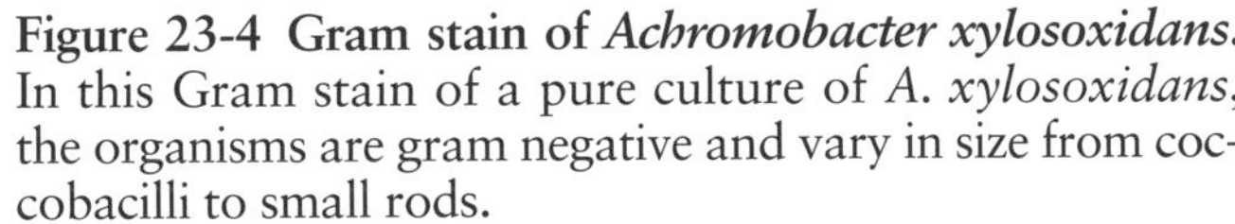

Figure 23-4 Gram stain of *Achromobacter xylosoxidans*. In this Gram stain of a pure culture of *A. xylosoxidans*, the organisms are gram negative and vary in size from coccobacilli to small rods.

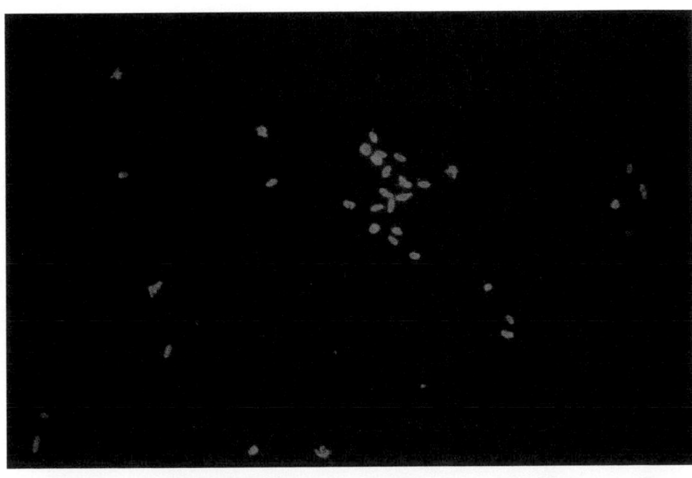

Figure 23-5 DFA stain for *Bordetella pertussis*. A smear of a nasopharyngeal specimen was directly stained with a fluorescein isothiocyanate-labeled antibody to *B. pertussis*. This smear was interpreted as positive for *B. pertussis*. The organisms shown appear as small coccobacilli that have a donut-like appearance, with the periphery of the cell staining darker than the center.

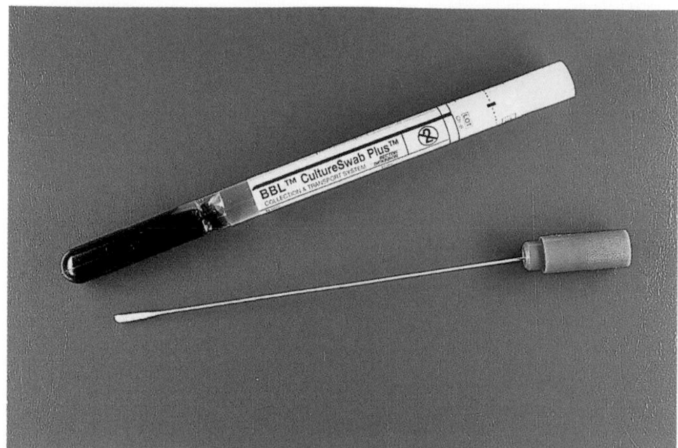

Figure 23-6 Charcoal-containing transport medium for the recovery of *Bordetella* species. Due to the fastidious nature of *Bordetella*, if specimens cannot be plated directly, a transport medium such as the one shown here is recommended. This transport medium contains charcoal to absorb toxins that may be present in the swab or specimen that can inhibit the growth of *Bordetella* spp., in particular *B. pertussis*.

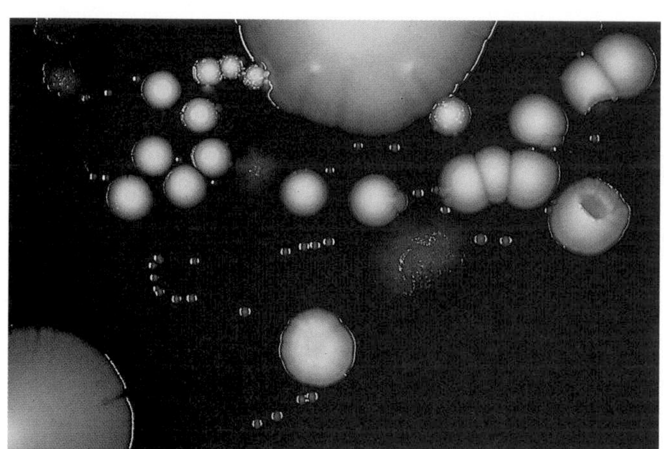

Figure 23-7 *Bordetella pertussis* on BGA. A nasopharyngeal swab was plated on BGA, which was incubated for 5 days under a humid 5% CO_2 atmosphere at 35°C. Shown here amid the normal flora, the colonies of *B. pertussis* are small and domed in shape, with the typical mercury drop-like appearance.

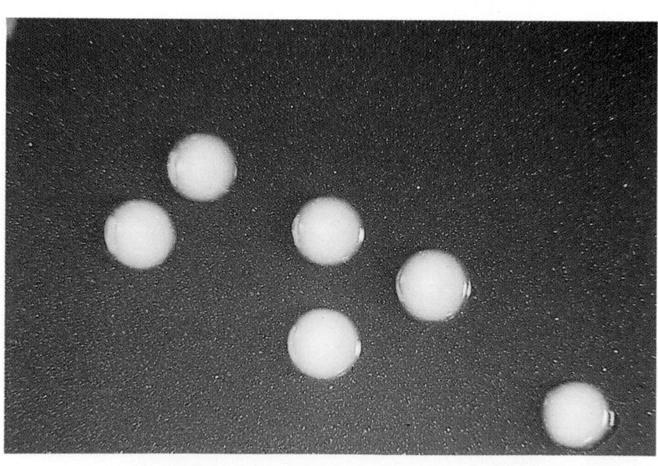

Figure 23-8 *Bordetella pertussis* on Regan-Lowe agar. Regan-Lowe medium contains horse blood and charcoal, which absorbs and neutralizes toxic substances that may be present in the agar. On this agar, colonies of *B. pertussis* have a pearly, opalescent sheen.

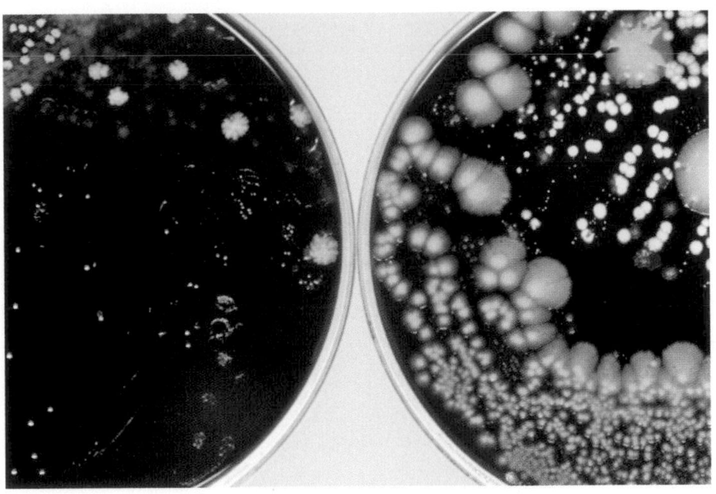

Figure 23-9 Culture of a nasopharyngeal specimen on BGA and Regan-Lowe agar. The culture plates were incubated for 5 days at 35°C under 5% CO_2. The BGA plate (right) permits the growth of normal respiratory flora, making the isolation of *B. pertussis* difficult. In contrast, on Regan-Lowe medium (left), which contains the antimicrobial agent cephalexin, the normal respiratory flora has been suppressed, making it easier to detect the small colonies of *B. pertussis*.

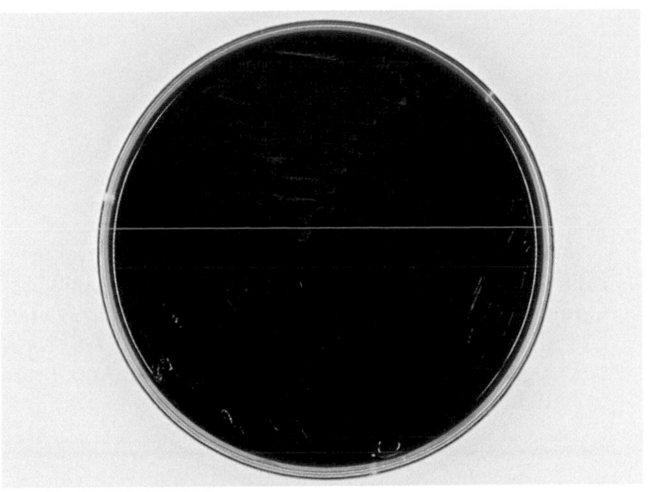

A

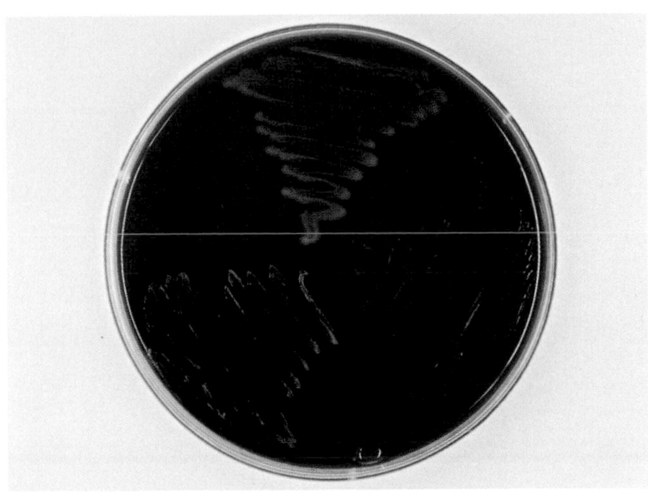

B

Figure 23-10 Three *Bordetella* species on BGA. The growth rates of the more common *Bordetella* spp. differ. Shown here is a BGA plate inoculated, in clockwise order, with *B. bronchiseptica* (top), *B. pertussis*, and *B. parapertussis*. This plate was incubated at 35°C under 5% CO_2 and photographed at 24 h (A) and 72 h (B) of incubation. At 24 h, visible colonies of *B. bronchiseptica* are present, in contrast to the 2 to 3 days required for *B. parapertussis* and the 4 days required for *B. pertussis* to show good growth.

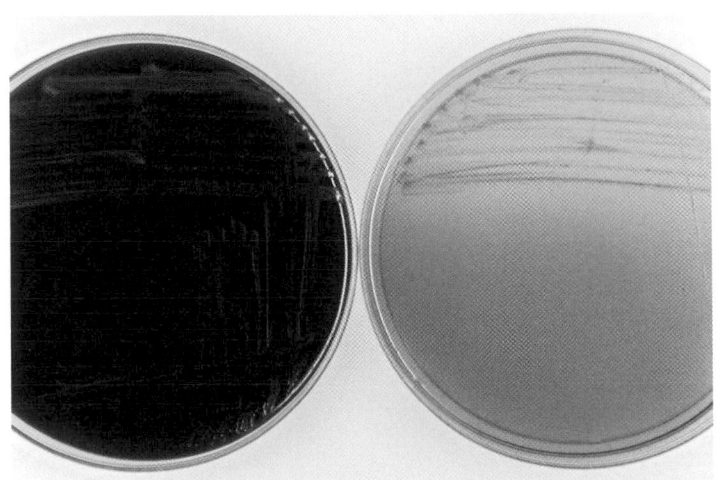

Figure 23-11 *Bordetella bronchiseptica* on blood agar and MacConkey agar. Unlike *B. pertussis*, *B. bronchiseptica* grows on both blood agar and MacConkey agar. On MacConkey agar, it is lactose negative.

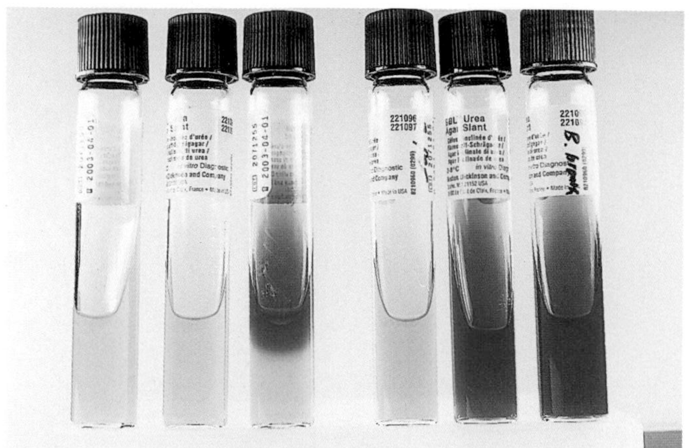

Figure 23-12 Comparison of three *Bordetella* species on urea agar slants. A key characteristic of *B. bronchiseptica* is its ability to rapidly hydrolyze urea. Positive reactions with this organism can be detected within 4 h of inoculation. *B. parapertussis* is also urease positive, but reactions may take up to 24 h to become positive. *B. pertussis* is urease negative. In the figure, the urea slants inoculated in the order (left to right) *B. pertussis*, *B. parapertussis*, and *B. bronchiseptica* were incubated for 4 h (left) and 24 h (right).

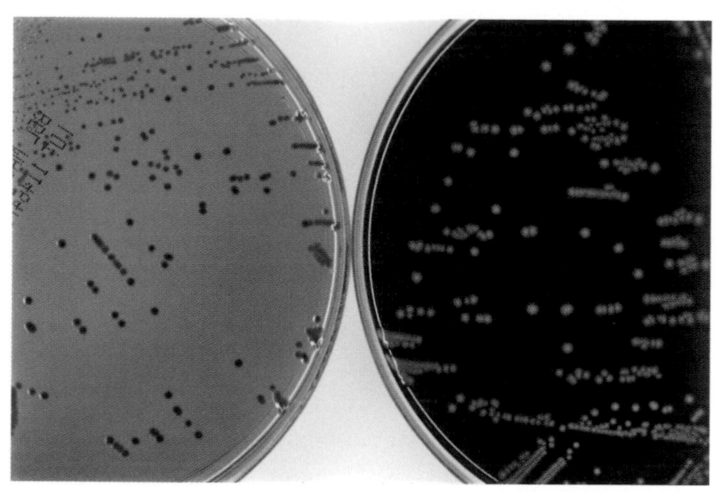

Figure 23-13 *Achromobacter xylosoxidans* on MacConkey and sheep blood agars. *Achromobacter* species grow well on both MacConkey and sheep blood agars. Shown is an isolate of *A. xylosoxidans* after overnight incubation at 35°C.

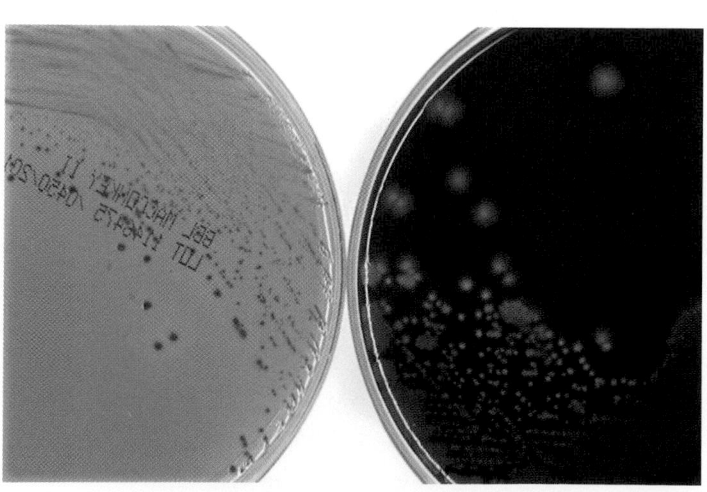

Figure 23-14 *Alcaligenes faecalis* on MacConkey and sheep blood agars. *A. faecalis* grows well on both MacConkey and sheep blood agars. A characteristic of this organism is the green discoloration surrounding the colony on sheep blood agar. The cultures shown were incubated overnight at 35°C.

Brucella 24

Four species of *Brucella*, *Brucella melitensis* (goats and sheep), *Brucella abortus* (cattle), *Brucella canis* (canines), and *Brucella suis* (swine), are human pathogens, while *Brucella neotomae* and *Brucella ovis* do not infect humans. The three marine species *Brucella delphini*, *Brucella pinnipediae*, and *Brucella cetaceae* can also cause disease in humans.

The host range for *Brucella* spp. includes mammals such as cattle, horses, goats, sheep, swine, dogs, coyotes, foxes, and rodents, while the marine species were isolated from seals, whales, and dolphins. These organisms have also been found in insects and ticks. Brucellosis is a zoonosis acquired by humans as a result of ingestion of, skin or mucosal contact with, or inhalation of infected material. Most of the 100 cases of brucellosis reported in the United States each year are due to consumption of unpasteurized dairy products.

The clinical presentation of brucellosis may include intermittent fever, chills, weakness, malaise, aches, sweating, and weight loss. The remittent fever, termed undulant fever, appears at regular intervals and may last for years in inadequately treated patients. Several organs, including the liver, spleen, bones, joints, genitourinary tract, central nervous system, lungs, heart, and skin, can be involved. Organs of the reticuloendothelial system are frequently affected. *Brucella* spp. are phagocytosed by monocytes and macrophages and carried to the lymph nodes, spleen, bone marrow, and liver, where they may form noncaseating granulomas that can be difficult to distinguish from sarcoidosis.

Members of the genus *Brucella* are aerobic, non-spore-forming, nonencapsulated, nonmotile, intracellular gram-negative coccobacilli that measure 0.5 to 0.7 μm by 0.6 to 1.5 μm. Specimens frequently submitted to the laboratory for diagnosis include blood, bone marrow, and biopsy specimens from the liver. Commercially available blood culture systems are reliable for the detection of *Brucella* spp., although the biphasic blood culture bottle, such as that containing Castañeda medium, appears to be the method of choice. Cultures should be held at 35°C under a 5 to 10% CO_2 atmosphere for a minimum of 21 days, and blind terminal subcultures are recommended. These organisms are catalase, oxidase, urease, and nitrate positive. Some species require complex media and CO_2 for growth (Table 24-1). Other tests that can be used to differentiate among the four clinically important species include urea hydrolysis, H_2S production, and dye sensitivity. *Brucella* spp. are classified as a type 3 biohazard and should be handled only by appropriately equipped laboratories. None of the commercially available identification systems can identify these bacteria.

Serological testing is recommended in all cases of suspected infection, since culture alone is not reliable. Antibody titers can persist for years, and therefore an increase in antibody titer is necessary to provide serological evidence of current disease. In general, a fourfold rise in antibody titer between two serum specimens collected at least a week apart is suggestive of current infection. Immunoglobulin M (IgM) antibodies appear first, followed by IgG 2 to 3 weeks later. Persistent antibody titers suggest poor response to the therapy, relapse, or chronic infections. Persistent IgG antibodies occur in 20 to 30% of treated and cured patients. Molecular techniques are becoming available for the detection and identification of this group of organisms.

Table 24-1 Differentiation of *Brucella* species[a]

Organism	Dye sensitivity		Urea hydrolysis	H_2S production	CO_2 requirement
	Basic fuchsin	Thionine			
B. melitensis	R	R	>90 min	None	0
B. abortus	R	S	>90 min	2–5 days	+/0
B. suis	S	R	<90 min	1–6 days	0
B. canis	S	R	<90 min	None	0

[a]R, resistant; S, susceptible; +, positive reaction; 0, negative reaction.

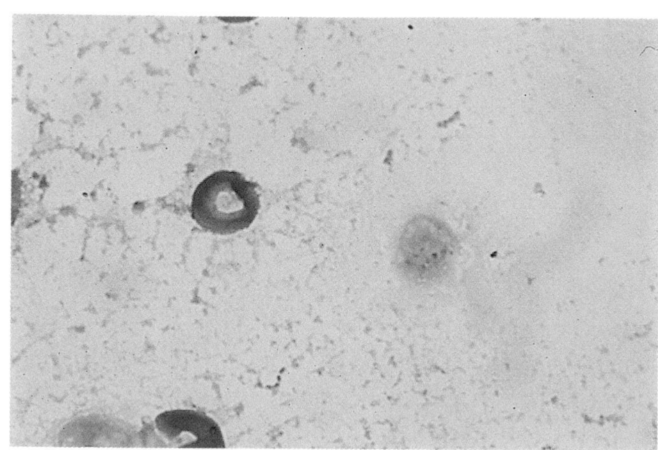
A

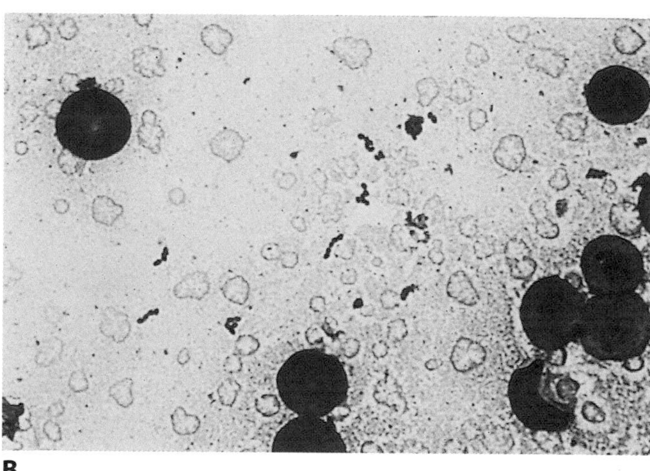
B

Figure 24-1 Gram stain of *Brucella* spp. (A) *Brucella* spp. are small, gram-negative coccobacilli that may have a "fine-sand" appearance. (B) A modified Gram stain with carbol fuchsin as the counterstain helps to better visualize these organisms. They are usually arranged singly, but pairs, short chains, and small groups can also be found.

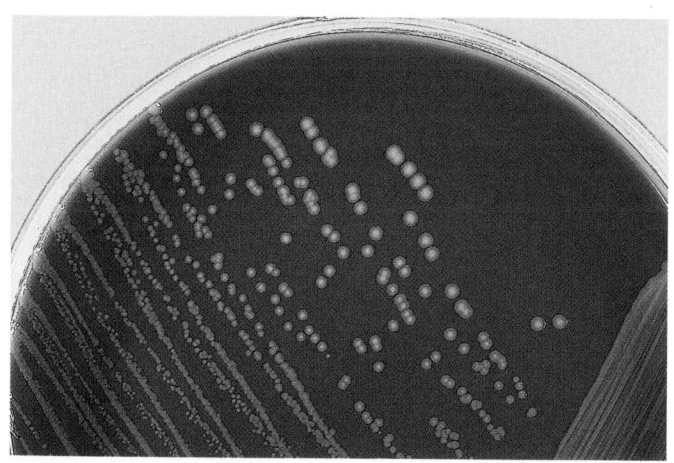

Figure 24-2 *Brucella abortus* on chocolate agar. Most *Brucella* spp. grow on chocolate agar, producing colonies that are small, round, raised, white to cream, and glistening. Cultures should be incubated at 35°C under 5 to 10% CO_2 for at least 7 days before being discarded.

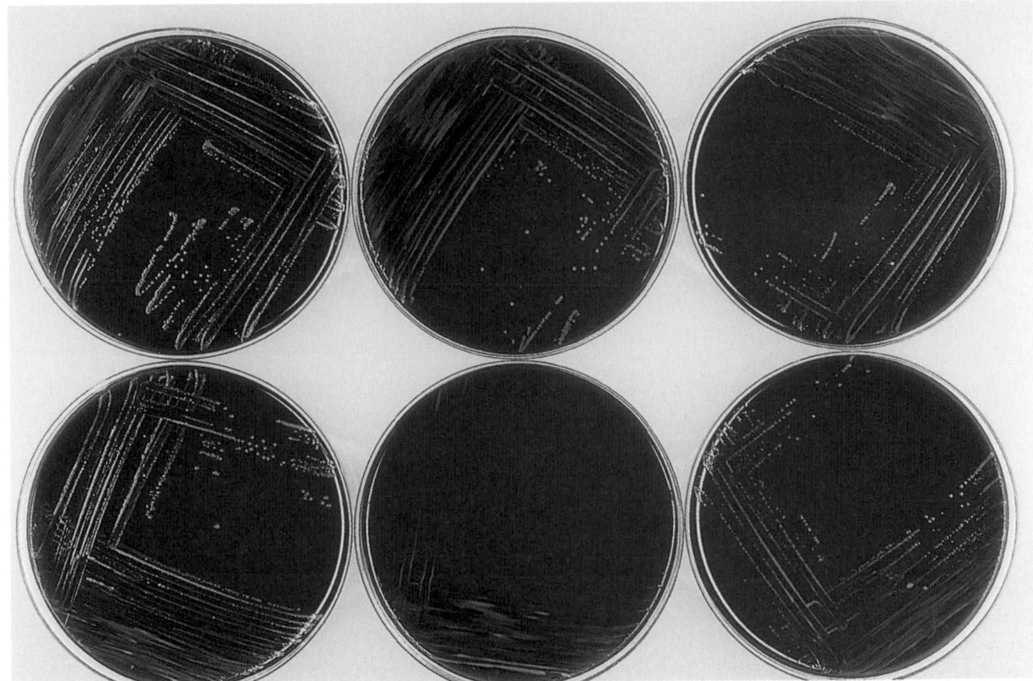

Figure 24-3 Enhancement of growth of *Brucella abortus* by CO_2. *B. abortus* grows better in the presence of CO_2, while the other *Brucella* spp. do not. The blood agar plates in the top row were incubated at 35°C under 5 to 10% CO_2, while the ones at the bottom were incubated in ambient air. From left to right, the organisms are *B. melitensis*, *B. abortus*, and *B. suis*.

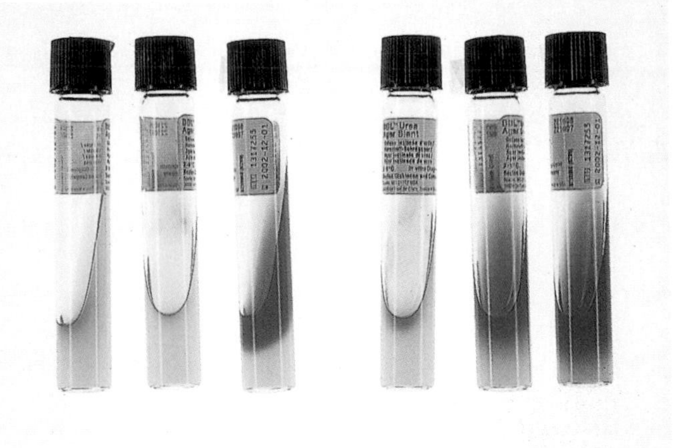

Figure 24-4 Urea hydrolysis by *Brucella* spp. *B. suis* and *B. canis* hydrolyze urea rapidly (in less than 1 h), whereas *B. melitensis* and *B. abortus* take longer or may be negative. In this figure, the three tubes on the left were incubated at 35°C for 1 h and those on the right were incubated for 24 h. From left to right, the organisms are *B. melitensis*, *B. abortus*, and *B. suis*, with the order repeated for the next three tubes.

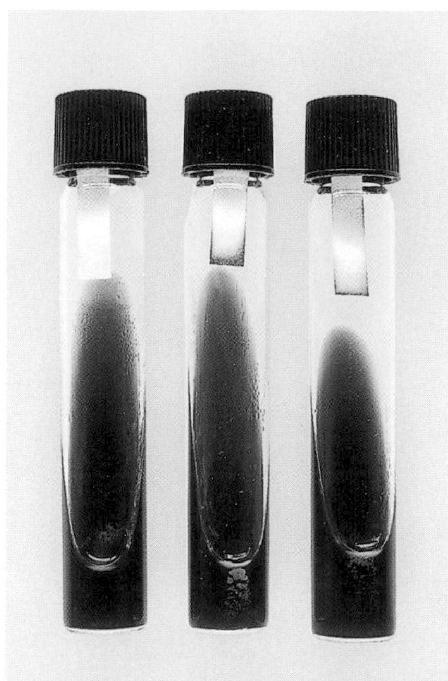

Figure 24-5 Production of H_2S by *Brucella* spp. To test for the production of H_2S, a *Brucella* slant is inoculated and a lead acetate paper strip is introduced into the tube so that it hangs down but does not touch the agar. The slant is then incubated at 35°C under 5 to 10% CO_2 for 6 days and is checked daily for blackening of the lead acetate. The paper strip should be replaced daily. *B. suis* produces a large amount of H_2S daily for the 6 days of observation, while *B. abortus* produces a moderate amount from days 2 to 5 and *B. melitensis* produces little if any. From left to right, cultures of *B. melitensis*, *B. abortus*, and *B. suis* are shown after 3 days of incubation.

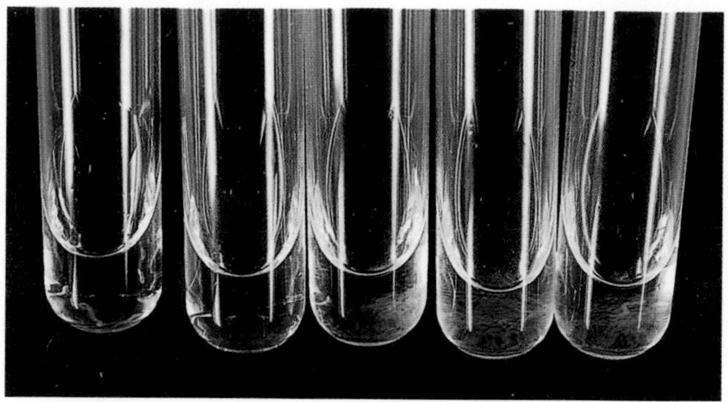

Figure 24-6 Serological testing for *Brucella* spp. Culture is not a very sensitive method for detecting *Brucella* spp. For this reason, it is recommended to use serum from a patient to perform a tube agglutination test that can detect antibody to *B. melitensis*, *B. abortus*, and *B. suis* but not *B. canis*. A single titer of ≥160 or a fourfold increase in antibody titer between two specimens collected 2 to 4 weeks apart is considered significant. Serial dilutions of the serum were incubated with the antigen and agglutination was observed in two tubes. The tube on the left is the negative control and the tube on the right the positive control. The antigen used in this assay was *B. abortus*.

Pasteurella 25

There are several species in the genus *Pasteurella*, of which *Pasteurella multocida*, *Pasteurella canis*, *Pasteurella dagmatis*, and *Pasteurella stomatis* can be isolated from humans.

P. multocida is the most common species found in human infections. Currently, there are three subspecies: *P. multocida* subsp. *multocida*, *P. multocida* subsp. *septica*, and *P. multocida* subsp. *gallicida*. This organism appears to be a commensal in the upper respiratory tracts of mammals and fowl and perhaps also of humans, in particular those with a chronic respiratory infection. Infections are frequently associated with animal bites, especially those from cats, and result in localized cellulitis and lymphadenitis. Pulmonary disease and systemic dissemination, including meningitis, may occur, particularly in immunocompromised patients and those with an underlying hepatic disease. *P. multocida* subsp. *multocida* is frequently isolated from respiratory infections and septicemia, while *P. multocida* subsp. *septica* is usually associated with wound infections.

Exudates from bites or scratches should be submitted to the laboratory for direct examination and culture. Blood and respiratory specimens for culture should be collected from patients with fever. *Pasteurella* spp. grow on chocolate and blood agars, producing small, gray, smooth, nonhemolytic colonies that may be mucoid. Several species of *Pasteurella*, including *P. multocida*, do not grow on MacConkey agar. Members of the genus *Pasteurella* are facultatively anaerobic, nonmotile, gram-negative, pleomorphic coccobacilli or bacilli. The majority of strains that are clinically significant are catalase, oxidase, alkaline phosphatase, and indole positive. Most of the species produce acid from fructose, glucose, mannose, and sucrose and reduce nitrates to nitrites.

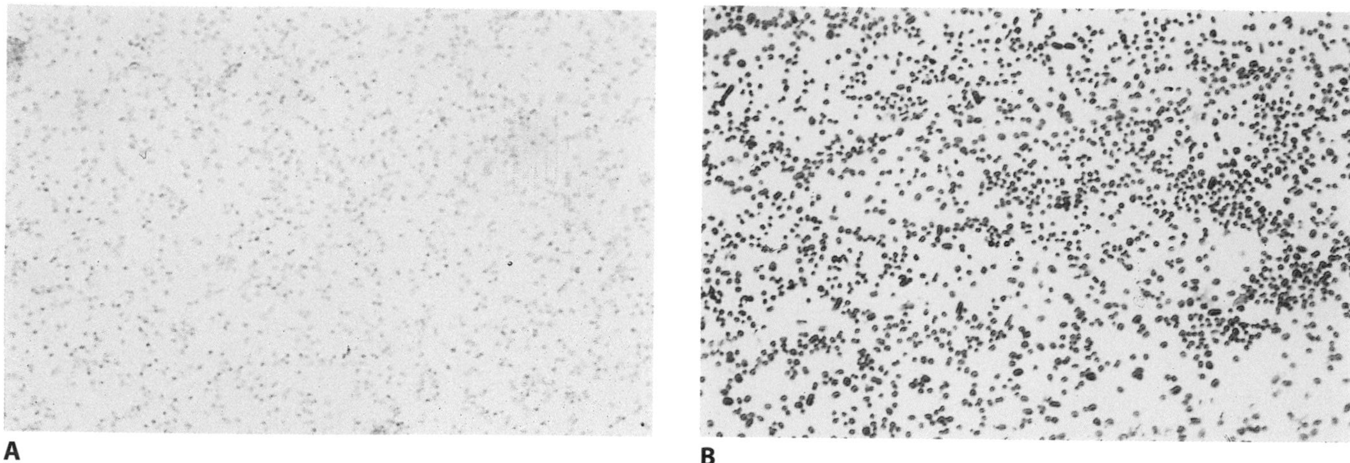

Figure 25-1 Gram stain of *Pasteurella multocida*. The specimens were counterstained with safranin (A) or carbol fuchsin (B). The pleomorphic structure of *P. multocida* is evident in both panels. These pleomorphic, gram-negative organisms may be coccobacillary, with ovoid, short bacilli measuring 0.5 to 1.0 μm, or filamentous; may have bipolar staining; and can occur singly, in pairs, or in short chains. A capsule is frequently observed in clinical isolates.

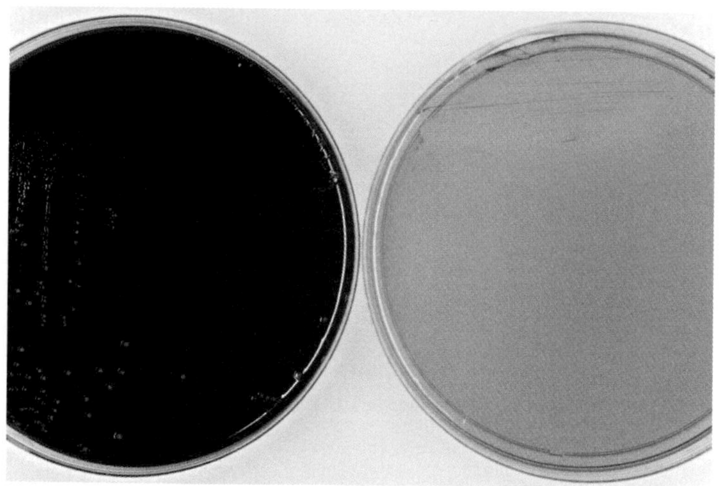

Figure 25-2 *Pasteurella multocida* on blood agar and MacConkey agar. *P. multocida* produces small (1- to 2-mm-diameter), gray colonies on blood agar (left) but does not grow on MacConkey agar (right). A characteristic odor, similar to that of *Escherichia coli*, results from the production of indole.

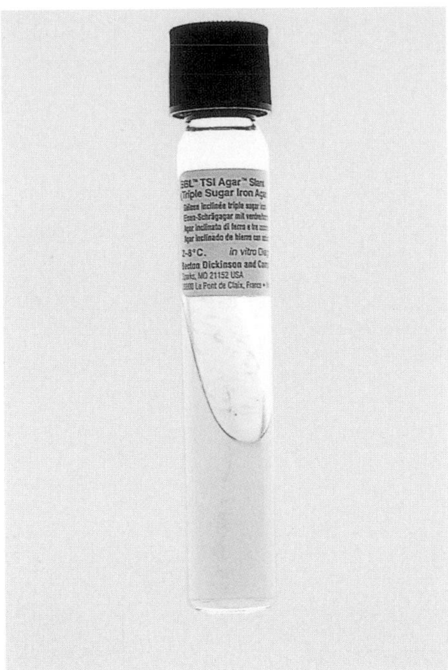

Figure 25-3 *Pasteurella multocida* in triple sugar iron agar. *P. multocida* produces a limited amount of acid from glucose, resulting in a weak acid reaction in the butt and slant of the triple sugar iron agar.

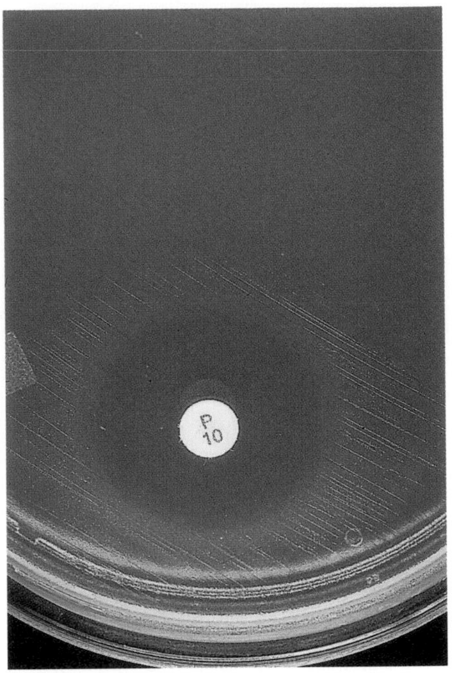

Figure 25-4 Susceptibility of *Pasteurella multocida* to penicillin. A 10-U disk of penicillin may be used to help in the identification of this organism. As shown here, a zone of inhibition of ≥15 mm is produced when a 0.5 McFarland suspension of *P. multocida* is plated on Mueller-Hinton agar.

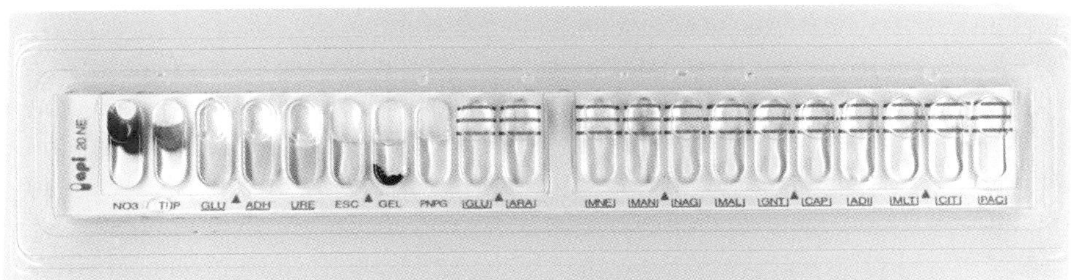

Figure 25-5 Identification methods for *Pasteurella multocida*. Shown here is the API 20NE (bioMérieux, Inc., Durham, NC), one of the kits available for the identification of nonfastidious, gram-negative bacteria that do not belong to the *Enterobacteriaceae*. This assay combines 8 conventional and 12 assimilation tests.

Bartonella and *Afipia*

26

Species of *Bartonella* associated with human infections include *Bartonella bacilliformis*, *Bartonella quintana*, *Bartonella henselae*, *Bartonella clarridgeiae*, *Bartonella vinsonii*, *Bartonella grahamii*, and *Bartonella elizabethae*. The genus *Afipia* includes *Afipia felis*, *Afipia broomeae*, *Afipia clevelandensis*, and several other unnamed genospecies.

While some of the species of the genus *Bartonella* have a global distribution, others are restricted to certain regions. *B. bacilliformis* is localized to the Andes because of the limited habitat of the sand fly vector, *Lutzomyia* (*Phlebotomus*) *verrucarum*. *B. bacilliformis* penetrates erythrocytes, which become fragile and are cleared by the reticuloendothelial system, resulting in severe anemia (Carrion's disease or Oroya fever) and a chronic nodular form (verruga peruana). *B. quintana* is transmitted by *Pediculus humanus*, the sucking louse, and has a worldwide distribution, particularly in areas with poor sanitary conditions. This organism causes the so-called trench fever or five-day fever, characterized by several episodes of acute fever and chills that can recur at 5-day intervals, accounting for the name of the disease. *B. quintana* can also produce bacillary angiomatosis, most often seen in patients with HIV-1 infection, consisting of vascular proliferation that involves the skin, subcutaneous tissues, liver, spleen, brain, lungs, and bones.

B. henselae is endemic throughout the world as a result of infection of the domestic cat; the flea *Ctenocephalides felis* appears to be the primary vector for cat-to-cat transmission. Cat scratch disease is caused mainly by *B. henselae*, although a few cases due to *B. clarridgeiae* and *A. felis* have been diagnosed. Approximately 25,000 cases of cat scratch disease are reported annually in the United States. Typically, following a cat bite or scratch, a pustule or papule appears at the site of inoculation accompanied by regional lymphadenopathy and fever. Bacillary peliosis due to *B. henselae* is more commonly seen in HIV-1-infected and immunocompromised patients and is characterized by the formation of cystic structures lined by endothelium in the liver and spleen. A Warthin-Starry silver stain of these lesions reveals clumps of bacilli. *B. henselae* and *B. quintana* can produce subacute endocarditis, particularly in elderly, homeless individuals and in those with cardiac valve replacement. *B. elizabethae* and *B. vinsonii* have also been isolated from individuals with endocarditis.

Blood and tissues are the specimens most frequently used for the isolation and detection of *Bartonella* and *Afipia* spp. *Bartonella* spp. are small (0.2 to 0.6 μm by 0.5 to 2.0 μm), curved, aerobic, gram-negative bacilli that grow only on enriched media containing blood. Of the human pathogens, *B. bacilliformis* grows better at 25 to 30°C, whereas *B. henselae*, *B. quintana*, and *B. elizabethae* prefer 35 to 37°C. Chocolate agar and Columbia agar supplemented with 5% sheep or rabbit blood are the preferred media for isolation. The use of liquid insect cell growth medium as a preenrichment step has increased the recovery of *Bartonella* spp. from clinical samples. Cultures should be held for a minimum of 2 to 3 weeks at 35 to 37°C under 5% CO_2. *B. henselae* produces two types of colonies. One is an irregular, raised, white, dry, rough "cauliflower-like" colony that appears to be embedded in the agar, and the other is a smaller form that is tan, circular, and moist and has a tendency to pit and adhere to the agar. Molecular techniques have so far been found to have limited sensitivity for the detection of *Bartonella* spp.; however, they can be used for the identification of the isolates.

Bartonella spp. are oxidase and urease negative, and they do not produce acid from carbohydrates. In contrast to *Bartonella* spp., *Afipia* spp. are urease and oxidase positive and most produce acid from D-xylose. *B. bacilliformis* and *B. clarridgeiae* are motile owing to a single flagellum. Although *B. henselae* and *B. quintana* do not have flagella, a "twitching" motion due to the pili can be observed when a wet mount preparation is examined.

Bartonella spp. can be identified by gas-liquid chromatography of their fatty acids. The MicroScan Rapid Anaerobe Panel (Siemens Healthcare Diagnostics, Deerfield, IL) gives a unique biotype for each species of *Bartonella*. Due to the difficulties in growing these organisms, several serological tests are frequently used for the diagnosis of *Bartonella* infections in humans. Immunofluorescence antibody assays, enzyme-linked immunosorbent assays, and Western blots have been used for the diagnosis of these infections. The results from these assays, however, are not easy to interpret since there is antigenic variability among *Bartonella* test strains and cross-reactivity can occur not only among different species of *Bartonella* but also with other pathogens such as *Chlamydia pneumoniae*, *Coxiella burnetii*, and *Rickettsia* spp. Therefore, the sensitivity and specificity reported for serological assays vary widely.

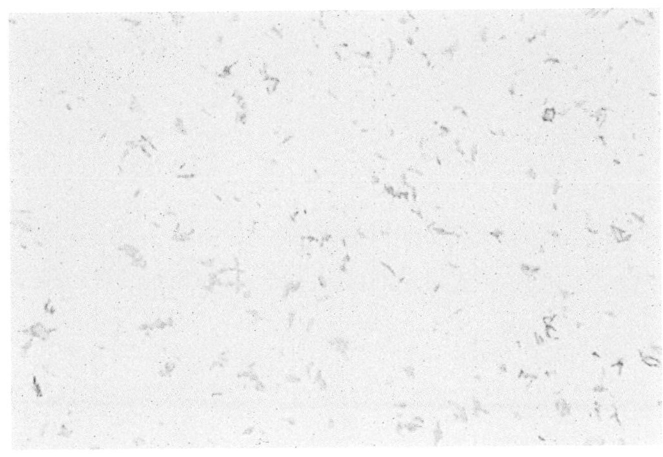

A

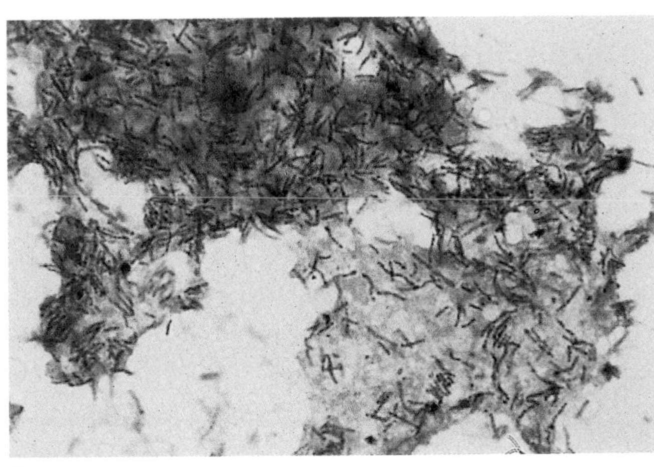

B

Figure 26-1 Gram stain of *Bartonella henselae*. (A) On a Gram stain with a safranin counterstain, *Bartonella* spp. appear as small, faintly stained, slightly curved, gram-negative bacilli. (B) Counterstaining with carbol fuchsin gives a more distinct morphology.

A

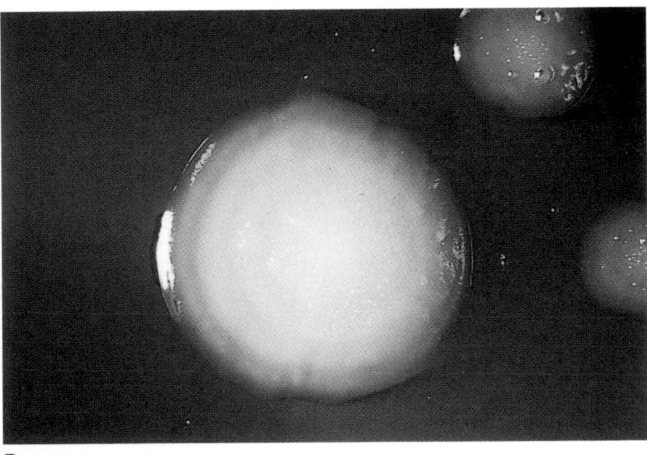

B

Figure 26-2 *Bartonella henselae* colonies. Large, white, irregular colonies with a cauliflower appearance, mixed with small, tan, moist colonies that pit the agar, can be observed after 5 to 7 days of incubation.

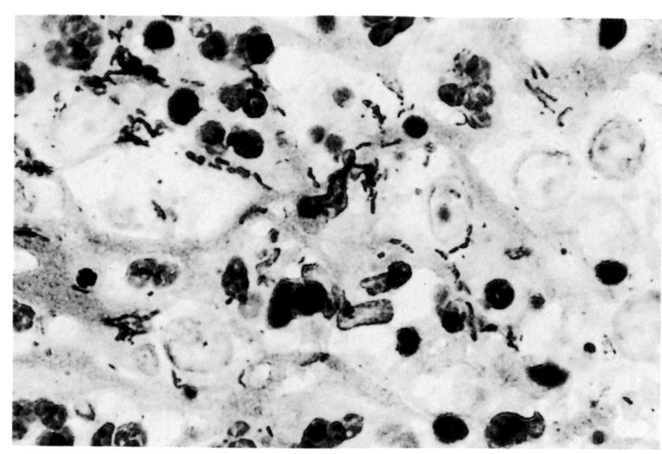

Figure 26-3 Warthin-Starry silver stain of a lymph node from a patient with cat scratch disease. *B. henselae* is present in this tissue section, predominantly surrounding blood vessels. The organisms appear as dark-brown, short bacilli, many of them in clumps.

Francisella 27

There are several species classified in the genus *Francisella*, including *Francisella philomiragia*, *Francisella novicida*, *Francisella noatunensis*, and *Francisella tularensis*. Three subspecies are included in the species *F. tularensis*: *F. tularensis* subsp. *tularensis* (type A), *F. tularensis* subsp. *holarctica* (type B), and *F. tularensis* subsp. *mediaasiatica*. *F. tularensis* subsp. *tularensis* occurs only in North America, *F. tularensis* subsp. *holarctica* can be found in the Old and the New Worlds, and *F. tularensis* subsp. *mediaasiatica* has been isolated only in Central Asia.

More than 100 species of vertebrates and invertebrates are natural reservoirs for these organisms. The most common sources of human infection with *F. tularensis* are wild rabbits, ticks, deerflies, and mosquitoes. The number of reported cases in the United States ranges from 100 to 200 per year, resulting in one to four deaths annually. This bacterium is extremely infectious, and only 10 organisms administered subcutaneously, or 25 by the respiratory route, are needed to cause infection. On the other hand, at least 10^8 bacteria must be ingested in order to produce an infection in the gastrointestinal tract. *F. turalensis* appears to be able to penetrate normal skin, although it may require microscopic breaks in the skin surface. Clinical specimens should be handled under Biosafety Level 2 conditions with standard precautions and transferred to Level 3 as soon as *F. tularensis* is suspected.

The clinical presentation is usually abrupt, with fever, chills, headache, and generalized pain. There are several distinct clinical forms including ulceroglandular (cutaneous ulcer with lymphadenopathy), glandular (lymphadenopathy only), oculoglandular (conjunctivitis with preauricular lymphadenopathy), oropharyngeal (upper respiratory and cervical lymphadenopathy), pneumonic, and typhoidal, with no localizing signs or symptoms. The most common presentation in the United States is the ulceroglandular form, resulting from tick bites and contact with infected animals. Following an incubation period of 3 to 10 days, a papule forms at the site of infection, eventually ulcerates, and is accompanied by regional lymphadenopathy. *F. philomiragia* is an opportunistic organism that causes infections mainly in immunocompromised patients, in particular those with chronic granulomatous disease, and in near-drowning individuals. In most near-drowning cases, the organism was isolated from sterile body fluids including the blood and cerebrospinal fluid. Fewer than 10 cases of *F. novicida* infection have been reported.

Organisms in the genus *Francisella* are small, pleomorphic, gram-negative bacilli that measure 0.2 μm by 0.2 to 1.0 μm and are obligately aerobic. Performing a direct Gram stain of tissues is not productive because the organisms are so small that they often cannot be distinguished from background material. Safranin is a poor counterstain. A direct fluorescent-antibody (DFA) test is available in some public health laboratories and at the Centers for Disease Control and Prevention. Immunohistochemical stains using monoclonal antibodies are useful for detecting *Francisella* in tissues. Specimens that are going to be amplified by PCR should be collected in guanidine isothiocyanate-containing buffer, which helps to preserve the DNA for several weeks.

Scrapings of ulcers and lymph node biopsy specimens are often submitted for culture. However, culture is not a very sensitive method. Isolation of this organism can be difficult due to its slow growth and specific nutritional requirements. The medium of choice in some reference labs is cystine heart agar supplemented with 9% chocolatized sheep blood (CHAB). Alternatively, chocolate agar supplemented with IsoVitaleX or buffered charcoal-yeast extract agar (BCYE) can be used. To prevent overgrowth by contaminating organisms in specimens such as ulcers and sputa, Thayer-Martin or modified Martin-Lewis media have also been used. The organism has been isolated from blood by using several commercial culture systems.

When grown at 35°C under 5% CO_2, colonies may take 2 to 5 days to appear. The colonies are small, bluish, smooth, and mucoid on cystine glucose blood agar and white to greenish and smooth on chocolate agar. On media containing blood, a small zone of alpha-hemolysis may appear around the colony. The organisms are oxidase negative, weakly catalase positive, and fairly inert biochemically and do not grow well, if at all, on MacConkey agar. For confirmation, a slide agglutination test with commercially available antiserum or a DFA test can be performed on a formalinized culture suspension. Nucleic acid amplification techniques have recently been developed for the detection and identification of *Francisella*. However, the most common approach for diagnosing these infections is by serological methods. Antibodies develop in most patients by 2 weeks after infection and can remain positive for more than 10 years. Immunoglobulin M antibodies can linger for many years and therefore do not imply an early or recent infection. Enzyme-linked immunosorbent assays and tube agglutination and microagglutination methods are available for the detection of antibodies to *Francisella*.

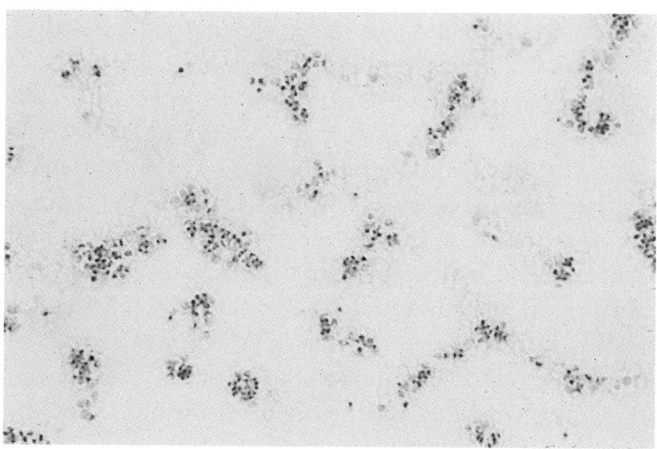

Figure 27-1 Gram stain of *Francisella tularensis*. *F. tularensis* is a minute, pleomorphic, gram-negative coccobacillus that may exhibit bipolar staining.

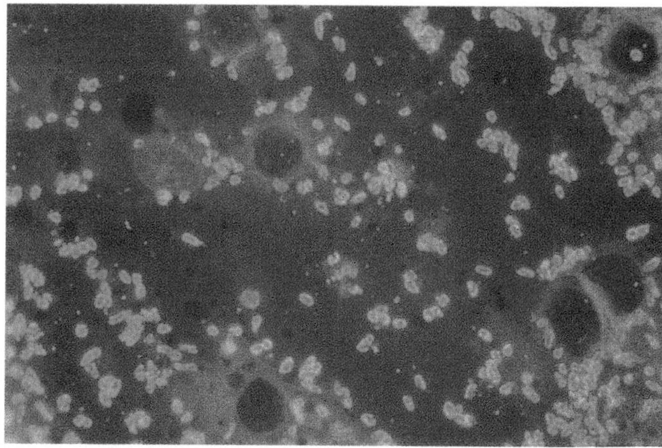

Figure 27-2 DFA staining of *Francisella tularensis*. A polyclonal rabbit antibody is available for the detection of *F. tularensis*. The pleomorphic structure of this organism is well documented here.

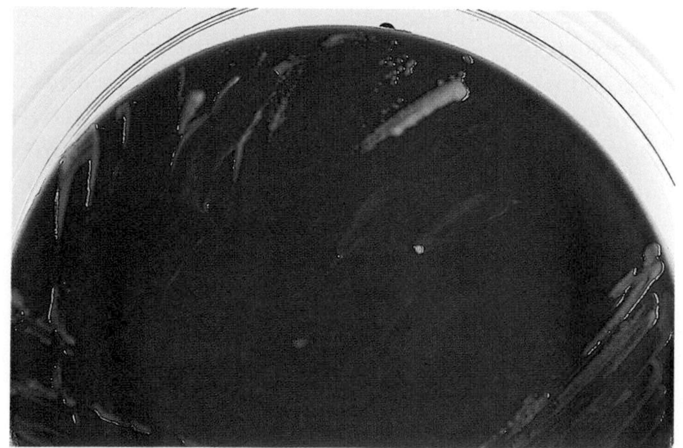

Figure 27-3 *Francisella tularensis* on modified Thayer-Martin agar. *F. tularensis* grows slowly, and 2 to 5 days may be needed before the colonies are visible. One of the advantages of utilizing modified Thayer-Martin medium is that it minimizes overgrowth by contaminating organisms. As shown here, the colonies are small, white-gray, smooth, and moist.

Introduction to Anaerobic Bacteria 28

Anaerobic bacteria are ubiquitous: they are commonly found in the environment, in soil as well as in water, and are also a major component of the indigenous microbial flora of animals. In humans, they can outnumber aerobic organisms by as much as 1,000:1. Anaerobes are commonly found on the mucosal surfaces of the gastrointestinal tract, the genitourinary tract, the oral cavity, and the upper respiratory tract. They are also part of the microflora of the skin. Under normal conditions, these organisms do not cause disease. However, the heavily colonized surfaces are portals of entry into tissues and the bloodstream. When anaerobic bacteria gain access to sterile body sites, they can become opportunistic pathogens and cause serious, sometimes fatal, infections.

Observations such as a foul odor, gas in the specimen, and black discoloration of blood-containing exudates can provide helpful clues to the presence of an anaerobic infection. Multiple bacteria and unique bacterial morphology in the direct Gram stain of clinical material can also provide presumptive evidence of the presence of anaerobes. Since most anaerobic infections arise in close proximity to mucosal surfaces, knowledge of the normal microbial flora of these sites provides critical information about the presumptive identification of the infectious agents. This is important because most anaerobic infections are usually polymicrobic, with a mixture of various aerobic, facultative, and anaerobic organisms. The presence of mixed bacterial flora, along with the slower growth of the anaerobes, often makes isolation and identification of significant organisms a difficult and time-consuming process.

SPECIMEN COLLECTION AND TRANSPORT

Specimen collection and transport are two of the most critical factors in successful laboratory isolation of anaerobic pathogens. In general, sterile aspiration is the best method to collect material from suspected anaerobic infections and also to avoid contamination with the indigenous flora. As an alternative, oxygen-free swabs are available; however, the use of swabs should be avoided whenever possible.

Immediately after collecting a specimen for anaerobic culture, it is important to provide protection from the lethal effects of oxygen during transport. Several options are available. Due to safety concerns, aspirates should not be left in the syringe but, rather, injected into an oxygen-free transport vial or tube such as in the prereduced anaerobically sterilized (PRAS) method of Hungate. Similar products, as well as various anaerobic swabs and anaerobic transport systems, are also commercially available. The agar gel transport swabs (Copan Diagnostics, Murrieta, CA) and the Vacutainer anaerobic transporter (BD Diagnostic Systems, Franklin Lakes, NJ) can be used for both specimen collection and transport. Regardless of the collection method or the transport system used, specimens for anaerobic culture should be sent to the laboratory for processing as soon as possible and should be cultured within 24 h for optimal recovery.

DIRECT DETECTION

Since the majority of anaerobic infections are polymicrobic and most anaerobes grow more slowly than aerobic and facultative bacteria, identification of anaerobic organisms is typically a laborious process and culture results are frequently delayed. Therefore, direct examination methods such as gross appearance (purulence, necrosis, or sulfur granules), odor (fetid or putrid), fluorescence under long-wave (366-nm) UV light, and Gram stain (unique anaerobic morphology) can give valuable clues to the presence of anaerobes.

The direct Gram stain of clinical material is one of the most important diagnostic procedures for the detection of anaerobes. It provides rapid, semiquantitative information about the relative amounts and types of organisms present in the specimen. Identification of multiple distinct morphotypes observed on the direct Gram stain is strong presumptive evidence of a mixed anaerobic infection. In some instances, it is possible to provide a presumptive anaerobic identification based on the Gram stain appearance. Anaerobic, gram-negative bacilli frequently stain faintly and irregularly with the conventional Gram stain method and thus can easily be overlooked when reading the smear. To enhance visualization of the gram-negative anaerobes, use of a modified Gram stain procedure, in which carbol fuchsin is used instead of safranin, is recommended. Since many of the clinically significant anaerobes have distinct microscopic morphologies, when the specimen source is correlated with Gram stain result it is possible to provide information that can serve as a guide to successful empirical therapy. For example, if large, boxcar-shaped, gram-positive bacilli with blunt ends are seen in the direct Gram stain of a specimen from an abdominal wound, one would suspect the presence of *Clostridium perfringens*, and the appropriate antimicrobial agent for this anaerobe can be selected. Refer to Table 28-1 for the characteristic Gram stain morphology of common anaerobes isolated from clinical specimens.

Table 28-1 Characteristics of anaerobes based on Gram stain morphology

Organism	Gram stain reaction and morphology
Actinomyces spp.	Branching, gram-positive bacilli
Clostridium perfringens	Large, gram-positive bacilli with blunt ends (boxcar shaped), no spores
Clostridium tetani	Gram-positive bacilli with round or oval terminal spores (drumstick or tennis racket shaped)
Propionibacterium spp.	Small, thin, pleomorphic, gram-positive bacilli
Bacteroides, *Porphyromonas*, or *Prevotella* spp.	Faintly staining, gram-negative coccobacilli
Fusobacterium nucleatum	Thin, gram-negative bacilli with tapered ends
Fusobacterium necrophorum or *Fusobacterium mortiferium*	Extremely pleomorphic, thin, gram-negative bacilli with bizarre shapes
Veillonella spp.	Very small, gram-negative cocci with a tendency to clump

SPECIMEN PROCESSING

Ideally, media used to culture anaerobes should never be exposed to oxygen, in order to avoid the production of toxic substances from the reduction of molecular oxygen. PRAS medium (Anaerobe Systems, Morgan Hill, CA) is made without exposure to oxygen, thus enhancing the recovery of anaerobes. As an alternative, primary anaerobic plates can be prereduced in an anaerobic jar or chamber for at least 24 h before use. For optimal recovery, media should be as fresh as possible. Growth is delayed and longer incubation is required when fresh media are not used.

Specimens from most anaerobic infections contain both facultative and anaerobic bacteria; therefore, a combination of enriched, selective, and differential media should be included in the primary medium setup to optimize growth, isolation, and presumptive identification of anaerobes. The following media are recommended: brucella blood agar or CDC anaerobe blood agar containing vitamin K_1 and hemin, bacteroides bile esculin agar, kanamycin-vancomycin-laked blood agar, and phenylethyl alcohol agar. Since thioglycolate broth supports the growth of both aerobic and anaerobic bacteria, it has limited value and serves primarily as a backup culture. For special situations, additional media such as egg yolk agar or cycloserine-cefoxitin-fructose agar can also be included in the primary isolation setup. Table 28-2 lists some of the recommended media and their use in the isolation of anaerobes from clinical specimens.

Anaerobic specimens should be processed in the laboratory as soon as possible by inoculating the appropriate media, immediately placing the inoculated plates into an oxygen-free environment, and incubating them at 35°C. Culture techniques include the use of anaerobic jars, anaerobic bags or pouches, and anaerobic chambers. The jars, bags, and pouches consist of a gas-impermeable container, a gas generator,

Table 28-2 Recommended media for anaerobic culture

Medium	Purpose
Primary isolation	
Brucella blood agar (BRU) (acceptable alternatives: CDC anaerobe blood agar, Schaedler blood agar, or enriched brain heart infusion blood agar)	Enriched with vitamin K_1 and hemin; nonselective; isolation of obligate and facultative anaerobes
Bacteroides bile esculin agar (BBE)	Selective and differential: gentamicin inhibits most aerobic organisms, 20% bile inhibits most anaerobes, and hydrolysis of esculin turns the medium brown; rapid isolation and presumptive identification of members of the *Bacteroides fragilis* group
Kanamycin-vancomycin-laked blood agar (KVLB) (acceptable alternatives: kanamycin-vancomycin blood agar or paromomycin-vancomycin blood agar)	Selective: kanamycin inhibits most facultative, gram-negative bacilli; vancomycin inhibits most gram-positive organisms as well as *Porphyromonas* spp.; and laked blood allows for early detection of pigmented *Prevotella* spp., often within 48 h
Phenylethyl alcohol agar (PEA)	Permits growth of both gram-positive and gram-negative anaerobes while inhibiting most *Enterobacteriaceae* including swarming *Proteus*
Thioglycolate broth (THIO)	Backup only
Special situations	
Cycloserine-cefoxitin-fructose agar (CCFA)	Selective and differential: used for the recovery and presumptive identification of *Clostridium difficile*
Egg yolk agar (EYA)	Differential: used when *Clostridium* spp. are suspected (lecithinase and lipase reactions)

and an indicator. When the generator is opened, carbon dioxide and hydrogen are produced. The hydrogen then combines with the oxygen to form water, and a carbon dioxide-rich environment is created. The use of an indicator such as methylene blue, which is blue when oxidized and white when reduced, verifies that the proper anaerobic atmosphere has been achieved and maintained. Due to high cost, space limitations, and lack of specimen volume, most clinical laboratories do not use anaerobic chambers. However, if proper specimen collection, transport, and processing have been observed, recovery of the clinically significant anaerobes appears to be comparable by all the methods. Anaerobes are most susceptible to oxygen exposure during their log phase of growth; therefore, anaerobic plates should be incubated for 48 h before initial examination. Negative cultures should be held for a minimum of 7 days.

IDENTIFICATION OF ANAEROBIC BACTERIA

Although identification of anaerobic bacteria is a labor-intensive process, preliminary grouping of anaerobes can be made by using Gram stain and colony morphology and susceptibility to special-potency antimicrobial disks. The three disks commonly used are vancomycin (5 μg), kanamycin (1 mg), and colistin (10 μg). A zone of inhibition of >10 mm is considered to indicate susceptibility for identification purposes. Refer to Table 28-3 for presumptive identification of anaerobes based on results obtained with special-potency antimicrobial disks. The vancomycin and colistin disks can also serve as an aid to determine the Gram reaction for anaerobic organisms that are easily overdecolorized. In general, gram-positive bacteria are susceptible to vancomycin and resistant to colistin, whereas gram-negative

Table 28-3 Presumptive identification of anaerobes based on special-potency antimicrobial disk results

	Result[a] with disk containing:		
Organism	Kanamycin (1 mg)	Vancomycin (5 μg)	Colistin (10 μg)
Bacteroides fragilis group	R	R	R
Bacteroides ureolyticus group	S	R	S
Fusobacterium spp.	S	R	S
Porphyromonas spp.	R	S	R
Veillonella spp.	S	R	S
Peptostreptococcus anaerobius	RS	S	R
Other anaerobic, gram-positive cocci	S	S	R
Anaerobic, gram-positive bacilli	V	S[b]	R

[a]R, resistant; S, susceptible; R^S, resistant, rarely susceptible; V, variable reaction.
[b]Rare *Lactobacillus* spp. and *Clostridium* spp. may be vancomycin resistant.

organisms are resistant to vancomycin. Other characteristics include hemolysis, pigment production, fluorescence, and simple tests such as indole, nitrate, and catalase, which can provide a presumptive identification of several clinically significant anaerobes. For definitive identification, a wide variety of techniques are available. They range from rapid minisystems to conventional PRAS biochemical tubes. In some instances, analysis of metabolic end products or cellular fatty acids may also be required. Mass spectrometry and molecular techniques have now been introduced as alternative approaches to identify anaerobes.

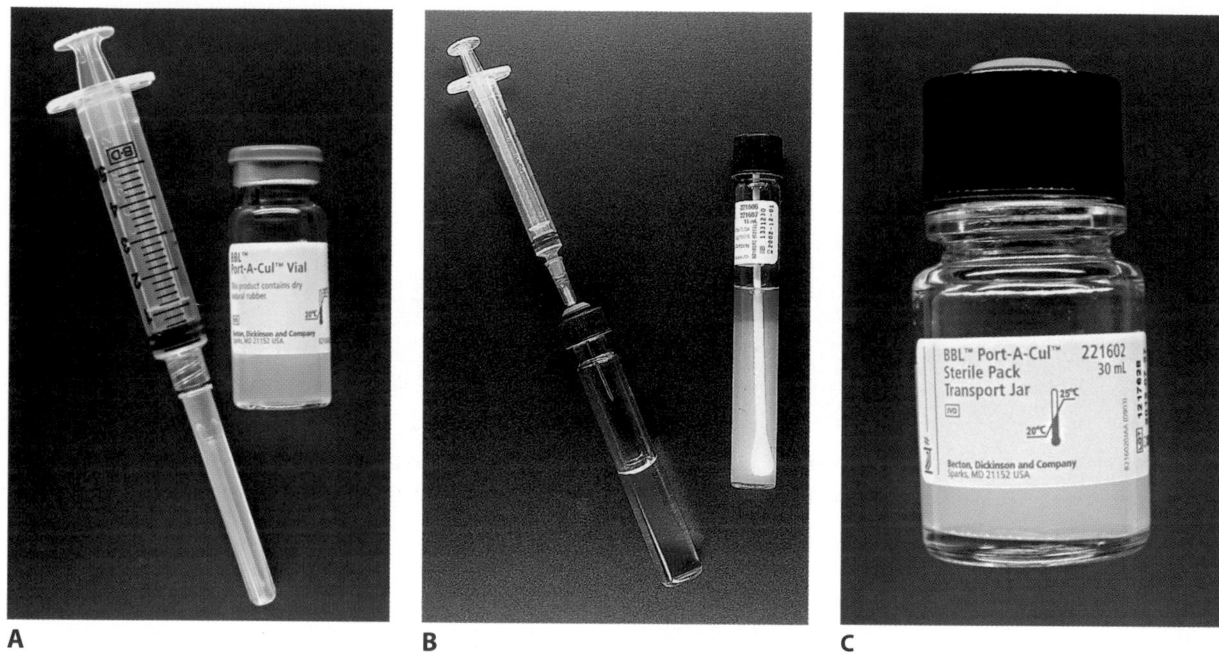

Figure 28-1 Anaerobic collection and transport. In general, the preferred method of obtaining material for anaerobic culture is by aspiration using a needle and syringe. An alternative collection method is the use of swabs. A variety of products are available to transport specimens and maintain viability of anaerobic organisms once the specimen is collected. (A) The Port-A-Cul Vial (BD Diagnostic Systems, Franklin Lakes, NJ) is used for fluid specimens, which are injected through the septum onto the solid agar surface. (B) Two similar products can be used to transport fluids, tissues, or specimens collected with a swab. As shown on the right, a swab specimen can be inserted directly into the Port-A-Cul Tube (BD Diagnostic Systems). Note the color change of the resazurin indicator at the top of the prereduced agar as a result of the oxidation of the medium when the screw cap is removed and the swab is inserted. The PRAS Anaerobic Transport Medium (Anaerobe Systems), shown on the left, has a screw cap containing a rubber septum. This allows for direct injection of aspirated material, thus avoiding oxidation. Small tissue samples and specimens collected using a swab can also be transported by removing the cap and inserting the specimen into the semisolid agar. (C) The Port-A-Cul Transport Jar (BD Diagnostic Systems) has a wide mouth with a screw cap, which allows for larger tissue or biopsy specimens to be directly inserted into the reduced holding medium.

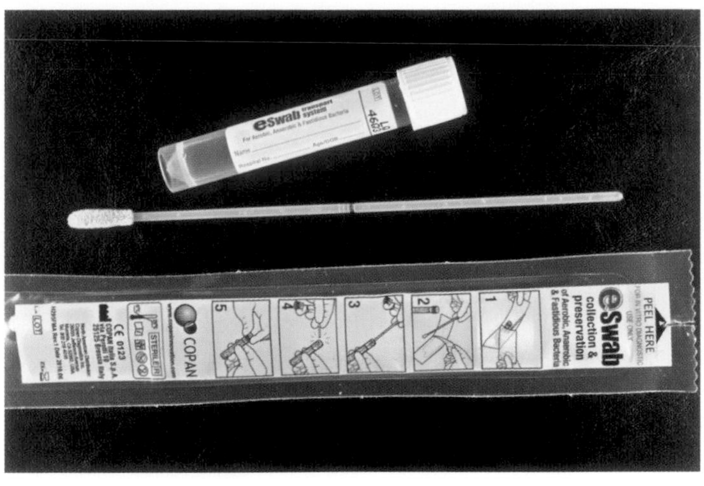

Figure 28-2 ESwab Collection and Transport System. ESwab (Copan Diagnostics) is a self-contained, liquid-based collection and transport system consisting of a Nylon Flocked Swab and 1 ml of modified liquid Amies. After specimen collection, the swab is placed into the tube, the applicator shaft is snapped, and the lid is screwed on tightly. The sample immediately elutes into the liquid medium, which allows for automated liquid handling. Aerobic, anaerobic, and fastidious bacteria maintain viability in ESwab for up to 48 h at room and refrigerator temperatures.

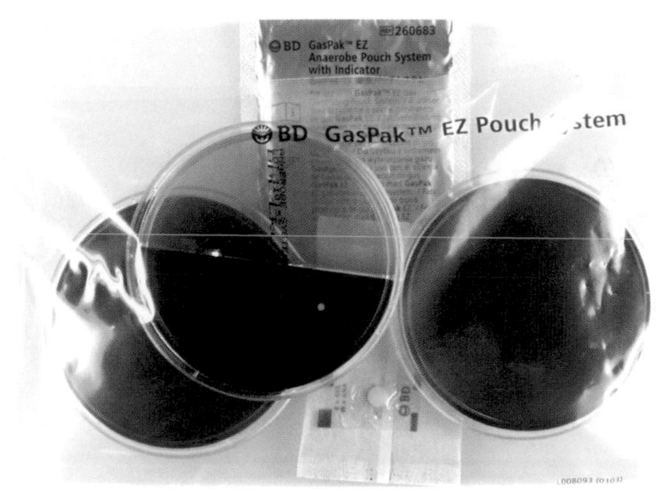

Figure 28-3 Anaerobic environment with the GasPak EZ Gas Generating Pouch System with indicator. The GasPak EZ Gas Generating Pouch System (BD Diagnostic Systems, Franklin Lakes, NJ) consists of a resealable pouch and a gas-generating sealed-reagent sachet, which becomes activated when removed from the outer wrapper. This system is convenient for the primary setup of anaerobic specimens or when only a small number of plates have been inoculated. After the plates are inoculated and placed into the bag along with activated sachet, the pouch is tightly sealed by pressing the zipper together. Carbon dioxide and hydrogen are released from the generator, producing an anaerobic environment. To ensure that anaerobic conditions have been maintained, the indicator is included and should remain white throughout the incubation.

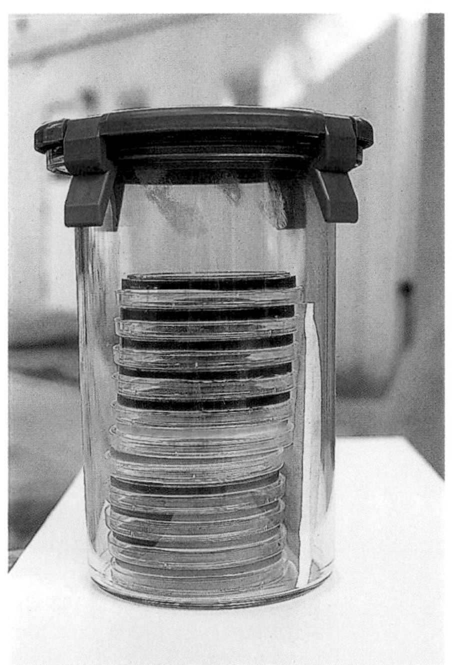

Figure 28-4 Anaerobic jar. Many types of anaerobic jars are commercially available. The standard round jar (EM Science, Gibbstown, NJ) can accommodate up to 12 plates and is commonly used in many laboratories. Inoculated plates are placed in the jar along with a gas-generating envelope and indicator strip. The container is sealed, and carbon dioxide and hydrogen are released from the envelope to produce anaerobic conditions.

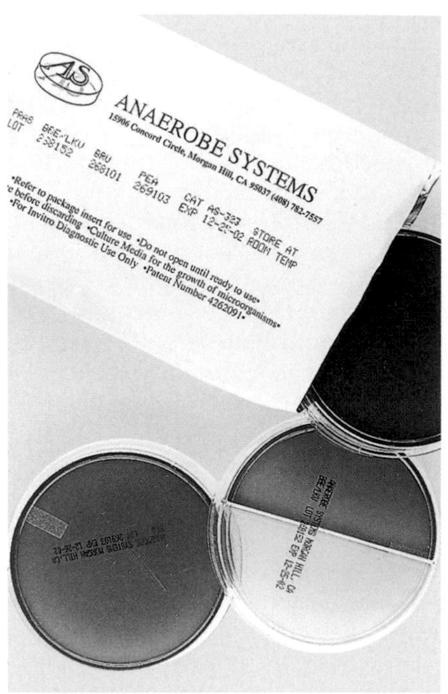

Figure 28-5 PRAS plated medium. PRAS medium is manufactured, packaged, shipped, and stored under anaerobic conditions. The primary anaerobic media pack shown here (Anaerobe Systems) contains enriched, selective, and differential media and includes brucella blood agar, phenylethyl alcohol agar, and a biplate with bacteroides bile esculin agar and kanamycin-vancomycin-laked blood agar. The plates are stored in a gas-impermeable foil pouch, which is opened at the time of specimen inoculation.

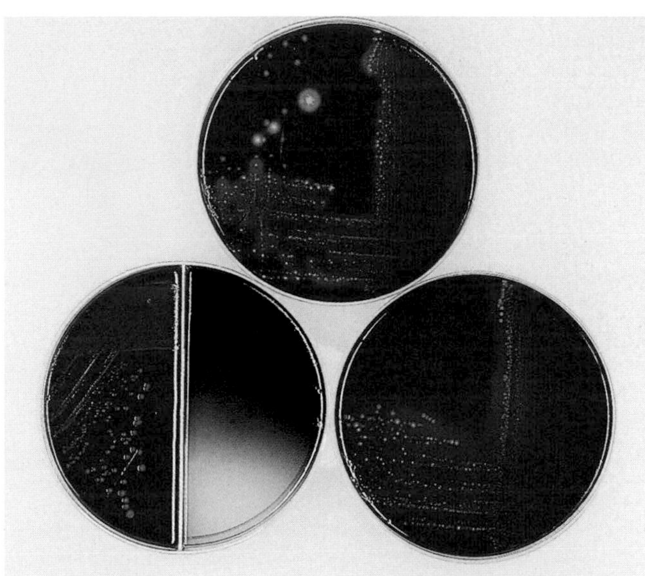

Figure 28-6 Growth of mixed aerobic and anaerobic organisms on primary media. Anaerobes are usually present in mixed culture. The combination of enriched, selective, and differential media included in the primary setup aids in evaluating cultures for the presence of anaerobes and may also provide a preliminary identification of anaerobic organisms. The culture shown is from a mixed infection with both aerobic and anaerobic bacteria. The brucella blood agar (top) is enriched and supports the growth of facultative and anaerobic bacteria, while the phenylethyl alcohol agar plate (bottom right) is selective and inhibits the growth of most members of the *Enterobacteriaceae*. A preliminary identification of the *Bacteroides fragilis* group can be made based on the growth on kanamycin-vancomycin-laked blood agar and bacteroides bile esculin agar and on the hydrolysis of esculin (biplate on the bottom left). Esculin hydrolysis by the *B. fragilis* group produces esculetin and dextrose. The esculetin reacts with the ferric ammonium citrate present in the medium, producing a dark brown to black complex. Note the browning of the medium around the colonies on the bacteroides bile esculin agar.

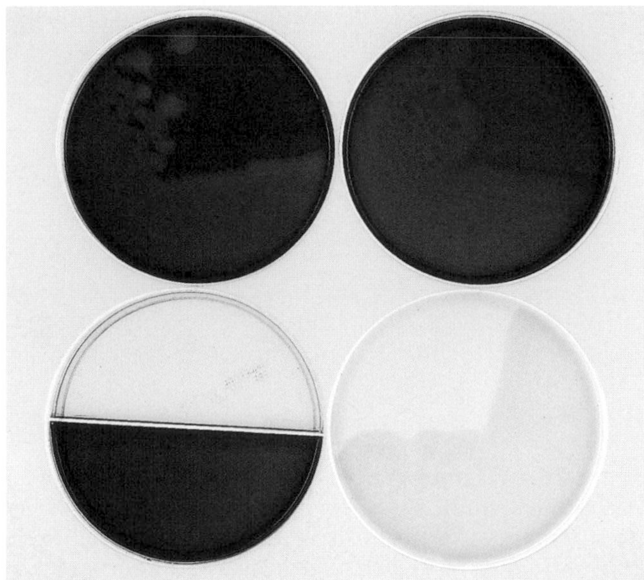

Figure 28-7 Egg yolk agar. When the Gram stain of a specimen shows the presence of leukocytes and large, gram-positive bacilli, suggesting a clostridial infection, egg yolk agar (EYA) should be included in the primary anaerobic media. Colony morphology, Gram reaction, and a positive lecithinase and/or lipase reaction can provide a rapid presumptive identification of some common clostridia. In the culture shown, note the double zones of beta-hemolysis on the brucella blood agar (top left) and the positive lecithinase reaction (opacity) on EYA (bottom right). The characteristic hemolysis and EYA reaction, along with the Gram stain and morphology, provide a presumptive identification of *Clostridium perfringens*.

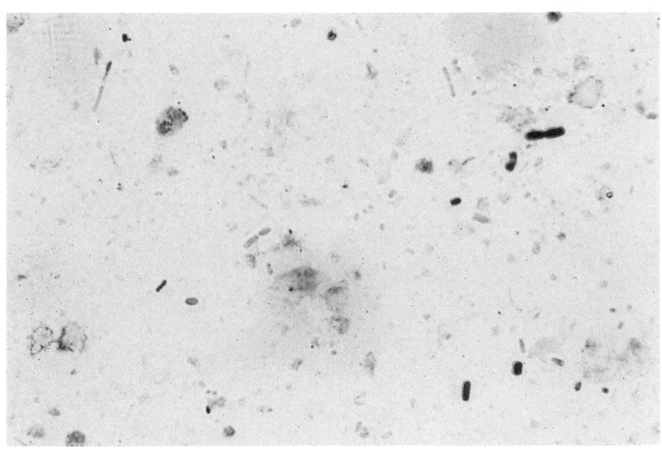

Figure 28-8 Gram stain of a mixed infection with suspected anaerobes. Most anaerobic infections are polymicrobic and include both aerobic and anaerobic organisms. In this Gram stain of a specimen from a foot abscess, multiple distinct morphotypes are present, including gram-negative bacilli and large, gram-positive bacilli. From the appearance of this Gram stain, there is strong presumptive evidence that anaerobes are present in this specimen. Note the large, gram-positive bacilli and the faintly staining gram-negative bacilli. The culture grew *Escherichia coli*, *Enterobacter* spp.; anaerobic, gram-negative bacilli; and a *Clostridium* sp.

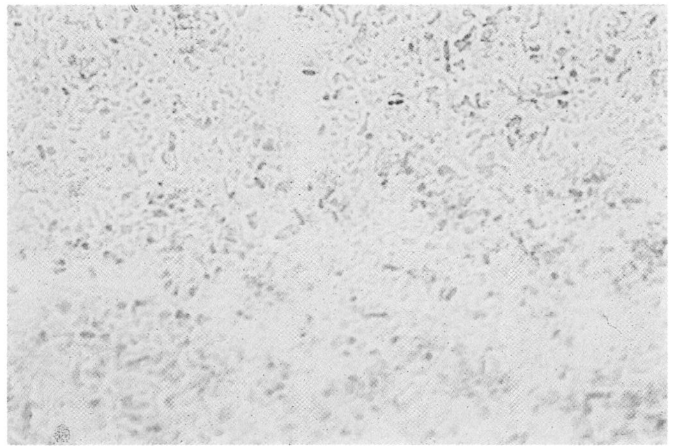

A

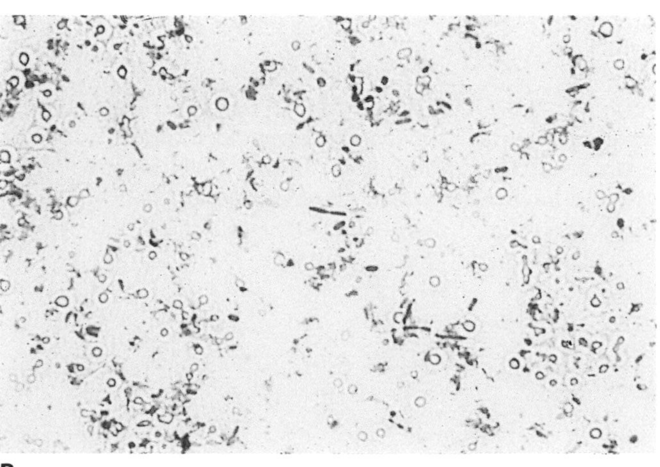

B

Figure 28-9 Gram stain of *Bacteroides fragilis*. In a Gram stain with safranin as the counterstain, gram-negative, anaerobic bacteria stain faintly and can be overlooked in direct smears of clinical specimens or in blood cultures. (A) Safranin was used as the counterstain in this Gram stain of a blood culture. The gram-negative bacilli are difficult to see. (B) Carbol fuchsin was used as the counterstain and the organism appears more prominent. *B. fragilis* was isolated from this blood culture.

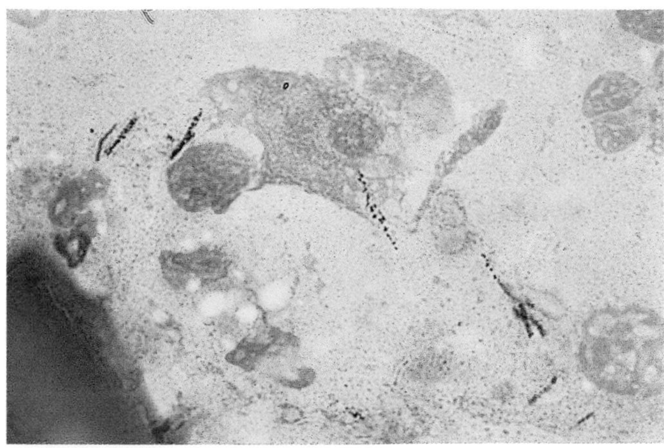

Figure 28-10 Gram stain of *Actinomyces israelii*. In the Gram stain shown, the branching, filamentous bacilli are typical of an *Actinomyces*-like organism. *Actinomyces* spp. are gram positive; however, their irregular staining may cause a beaded or banded appearance. *A. israelii* was isolated from this culture.

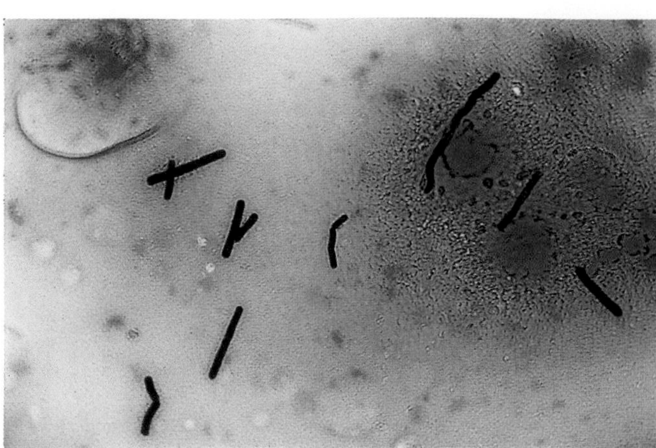

Figure 28-11 Gram stain of *Clostridium perfringens*. This Gram stain of a positive blood culture shows large, boxcar-shaped, gram-positive bacilli with no spores, which is typical of *C. perfringens*. Cells can occur singly or in pairs and are 0.6 to 2.4 μm by 1.3 to 19.0 μm.

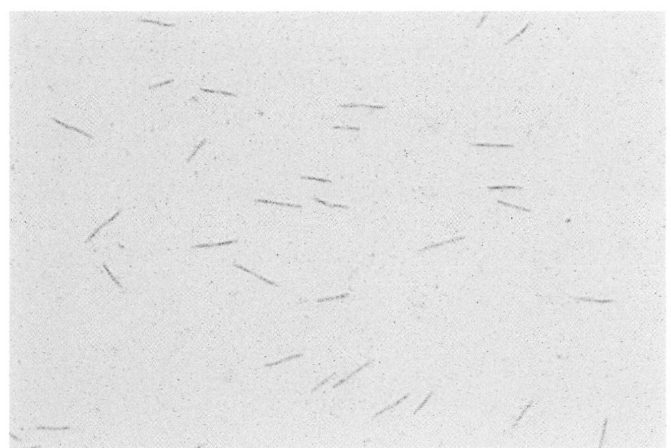

Figure 28-12 Gram stain of *Fusobacterium nucleatum*. As shown here, *F. nucleatum* organisms appear as thin, gram-negative bacilli that are 0.4 to 0.7 μm by 3 to 10 μm and have tapered or pointed ends.

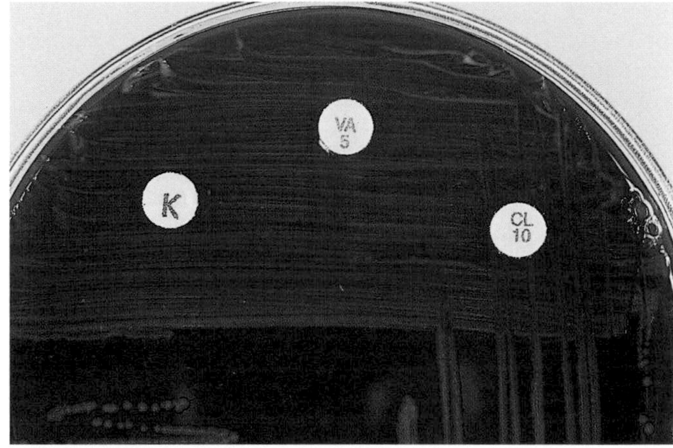

Figure 28-13 Disk pattern of the *Bacteroides fragilis* group. Special-potency antibiotic disks can be used to aid in the preliminary grouping of anaerobes and can also serve as a check for the appropriate Gram reaction. In general, gram-negative organisms are resistant to vancomycin, while gram-positive organisms are susceptible to vancomycin and resistant to colistin. As shown, the *B. fragilis* group is resistant to all three of the antibiotics: kanamycin (1 mg), vancomycin (5 μg), and colistin (10 μg).

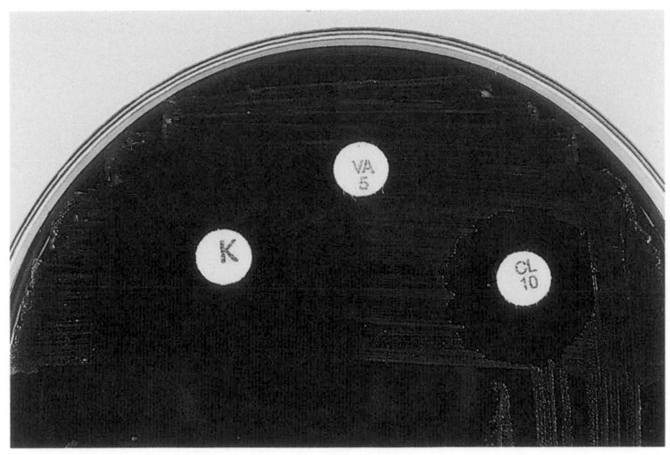

Figure 28-14 Disk pattern of *Fusobacterium* spp. The disk pattern shown, kanamycin and colistin susceptible and vancomycin resistant, is typical of *Fusobacterium* spp.

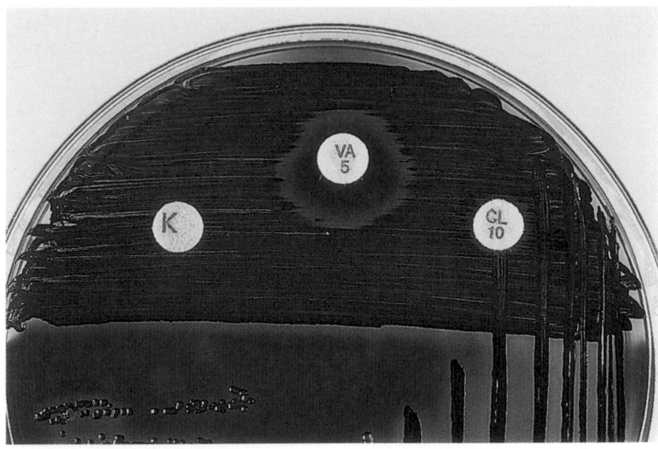

Figure 28-15 Disk pattern of *Porphyromonas* spp. Unlike other gram-negative organisms, *Porphyromonas* spp. are susceptible to vancomycin. The organism shown here is kanamycin and colistin resistant (with a zone of inhibition of <10 mm in diameter) but vancomycin susceptible, which is characteristic of *Porphyromonas* spp.

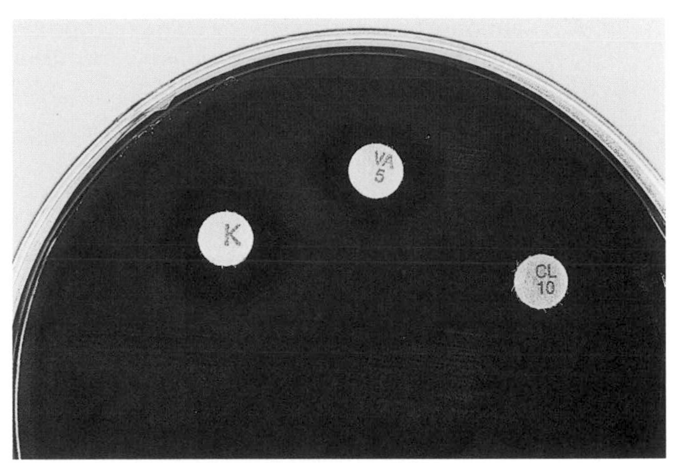

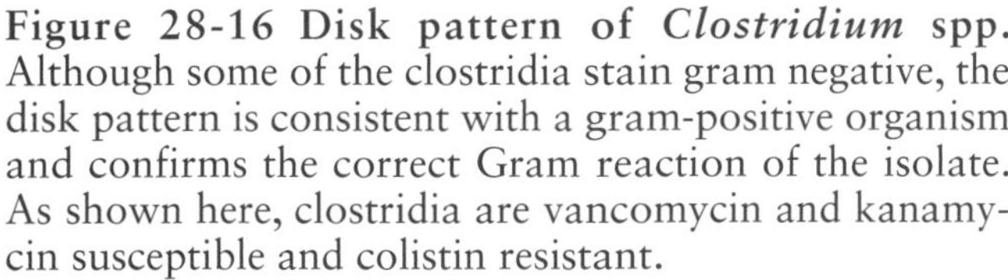

Figure 28-16 Disk pattern of *Clostridium* spp. Although some of the clostridia stain gram negative, the disk pattern is consistent with a gram-positive organism and confirms the correct Gram reaction of the isolate. As shown here, clostridia are vancomycin and kanamycin susceptible and colistin resistant.

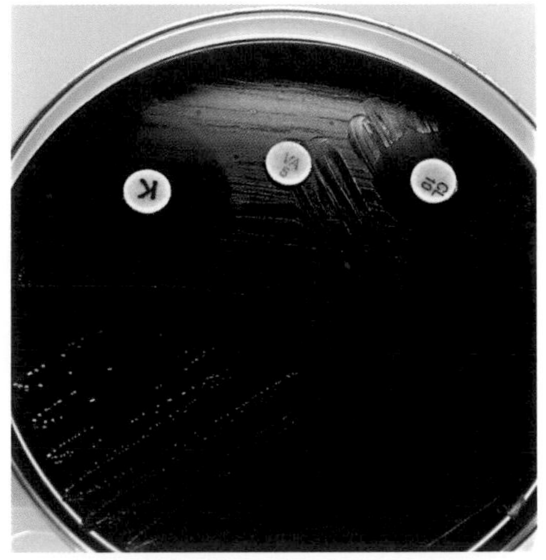

Figure 28-17 Disk pattern of *Veillonella* spp. Although *Veillonella* spp. are gram-negative cocci, they can retain some of the crystal violet stain and appear gram variable. However, their disk pattern, as shown here, is consistent with that of a gram-negative organism. They are vancomycin resistant and kanamycin and colistin susceptible.

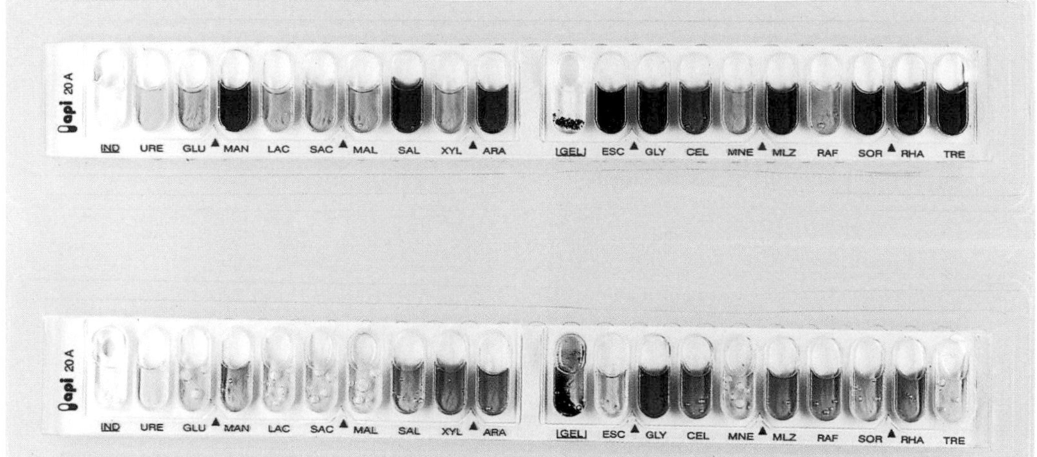

Figure 28-18 Biochemically based minisystem for identification of anaerobic organisms. There are several commercially available systems for the identification of anaerobic organisms. The API 20A (bioMérieux, Inc., Durham, NC) was one of the first alternatives to conventional tube media and uses many of the same tests. A bacterial suspension equivalent to a no. 3 McFarland standard is prepared and used to inoculate the strip, which consists of 20 microtubes. The strip is then incubated anaerobically at 35°C for 24 to 48 h, depending on the growth rate of the anaerobic organism. Similar to other API products, the 20A, along with the catalase reaction and three morphological characteristics (presence of spores, Gram reaction, and morphology), creates a numerical profile that is used to identify the organism. The two organisms shown are *Clostridium perfringens* (top) and *Bacteroides fragilis* (bottom).

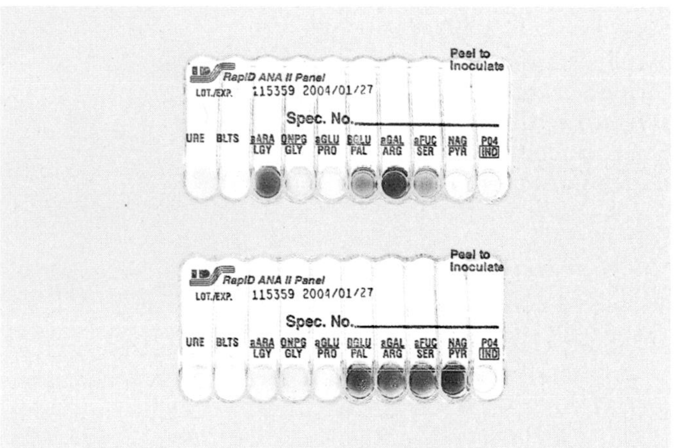

Figure 28-19 Preexisting enzyme-based minisystem for anaerobic identification. The RapID ANA II (Thermo Scientific, Waltham, MA) is a micromethod employing both conventional and chromogenic substrates for the identification of clinically significant anaerobes. The test is based on the presence of preexisting enzymes and does not require growth of the organism. A bacterial suspension equivalent to a no. 3 McFarland standard is prepared and used to inoculate the panel, which is then incubated aerobically at 35°C for 4 h. The panel contains 10 reaction wells, 8 of which are bifunctional, containing 2 separate tests in the same well, thereby providing a total of 18 tests. To provide both test results, the bifunctional tests are read before and again after the addition of reagents. The two organisms shown are *Clostridium perfringens* (top) and *Bacteroides fragilis* (bottom).

Clostridium

29

The genus *Clostridium* includes obligate anaerobic, gram-positive bacilli that can form spores. There are more than 200 species and subspecies; however, the number associated with human infections is limited. These organisms are ubiquitous in nature, widely distributed in soil, and frequent inhabitants of the intestinal tract. Some of the most common *Clostridium* spp. isolated from human specimens are *Clostridium perfringens*, *Clostridium clostridioforme*, *Clostridium innocuum*, *Clostridium ramosum*, *Clostridium difficile*, *Clostridium butyricum*, and *Clostridium cadaveris*. The characteristics of these and other *Clostridium* spp. are outlined in Table 29-1.

C. perfringens is the species most frequently isolated from clinical specimens and causes a variety of infections, including the majority of clostridial bacteremias. *C. perfringens* type A is associated with food-borne gastroenteritis that often results from eating improperly cooked meat or meat products. Diarrhea and abdominal cramps usually appear 7 to 15 h after ingestion of the contaminated food as a result of the enterotoxin produced by the organism. Like other *Clostridium* spp., such as *Clostridium novyi*, *Clostridium septicum*, and *Clostridium histolyticum*, this organism produces alpha-toxin, which may result in myonecrosis (gas gangrene), a life-threatening condition. *C. perfringens* type C may be part of the normal flora. However, strains that produce beta-toxin can cause enteritis necroticans, a severe disease of the small bowel that usually occurs in children.

C. difficile is the cause of antibiotic-associated diarrhea and pseudomembranous colitis. This organism is a member of the normal flora in 30% of neonates. Carriage rates range from 3 to 5% in healthy adults but increase to 20 to 30% in sedentary patients. Both nontoxigenic and toxigenic strains can be found in the hospital environment; however, only toxigenic strains are associated with disease. Of these, most produce toxins A and B, but some produce only toxin B. Both toxins appear to be important in the pathogenesis of the disease and can induce cytopathic effects in cell culture.

Clostridium botulinum produces seven different types of neurotoxin. Types A, B, E, and F are the principal causes of botulism in humans. Four categories of clinical botulism are currently recognized: (i) food-borne botulism, resulting from the ingestion of preformed toxin; (ii) wound botulism, resulting from the production of toxin by *C. botulinum* growing in the wound; (iii) infant botulism, in which the toxin is formed by *C. botulinum* colonizing the intestinal tract (in these cases, breast-feeding and ingestion of honey are potential sources of the spores); and (iv) botulism due to colonization of the intestine in older children and adults.

Tetanospasmin, the toxin elaborated by *Clostridium tetani*, is the cause of the clinical manifestations of tetanus. This toxin binds to components of the neuroexocytotic apparatus, blocking inhibitory impulses to the motor neurons. As a result, *C. tetani* produces spastic paralysis, in contrast to *C. botulinum*, which produces flaccid paralysis.

Bacteremia due to *C. septicum* is commonly associated with neoplasias, particularly colon and breast cancer, leukemia, and lymphoma. Patients infected with this

Table 29-1 Characteristics of *Clostridium* spp.

Organism	Colony morphology	Gram stain and spores	Other characteristic(s)
Group 1: saccharolytic, proteolytic			
C. bifermentans	Gray-white; scalloped edge; chalk-white colonies on egg yolk agar	Gram-positive bacilli often in chains; subterminal spores and many free spores	Indole positive, lecithinase positive, urease negative
C. botulinum	Gray-white; irregular; usually beta-hemolytic	Gram-positive bacilli singly or in pairs; oval, subterminal spores cause swelling of the cells	
C. cadaveris	White-gray; entire or slightly irregular and raised	Gram-positive bacilli; oval terminal spores	Spot indole positive, DNase positive
C. difficile	Creamy yellow-gray-white; irregular; coarse or mosaic internal structure; fluoresces chartreuse on cycloserine-cefoxitin-fructose agar, C. difficile selective agar, or CDC agar under UV light	Straight, gram-positive bacilli often in short chains; rare oval, subterminal spores and free spores	Mannitol weak positive, esculin hydrolysis positive, horse stable odor
C. perfringens	Gray-yellow; circular; entire; glossy; translucent with double zone of beta-hemolysis	Gram-positive, boxcar-shaped bacilli, singly or in pairs; central to subterminal, oval spores that swell the cell but are rarely seen	Lecithinase positive, reverse CAMP positive
C. septicum	Gray, translucent; swarms like Medusa heads; beta-hemolytic	Pleomorphic, gram-positive bacilli; may produce long filaments and turn gram- negative in old cultures; rare spores are oval and subterminal, swelling the cell	Sucrose negative, DNase positive
C. sordellii	Large; gray-white; scalloped edge	Large, gram-positive bacilli; subterminal or free spores, often in chains	Indole positive, lecithinase positive, urease positive
C. sporogenes	Medusa head shape; may swarm	Gram-positive bacilli; abundant oval, subterminal spores and many free spores	Lipase positive, esculin hydrolysis positive
Group 2: saccharolytic, nonproteolytic			
C. baratii	Double zone of hemolysis	Boxcar-shaped bacilli; rare spores	Lecithinase positive
C. butyricum	Large; irregular; mottled to mosaic internal structure	Gram-positive bacilli; subterminal spores	Ferments many carbohydrates
C. clostridioforme	Small; convex; entire edge; irregular; greening of agar around colonies	Long, thin, gram-negative bacilli; tapered ends; spores are rare	Lactose positive, β-*N*-acetylglucosaminidase negative
C. glycolicum	Gray-white; entire to scalloped edge; convex	Gram-positive bacilli; subterminal and free spores	DNase positive
C. innocuum	Gray-white to brilliant greenish colonies; mosaic internal structure	Gram-positive bacilli; rare terminal spores may be difficult to find	Mannitol positive, lactose negative, maltose negative, nonmotile
C. ramosum	Resembles *Bacteroides fragilis* but usually has a slightly irregular edge	Gram-variable, palisading, slender bacilli; spores are rare, round or oval, and terminal	Mannitol positive, nonmotile
C. tertium	White-gray; irregular margins	Gram variable with terminal spores when incubated anaerobically	Aerotolerant
Group 3: asaccharolytic			
C. tetani	Gray, translucent; irregular to rhizoid; may form a film over entire agar surface; narrow zone of beta-hemolysis	Gram-positive cells that turn gram negative after 24 h in culture; singly or in pairs; spores oval and terminal with tennis racket or drumstick appearance	

organism are also frequently neutropenic, and it is very important to diagnose this infection rapidly in order to implement adequate therapy. The ileocecal region of the intestinal tract appears to be the portal of entry for this bacterium into the blood. *Clostridium tertium* can also cause bacteremia in patients with malignancies, acute pancreatitis, and neutropenic enterocolitis. In cases of suspected enterocolitis with myonecrosis due to *C. septicum*, cultures of blood and feces and a tissue biopsy specimen should be submitted for diagnosis.

Anaerobic methods should be used for specimen collection, transportation, and storage of these bacteria. Collection of tissue specimens from several sites is recommended for culture, and direct examination of the specimen by Gram stain is important for a rapid presumptive clinical diagnosis. For the foodborne diseases produced by *C. perfringens*, specimens should be referred to a public health laboratory. In the case of suspected *C. botulinum* infection, the state health department or Centers for Disease Control and Prevention should be immediately notified and the appropriate specimens should be submitted for culture and toxin determination.

A liquid stool specimen is recommended for the isolation of *C. difficile* by culture, particularly since this organism can be recovered from asymptomatic individuals. Only strains that carry the pathogenicity locus (PaLoc) have the genes for toxins A and B. For toxin detection, tissue culture or enzyme immunoassays (EIAs) can be used. Tissue culture was considered the gold standard for the detection of toxin B but has now been replaced by nucleic acid tests. EIAs, which can detect both toxins A and B, are widely employed due to their rapidity and ease of use; however, EIAs are less sensitive and specific than tissue culture. Other methods include the simultaneous detection by EIA of the *C. difficile* glutamate dehydrogenase (GDH) antigen in combination with toxins A and B. The GDH assay has high sensitivity but low specificity because it cannot distinguish toxigenic from nontoxigenic isolates. Therefore, the EIA results for both GDH and toxins A and B are necessary for final interpretation. DNA-based methods that detect the presence of the toxin genes are now considered the gold standard in the clinical laboratory for the detection of *C. difficile*. The DNA methods have high sensitivity and specificity for the detection of the toxin A and B genes (*tcdA* and *tcdB*) and are rapid. They should be performed only on stool specimens from patients with diarrhea since 5 to 10% of the normal population are asymptomatic carriers of the toxigenic strains. In these individuals, the toxigenic *C. difficile* strain is present; thus the toxin gene can be detected, but the protein is not expressed. Currently, the drawbacks of the DNA assays are that they are expensive and require specialized equipment.

Gas gangrene is a clinical emergency and requires immediate treatment. Therefore, a Gram stain of a wound may be extremely helpful in diagnosing cases of infections due to *Clostridium* spp. Although clostridia are commonly associated with polymicrobial abdominal flora, the characteristic morphology of some species and the presence of spores are helpful in providing an initial diagnosis until culture confirmation is obtained. Typically gram-positive bacilli with or without spores are detected. When produced, spores can be spherical to ovoid; are located terminally, subterminally, or centrally; and may or may not cause swelling of the cell. Most clostridia are straight or curved, gram-positive bacilli; however, there is great variation in morphology and staining characteristics. Cells can range from 0.5 to 2.4 μm in width and 1.3 to 35 μm in length and thus can appear coccoid to filamentous with rounded, tapered, or blunt ends. Single cells, pairs, or chains of different lengths can be observed. The Gram stain characteristics of the *Clostridium* spp. most commonly isolated from clinical specimens are summarized in Table 29-1.

Most species of clostridia grow well on the anaerobic media routinely used in the clinical laboratory. Specimens should be plated on CDC anaerobe blood agar or other suitable enriched, nonselective anaerobic blood agar medium and anaerobic phenylethyl alcohol blood agar. Cycloserine-cefoxitin-fructose agar (CCFA; Anaerobe Systems, Morgan Hill, CA) is a selective and differential medium for the isolation and presumptive identification of *C. difficile*. Formation of spores can be enhanced by growing the specimen in a chopped-meat broth at 30°C, except for *C. perfringens*, which sporulates better at 37°C. For specimens from wounds and abscesses, adding egg yolk agar to the routine primary media will facilitate early presumptive identification of *Clostridium* species. For definitive identification, analysis of metabolic products or cellular fatty acids may be required. However, a presumptive identification can be made for most clostridia isolated from clinical specimens based on Gram stain, colony morphology, aerotolerance, a few biochemical reactions, and characteristics on differential media.

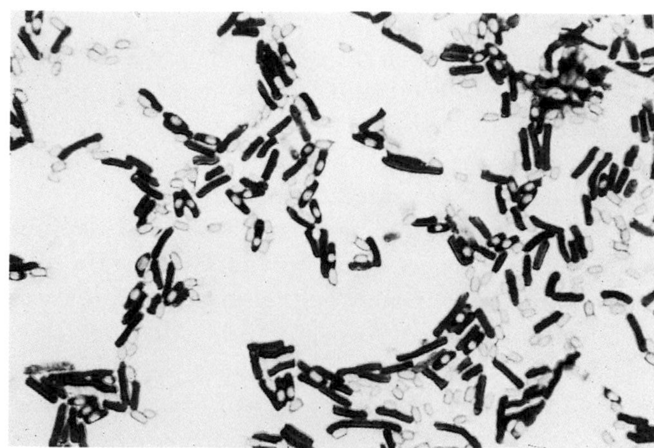

Figure 29-1 Gram stain of *Clostridium bifermentans*. *C. bifermentans* is a gram-positive bacillus measuring 0.6 to 1.9 μm by 1.6 to 11 μm and can be found singly or in short chains. The spores are oval, do not swell the cell, and can be central or subterminal.

A

B

Figure 29-2 Culture of *Clostridium bifermentans* on CDC agar. White-gray or translucent, flat colonies with irregular scalloped margins are produced by *C. bifermentans* on CDC agar.

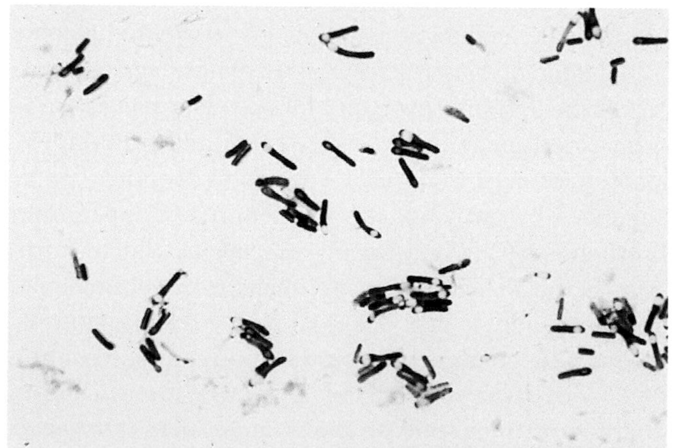

Figure 29-3 Gram stain of *Clostridium botulinum*. *C. botulinum* usually appears as single straight or curved, gram-positive bacilli. The bacilli sporulate readily on most media and have oval, subterminal spores that cause swelling of the cells.

Figure 29-4 *Clostridium botulinum* on CDC agar. Colonies of *C. botulinum* are gray-white or translucent, flat or raised, circular to irregular, and with a small zone of beta-hemolysis. Phenotypically they cannot be differentiated from *C. sporogenes*, and a mouse toxin neutralization assay, gel electrophoresis, or other tests are necessary for a definitive identification.

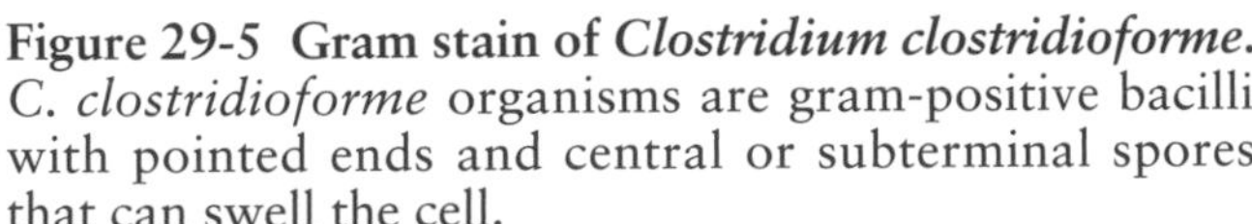

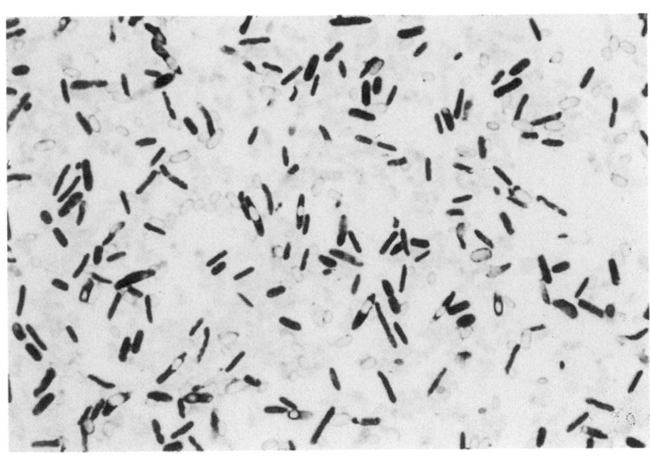

Figure 29-5 Gram stain of *Clostridium clostridioforme*. *C. clostridioforme* organisms are gram-positive bacilli with pointed ends and central or subterminal spores that can swell the cell.

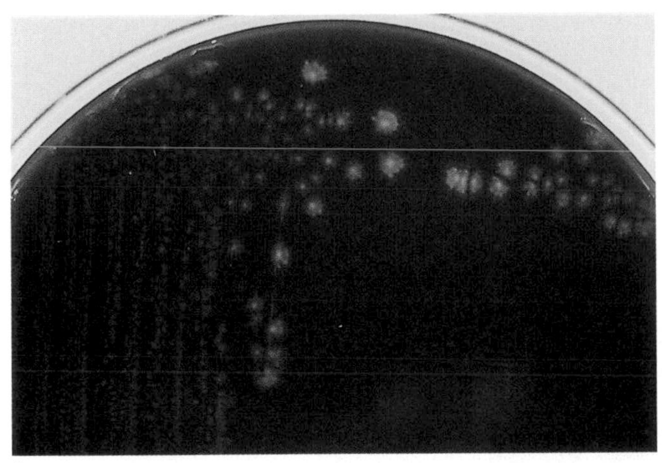

A

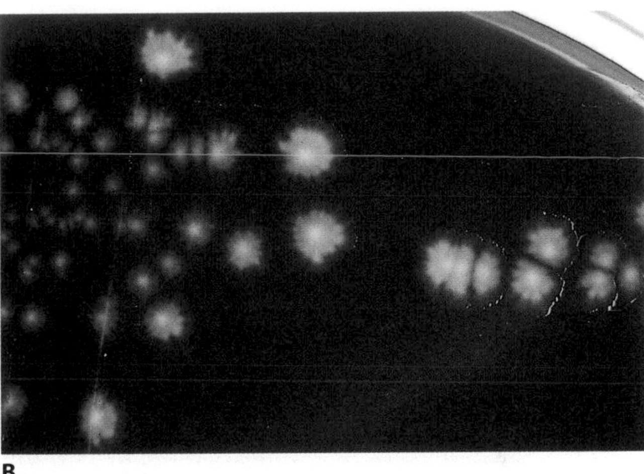

B

Figure 29-6 *Clostridium clostridioforme* on CDC agar. This organism forms nonhemolytic colonies that are white-gray with opaque centers and translucent, mottled, irregular edges.

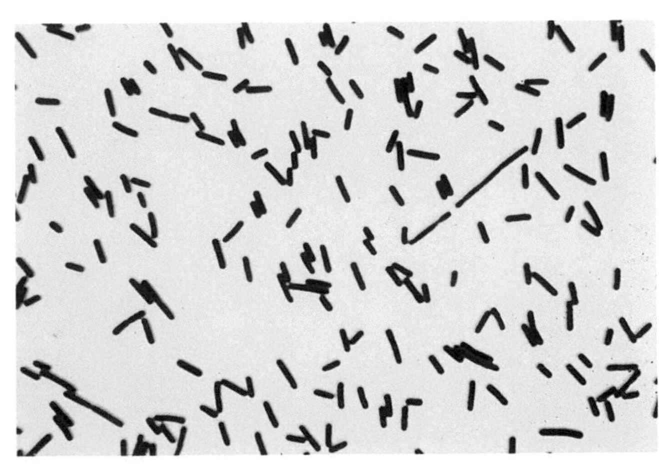

Figure 29-7 Gram stain of *Clostridium difficile*. *C. difficile* is a straight, gram-positive bacillus that measures 0.5 to 2.0 μm by 3 to 15 μm and often forms short chains aligned end to end. It can produce spores that are oval and subterminal and that cause swelling of the cells.

A

B

Figure 29-8 ***Clostridium difficile*** **on CDC agar.** Colonies of *C. difficile* are gray to white, opaque, matte to glossy, flat, round, occasionally rhizoid, and nonhemolytic. They have a distinctive odor commonly described as "horse manure."

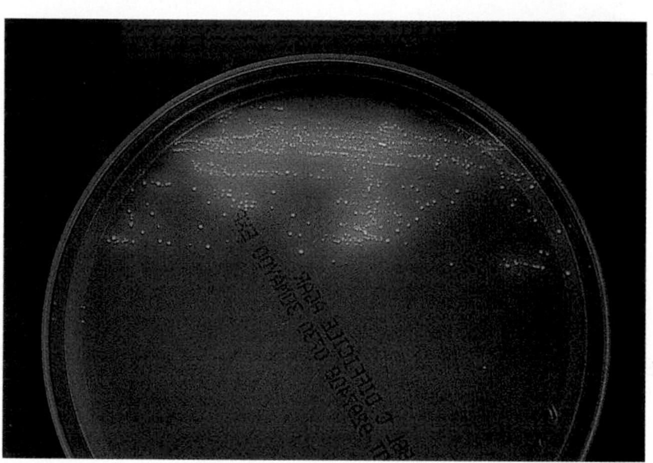

Figure 29-9 ***Clostridium difficile*** **on CDC agar, examined under UV light.** As shown here, colonies of *C. difficile* fluoresce chartreuse under UV light.

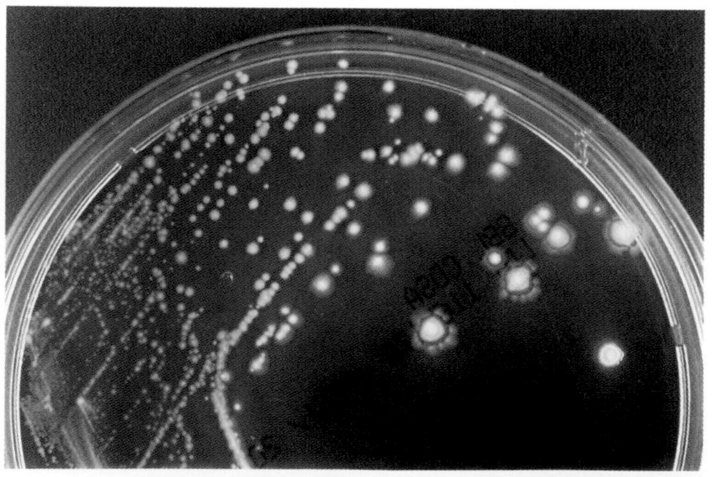

Figure 29-10 ***Clostridium difficile*** **on BBL** ***Clostridium difficile*** **Selective Agar.** BBL *Clostridium difficile* Selective Agar (BD Diagnostic Systems, Franklin Lakes, NJ) is a selective and differential medium developed for the isolation of *C. difficile*. Large colonies with a yellow color characteristic of *C. difficile* are shown. As growth of *C. difficile* occurs, the pH of the medium increases, causing the neutral red indicator to turn yellow. Due to intestinal colonization, laboratory confirmation of the diagnosis of *C. difficile*-induced diarrhea depends on verifying toxin production. Colonies from this agar are subcultured to a broth, and the filtered liquid can be used to perform the cytotoxin assay.

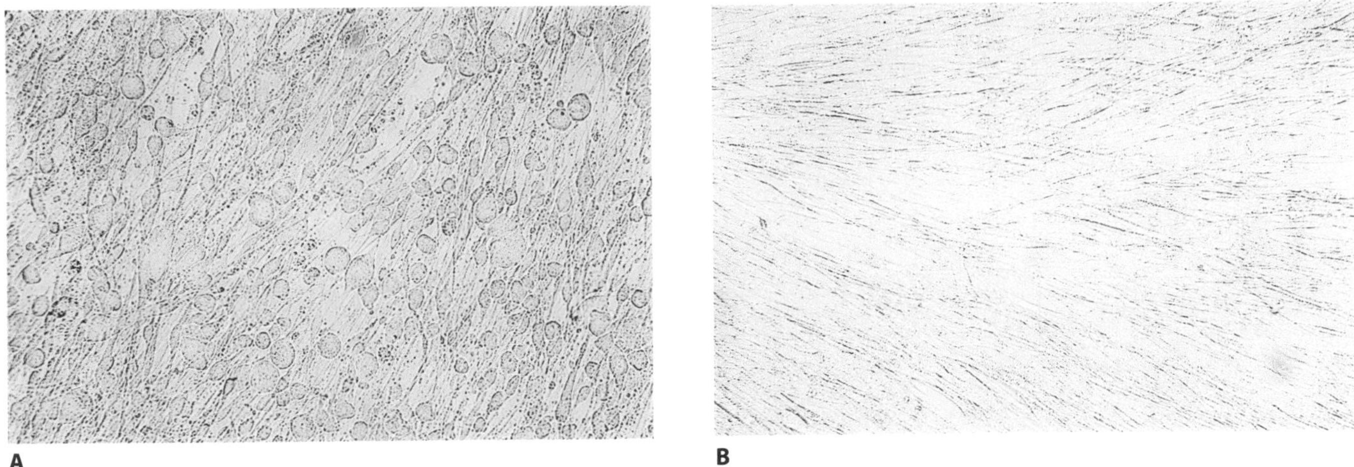

Figure 29-11 Cytotoxin neutralization assay for *Clostridium difficile* with MRC-5 cells. Cytotoxin neutralization can be used to detect the presence of *C. difficile* toxin B, since this bacterium is frequently isolated from asymptomatic individuals and toxigenic isolates are the only pathogenic strains. To perform this test, before being placed on a tissue culture monolayer, an aliquot from the fecal supernatant is incubated with antiserum that neutralizes toxin B. A second fecal aliquot is placed directly onto the cell monolayer. A positive specimen produces a cytopathic effect on the directly inoculated monolayer (A), while no cytopathic effect is detected on the control monolayer, in which neutralizing antiserum to toxin B was added (B). Toxin detection and neutralization using a tissue culture cytotoxin assay was considered to be the gold standard for the laboratory identification of pathogenic *C. difficile*. Currently, molecular techniques are the preferred method.

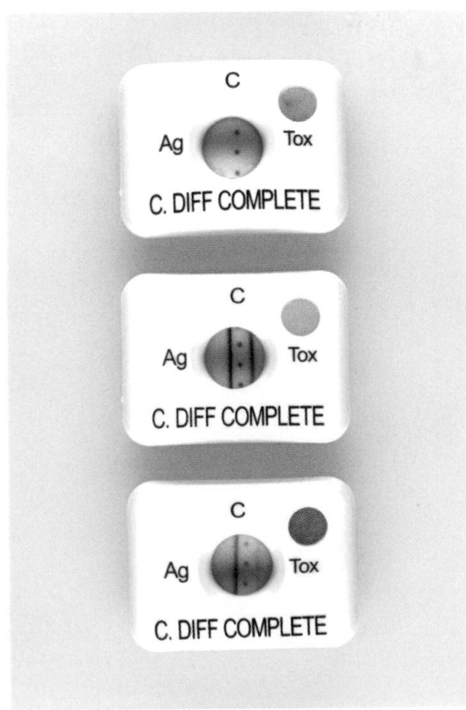

Figure 29-12 Detection of *Clostridium difficile* GDH and toxins A and B by EIA. The Wampole *C. diff* Quik Chek Complete assay (TechLab, Inc., Blacksburg, VA) simultaneously detects the presence of GDH, an antigen unique to *C. difficile*, and toxins A and B by using specific antibodies for these three components. The GDH test is highly sensitive but lacks specificity because there are strains of *C. difficile* that are not toxigenic. The assay for toxins A and B is highly specific but not very sensitive. The blue dots in the middle of the reaction window represent the internal controls. These dots need to be positive to be able to interpret the results. A blue line on the "Ag" and "Tox" sides indicates that the antigen and the toxins (A and/or B), respectively, are positive. In this figure, the top reaction is negative for both the antigen and the toxins, the middle card is positive for both, and the bottom is positive for the antigen and negative for the toxins.

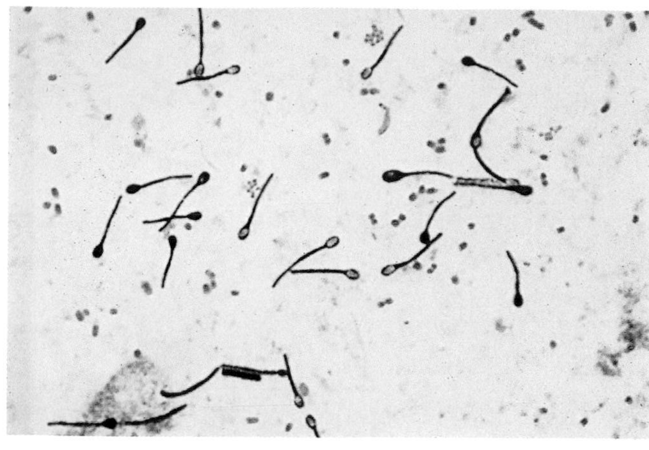

Figure 29-13 Gram stain of *Clostridium paraputrificum* from a blood culture. The organisms appear here as long, thin, straight or slightly curved, gram-positive bacilli, 0.5 to 1.5 μm by 2.0 to 20 μm, that can also easily stain gram negative, with oval, terminal spores that swell the cells. In the background, a small, gram-negative bacillus with bipolar staining can be observed.

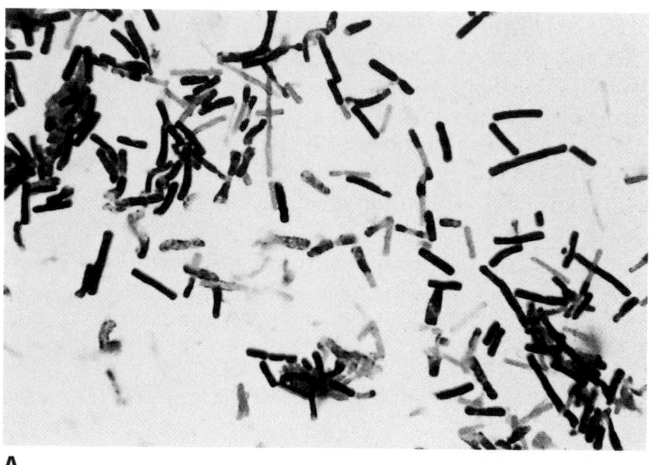

A

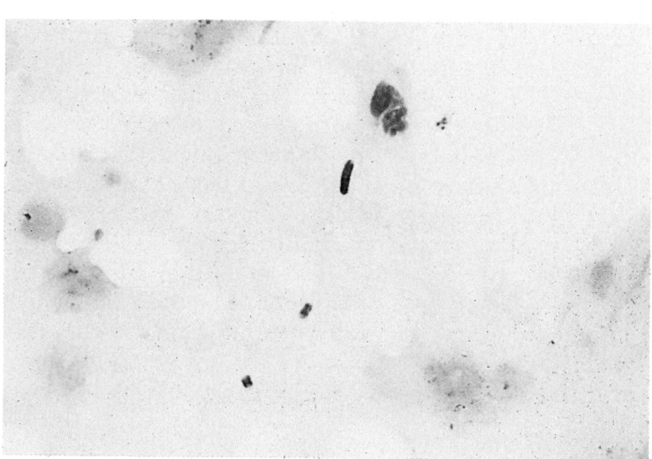

B

Figure 29-14 Gram stain of *Clostridium perfringens* from a culture and from a patient with necrotizing fasciitis. (A) *C. perfringens* organisms in culture are gram-positive bacilli with blunt ends, described as boxcar shaped, usually 2 to 4 μm long by 0.8 to 1.5 μm in diameter. Some of the cells in this preparation are gram negative, and no spores are present. Spores are rarely seen in vivo or in vitro; when found, they are large, oval, and central or subterminal in location and cause the cell to swell. Young cultures often have short, coccoid cells, while older cultures contain longer, filamentous cells. (B) Direct Gram stains from tissues from patients with gas gangrene are characterized in general by the absence of inflammatory cells and the presence of boxcar-shaped, gram-variable bacilli.

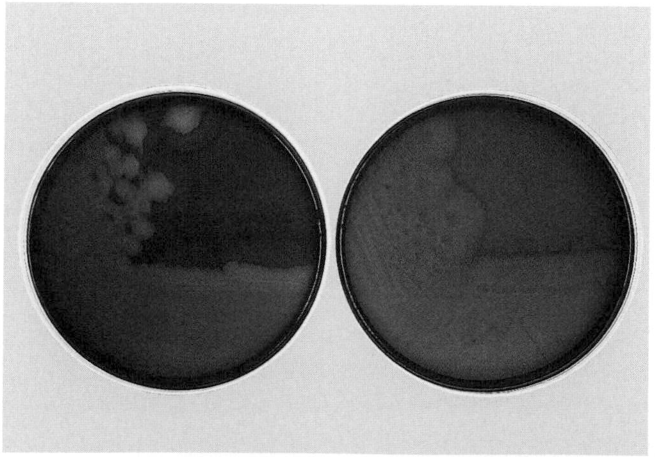

Figure 29-15 *Clostridium perfringens* on brucella agar (left) and phenylethyl alcohol agar (right). A double zone of hemolysis can be seen surrounding the colonies. The smaller zone of complete hemolysis is produced by a theta-toxin, a heat- and oxygen-labile toxin, while the outer zone of partial hemolysis is produced by phospholipase C, an alpha-toxin that is also responsible for the lecithin hydrolysis shown in Fig. 29-16.

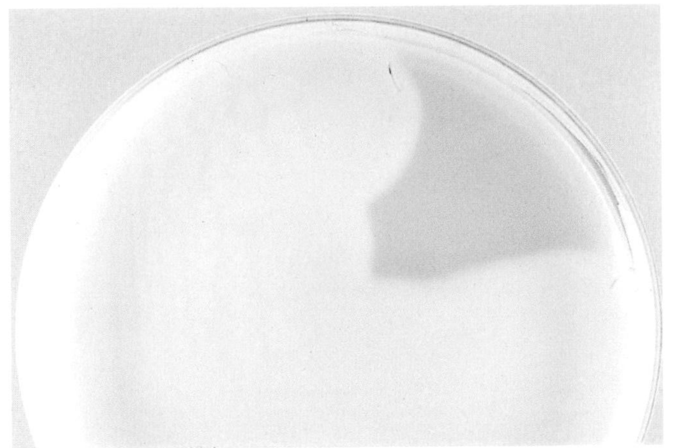

Figure 29-16 ***Clostridium perfringens*** **on egg yolk agar.** On egg yolk agar, *C. perfringens* is lecithinase positive, as seen by the zone of opacity surrounding the colony. This effect is produced by phospholipase C, also called alpha-toxin, which hydrolyzes the lecithin. This opacity is not a surface phenomenon but, rather, is in the medium itself due to the precipitation of complex fats.

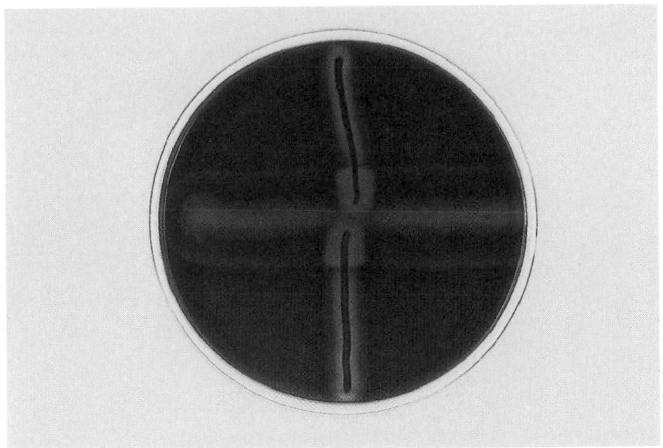

Figure 29-17 Reverse CAMP test for identification of ***Clostridium perfringens.*** More than 95% of *C. perfringens* strains produce a positive reverse CAMP test. To perform this test, a CDC anaerobe blood agar plate is inoculated down the center with a single streak of *Streptococcus agalactiae* (group B streptococcus), which produces a diffusible extracellular protein (CAMP factor) that can act synergistically with the *C. perfringens* alpha-toxin to lyse erythrocytes. The suspected isolate of *C. perfringens* is inoculated perpendicularly to, but not touching, the *Streptococcus* streak, and the plate is incubated anaerobically for 24 to 48 h. As shown in this figure, development of an arrowhead of hemolysis with the tip coming from the *Streptococcus* strain toward the *Clostridium* strain indicates a positive test.

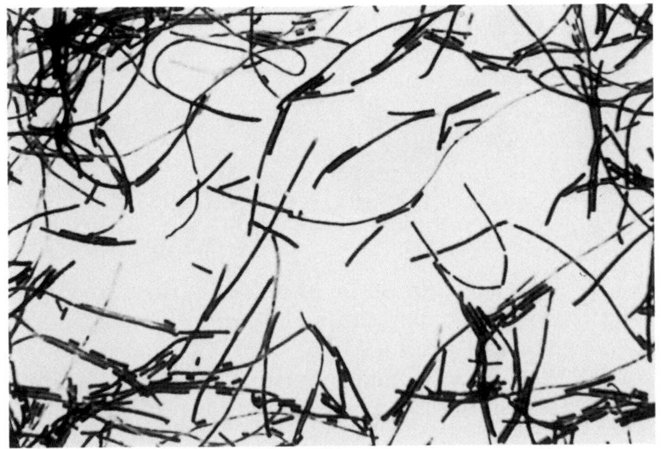

Figure 29-18 Gram stain of ***Clostridium ramosum.*** *C. ramosum* organisms are gram-variable, straight or curved bacilli that frequently produce short chains, V-shaped arrangements, and long filaments. They are thinner than most clostridia, varying from 0.5 to 0.9 μm in diameter and 2.0 to 13 μm in length. Spores are rarely produced; when present, they are small, round, and usually terminal, causing swelling of the cell. *C. ramosum* is one of the clostridia most frequently isolated from clinical specimens, particularly following abdominal trauma.

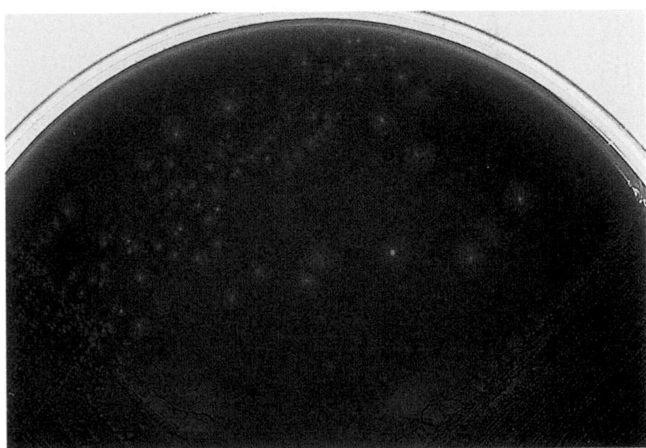

Figure 29-19 ***Clostridium ramosum*** **on CDC agar.** Colonies of *C. ramosum* are small, gray-white or translucent, smooth, irregular with scalloped margins, and nonhemolytic.

Figure 29-20 Antimicrobial susceptibility testing of *Clostridium ramosum*. As shown here, *C. ramosum* is one of the few anaerobic organisms resistant to rifampin (RA).

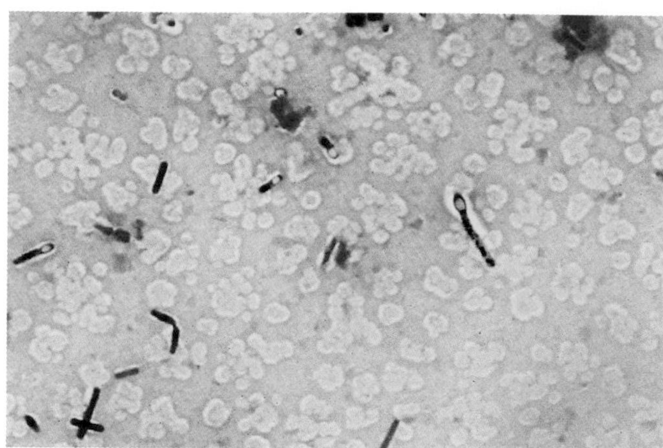

Figure 29-21 Gram stain of *Clostridium septicum* from a blood culture. In young cultures, this organism appears gram positive; however, it becomes gram negative with age and often stains unevenly. The bacilli are straight or curved and may occur singly or in pairs. The spores swell the cell, are oval, and have a subterminal location, as shown here.

Figure 29-22 *Clostridium septicum* on CDC agar. *C. septicum* produces a typical colony that is gray, glossy, translucent, and beta-hemolytic, with a rhizoid margin resembling a "Medusa head." As shown here, colonies can swarm in less than 24 h, forming an invisible film over the agar surface.

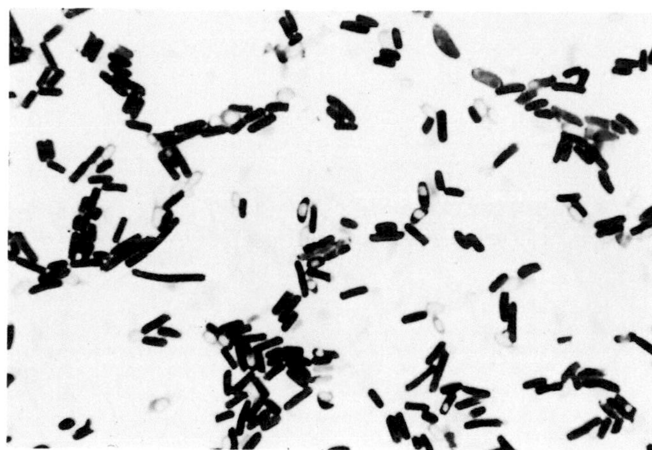

Figure 29-23 Gram stain of *Clostridium sordellii*. On prolonged incubation under anaerobic conditions, *C. sordellii* can produce oval, central to subterminal spores that cause a slight swelling of the cells. Free spores are also observed in some preparations.

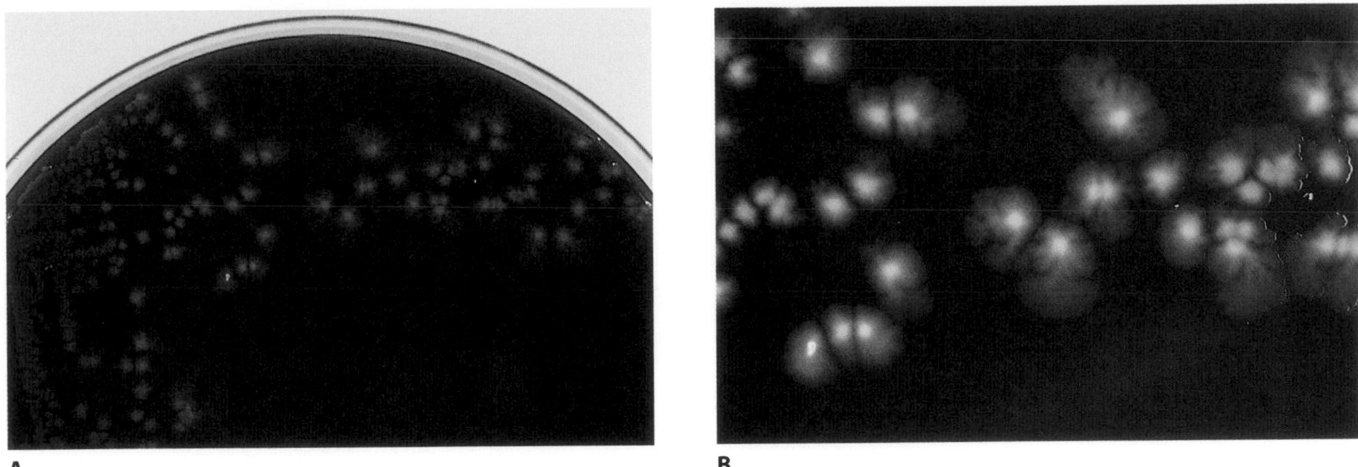

Figure 29-24 ***Clostridium sordellii*** **on CDC agar.** On CDC agar, colonies of *C. sordellii* appear white or gray and chalk-like, opaque to translucent, with lobate edges.

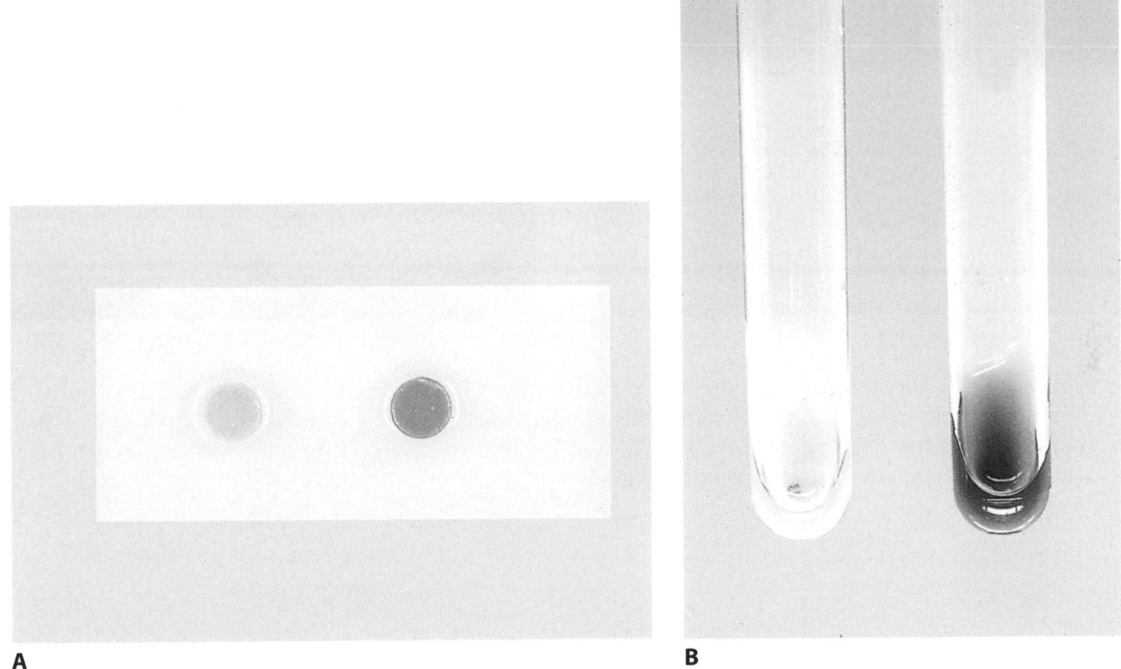

Figure 29-25 Urea and indole reactions of ***Clostridium sordellii*****.** *C. sordellii* is one of the few clostridia that gives positive indole (A) and urea (B) reactions. On both images, the negative reaction is on the left and the positive reaction is on the right.

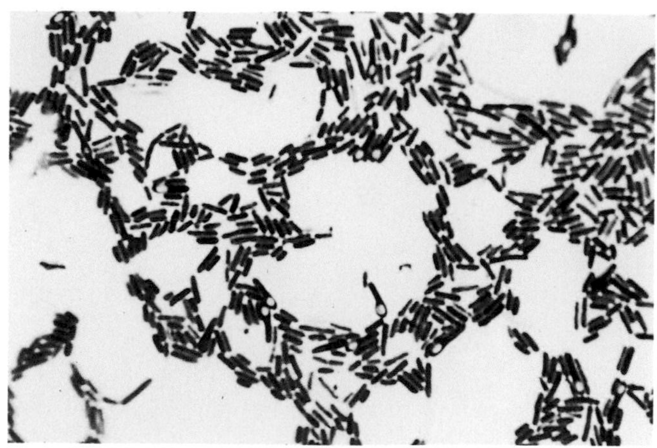

Figure 29-26 Gram stain of *Clostridium sporogenes*. *C. sporogenes* is one of the smaller species within the genus, with cells varying from 0.3 to 1.4 μm by 1.3 to 16 μm. They occur singly and readily produce oval, subterminal spores that swell the cell.

A

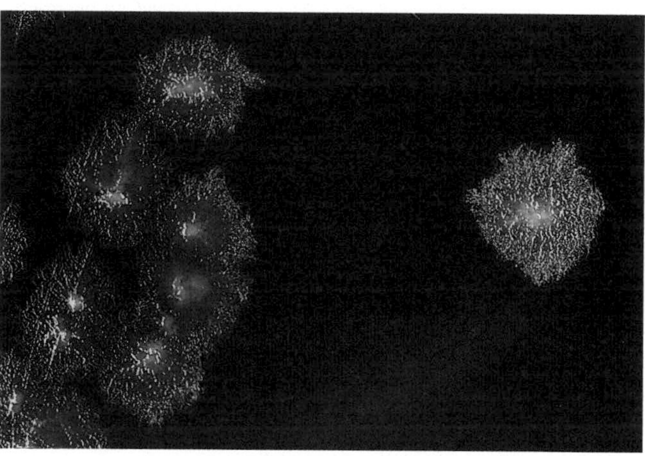

B

Figure 29-27 *Clostridium sporogenes* on CDC agar. Colonies of *C. sporogenes* are moist, white, and opaque at the center, with rhizoid edges that, within 4 to 6 h, form Medusa heads that attach firmly to the agar. By 24 to 48 h of incubation, the colony may swarm, becoming a heavy film of growth that covers the plate.

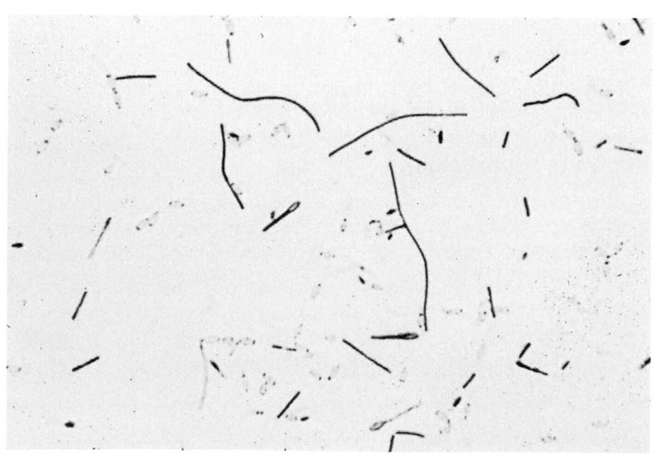

Figure 29-28 Gram stain of *Clostridium tertium* from a blood culture. The bacilli are long, thin, and gram variable and have large, oval, terminal spores that cause marked swelling of the cells.

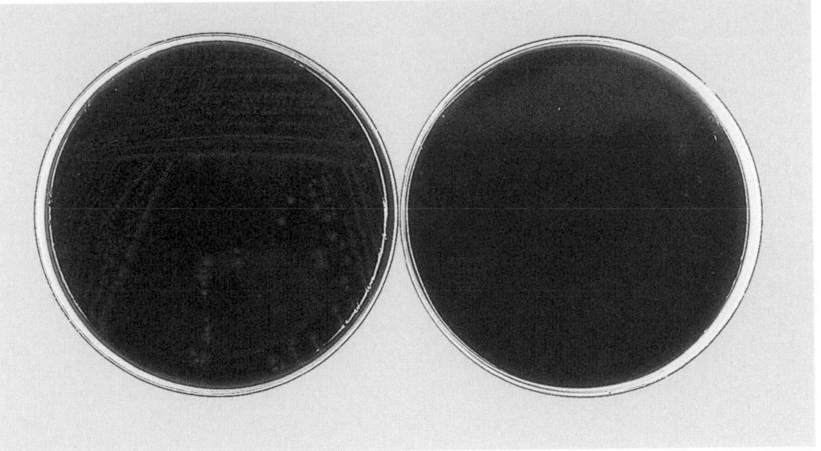

Figure 29-29 *Clostridium tertium* on CDC agar under anaerobic (left) and aerobic (right) conditions. As shown here, *C. tertium* is one of the few aerotolerant species of *Clostridium* found in clinical specimens. *C. tertium* can easily be confused with non-spore-forming, gram-negative bacilli or with *Bacillus* spp. This species can be differentiated from *Bacillus* spp. based on sporulation requirements, with *C. tertium* sporulating only under anaerobic conditions and *Bacillus* producing spores only under aerobic conditions.

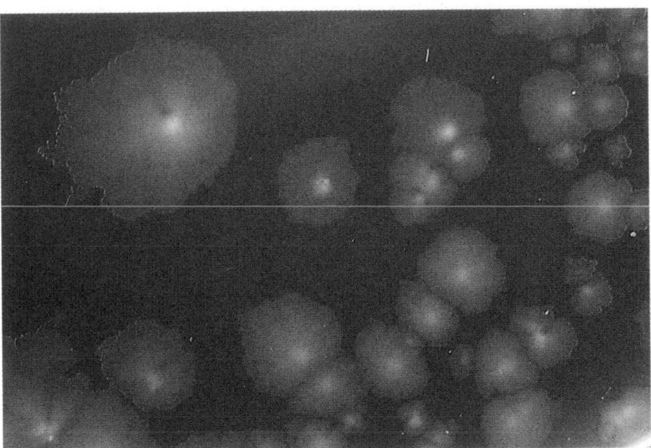

Figure 29-30 *Clostridium tertium* on CDC agar. Colonies of *C. tertium* measure 2 to 4 mm in diameter and are white to gray, opaque to translucent, and circular with irregular edges. Hemolysis is variable, and there are alpha-hemolytic, beta-hemolytic, and nonhemolytic strains.

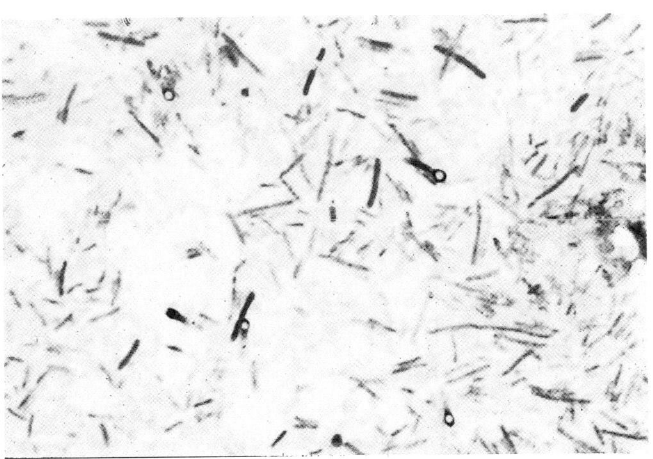

Figure 29-31 Gram stain of *Clostridium tetani*. This preparation shows gram-positive bacilli singly and in pairs, with round spores that are located in the terminal region, giving a tennis racket- or drumstick-like appearance. Initially the cells appear gram positive, but after 24 h of incubation, they readily stain gram negative.

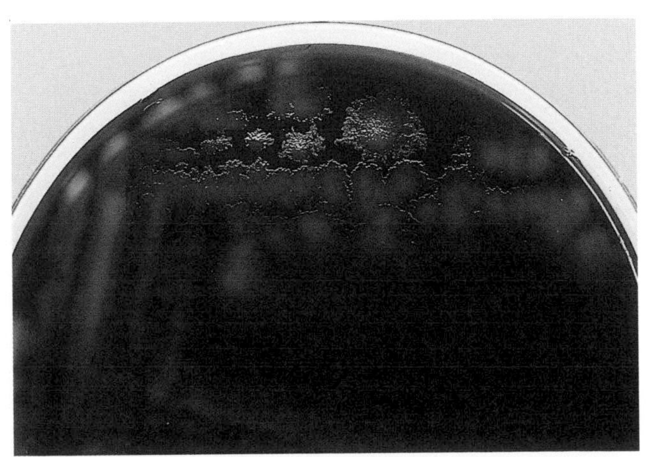

Figure 29-32 Culture of *Clostridium tetani* on CDC agar. Colonies of *C. tetani* are 4 to 6 μm in diameter, gray, translucent, and flat with an irregular to rhizoid margin and may swarm on the agar surface. A small zone of beta-hemolysis can be observed around the colonies. *C. tetani* is generally found mixed with other organisms in wounds and is often very fastidious and difficult to grow.

Peptostreptococcus, Finegoldia, Anaerococcus, Peptoniphilus, Propionibacterium, Lactobacillus, Actinomyces, and Other Non-Spore-Forming, Anaerobic Gram-Positive Bacteria

30

ANAEROBIC GRAM-POSITIVE COCCI

The obligate anaerobic, gram-positive cocci include cocci that do not produce spores and sometimes appear as elongated coccobacilli. A recent major change in taxonomy resulted in the reclassification of many anaerobic cocci and the proposal of several new genera. The anaerobic gram-positive cocci now include *Anaerococcus*, *Atopobium*, *Coprococcus*, *Finegoldia*, *Gallicola*, *Gemella*, *Peptococcus*, *Peptoniphilus*, *Peptostreptococcus*, *Ruminococcus*, and *Sarcina*. *Parvimonas* has been proposed to replace *Micromonas*. The only species remaining in the genus *Peptococcus* is *Peptococcus niger*, and the only two *Peptostreptococcus* species are *Peptostreptococcus anaerobius* and *Peptostreptococcus stomatis*. The three species most commonly found in clinical specimens are *Finegoldia magna*, *P. anaerobius*, and *Parvimonas micra* (*Micromonas micros*). *Ruminococcus* and *Coprococcus*, which are members of the normal fecal flora; the obligately anaerobic *Streptococcus pleomorphus* and *Streptococcus hansenii*; and *Peptococcus niger* are rarely isolated from clinical specimens.

The anaerobic gram-positive cocci are found in humans and animals as members of the normal flora of the skin, oropharynx, and upper respiratory tract, as well as the gastrointestinal and genitourinary tracts. For the most part they are considered opportunistic pathogens. They have been isolated from head and neck infections, including chronic otitis media and sinusitis, periodontitis, pneumonia, and brain abscesses. Anaerobic gram-positive cocci have also been recognized for many years as causes of genital infections, including postpartum endometritis, tubo-ovarian abscesses, pelvic inflammatory disease, septic abortions, and chorioamnionitis. Bacteremia is a complication that is not uncommon following gynecological or obstetric infections. However, bacteremia with anaerobic gram-positive cocci is less severe than bacteremia caused by *Bacteroides*, which is often fatal. In patients with a perforated bowel, appendicitis, penetrating trauma including surgery, or cancer, mixed infections with other anaerobes, *Enterobacteriaceae*, and *Enterococcus* spp. are common and can lead to an intra-abdominal abscess.

Gram stains of clinical material can be useful in detecting the presence of mixed infections and can also provide presumptive evidence of certain anaerobes; however, this method is of little value in differentiating anaerobic from aerobic and facultative, gram-positive cocci. The anaerobic gram-positive cocci can vary in size from 0.3 to 1.6 μm, and changes in staining characteristics and morphology may occur as a result of growth on different media and with the age of the organism. This makes the interpretation of the Gram stain difficult. When gram-negative or gram-variable staining is observed, the KOH solubility test (string test), the LanaGram using L-alanine-*p*-nitroanilide reagent (Hardy Diagnostics, Santa Maria, CA), and susceptibility to vancomycin (5-μg disk) can be helpful in differentiating gram-positive and gram-negative organisms.

In clinical specimens, it can also be difficult to identify microaerophilic streptococci, which may only grow on primary anaerobic media but will subsequently grow in 5 to 10% CO_2 upon repeat subculture. A metronidazole

(5-μg) disk test can be used as an inexpensive but effective technique to differentiate microaerophilic organisms from anaerobic gram-positive cocci. Microaerophilic strains show no inhibition of growth, while anaerobic gram-positive cocci demonstrate a zone of inhibition of at least 15 mm around the metronidazole disk.

F. magna cells are 0.7 to 1.2 μm in diameter and appear in pairs, clusters, or a tightly packed arrangement. Colonies are minute to 0.5 mm in diameter, circular, dull, smooth, and nonhemolytic. *P. micra* (*M. micros*) colonies are minute to 1 mm in diameter, convex, and dull. The cells are similar in appearance to those of *F. magna* but are smaller (0.3 to 0.7 μm in diameter) and usually form short chains. Since different growth conditions result in strain variability, differentiation of the two species is subjective when based on their cellular morphology alone.

Colonies of *P. anaerobius* are usually larger and vary in diameter from 0.5 to 2 mm. They are gray-white and nonhemolytic and may have a pungently sweet odor. The cells are 0.5 to 0.6 μm in diameter, and in young cultures they may appear as elongated cocci in chains. A presumptive identification can be made based on sodium polyanethol sulfonate (SPS) susceptibility.

Peptoniphilus asaccharolyticus produces colonies that may be yellow or gray and translucent. They can vary from minute to 2 mm in diameter, and on Gram stain they may be arranged in pairs, tetrads, or clumps. Older cells may appear gram negative. A presumptive identification can be reported if the anaerobic gram-positive cocci are isolated from a human clinical specimen and are SPS resistant and indole positive. *Peptoniphilus indolicus*, which is also indole positive, is rarely isolated from clinical specimens.

Indole, urease, catalase, and the inhibition of growth by SPS are rapid key tests that aid in the presumptive identification of some anaerobic gram-positive cocci (Table 30-1). The ability of rapid commercial systems to accurately identify the members of this group ranges from 15% for *Anaerococcus prevotii* to 90 to 100% for *P. micra*, *F. magna*, *P. asaccharolyticus*, and *P. anaerobius*. Although biochemical tests may be helpful, identification based on the results of these tests alone should be considered presumptive. Chromatographic analysis of metabolic fatty acids is required for definitive species identification.

ANAEROBIC, NON-SPORE-FORMING, GRAM-POSITIVE BACILLI

The anaerobic, non-spore-forming, gram-positive bacilli comprise a diverse group varying from obligate to facultatively anaerobic organisms. In recent years there have been significant taxonomic changes, and currently the group includes the traditional genera *Actinomyces*, *Bifidobacterium*, *Eubacterium*, *Lactobacillus*, *Mobiluncus*, and *Propionibacterium*, as well as the new genera *Actinobaculum*, *Anaerofustis*, *Anaerotruncus*, *Arcanobacterium*, *Atopobium*, *Bulleidia*, *Catenibacterium*, *Collinsella*, *Cryptobacterium*, *Dorea*, *Eggerthella*, *Filifactor*, *Flavonifractor*, *Gordonibacter*, *Holdemania*, *Mogibacterium*, *Olsenella*, *Paraeggerthella*, *Parascardovia*, *Propioniferax*, *Propionimicrobium*, *Pseudoramibacter*, *Roseburia*, *Scardovia*, *Shuttleworthia*, *Slackia*, *Solobacterium*, *Turicibacter*, and *Varibaculum*.

Humans and animals are the natural habitat of these organisms. *Actinomyces* and *Atopobium* spp. are found in the mouth and upper respiratory tract. *Bifidobacterium* and *Eubacterium* spp. are usually present in the mouth and are found in large numbers in the intestinal tract. *Lactobacillus* spp. are widely distributed throughout the body, including the mouth and the intestinal and genital tracts. *Mobiluncus* spp. normally inhabit the genital tract, and *Propionibacterium* spp. can be isolated from the skin, conjunctiva, oral cavity, and large intestine. Of the newly described genera, most have been recovered from the human oral cavity, while *Collinsella*, *Catenibacterium*, and *Holdemania* have been recovered from feces.

Table 30-1 Characteristics of the most commonly isolated anaerobic gram-positive cocci[a]

Species	SPS	Indole	Urease	Cells of ≥0.6 μm	Gram stain morphology
Finegoldia magna	R	0	0	+	Cocci are large; arranged in pairs, tetrads, and clusters
Parvimonas micra (*Micromonas micros*)	R	0	0	0	Cocci are small; arranged in pairs, chains, and clusters
Peptoniphilus asaccharolyticus	R	+	0	0	Cells stain poorly; cocci are uniform in size and clump
Peptostreptococcus anaerobius	S	0	0	0	Cocci are pleomorphic; arranged in chains

[a] +, positive reaction; 0, negative reaction; S, susceptible; R, resistant.

These organisms are opportunistic pathogens that seldom cause infections alone but are most often found in polymicrobic infections throughout the body, provided that suitable conditions for colonization and penetration exist. Actinomycosis is a chronic granulomatous infection that can result in abscess formation with draining sinuses. The purulent discharge frequently contains sulfur granules, which are masses of bacteria cemented together by a polysaccharide-protein complex and calcium phosphate, with colors ranging from white to yellow-brown. The presence of sulfur granules is considered diagnostic. If the granules are large enough, they can be crushed and observed microscopically (magnification, ×100) by the wet-mount technique. Sulfur granules have characteristic club-shaped masses of filaments radiating from the granules. If they are Gram stained, gram-positive branched and unbranched filaments are seen. When sulfur granules are present, they should be rinsed with sterile broth, crushed, and inoculated onto anaerobic media. The Brown-Brenn stain facilitates the detection of sulfur granules in histological preparations. Staining of tissue specimens with hematoxylin and eosin shows that the periphery of the granules has eosinophilic clubs. Besides *Actinomyces*, other organisms such as *Nocardia*, *Streptomyces*, and *Staphylococcus* can also produce granules with clubs. Actinomycosis can occur in the brain, the lower respiratory tract, and the genital tract, especially in infections related to intrauterine devices; however, the most common infections occur in cervicofacial regions in males. Although *Actinomyces israelii* is the species most frequently isolated from human actinomycosis, other species of *Actinomyces*, as well as *Propionibacterium propionicum*, may also be etiological agents.

Propionibacterium spp. can cause infections of the skin, conjunctiva, bone, joints, and central nervous system. Infections are often associated with surgical procedures or foreign bodies such as prosthetic valve and ventriculoatrial shunt implants. In addition, *Propionibacterium acnes* plays a significant role in acne vulgaris. Other members of this group of anaerobes are generally nonpathogenic. Although *Eubacterium* and *Bifidobacterium* spp. are rarely encountered in clinical specimens, *Eubacterium* spp. have been isolated in mixed cultures from wounds and abscesses and *Bifidobacterium dentium*, one of the few species in this genus with pathogenic potential, has been isolated from dental caries and from other clinical material. *Lactobacillus* spp. are rarely involved in human infection but have been isolated from cases of bacteremia and endocarditis, particularly in immunocompromised patients. The pathogenicity of *Mobiluncus* spp. is not well defined; however, it is generally thought to play a role in bacterial vaginosis.

Actinomyces spp. can vary from straight or slightly curved bacilli (0.2 to 1.0 μm) to slender filaments with true branching. The cells may have swollen, clubbed, or clavate ends and may occur singly or in pairs with a diphtheroidal arrangement or may be pleomorphic. They are gram positive, but their irregular staining can result in a beaded or banded appearance. A modified acid-fast stain can be used to differentiate *Actinomyces* spp. from *Nocardia* spp., which are partially acid fast. *A. israelii* is noted for its branching filaments on Gram stain and also for its colony morphology. All *Actinomyces* spp. are microaerophilic, with the exception of *Actinomyces meyeri*, which is an obligate anaerobe. They are slow growers, requiring at least 48 h for colonies to appear on primary culture. Young colonies commonly have branching filaments radiating from a central point, giving the appearance of "spider colonies." As the colonies mature, they become rough and umbonate with undulate edges, resulting in a "molar tooth" appearance. Other *Actinomyces* spp. can produce colonies ranging from smooth and circular to granular or "raspberry-like." Most colonies are gray-white and opaque. Catalase, urease, and pigment production are helpful in species determination. With the exception of *Actinomyces viscosus*, most *Actinomyces* spp. are catalase negative. *Actinomyces odontolyticus* produces a red pigment, and *Actinomyces naeslundii* and *A. viscosus* are urea positive. The biochemical reactions of several newer species are based on a single strain. As a result, discrepancies in some biochemical tables differentiating the *Actinomyces* spp. may appear.

Bifidobacterium spp. can be diphtheroid to filamentous with pointed, club-shaped or slightly bifurcated ends and may appear to be branching; however, they are generally larger than the cells of *Actinomyces* spp. and *Propionibacterium* spp. They can occur singly, in chains, or in a palisade arrangement. Colonies are entire, convex, and white to cream. *Bifidobacterium* spp. are catalase, indole, and nitrate negative but positive for esculin hydrolysis.

Eubacterium spp. vary from uniform to pleomorphic bacilli. They may be coccoid, diphtheroidal, or filamentous and can be thin to plump. They are generally arranged in pairs, short chains, or sometimes small clumps. The colonies are small, ranging from punctiform to 2 mm; entire; circular; and translucent to slightly opaque. They are biochemically inactive. *Eggerthella lenta* (formerly called *Eubacterium lentum*)

Table 30-2 Characteristics of the anaerobic, non-spore-forming, gram-positive bacilli[a]

Species	Aerotolerance	Catalase	Indole	Nitrate	Esculin	Motility	Urea	Pigment
Actinomyces spp.								
A. israelii	(+)	0	0	+	+	0	0	0
A. meyeri	0	0	0	V	0	0	0	0
A. naeslundii	+	0	0	+	V	0	+	0
A. odontolyticus	+	0	0	+	V	0	0	+
A. viscosus	+	+	0	+	V	0	V	0
Propionibacterium spp.								
P. acnes	+	+	+	+	0	0	0	0
P. propionicum	0	0	0	+	0	0	0	0
Bifidobacterium spp.	V	0^+	0	0	$+^0$	0	0	0
Eubacterium spp.	0	0^+	0^+	0	V	0	0	0
Lactobacillus spp.	V	0	0	0^+	V	0	0	0
Mobiluncus spp.	0	0	0	V	0	+	0	0

[a]+, positive reaction; $+^0$, most strains positive, some negative; (+), better growth in anaerobic conditions; 0, negative reaction; 0^+, most strains negative, some weakly positive; V, variable reaction.

is the species most commonly isolated from clinical specimens.

Lactobacillus spp. are gram-positive bacilli that vary from long and slender with straight sides to slightly bent or coryneform coccobacilli. The length of the cell and the degree of curvature is based on the age of the culture, the medium, and the oxygen tension. Most *Lactobacillus* spp. isolated from clinical specimens are microaerophilic, but some are obligate anaerobes. They can usually be identified by their Gram stain morphology, negative catalase reaction, and production of lactic acid from the metabolism of glucose.

Mobiluncus spp. are strict anaerobes. On Gram stain they appear as curved bacilli and consistently stain gram negative or gram variable; however, their cell wall lacks lipopolysaccharide and is structurally similar to that of gram-positive organisms. The motility of *Mobiluncus* spp. distinguishes them from other anaerobic, non-spore-forming, gram-positive bacilli. Two species, *Mobiluncus mulieris* and *Mobiluncus curtisii*, are now recognized. *M. curtisii* is a curved, gram-variable bacillus with pointed ends and measures 1.7 μm in length, while *M. mulieris* is gram negative and longer, measuring 2.9 μm. Both are oxidase, catalase, and indole negative.

Propionibacterium spp. are pleomorphic bacilli and sometimes have a false branching or beaded appearance. They can contain metachromatic granules and appear club shaped or have a "Chinese letter" configuration. The most common clinical isolate is *P. acnes*, which characteristically grows as a small, white, shiny to opaque, convex colony with an entire edge. Presumptive identification can be made based on positive catalase and indole reactions.

Aerotolerance, Gram stain, colony morphology, fluorescence under long-wave UV light, pigment production, and biochemical reactions such as nitrate, catalase, indole, and esculin can be useful in the presumptive identification of the more commonly isolated or clinically important anaerobes in this group (Table 30-2). For instance, a catalase-positive organism is probably *Propionibacterium* or *A. viscosus*. An indole-positive organism is likely to be *Propionibacterium*, and with a positive nitrate test one can generally rule out *Bifidobacterium* and *Lactobacillus* spp. Most *Actinomyces* and *Propionibacterium* spp. are facultatively anaerobic or microaerophilic, while only a few *Eubacterium* strains tolerate oxygen. Although colony morphology, cell morphology, and rapid biochemical tests may be useful for presumptively grouping the non-spore-forming, anaerobic gram-positive bacilli into genera, these characteristics may be variable, and analysis of metabolic end products and molecular methods may be necessary for definitive species identification.

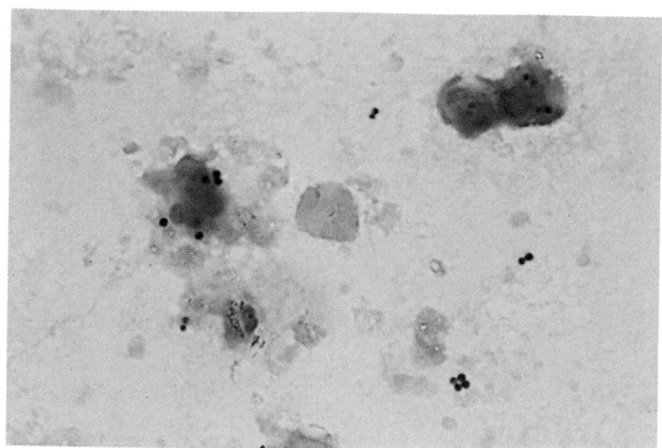

Figure 30-1 Gram stain of a specimen from a femur infected with aerobic and anaerobic gram-positive cocci. Although the Gram stain can be very useful in suggesting the presence of anaerobes and also in providing a presumptive identification of certain anaerobic organisms, it cannot differentiate between aerobic and anaerobic cocci. In this Gram stain of a specimen from a lesion in the femur, all of the cocci look similar. The culture grew *Staphylococcus aureus* and anaerobic gram-positive cocci.

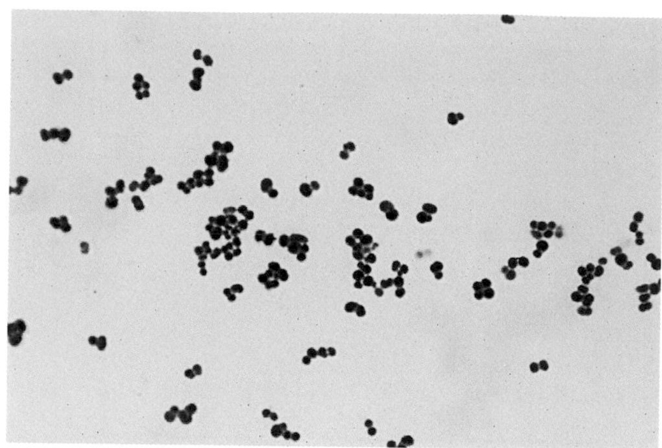

Figure 30-2 Gram stain of *Finegoldia magna*. *F. magna* cells are gram-positive cocci in pairs or clusters, measuring 0.7 to 1.2 μm.

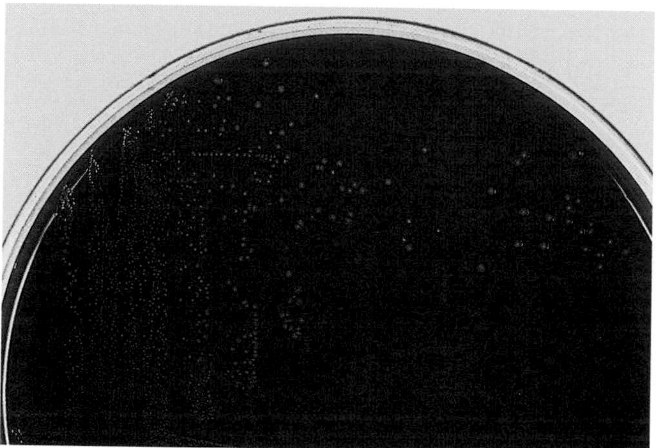

Figure 30-3 *Finegoldia magna* on CDC agar. After 48 h, colonies of *F. magna* are minute to 0.5 mm in diameter, circular, dull, smooth, and nonhemolytic.

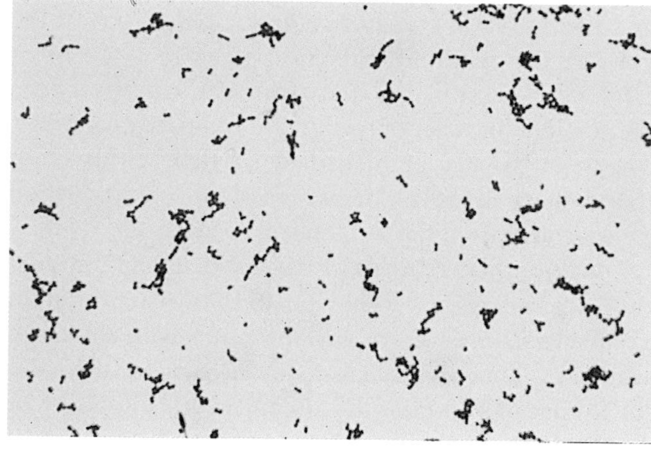

Figure 30-4 Gram stain of *Parvimonas micra* (*Micromonas micros*). *P. micra* is among the smallest of the anaerobic gram-positive cocci. The cells measure 0.3 to 0.7 μm and usually form pairs or short chains.

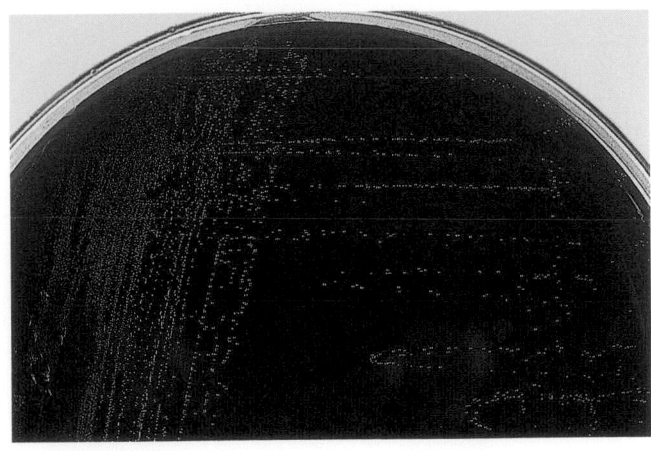

Figure 30-5 *Parvimonas micra* (*Micromonas micros*) on CDC agar. *P. micra* colonies are circular, convex, white to translucent gray, and opaque. After 48 h of incubation, the colonies are minute to 1 mm in diameter.

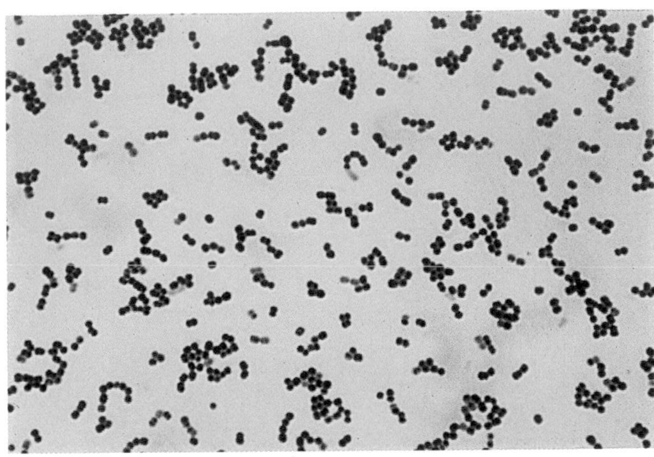

Figure 30-6 Gram stain of *Peptostreptococcus anaerobius*. *P. anaerobius* cells are fairly large, gram-positive cocci measuring 0.5 to 0.6 μm in diameter. As shown here, the cells often elongate and occur in pairs and chains.

Figure 30-7 *Peptostreptococcus anaerobius* on CDC agar. Colonies of *P. anaerobius* are circular, entire, gray to white, and opaque. They vary in diameter from 0.5 to 2 mm after 48 h of incubation; they are larger than most other anaerobic gram-positive cocci. Another characteristic is the sweet, fetid odor associated with this organism.

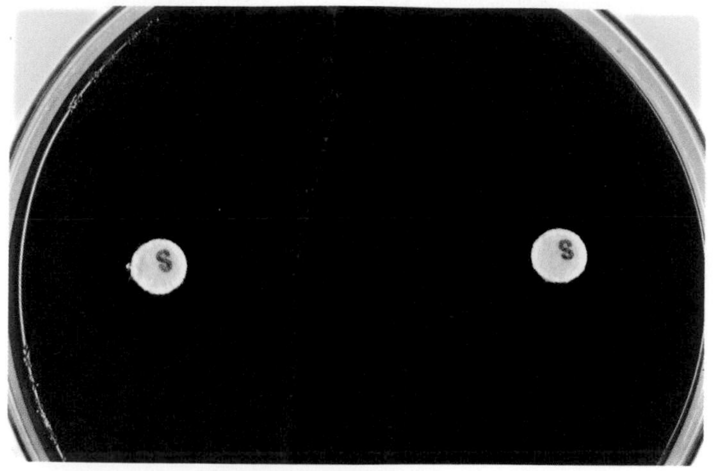

Figure 30-8 SPS disk test. As shown here, an SPS disk is added to a heavily inoculated subculture plate and incubated anaerobically for 48 h. If the organism is susceptible to SPS, there will be a zone of inhibition (≥12 mm) around the disk. The organism on the right is susceptible, and the one on the left is resistant. The disk test is especially valuable for presumptive identification of *P. anaerobius*, which is susceptible to SPS.

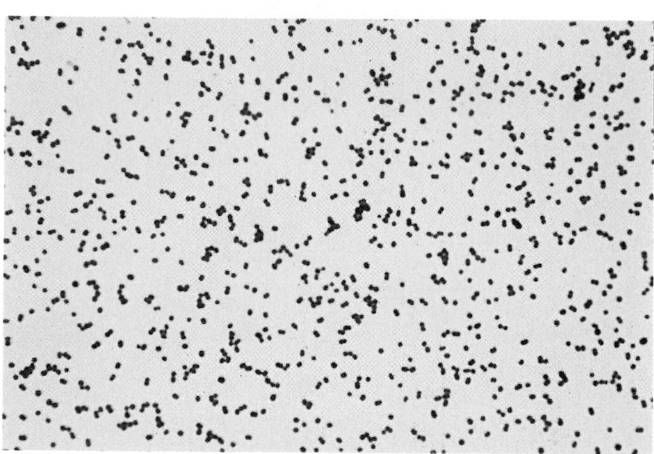

Figure 30-9 Gram stain of *Peptoniphilus asaccharolyticus*. *P. asaccharolyticus* cells are cocci measuring 0.5 to 1.6 μm and can be seen in pairs, tetrads, or irregular clumps. As shown here, they may have a tendency to stain gram negative.

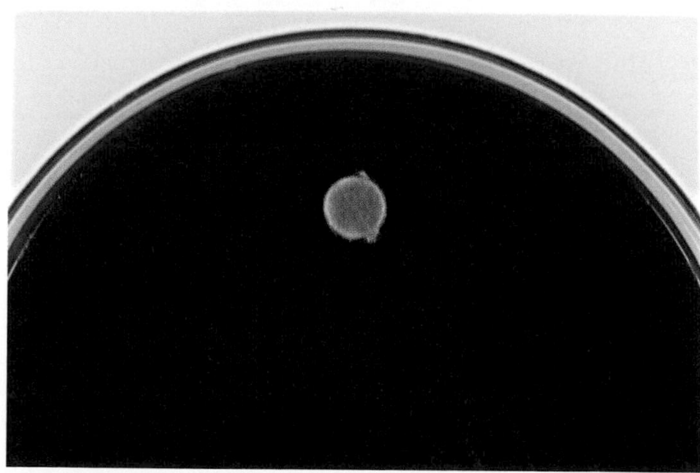

Figure 30-10 Spot indole test used for presumptive identification of *Peptoniphilus asaccharolyticus*. The spot indole test can be performed by placing a blank disk in the area of heavy growth on a subculture plate. After 48 h of incubation under anaerobic conditions, one drop of 1% *p*-dimethylaminocinnamaldehyde is added to the disk. The disk becomes blue to green if the organism produces indole, whereas a pink to orange color indicates a negative test. Anaerobic gram-positive cocci isolated from human clinical specimens can presumptively be identified as *P. asaccharolyticus* if they are SPS resistant and indole positive. *P. indolicus*, the other anaerobic gram-positive coccus that is indole positive, is rarely isolated from clinical specimens.

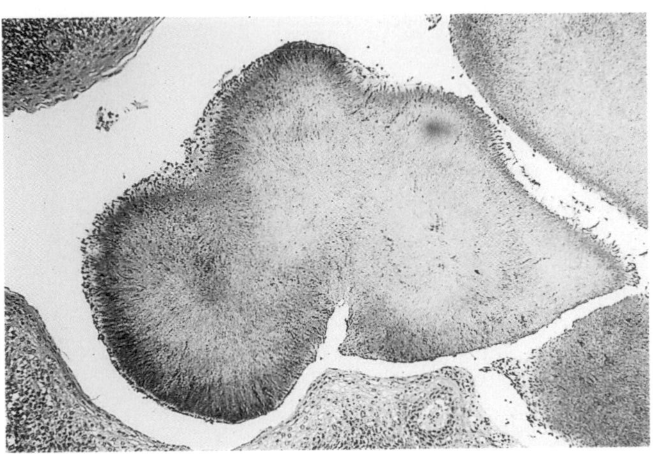

Figure 30-11 Hematoxylin and eosin stain of a sulfur granule from the tonsils. Sulfur granules are a conglomeration of microorganisms that form only in vivo and are usually yellow but can also be white, gray, or brown. Sulfur granules range in size from less than 0.1 mm to up to 3 to 5 mm. The granule is composed of delicate branched and beaded filaments embedded in an amorphous material that is brittle, cracks easily, and has essentially the same composition as organisms grown in vitro. In the periphery it is possible to see, at high magnification, the radially oriented filaments terminating in clubs or enlargements; as a result, the name "ray fungus" was used in the past. The Brown-Brenn modification of the Gram stain demonstrates that the filaments are gram positive. These granules are usually surrounded by acute and chronic inflammatory cells.

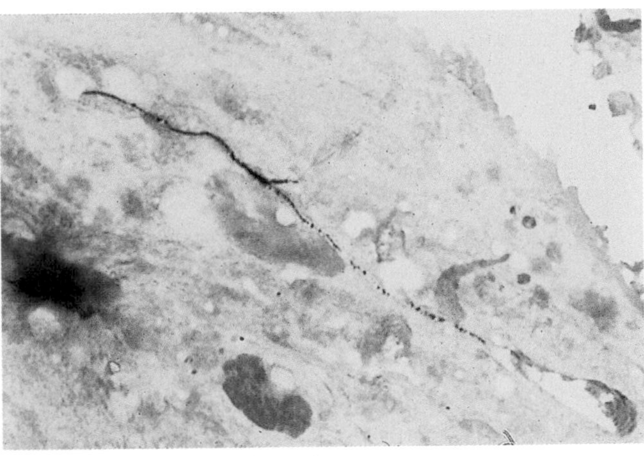

Figure 30-12 Gram stain of *Actinomyces israelii*. *A. israelii* cells are gram-positive bacilli that can appear club shaped, diphtheroid-like, or as slender filaments with various degrees of true branching. Short filaments can be 1.5 to 5 μm in length, while longer filaments can be 10 to 50 μm or longer. Although *A. israelii* is gram positive, irregular staining is common and gives rise to a beaded appearance.

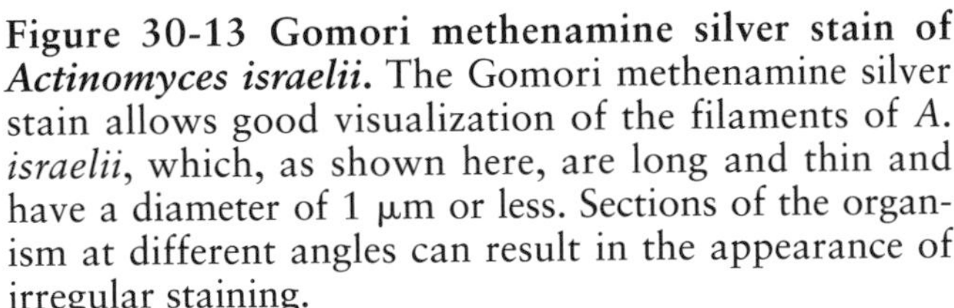

Figure 30-13 Gomori methenamine silver stain of *Actinomyces israelii*. The Gomori methenamine silver stain allows good visualization of the filaments of *A. israelii*, which, as shown here, are long and thin and have a diameter of 1 μm or less. Sections of the organism at different angles can result in the appearance of irregular staining.

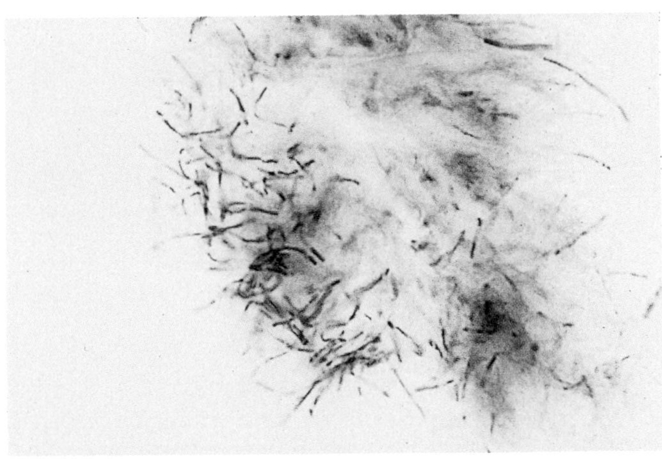

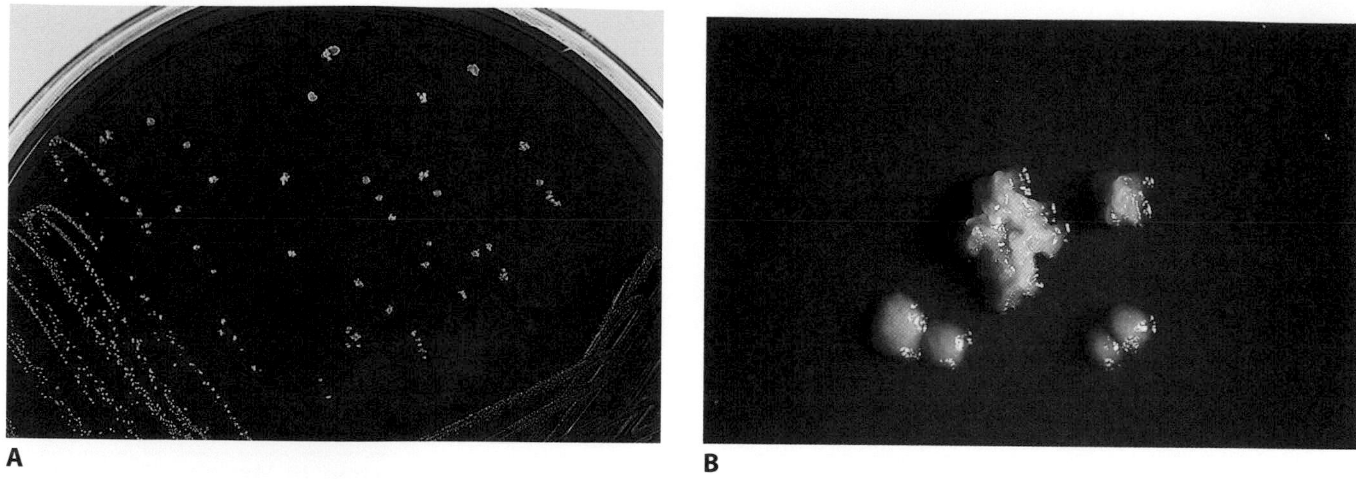

Figure 30-14 Young colonies (A) and mature colonies (B) of *Actinomyces israelii* on CDC agar. *A. israelii* is microaerophilic and slow growing, often requiring more than 48 h for growth to appear on primary culture. (A) Young colonies of *A. israelii* grown on CDC agar for 72 h appear as small colonies that are spider-like in appearance. (B) After incubation for 7 days, the colonies are opaque and cream or gray-white and have a "molar tooth" morphology, which is typical of *A. israelii*.

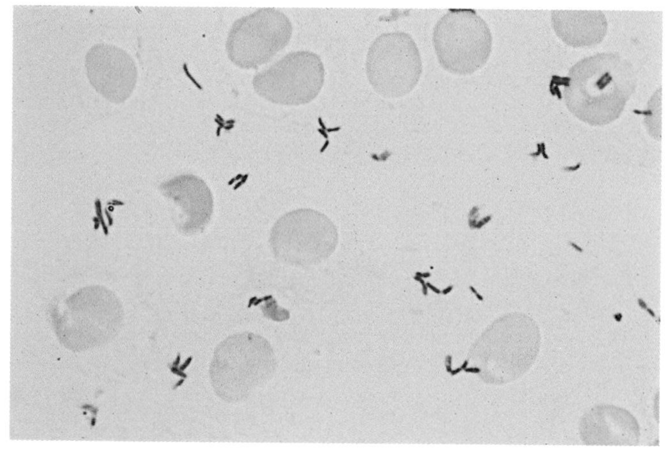

Figure 30-15 Gram stain of *Actinomyces odontolyticus*. *A. odontolyticus* cells are variable in morphology. This gram-positive bacillus can be small and club shaped or have bifurcated ends. It can also appear as thin filaments. As shown in this Gram stain of a blood culture sample, *A. odontolyticus* cells are pleomorphic, with small bacilli and thin filaments present.

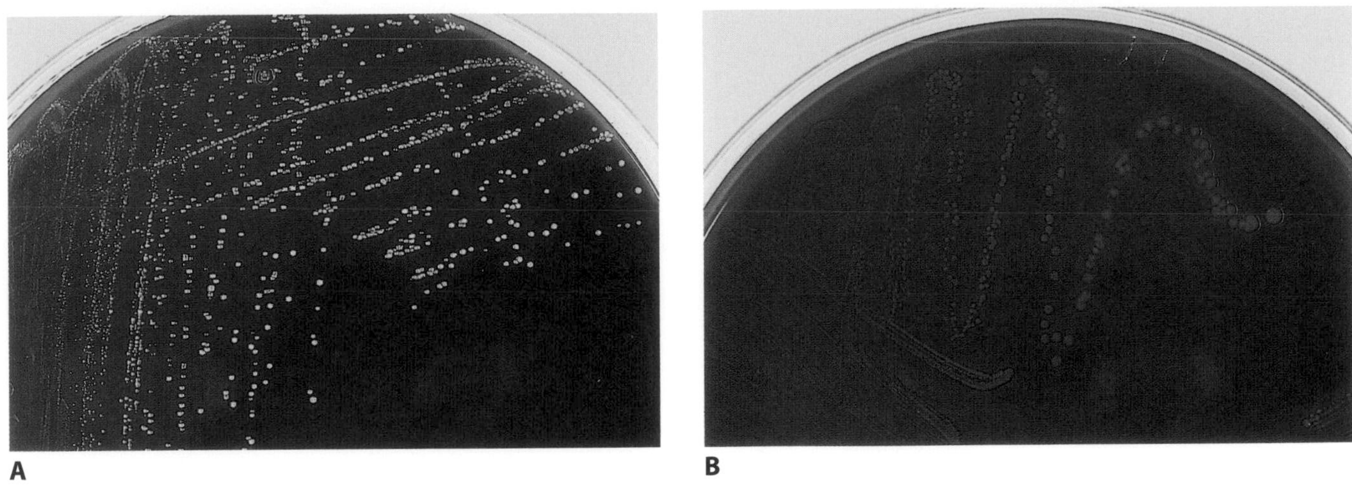

Figure 30-16 ***Actinomyces odontolyticus*** **on CDC agar.** (A) After 48 h, *A. odontolyticus* forms small, opaque, white colonies. (B) The colonies may produce a pink pigment when incubation is extended from 4 to 10 days.

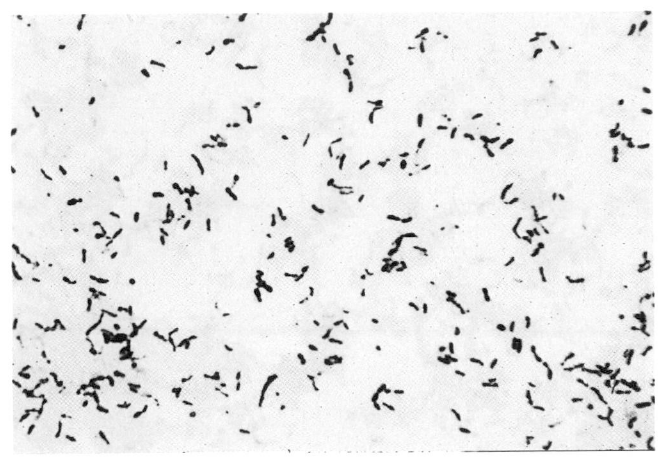

Figure 30-17 Gram stain of *Propionibacterium acnes* from a blood culture. The morphology of *P. acnes* may vary considerably. Cells can measure 0.5 to 0.8 μm by 1.5 μm. They can be diphtheroidal or club shaped with round or tapered ends and can be coccoidal or branching. The "Chinese letter" configuration is common.

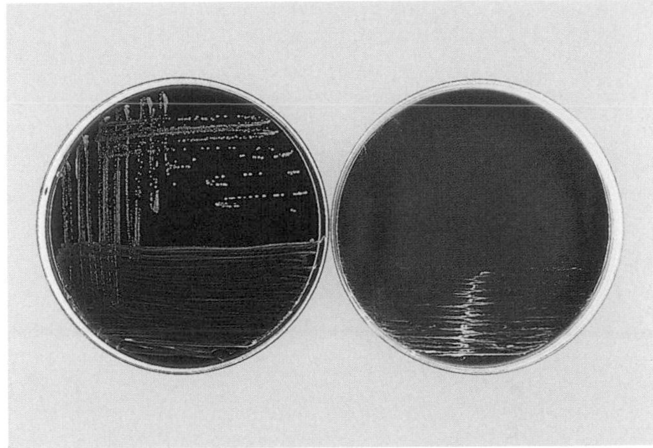

Figure 30-18 Aerotolerance of *Propionibacterium acnes*. Like many species of *Actinomyces*, *P. acnes* is microaerophilic. In the cultures shown, *P. acnes* was grown for 48 h on chocolate agar incubated at 35°C in 5 to 10% CO_2 (right) and for 48 h on CDC agar incubated anaerobically (left). Although the organism is able to grow under both conditions, enhanced growth is seen when it is grown anaerobically.

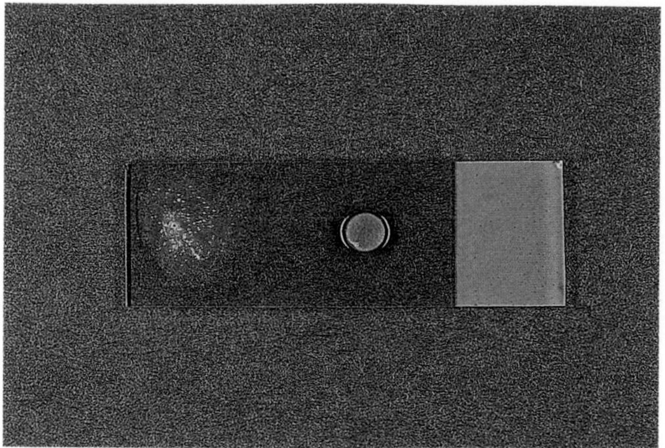

Figure 30-19 Indole and catalase tests for presumptive identification of *Propionibacterium acnes*. A presumptive identification of *P. acnes* can be made if an anaerobic gram-positive bacillus has a pleomorphic, diphtheroid morphology and is indole positive, as indicated by the blue disk (right), and catalase positive, as shown by the bubbles produced when the organism is added to a drop of hydrogen peroxide (left).

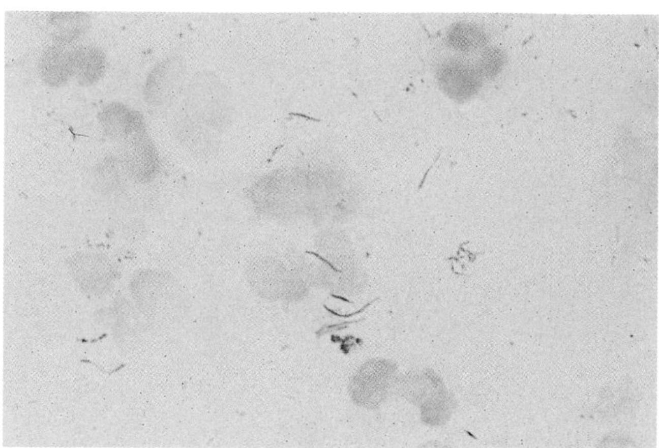

Figure 30-20 Gram stain of *Bifidobacterium dentium*. The cell morphology of *B. dentium* is pleomorphic and can vary from short, thin bacilli with pointed ends to long cells with slight bends and protuberances with club-shaped ends or branching with or without one bifurcated end, or they may appear coccoidal. They occur singly, in chains, or in palisade arrangements.

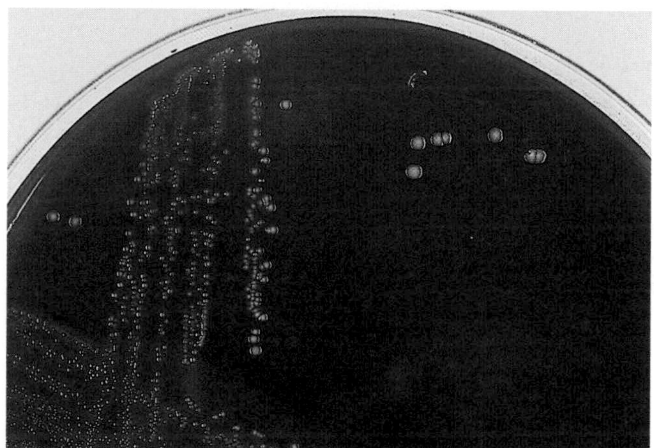

Figure 30-21 *Bifidobacterium dentium* on CDC agar. This culture of *B. dentium* was grown for 48 h on CDC agar. The colonies are entire and cream to white with a smooth, glistening, soft consistency.

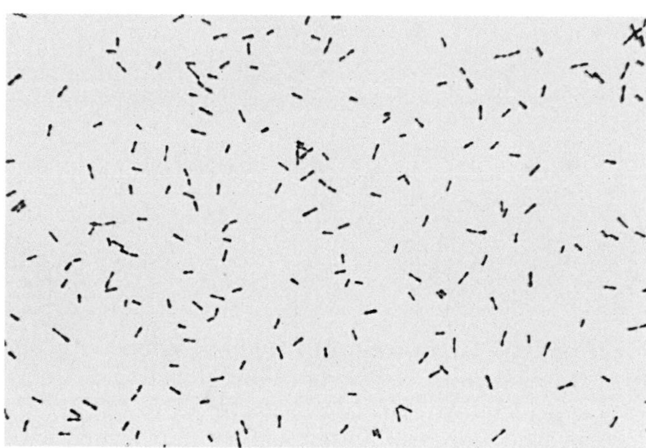

Figure 30-22 Gram stain of *Eggerthella lenta*. *E. lenta* cells are small, pleomorphic bacilli measuring 0.2 to 0.4 μm by 0.2 to 2.0 μm. As shown here, they may be diphtheroidal and occur singly, in pairs, or in short chains.

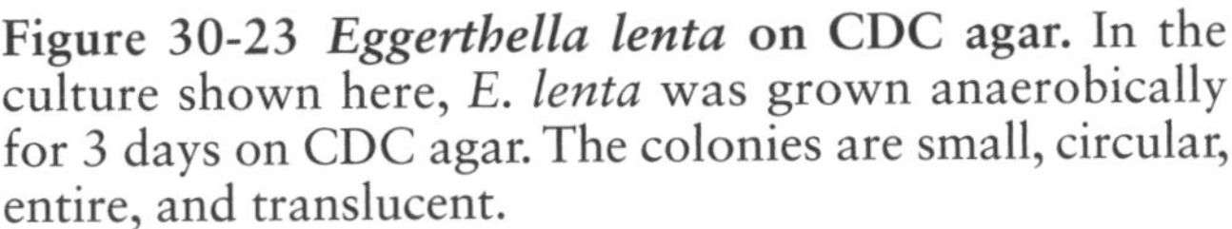

Figure 30-23 *Eggerthella lenta* on CDC agar. In the culture shown here, *E. lenta* was grown anaerobically for 3 days on CDC agar. The colonies are small, circular, entire, and translucent.

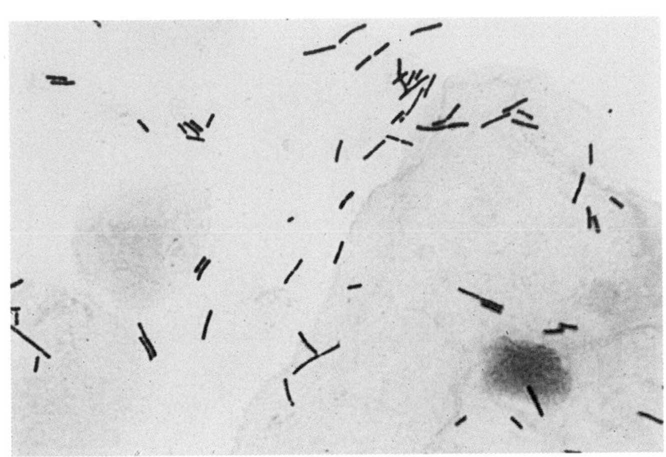

Figure 30-24 Gram stain of *Lactobacillus* spp. The Gram stain shown is from a vaginal specimen. Note the slender, gram-positive bacilli with parallel sides and blunt ends, which is typical of *Lactobacillus* spp.

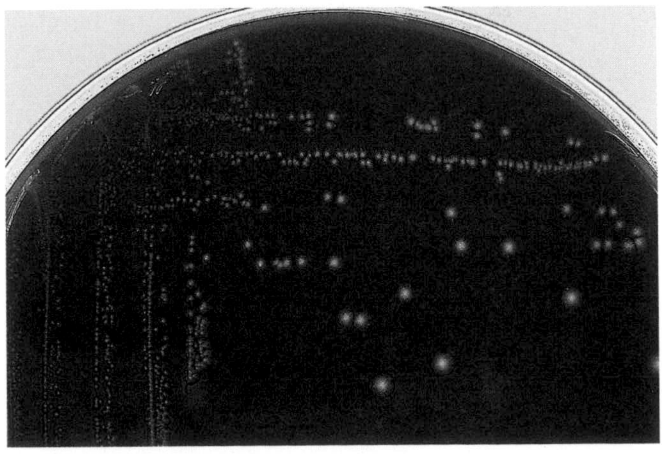

Figure 30-25 *Lactobacillus* spp. on CDC agar. After 72 h, anaerobic *Lactobacillus* spp. produce colonies, measuring 2 to 5 mm in diameter, that are convex, entire, smooth, opaque, and nonpigmented.

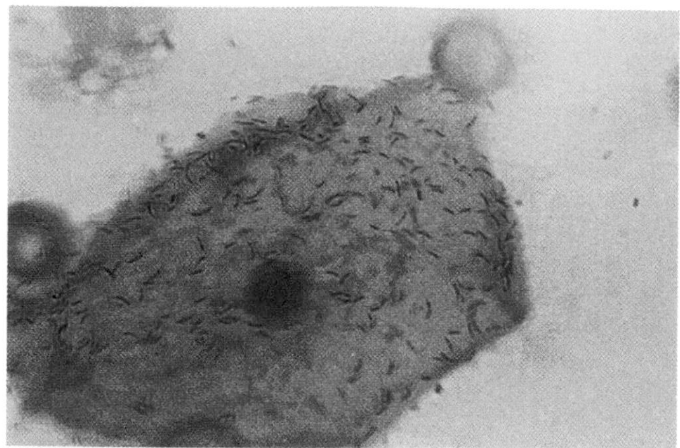

Figure 30-26 Gram stain of *Mobiluncus* spp. Since routine vaginal cultures for the isolation of *Mobiluncus* spp. are costly, time-consuming, and often not clinically useful, an acceptable alternative is the use of the direct Gram stain to provide a presumptive identification. As shown here, *Mobiluncus* spp. appear as curved bacilli, which consistently stain gram negative or gram variable. The absence of lipopolysaccharide in their cell wall and their structural similarity to gram-positive organisms keep them in this group. Their motility distinguishes them from other anaerobic, non-spore-forming, gram-positive bacilli.

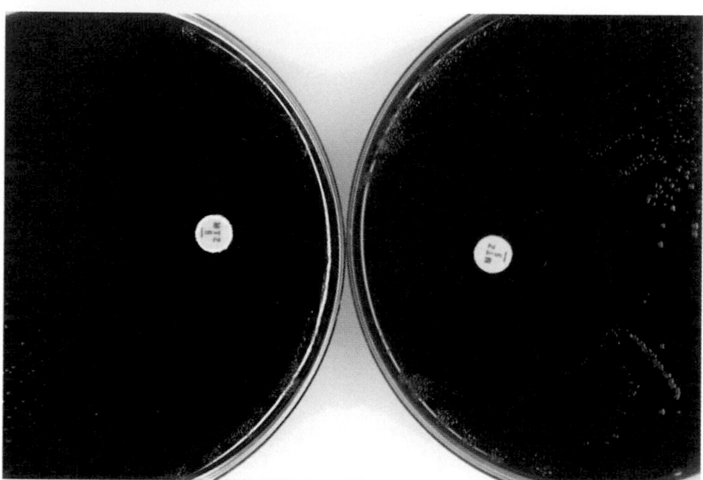

Figure 30-27 Metronidazole disk test. Anaerobic gram-positive cocci can be reliably differentiated from microaerophilic strains by applying a 5-μg metronidazole disk to the inoculated plate and incubating for 48 h. Microaerophic strains will show no inhibition, whereas anaerobic cocci will demonstrate a zone of inhibition of ≥15 mm. The organism on the right is *Peptostreptococcus anaerobius*, an obligate anaerobic coccus, and the organism on the left is *Streptococcus sanguinis*, which is microaerophilic.

Bacteroides, *Porphyromonas*, *Prevotella*, *Fusobacterium*, and Other Anaerobic Gram-Negative Bacteria

31

As a result of nucleic acid analysis, the taxonomy of the anaerobic, gram-negative bacteria continues to evolve, with old species being renamed and new species being added. Apart from *Campylobacter* and *Capnocytophaga*, which are discussed in other chapters, *Bacteroides*, *Porphyromonas*, *Prevotella*, and *Fusobacterium* are the clinically important genera. The anaerobic gram-negative cocci include the genera *Acidaminococcus*, *Anaeroglobus*, *Megasphaera*, and *Veillonella*. Of these, *Veillonella* is the genus most commonly isolated from clinical specimens. Anaerobic gram-negative bacteria are part of the normal flora of the mouth and the upper respiratory, gastrointestinal, and genitourinary tracts of humans and animals. As a result of disease or trauma, they can migrate from their endogenous locations into normally sterile sites.

Although the taxonomic position of several species remains uncertain, the genus *Bacteroides* includes the *Bacteroides fragilis* group and closely related species, which hydrolyze esculin, grow in 20% bile, and are nonmotile. Although there are currently 23 species listed within the *B. fragilis* group, those species most commonly encountered in clinical specimens are *B. fragilis*, *Bacteroides thetaiotaomicron*, *Bacteroides ovatus*, and *Bacteroides capillosus*. Clinically, the *B. fragilis* group is important because of the frequent involvement of its members in infections and their resistance to antimicrobial agents. *B. fragilis* and *B. thetaiotaomicron* are the two species within the group that are most often isolated as pathogens, and *B. fragilis* is the most common anaerobe that causes bacteremia. These organisms can also cause abscesses, which are mainly intra-abdominal, perineal, and perirectal, as well as other soft tissue infections such as foot and decubitus ulcers. Bites or trauma can result in life-threatening diseases resulting from a *B. fragilis* infection.

The pigmented *Prevotella* spp. most frequently encountered in clinical specimens include *Prevotella corporis*, *Prevotella denticola*, *Prevotella intermedia*, *Prevotella loescheii*, and *Prevotella melaninogenica*. Through the use of 16S rRNA gene sequencing, the number of *Prevotella* spp. has increased and 12 new species have been isolated from humans. Although most commonly found in the oral cavity, *Prevotella bivia* and *Prevotella disiens* have been associated with genitourinary tract infections, and *P. intermedia* (formerly *Bacteroides intermedius*) has been recovered from various infection sites.

Of the 17 current *Porphyromonas* spp., *Porphyromonas asaccharolytica*, *Porphyromonas bennonis*, *Porphyromonas catoniae*, *Porphyromonas endodontalis*, *Porphyromonas gingivalis*, *Porphyromonas somerae*, and *Porphyromonas uenonis* are the ones most frequently isolated from clinical specimens. With the exception of *P. catoniae*, they are pigmented, asaccharolytic, and generally considered pathogens.

A majority of the chronic infections involving the sinuses, ears, and periodontal region are polymicrobic and predominantly anaerobic. *Prevotella* spp., *Porphyromonas* spp., *Fusobacterium* spp., and *Bacteroides* spp. other than *B. fragilis* are the organisms most commonly isolated from these sites. These organisms also cause brain abscesses, typically in patients with a history of chronic sinusitis or otitis. Infections of the female genital tract, including endometritis and pelvic inflammatory disease, usually involve mixtures of anaerobes including *P. bivia* and *P. disiens*.

Fusobacterium nucleatum is the *Fusobacterium* species most frequently isolated from clinical specimens, including those obtained from the upper respiratory, genital, and gastrointestinal tracts. *Fusobacterium necrophorum* is associated with Lemierre's syndrome (necrobacillosis) and can cause severe peritonsillar abscesses that sometimes lead to neck infections, jugular vein thrombophlebitis, and bacteremia, while *Fusobacterium mortiferum* and *Fusobacterium varium* are associated with intra-abdominal infections.

The anerobic, gram-negative cocci account for only a small portion of the anaerobic bacteria isolated from human clinical specimens. Of the genera *Veillonella*, *Acidaminococcus*, *Megasphaera*, *Anaeroglobus*, and *Negativicoccus*, *Veillonella* is the only genus of clinical significance and *Veillonella parvula* is the species most commonly isolated from clinical specimens. Although *Veillonella* spp. are frequently isolated from polymicrobic cultures, they are rarely identified as the only etiological agent in serious infections. *Veillonella atypica*, *Veillonella dispar*, and *V. parvula* are found in the oral cavity and can cause infections of the head and neck, respiratory tract, and bite wounds.

To isolate and characterize these organisms, specimens must be collected and transported anaerobically for optimal recovery. Direct examination of the clinical material is also important in the initial determination of the presence of anaerobes. When preparing the direct smear, use of carbol fuchsin as the counterstain in the Gram stain procedure will enhance staining of the gram-negative anaerobes. For primary isolation, a combination of selective and differential media is used. In general, it is recommended that nonselective media such as brucella or CDC anaerobe blood agar containing vitamin K_1 and hemin, kanamycin-vancomycin-laked blood (KVLB) agar, and bacteroides bile esculin (BBE) agar be used. This combination of media will facilitate the isolation and presumptive identification of the *B. fragilis* group and *Bilophila* spp.

Most of the clinically significant anaerobic gram-negative bacilli can be placed in broad groups, and some can be presumptively identified by using the special-potency antibiotic disks, vancomycin (5 μg), kanamycin (1 mg), and colistin (10 μg), along with a few simple tests such as growth in bile and indole, nitrate, urea, and pigment production. The characteristics that differentiate the most common clinical species are listed in Table 31-1, and the characteristics of the most common species in the *B. fragilis* group are listed in Table 31-2. Many of these tests were incorporated into the three Presumpto Quad plates developed at the Centers for Disease Control and Prevention (CDC) to aid in the identification of anaerobic bacteria. Anaerobic Gram-Negative ID Quad (Thermo Scientific Remel Products, Lenexa, KS) most closely corresponds to CDC Presumpto Plate 1. It contains kanamycin, esculin, bile, and tryptophan and is helpful in identifying *Bacteroides* and *Fusobacterium* spp. Definitive identification of most anaerobic gram-negative bacilli requires additional biochemical tests, metabolic end-product analysis, or characterization of cell wall fatty acids. Molecular methods for identification are not yet standardized and are not commercially available.

Table 31-1 Characteristics of the most common anaerobic gram-negative bacilli isolated from clinical specimens[a]

Species	Cell morphology	Vancomycin (5 μg)	Kanamycin (1 mg)	Colistin (10 μg)	Growth in 20% bile	Catalase	Indole	Nitrate	Urea	Pigment
Bacteroides spp.										
B. fragilis group	Short	R	R	R	+	V	V	0	0	0
Other *Bacteroides* spp.	Variable	R	R	V	V	V	V	0	0	0
Fusobacterium spp.										
F. mortiferum	Pleomorphic with large round bodies	R	S	S	+	0	0	0	0	0
F. necrophorum	Pleomorphic	R	S	S	V	0	+	0	0	0
F. nucleatum	Slender, long	R	S	S	0	0	+	0	0	0
F. varium	Large with rounded ends	R	S	S	+	0	V	0	0	0
Pigmented species										
Prevotella spp.	Coccobacillary	R	R^S	V	0	0	V	0	0	+
Porphyromonas spp.	Variable	S	R	R	0	V	V	0	0	+[b]
Veillonella spp.	Small cocci	R	S	S	0	V	0	+	0	0

[a]S, susceptible; R, resistant; R^S, resistant, rarely susceptible; +, positive reaction; V, variable reaction; 0, negative reaction.

[b]*P. catoniae* is the only nonpigmented *Porphyromonas* sp.

Table 31-2 Characteristics of the most common species within the *B. fragilis* group[a]

Species	Esculin hydrolysis	Catalase	Indole	Arabinose	Salicin
B. fragilis	+	+	0	0	0
B. ovatus	+	+	+	+	+
B. thetaiotaomicron	+	+	+	+	0
B. vulgatus	0	0	0	+	0

[a]+, positive reaction; 0, negative reaction.

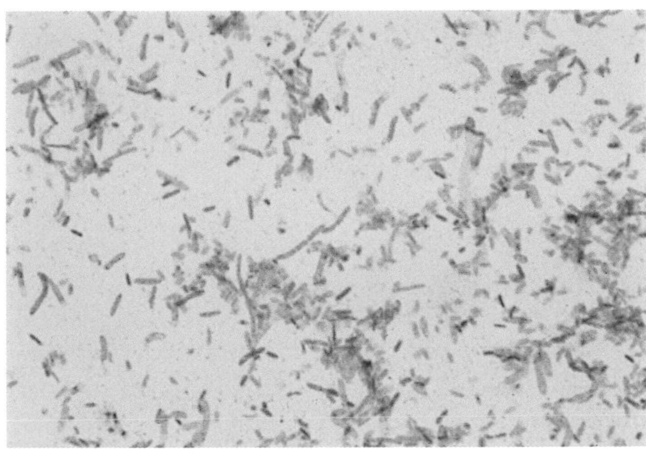

Figure 31-1 Gram stain of *Bacteroides fragilis* using carbol fuchsin as the counterstain. The members of the *B. fragilis* group are irregularly staining, pleomorphic, gram-negative bacilli that vary in length. They can appear elongated or as coccobacilli and occur singly or in pairs. Staining is enhanced when carbol fuchsin is used as the counterstain in the Gram stain procedure.

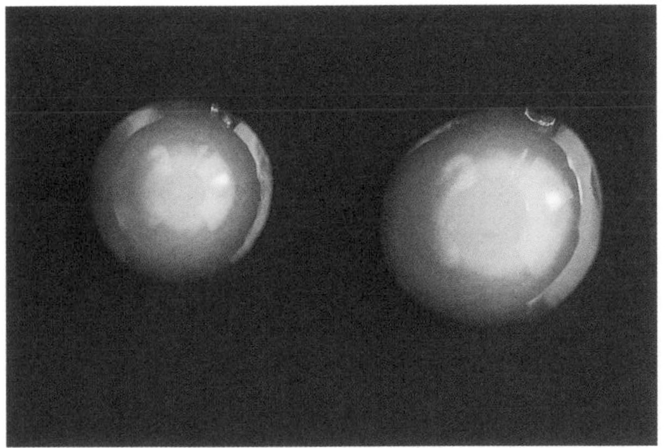

A

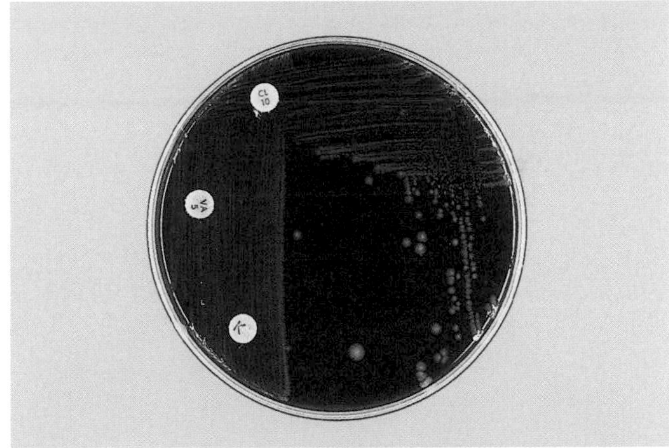

B

Figure 31-2 *Bacteroides fragilis* growing on CDC agar (A) and presumptive identification of the *B. fragilis* group by using special-potency antimicrobial disks (B). After 48 h of incubation, colonies of *B. fragilis* on CDC agar are 1 to 3 mm in diameter, circular, entire, convex, and gray to white. Hemolysis can vary, with some strains exhibiting beta-hemolysis. (A) When *B. fragilis* colonies are viewed by obliquely transmitted light, concentric rings or whorls are visible. (B) The *B. fragilis* group is characterized by resistance (a zone diameter of 10 mm or less) to all three special-potency antimicrobial disks: kanamycin (1 mg), vancomycin (5 μg), and colistin (10 μg).

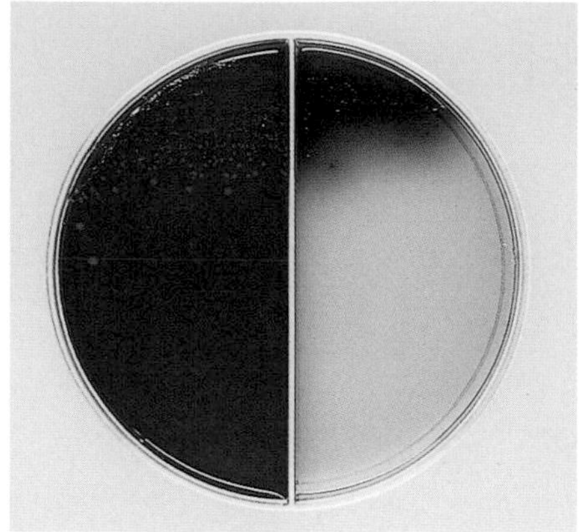

Figure 31-3 ***Bacteroides fragilis*** **on KVLB agar and BBE agar.** These organisms are not inhibited by kanamycin and vancomycin and thus exhibit good growth on KVLB agar (left). Another characteristic is their ability to grow in 20% bile and hydrolyze esculin, causing browning of the BBE agar (right).

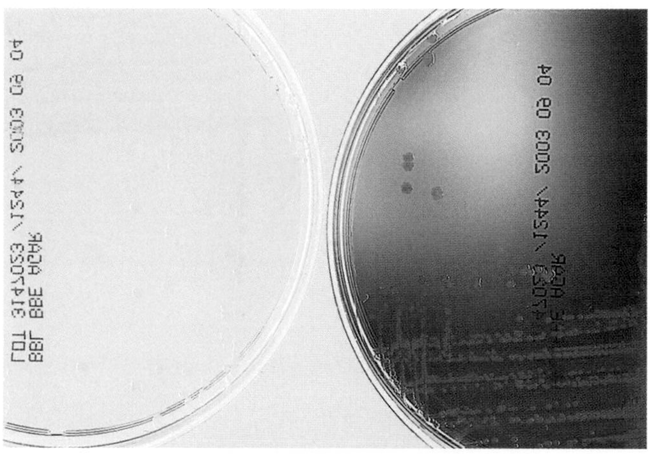

Figure 31-4 ***Bacteroides fragilis*** **and** ***Bacteroides vulgatus*** **on BBE agar.** A characteristic shared by members of the *B. fragilis* group is their ability to grow in 20% bile and hydrolyze esculin. *B. vulgatus* is the exception. While it can grow in bile, it cannot hydrolyze esculin. Note the dark colonies of *B. fragilis* and the blackening of BBE agar (right), in contrast to the growth of, but lack of esculin hydrolysis by, *B. vulgatus* (left).

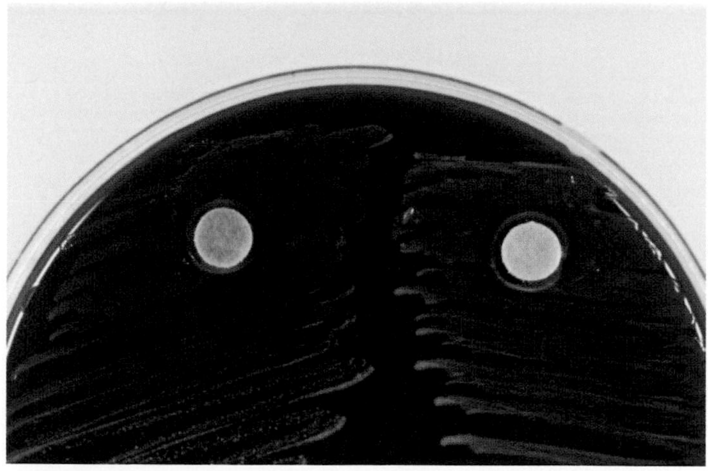

Figure 31-5 Spot indole test. The spot indole test can be performed directly on a pure culture by placing a sterile blank disk on an area of heavy growth. After several minutes, one drop of 1% *p*-dimethylaminocinnamaldehyde is added to the disk. The disk turns blue to green if the organism produces indole. As shown here, *Bacteroides thetaiotaomicron* gives a positive reaction (left) while *Bacteroides fragilis* gives a negative reaction (right). The spot indole can be a useful rapid test for identifying species within the group.

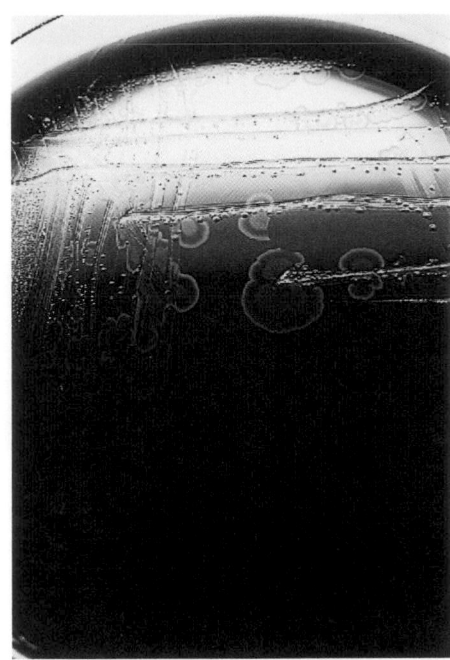

Figure 31-6 *Bacteroides ureolyticus* on CDC agar. *B. ureolyticus* is slow growing; its colonies are small and translucent to transparent and measure 1 mm in diameter. As shown here, the colony morphology is variable. Note the smooth, circular, and convex colonies as well as the spreading colonies. In some areas, pitting of the agar can also be observed.

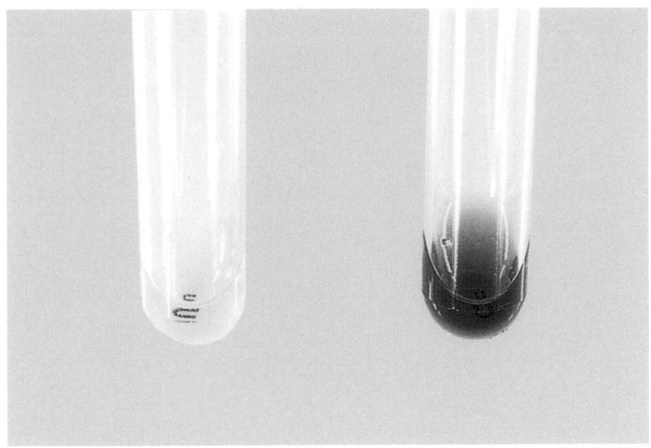

Figure 31-7 Urea test for the presumptive identification of *Bacteroides ureolyticus*. The BBL Taxo urea differentiation disk (BD Diagnostic Systems, Franklin Lakes, NJ) can be used as a rapid method of determining urea hydrolysis. A suspension of the organism is prepared in 0.5 ml of sterile water. On addition of a urea disk, the bacterial suspension is incubated aerobically for up to 4 h. A color change to pink indicates a positive reaction. Positive urease production is an important test used to differentiate *B. ureolyticus* (right) from other anaerobic gram-negative, pitting bacilli such as *Campylobacter gracilis* (left).

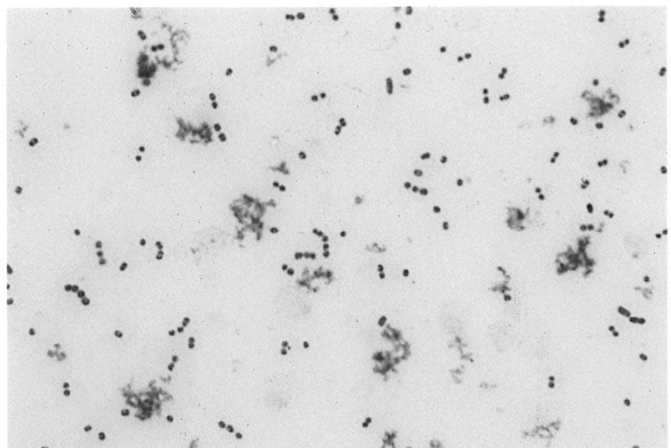

Figure 31-8 Gram stain of *Prevotella melaninogenica* with carbol fuchsin as the counterstain. The Gram stain morphology of *Prevotella* spp. is similar to that of *Bacteroides* spp. *Prevotella* organisms are small, gram-negative bacilli or coccobacilli measuring 0.5 to 0.8 μm by 0.9 to 2.0 μm. Note the almost spherical appearance of the cells, which are arranged in pairs and short chains. The blood culture shown here grew *P. melaninogenica*.

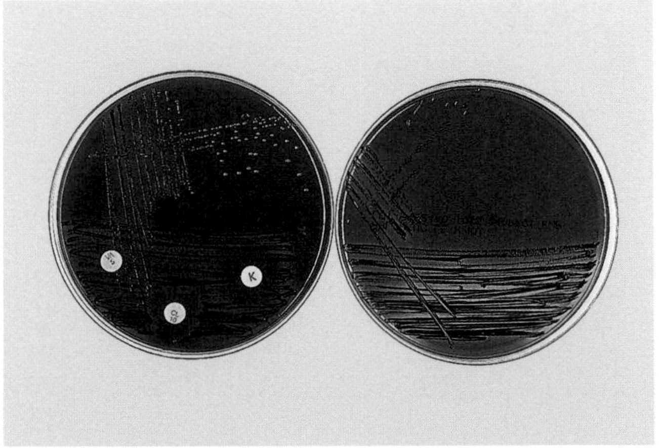

Figure 31-9 *Prevotella corporis* on CDC agar and KVLB agar. Colonies of *P. corporis* are shown after 72 h of growth on CDC agar (left) and KVLB agar (right). The disk pattern for *Prevotella* spp., unlike the *B. fragilis* group, is kanamycin and vancomycin resistant but either resistant or susceptible to colistin. Note the enhanced pigment production on KVLB agar.

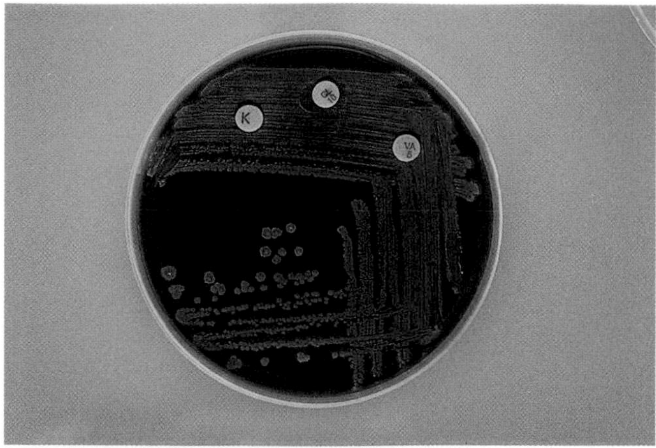

Figure 31-10 Fluorescence of a *Prevotella* species growing on CDC agar. Many *Prevotella* strains require up to 3 weeks for pigment to appear. However, fluorescence can be detected within 48 to 72 h by exposing the colonies to long-wave UV light. Note the typical brick-red fluorescence of this pigment-producing *Prevotella* species.

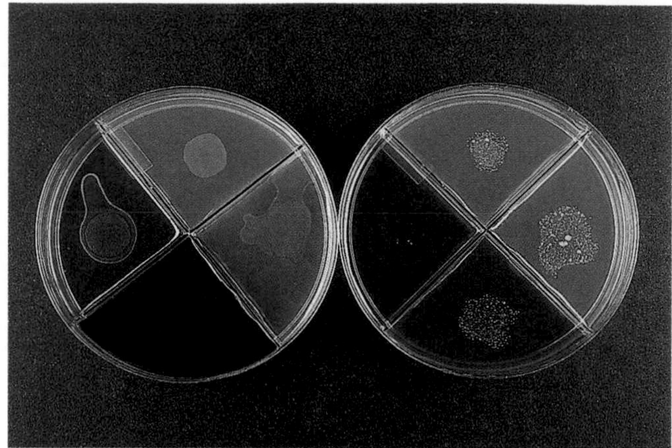

Figure 31-11 Anaerobic Gram-Negative ID Quad. The Anaerobic Gram-Negative ID Quad system corresponds to CDC Presumpto Plate 1 and contains the following media: quadrant I, kanamycin agar (top); quadrant II, Lombard-Dowell agar for detection of indole (right); quadrant III, esculin agar for detection of esculin hydrolysis and catalase activity (bottom); and quadrant IV, bile agar (left). The Quad plates shown were inoculated with *B. fragilis* and *P. melaninogenica*. *B. fragilis* (left Quad plate) grows on kanamycin agar (top), hydrolyzes esculin (bottom), and grows on bile agar (left), while *P. melaninogenica* (right Quad plate) grows on the kanamycin agar, does not hydrolyze esculin, and cannot grow in bile. *B. fragilis* is catalase positive and *P. melaninogenica* is catalase negative, and both organisms are indole negative.

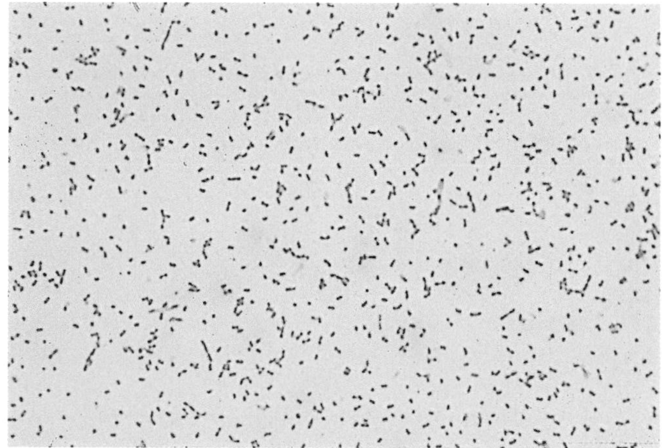

Figure 31-12 Gram stain of *Porphyromonas* sp. from CDC agar with a carbol fuchsin counterstain. *Porphyromonas* sp. is a gram-negative bacillus measuring 0.4 to 0.6 μm by 1 to 2 μm. Longer cells are occasionally present, and shorter, almost spherical cells can be seen when the organism is grown on solid media, as in this Gram stain of a 48-h culture of *Porphyromonas* sp.

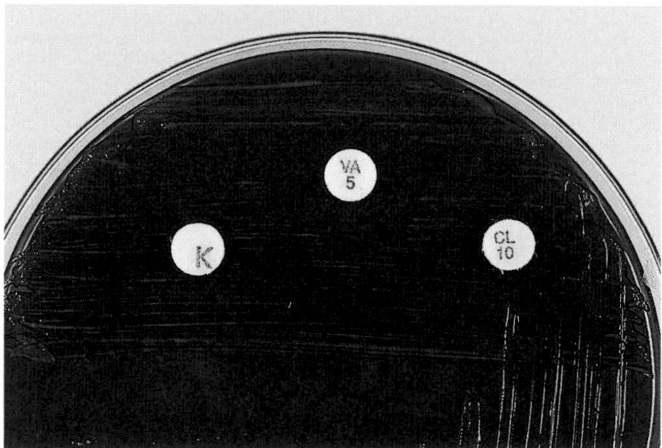

Figure 31-13 *Porphyromonas* spp. on CDC agar. Unlike *Prevotella*, *Porphyromonas* is susceptible to vancomycin and resistant to kanamycin and colistin.

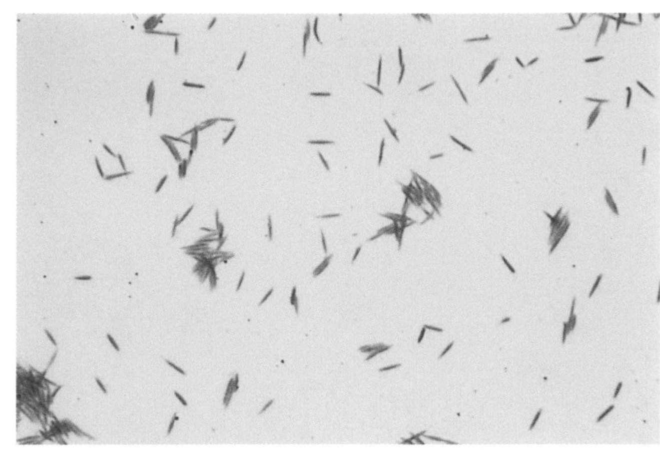

Figure 31-14 Gram stain of *Fusobacterium nucleatum* with a carbol fuchsin counterstain. *F. nucleatum* appears as long, thin, gram-negative bacilli with tapered ends. It is the only *Fusobacterium* sp. that consistently demonstrates this fusiform morphology.

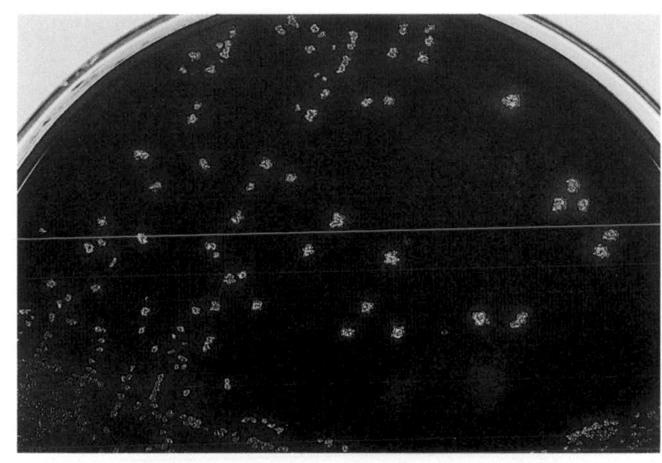

Figure 31-15 *Fusobacterium nucleatum* on CDC agar. *F. nucleatum* produces small, irregularly shaped colonies (often described as "bread crumbs") with greening of the agar.

Figure 31-16 Fluorescence of *Fusobacterium* spp. *Fusobacterium* fluoresces chartreuse when exposed to long-wave UV light.

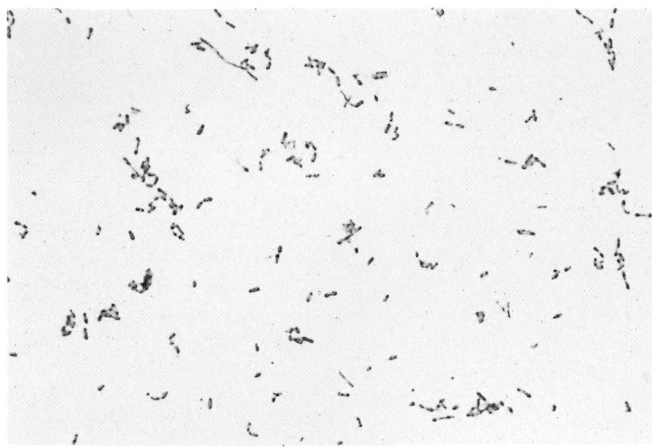

Figure 31-17 Gram stain of *Fusobacterium necrophorum* with a carbol fuchsin counterstain. *F. necrophorum* bacteria are pleomorphic, long, gram-negative bacilli, measuring 0.5 to 0.7 μm by 10 μm, with round or tapered ends. They can vary from coccoid to long filaments depending on the medium and age of the culture. Filamentous forms are more common in broth cultures, whereas rod-like forms are frequently seen in older cultures or when the organism is grown on agar, as shown here.

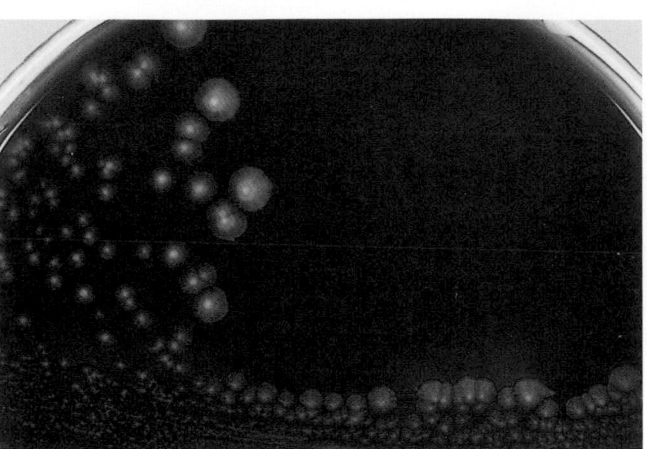

Figure 31-18 *Fusobacterium necrophorum* on CDC agar. After 48 h of incubation, *F. necrophorum* produces umbonate, circular, glistening, white to tan colonies on CDC agar.

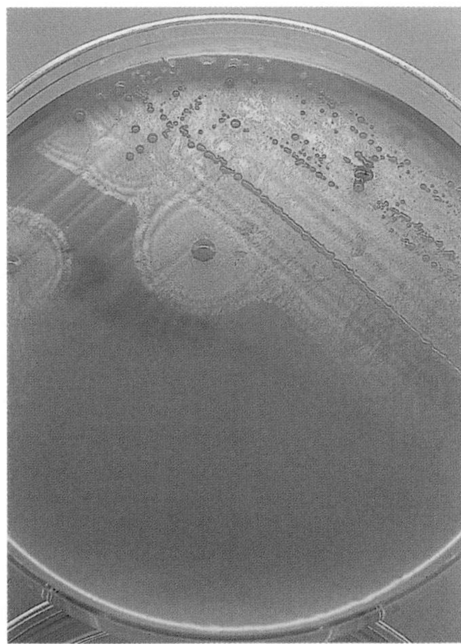

Figure 31-19 *Fusobacterium necrophorum* on egg yolk agar. As shown here, *F. necrophorum* is lipase positive. Note the mother-of-pearl sheen on the surface of the egg yolk agar.

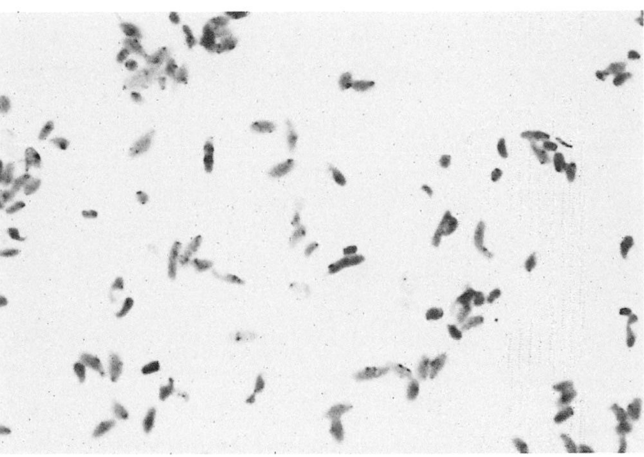

Figure 31-20 Gram stain of *Fusobacterium mortiferum* with a carbol fuchsin counterstain. Cells of *F. mortiferum* are 0.8 to 1.0 μm by 1.5 to 10 μm and appear as gram-negative bacilli. Note the extreme pleomorphism and irregular staining.

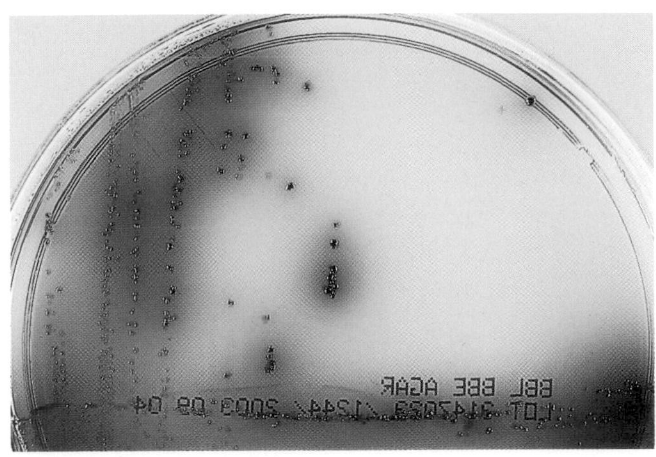

Figure 31-21 ***Fusobacterium mortiferum*** **on BBE agar.** Because *F. mortiferum* is bile tolerant and hydrolyzes esculin, it can be mistaken for a member of the *B. fragilis* group. Note the growth of dark colonies and blackening of the BBE agar.

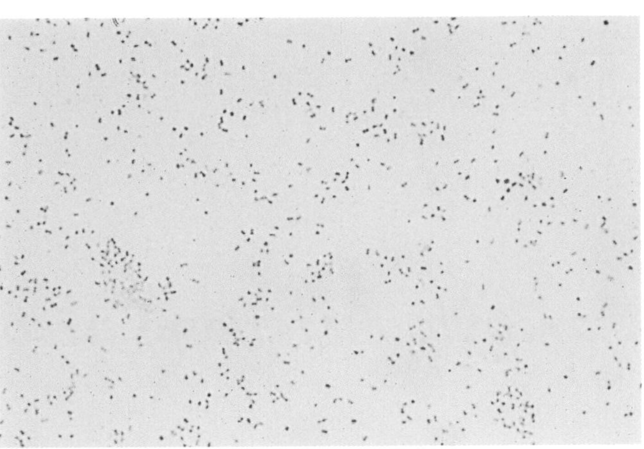

Figure 31-22 Gram stain of ***Veillonella*** **spp.** *Veillonella* spp. are tiny, gram-negative cocci, measuring 0.3 to 0.5 μm in diameter. They may appear as diplococci or in short chains or clumps.

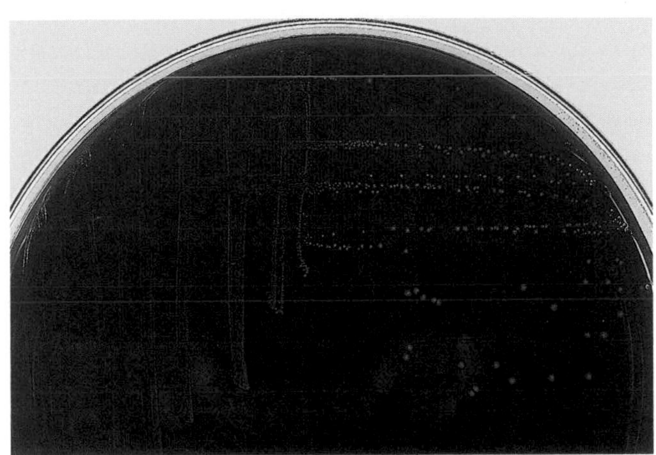

Figure 31-23 ***Veillonella parvula*** **on CDC agar.** After 48 h of incubation, *Veillonella* colonies are small, measuring 1 to 3 mm in diameter; entire; opaque; and nonhemolytic.

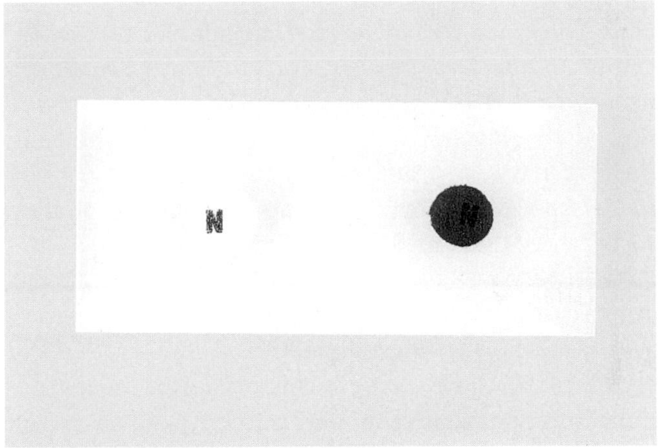

Figure 31-24 Nitrate disk test. The nitrate disk is a miniature version of the conventional tube nitrate reduction test used for identification of aerobic bacteria. The disk is placed on the heavily inoculated first quadrant of a culture, which is incubated anaerobically for 24 to 48 h. One drop each of nitrate reagent A (*N*,*N*-dimethyl-naphthylamine) and reagent B (sulfanilic acid) are added to the disk. A positive reaction is indicated by the development of a red color (right), indicating that the nitrate was reduced to nitrite. If the test is negative, no color develops (left). Similar to the conventional test, zinc dust can be added if the initial result is negative, to determine if nitrate was reduced beyond nitrite. The nitrate test can be use to presumptively identify anaerobic gram-negative bacilli such as *B. ureolyticus* and tiny, anaerobic gram-negative cocci such as *Veillonella* spp.

Campylobacter and *Arcobacter* 32

Three genera, *Campylobacter*, *Arcobacter*, and *Sulfurospirillum*, are included in the family *Campylobacteraceae*. The genus *Campylobacter* includes 22 species, the genus *Arcobacter* 7 species, and the genus *Sulfurospirillum* 6 species. While organisms in the genera *Campylobacter* and *Arcobacter* cause infections in humans, those in the genus *Sulfurospirillum* do not. *Campylobacter* spp. are primarily zoonotic, affecting poultry, cattle, sheep, pigs, and domestic animals.

Campylobacter jejuni (*C. jejuni* subsp. *jejuni*) is recognized as the most common bacterial enteric pathogen in the world; approximately 2 million cases occur yearly in the United States. This organism causes sporadic infections during summer and early fall as a result of ingestion of improperly handled food, primarily poultry products, raw milk, and water. Two age groups are frequently affected: young children and adults aged 20 to 40 years. The clinical presentation ranges from asymptomatic to severe cases with fever, abdominal cramps, and diarrhea that may be bloody and may last for several days or weeks. Relapses are observed in 5 to 10% of cases. The most severe presentations occur in immunocompromised patients and in the elderly. Extraintestinal involvement and chronic sequelae occur in certain cases; they include bacteremia, arthritis (Reiter's syndrome), bursitis, meningitis, endocarditis, and abortion. A clinical presentation similar to acute appendicitis may result in unnecessary surgery. *C. jejuni* is the most common infectious agent associated with Guillain-Barré syndrome.

Campylobacter coli produces the same clinical picture as *C. jejuni* and probably accounts for 5 to 10% of the cases of diarrhea due to campylobacters. In underdeveloped countries, *C. coli* may be a more common pathogen than *C. jejuni*. *Campylobacter fetus* subsp. *fetus* causes bacteremia and extraintestinal infections, particularly in individuals with underlying diseases or in those who are pregnant or immunocompromised. *Campylobacter lari* and *Campylobacter upsaliensis* have also been isolated from patients with diarrhea and bacteremia. Two of the four species of *Arcobacter*, *Arcobacter butzleri* and *Arcobacter cryaerophilus*, have been isolated from humans with diarrhea and bacteremia.

For direct examination of specimens suspected of harboring *Campylobacter*, the use of carbol fuchsin or aqueous basic fuchsin as the counterstain in the Gram stain is recommended. Organisms in the genus *Campylobacter* are gram-negative, curved, "seagull wing"-shaped, motile, non-spore-forming bacilli that measure 0.2 to 0.9 μm wide by 0.5 to 5.0 μm long. They have a typical "darting" motility, resulting from a single polar flagellum, when observed under phase-contrast microscopy. Stool specimens may show polymorphonuclear leukocytes.

There are several commercially available antigen tests for the detection of *Campylobacter* in stool samples. Compared with culture, the sensitivity of these assays ranges from 80 to 96%, and although their specificity is usually >97%, they have poor positive predictive values due to the relatively low incidence of this infection. Nucleic acid detection techniques are not yet commercially available.

Campylobacters are microaerophilic, although some strains grow both aerobically and anaerobically.

Some species of *Campylobacter*, such as *Campylobacter sputorum*, *Campylobacter concisus*, and *Campylobacter mucosalis*, require a gas mixture with more than 2% hydrogen for growth and isolation. Most of these organisms can grow at 42°C. Members of the genus *Arcobacter* are referred to as aerotolerant campylobacters because they can grow in the presence of atmospheric concentrations of oxygen. These organisms grow at temperatures ranging from 15 to 37°C but do not grow at 42°C. Other characteristics useful in distinguishing them from *Campylobacter* spp. include hydrolysis of indoxyl acetate and inability to hydrolyze hippurate.

Several types of media can be used to recover these organisms from clinical specimens. Charcoal cefoperazone deoxycholate agar (Oxoid Inc. North America, Nepean, Ontario, Canada) and charcoal-based selective medium (Oxoid Inc.) are recommended for isolation. The *Campylobacter* blood agar plate (Campy BAP) contains a brucella agar base, sheep blood, and a combination of the following antibiotics: vancomycin, trimethoprim, polymyxin B, amphotericin B, and cephalothin. For optimal recovery, the inoculated plates should be incubated in a microaerobic environment containing 5 to 7% O_2, 5 to 10% CO_2, and 80 to 90% N_2. These conditions can be achieved by using commercially available microaerobic gas generator packs. It should be noted, however, that the candle jar does not provide these conditions. In cases where *C. jejuni* is suspected, the plates should be incubated at 42°C to favor the growth of the organism and suppress the growth of the intestinal flora. On the other hand, if *C. fetus* subsp. *fetus* is suspected, the plates should be incubated at 37°C. *C. upsaliensis* is susceptible to the antibiotics used to isolate campylobacters, and as a result it is not recovered on these media.

In addition to the typical Gram stain morphology, growth characteristics at different temperatures and under different atmospheric conditions, darting motility, catalase and oxidase production, hippurate hydrolysis, indoxyl acetate hydrolysis, production of H_2S, and susceptibility to antibiotics are the most useful tests for identification of campylobacters. Molecular techniques for isolation and identification are currently under development.

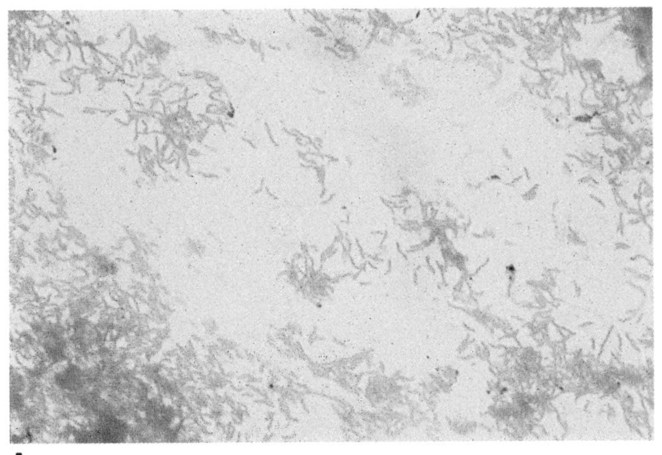

A

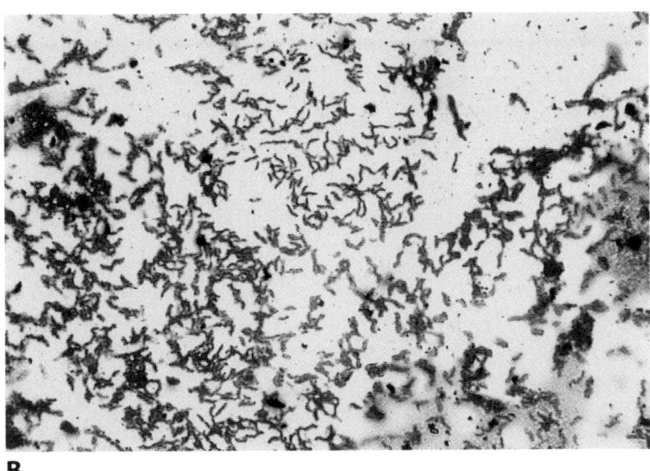

B

Figure 32-1 Gram stain of *Campylobacter jejuni* counterstained with safranin (A) and carbol fuchsin (B). Campylobacters are slender, long, curved, pleomorphic, gram-negative bacilli. As shown here, short chains of organisms have a typical "seagull wing" appearance. Safranin, as used in the routine Gram stain, results in very faint staining of these organisms. The morphology of *C. jejuni* is better defined on a Gram stain counterstained with carbol fuchsin rather than safranin.

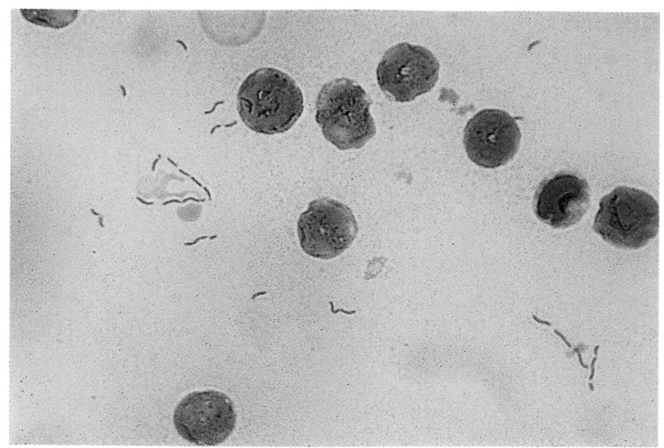

Figure 32-2 Gram stain of *Campylobacter fetus* from a blood culture. *C. fetus* frequently causes bacteremia and extraintestinal infections in immunocompromised patients.

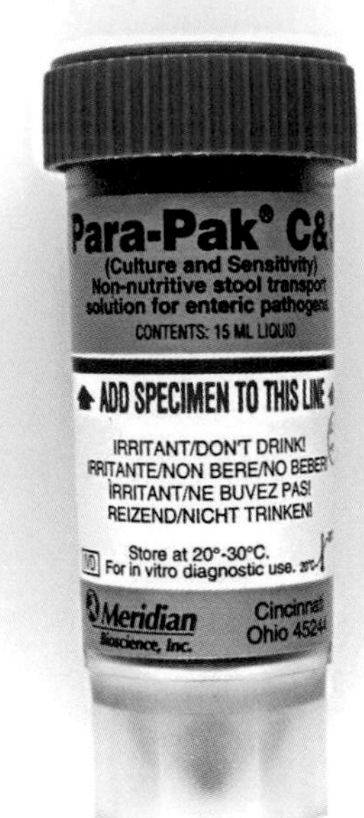

Figure 32-3 Para-Pak C&S. The Para-Pak C&S (Culture and Sensitivity; Meridian Bioscience, Inc., Cincinnati, OH) is a system for the collection and transportation of bacterial enteric pathogens including *Campylobacter* spp. The 30-ml plastic vial contains 15 ml of modified Cary-Blair transport medium and uses phenol red as an indicator. This isotonic, nonnutritive medium preserves the viability of enteric pathogens and minimizes the overgrowth by commensal organisms. A change in color of the medium from red to yellow indicates overgrowth and improper storage of the specimen.

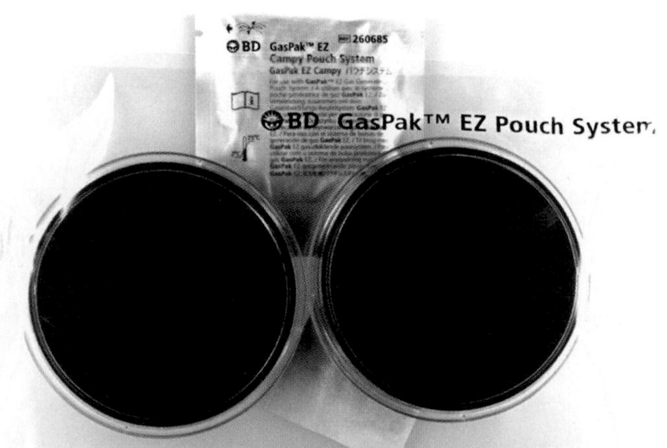

Figure 32-4 GasPak EZ Gas Generating Pouch System. The GasPak EZ Gas Generating Pouch System (BD Diagnostic Systems, Franklin Lakes, NJ) shown here provides an atmosphere suitable for the growth of campylobacters. The GasPak gas-generating sachet contains all the components needed to produce specific atmospheric conditions to optimize the recovery of *Campylobacter* spp. Two petri dishes can be inserted into the pouch for incubation.

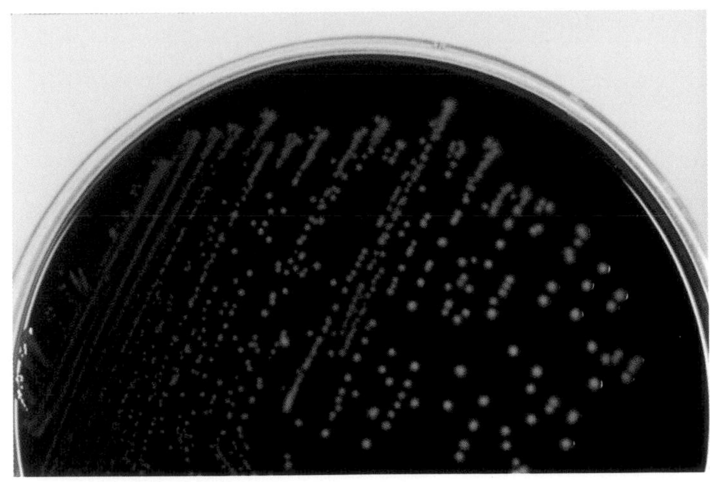

Figure 32-5 *Campylobacter jejuni* on Campy CSM medium. The charcoal-based selective CSM agar (Quebact Laboratories Inc., Montreal, Canada) is a blood-free medium useful for the isolation of *C. jejuni*. This medium has cefoperazone, vancomycin, and cycloheximide to inhibit the growth of other fecal organisms. As shown in this figure, *C. jejuni* produces white-gray, glistening, round colonies on CSM agar.

Figure 32-6 *Campylobacter jejuni* on Campy BAP medium. On Campy BAP agar, the colonies of *C. jejuni* may be gray and flat, although some are raised, irregular, dry or moist, "runny looking," and spreading along the streak lines.

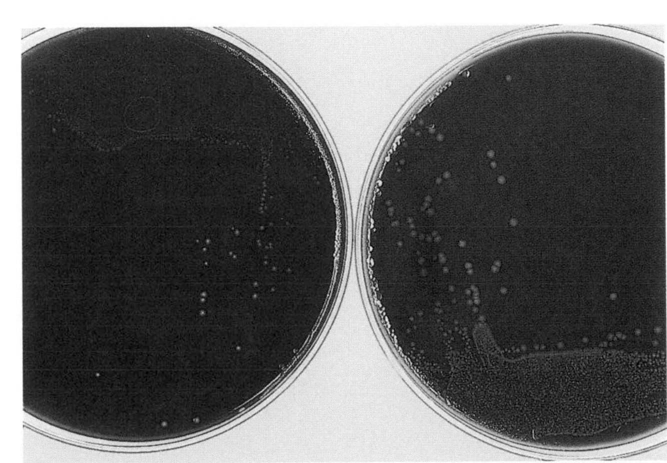

Figure 32-7 *Campylobacter fetus* on blood agar (left) and chocolate agar (right). *C. fetus* is not a thermophilic organism. Media should be incubated at 37°C under microaerophilic conditions. As shown here, *C. fetus* grows better on chocolate agar than on blood agar and forms colonies that are gray and flat and measure 1 to 2 mm in diameter after 48 h of incubation.

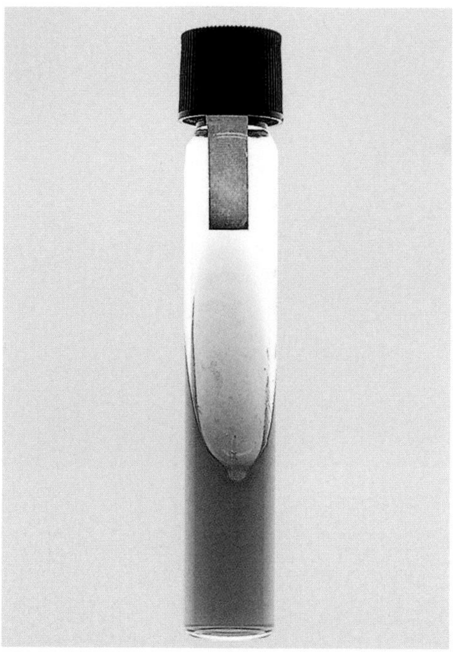

Figure 32-8 ***Campylobacter jejuni*** **on a triple sugar iron (TSI) slant with a lead acetate strip.** *C. jejuni* gives a positive H_2S reaction on lead acetate paper but is nonreactive for H_2S production on a TSI agar slant. *C. fetus* subsp. *fetus* and *C. fetus* subsp. *venerealis* give the same type of reaction. In contrast, *C. sputorum* and *C. mucosalis* give positive H_2S reactions on a TSI agar slant.

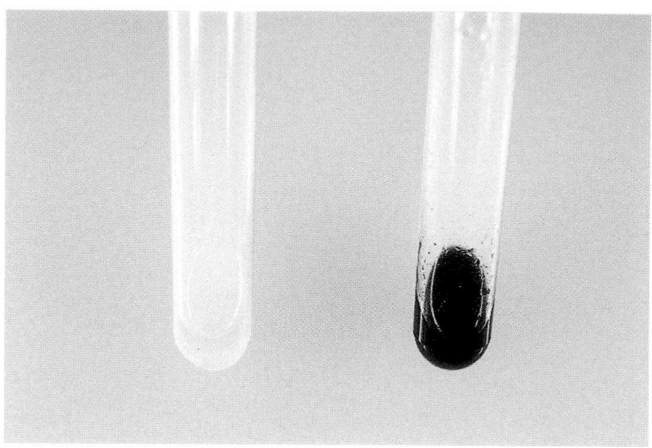

Figure 32-9 Hippurate hydrolysis test for ***Campylobacter jejuni.*** *C. jejuni* is the only *Campylobacter* species that hydrolyzes hippurate (right tube; the left tube is a control). This is an important characteristic in its differentiation from *C. coli.*

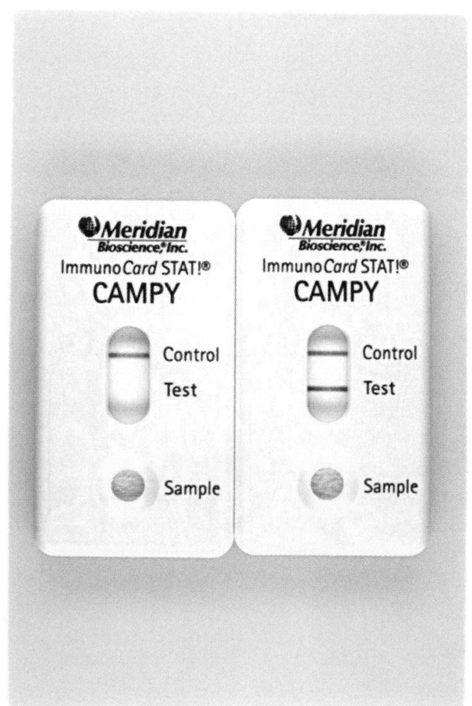

Figure 32-10 Immuno*Card* STAT! Campy. The Immuno*Card* STAT! Campy (Meridian Biosciences, Inc.) is a rapid assay for the detection of *Campylobacter* antigens in stools. This immunochromatographic test uses monoclonal antibodies specific for an antigen present in both *C. jejuni* and *C. coli.* The stool sample is added to a diluent buffer and applied to the sample port. When the sample moves through the card, the *Campylobacter* antigen binds to the monoclonal antibody-colloidal gold conjugate. A capture monoclonal antibody bound to the membrane in the central window of the device binds the antigen–*Campylobacter* antibody–colloidal gold complex, resulting in a pink-red line. The control line of the assay shows that the sample has migrated through the device and that the test reagents are working.

33 *Helicobacter*

There are more than 30 *Helicobacter* species, and several of them, such as *Helicobacter pylori*, *Helicobacter fennelliae*, and *Helicobacter cinaedi*, are human pathogens. The gastric helicobacters include *H. pylori* and affect the stomach, while the enterohepatic helicobacters, such as *H. fennelliae*, are found in the intestine but rarely cause infections in humans.

In developed countries, 30 to 60% of the adult population is colonized with *H. pylori*, while in emerging countries, the prevalence is 70 to 90%. Most of the infections are acquired during childhood by the oral-oral or the fecal-oral route. In addition to humans, *H. pylori* can infect animals including monkeys, cats, dogs, cattle, swine, horses, rodents, chickens, dolphins, and whales. *H. pylori* can cause a wide range of clinical manifestations. It has been associated with chronic gastritis, peptic ulcer, gastric adenocarcinoma, and a B-cell mucosa-associated lymphoid tissue lymphoma. Interestingly, colonization with *H. pylori* may offer some protection against gastroesophageal reflux and adenocarcinomas of the lower esophagus and gastric cardia. *H. fennelliae* and *H. cinaedi* have been isolated from the feces of patients with AIDS, and they may cause proctitis, enteritis, and bacteremia.

H. pylori is a gram-negative, spiral, curved or straight, flagellated, microaerophilic bacillus measuring 1 to 10 μm in length by 0.3 to 0.6 μm in width. The spiral shape is frequently observed in gastric biopsy specimens; however, when cultured on solid media, the bacterium can have a rod-like shape that on prolonged incubation may assume a coccoid form.

The typical specimen for culture is a gastric biopsy specimen, and *H. pylori* requires complex media for growth. Chocolate agar, brain heart infusion, and brucella agar, supplemented with horse or rabbit blood, are good nonselective media, while Thayer-Martin agar, Pylori agar, and Dent's medium have been used as selective media. Colonies from primary cultures usually appear in 3 to 5 days at 37°C in a humid atmosphere with low levels of oxygen (5 to 10%) and increased levels of carbon dioxide (5 to 12%), and they are small (1 to 2 mm in diameter), translucent, and nonhemolytic.

Presumptive identification of *H. pylori* should be based on Gram stain characteristics and positive catalase, oxidase, and rapid urease reactions (Table 33-1). *H. cinaedi* and *H. fennelliae* are oxidase and catalase positive but urease negative. Susceptibility to nalidixic acid and the ability to reduce nitrate can also be used to differentiate between *Helicobacter* species.

A gastric biopsy specimen can be cultured, as described above, and can also be tested by the *Campylobacter*-like organism (CLO) test. In this test, the specimen is placed in a gel that contains urea. The urease produced by the *H. pylori* rapidly hydrolyzes the urea, yielding ammonia, which results in a change in the color of the indicator. Histological examination using hematoxylin and eosin, special stains such as a modified Giemsa, or the Warthin-Starry silver stain can also be used for identification of *H. pylori* in gastric biopsy specimens. Currently, histological examination is the gold standard for the diagnosis of an *H. pylori* infection.

There are several approaches that do not require an endoscopy for diagnosis of an infection with *H. pylori*. These include serological testing, the urea breath test (UBT), and stool antigen detection. Immunoglobulin G antibodies may persist for several months after eradication of the organism. Thus, serological testing cannot be used to establish the presence of a current infection, although for untreated symptomatic patients the specificity of this assay is very high. In successfully treated patients, there should be a significant decline of antibody titers over a period of 6 to 12 months. However, this test is not recommended for posttreatment follow-up. To perform the UBT, the patient drinks urea labeled with ^{13}C or ^{14}C and the amount of labeled CO_2 exhaled, resulting from the hydrolysis of the urea by *H. pylori* urease, is quantitated. To perform direct detection tests, stool specimens can be tested for *H. pylori* using nucleic acid amplification techniques, enzyme-linked immunosorbent assays, or similar methods. Antigen detection tests can help in the diagnosis of *H. pylori* infections, and if the UBT is not available, they can be used for confirmation of eradication following treatment.

Table 33-1 Biochemical reactions of *Helicobacter* species[a]

Species	Oxidase	Catalase	Urease	Nitrate reduction	Nalidixic acid
H. pylori	+	+	+	0	R
H. cinaedi	+	+	0	+	S
H. fennelliae	+	+	0	0	S

[a]R, resistant; S, susceptible; +, positive reaction; 0, negative reaction.

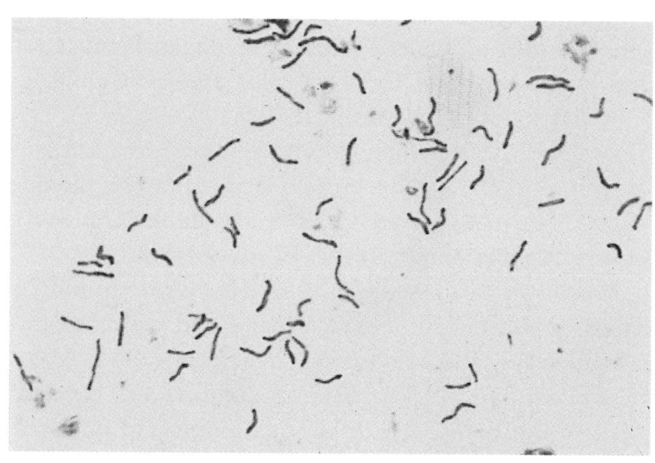

Figure 33-1 Gram stain of *Helicobacter pylori* grown on Thayer-Martin medium. As shown here, *H. pylori* is a gram-negative bacillus, with an S-shaped, "seagull wing" appearance.

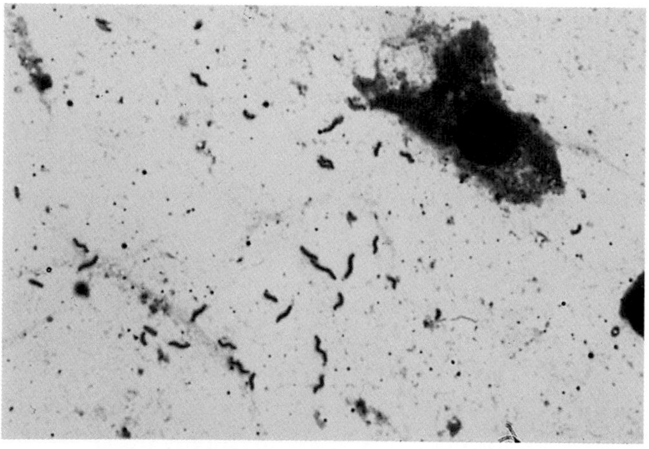

Figure 33-2 Gram stain of a touch preparation from a gastric biopsy specimen positive for *Helicobacter pylori*. Touch preparations of gastric biopsy material do not require fixation and thus can provide a rapid diagnosis. These preparations are made by simply pressing the fresh biopsy tissue against a glass slide. To enhance the staining of the organisms, the sample in this figure was counterstained with carbol fuchsin.

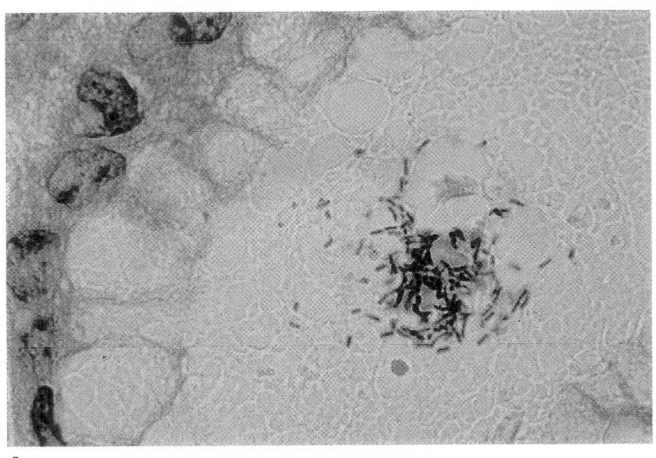

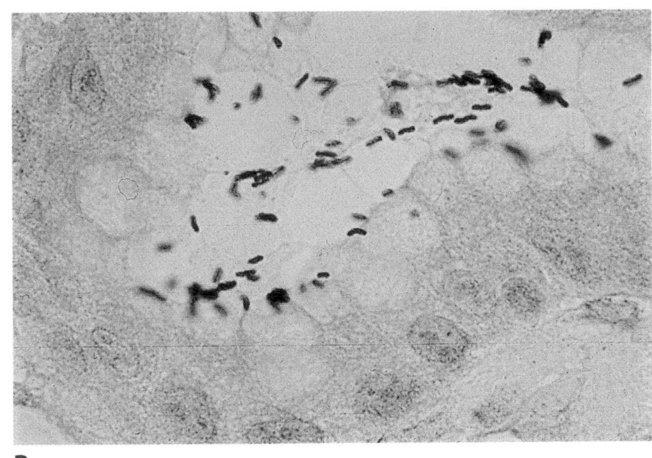

A B

Figure 33-3 Gastric biopsy specimen for *Helicobacter pylori* stained with Giemsa (A) and Warthin-Starry silver (B) stain. To facilitate the visualization of the bacteria, this gastric biopsy specimen was stained with Giemsa or Warthin-Starry silver stain. *H. pylori* can readily be detected as slender, curved bacilli in these gastric biopsy specimens.

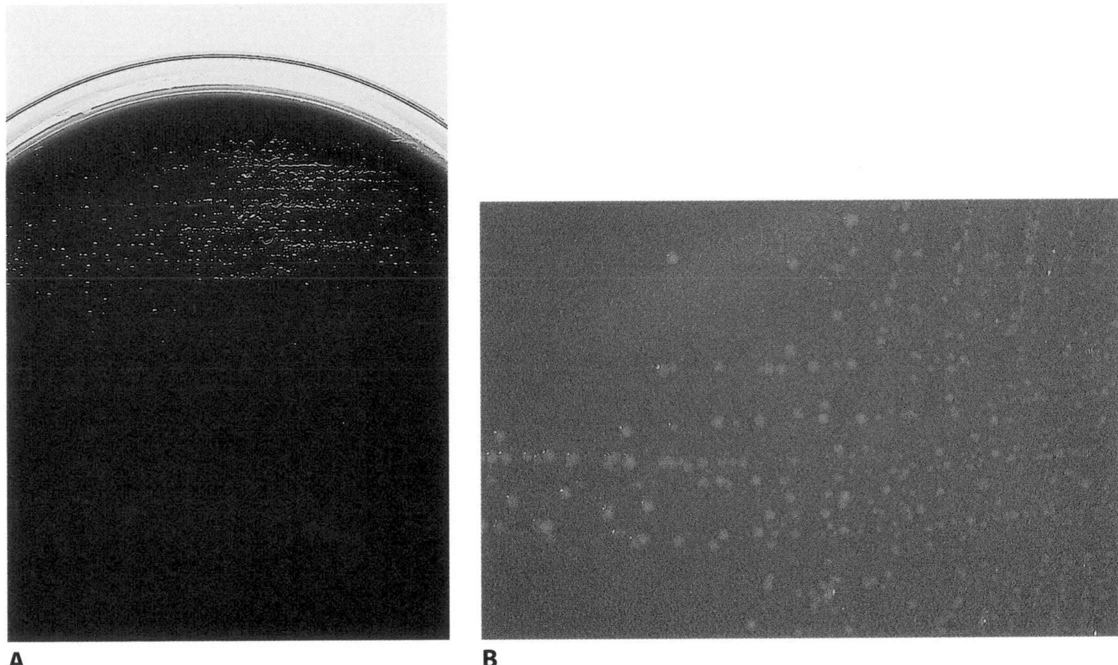

A B

Figure 33-4 *Helicobacter pylori* on Thayer-Martin medium. Colonies of *H. pylori* may require 4 to 7 days of incubation. As shown here, the colonies are small, round, and translucent.

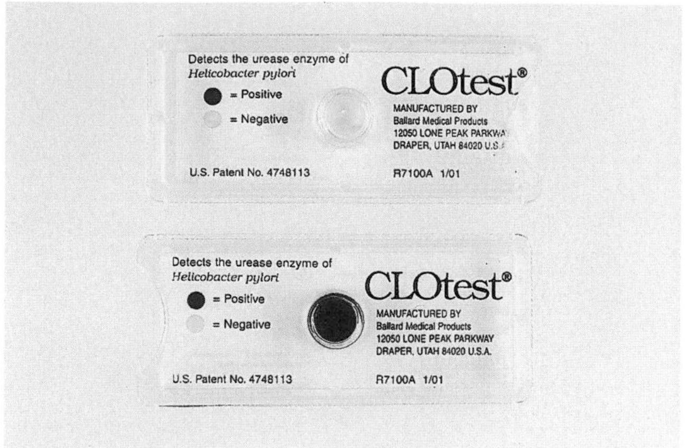

Figure 33-5 The CLO test for gastric biopsy tissue. *H. pylori* produces large amounts of urease that can be detected rapidly by placing a tissue biopsy specimen on a medium containing urea. A pH indicator included in the CLO test (Ballard Medical Products, Draper, UT) makes the medium turn magenta if urease is present (bottom), while the control remains yellow (top).

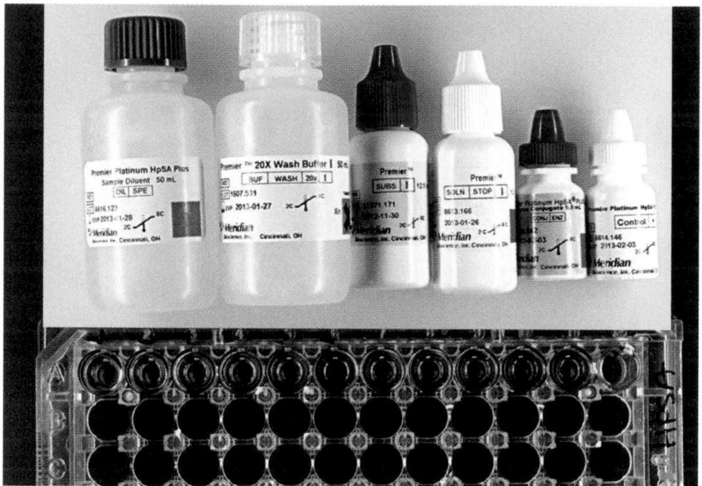

Figure 33-6 Detection of *Helicobacter pylori* antigen by an enzyme immunoassay. Stool specimens can be tested for the presence of *H. pylori* antigen by enzyme immunoassays such as the Premier Platinum HpSA Plus (Meridian Bioscience, Inc., Cincinnati, OH). In this test, the qualitative detection of *H. pylori* antigen in human feces is based on the use of monoclonal antibodies.This assay is highly specific and sensitive and has the advantage that no invasive procedures are needed to obtain the specimen. It can be used for diagnostic purposes and also to monitor the response to antimicrobial therapy. A rapid antigen detection test, the Immuno*Card* STAT! HpSA, is available from the same company.

Chlamydia

34

Members of the genus *Chlamydia* are obligate intracellular bacteria. Three species are human pathogens: *Chlamydia trachomatis*, *Chlamydia pneumoniae*, and *Chlamydia psittaci*. There has been a proposal to divide this genus into *Chlamydia* and *Chlamydophila*, with both *C. pneumoniae* and *C. psittaci* placed in the genus *Chlamydophila*. However, since this remains controversial, in this chapter a single genus, *Chlamydia*, will be used.

All *Chlamydia* spp. exist in two main forms, the elementary body (EB) and the reticulate body (RB). The EB, which is 0.3 μm in size, is the extracellular, infective, "spore-like" form of this organism. Once the EB enters a susceptible host cell, it becomes located in a cytoplasmic inclusion and undergoes a structural and metabolic conversion to an RB, which is about three times the size of an EB. The RB is metabolically active and undergoes binary fission. At some point in its maturation, the RB condenses, eventually reorganizing back into an EB. Depending on the species and the culture conditions, in vitro this cycle can take 36 to 72 h. Once the cycle is complete, the infected host cell releases the EBs, which can then initiate another round of infection.

The three species differ in their epidemiology and disease spectrum. Members of the species *C. trachomatis* can be divided into different serotypes, A though K, Ba, and L1, L2, and L3, based primarily on antigenic differences in the major outer membrane protein (MOMP). These different serotypes are also associated with a particular clinical presentation. *C. trachomatis* is the leading cause of preventable blindness in the world. Blindness resulting from trachoma usually occurs in underdeveloped countries. The scarring of the eyelid and conjunctiva, as well as the pannus, resulting in blindness is thought to be due to both immune and mechanical damage to the host from repeated exposure and infection by this pathogen. More commonly, serotypes A, B, Ba, and C can be isolated from the eye in settings of endemic trachoma. In developed countries, *C. trachomatis* is the leading cause of sexually transmitted bacterial disease, causing infection primarily of the urethra and cervix. Infants born to infected mothers may be exposed to this organism at birth, and ocular and respiratory infections may result. In addition, females may develop pelvic inflammatory disease after contracting a *C. trachomatis* genital infection, with infertility as a sequela. Individuals may also develop conjunctivitis and pharyngitis through contact with infected secretions. The most common serotypes isolated from genital infections are D through K. Lymphogranuloma venereum, a more systemic and aggressive sexually transmitted infection, is caused by serotypes L1, L2, and L3. While not common in the United States, this infection is prevalent in Africa.

C. pneumoniae is transmitted between humans via respiratory secretions. This organism is a common cause of community-acquired pneumonia and has been found in focal outbreaks, for example, in boarding schools and military camps. It has also been implicated as a contributing factor to chronic diseases such as asthma, atherosclerosis, strokes, Alzheimer's disease, and multiple sclerosis. However, the role, if any, this pathogen plays in these chronic conditions is controversial since a causal relation has not been proven.

C. psittaci is primarily an animal pathogen, with humans acquiring the infection as a zoonosis. Domestic birds are the primary reservoir of human exposure to *C. psittaci*. The main manifestation of an infection by this organism in humans is pneumonia, which can develop into a fatal systemic infection.

Several laboratory methods are available to aid in the diagnosis of a *Chlamydia* infection. Until the introduction of nucleic acid amplification tests (NAATs), the gold standard for the laboratory diagnosis of *Chlamydia* was cell culture; however, today NAATs are the preferred methods. For culture, specimens are usually obtained with a swab to optimize the collection of infected epithelial cells. The specimens are then transported in a holding medium such as 2-sucrose phosphate (2-SP). Commonly used host cells for the isolation of *C. trachomatis* and *C. psittaci* include HeLa and McCoy cells; while both cell lines also support the growth of *C. pneumoniae*, some investigators prefer to use either HEp-2 or HL cells to isolate this species. There is no standard isolation procedure, but most methods rely on infecting cells raised in either shell vials or microtiter plates. Centrifugation, DEAE pretreatment of cell monolayers, addition of a eukaryotic cell protein synthesis inhibitor (e.g., cycloheximide), and blind passage or repeated centrifugation are common methods used to enhance the recovery of *Chlamydia*. In general, cultures are incubated for 48 to 72 h, or up to 7 days if a blind pass is used before the cultures are examined. The most sensitive stains used to detect inclusions in infected cell monolayers consist of fluorescence-tagged monoclonal antibodies directed at either the lipopolysaccharide, which will detect all three species of *Chlamydia*, or the MOMP, which detect *C. trachomatis*. In a positive culture, intracellular cytoplasmic inclusions are present. Because of the fastidious nature of *Chlamydia*, the sensitivity of culture is lower than that of NAATs. However, in medical-legal cases, culture remains the method of choice because of its high specificity compared with amplification methods.

As mentioned above, NAATs are the most common methods employed for the laboratory diagnosis of *C. trachomatis* infections. This is due to the relative high sensitivity and specificity of the commercially available methods and the ability to test urine and self-collected vaginal samples; therefore, specimen collection is more convenient for both males and females. In addition, NAATs lend themsleves to automation, thus facilitating high-volume testing.

Other rapid methods for the diagnosis of a *C. trachomatis* infection include a direct fluorescent-antibody stain (DFA) and enzyme immunoassays (EIAs). Both types of assays have low sensitivities compared with culture and NAATs. Compared with culture, the sensitivity of these assays, depending on many variables including the population examined and the culture technique used for comparison, has been reported to vary from 50 to 90%. The DFA, however, has been found to be useful in the diagnosis of neonatal conjunctivitis, where the organism burden is high. For the diagnosis of *C. pneumoniae* and *C. psittaci*, alternatives to culture are not commercially available; however, NAATs have been used in research settings.

Serological testing has been used as an epidemiological tool to investigate *Chlamydia* infections. The microimmunofluorescence assay (MIF) is the gold standard of *Chlamydia* serological testing. In this assay, preparations of formalin-fixed EBs are used as the antigen. Individual fluorescent EBs are interpreted as a positive test. This assay suffers from reproducibility problems due to the reagents and the subjectivity inherent in reading the results. EIA and inclusion immunofluorescence assays have been developed, but their use has been limited. An additional limitation of serological tests for *Chlamydia* is the lack of definition of an acute versus a past or chronic infection.

Figure 34-1 Positive cell culture for *Chlamydia trachomatis*. HeLa 229 cells propagated in shell vials were inoculated with a cervical specimen that was transported at 4°C in 2-SP medium. The shell vials were centrifuged for 1 h at 1,000 × *g* at 35–37°C. After centrifugation, cycloheximide (1 μg/ml) was added to the culture, which was then incubated for 48 h at 35–37°C. The monolayer was then fixed with ethanol and stained with a monoclonal antibody to the MOMP of *C. trachomatis*. A single large, apple-green fluorescent intracytoplasmic inclusion, against the red background of the Evans blue counterstain, can be seen taking up the majority of the host cytoplasm of the infected cell.

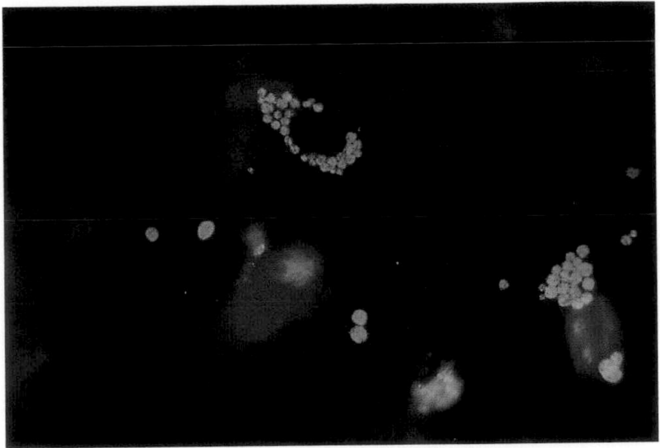

Figure 34-2 Positive cell culture for *Chlamydia pneumoniae*. HEp-2 cell monolayers in shell vials were inoculated with a throat specimen transported in 2-SP medium. Prior to inoculation, the cells were treated with DEAE-dextran (30 μg/ml). The culture was centrifuged for 1 h at 1,000 × *g* at 35–37°C. After the centrifugation, cycloheximide (1 μg/ml) was added to the culture, which was incubated for 72 h at 35–37°C. The monolayer was fixed with ethanol and stained with a genus-specific lipopolysaccharide monoclonal antibody tagged with fluorescein isothiocyanate. *C. pneumoniae* takes longer than *C. trachomatis* to complete its intracellular developmental cycle and tends to form multiple distinct inclusions within a single cell. The inclusions appear bright apple green against the red background of the Evans blue counterstain. The microscopic field shown contains cells with multiple inclusions.

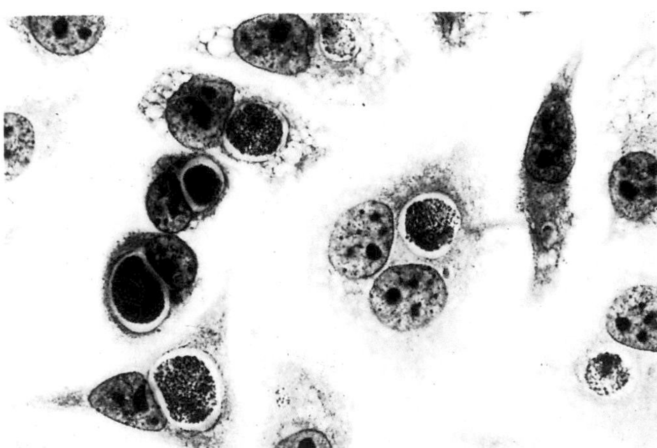

Figure 34-3 Giemsa stain of a positive *Chlamydia trachomatis* culture. McCoy cells were infected as described in Fig. 34-1 with conjunctival scrapings from a 3-day-old infant. After 48 h, the culture was fixed with methanol and stained with Giemsa stain. The infected cells have a distinct intracytoplasmic inclusion, which is dark purple with a halo. These inclusions often appear to be pushing the nucleus to the periphery of the cell. Giemsa stain has also been used successfully to stain direct smears of conjunctival scrapings, especially from young infants, to detect *C. trachomatis*-infected cells.

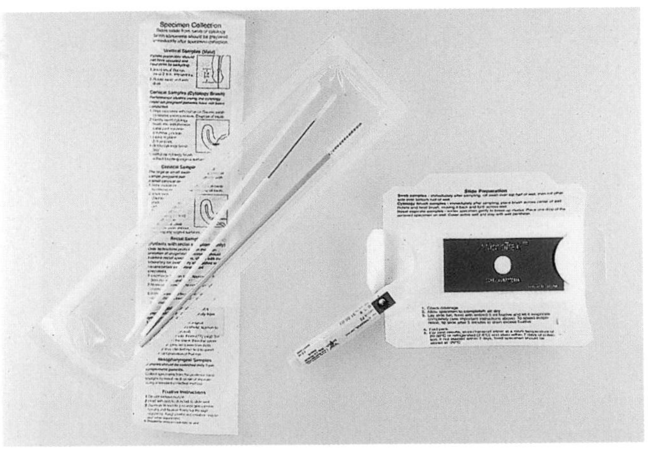

Figure 34-4 DFA smear collection kit for *Chlamydia trachomatis*. Collection kits for the DFA assay are commercially available. The kit shown contains a cytobrush, a regular Dacron swab and a mini-tip swab for the collection of a urethral specimen, a glass slide, a slide holder, and fixative.

Figure 34-5 Positive DFA test for *Chlamydia trachomatis*. The DFA test was one of the first commercially available tests to aid in the laboratory diagnosis of infections caused by *C. trachomatis*. To perform the DFA test, cell scrapings of the affected area are obtained to optimize the collection of epithelial cells. Smears are prepared, fixed, and stained with a monoclonal antibody to either the lipopolysaccharide or the MOMP of *C. trachomatis*. The smear is examined for apple-green fluorescing EBs or RBs. In the example shown, both the larger RBs and smaller EBs can be seen. The host epithelial cells appear red due to the incorporation of Evans blue dye into the stain. Rarely is an intact cell containing an inclusion seen with this test. This test can be performed within 1 h, making it one of the most rapid *Chlamydia* assays.

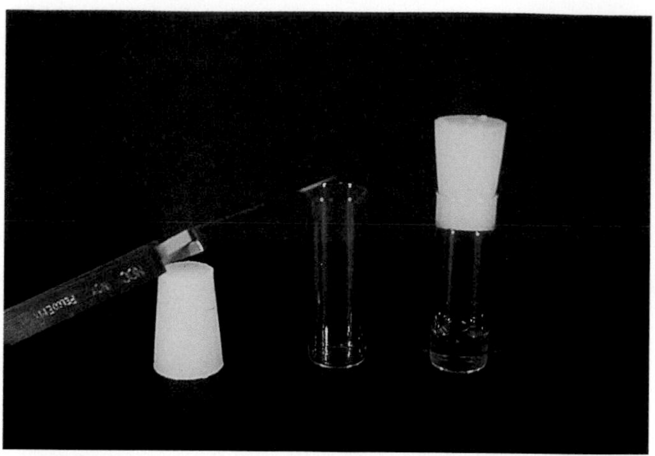

Figure 34-6 Shell vial used for a *Chlamydia* culture. Host cells to be used for a *Chlamydia* culture are grown either on a standard microtiter plate or on a sterile round coverglass that fits in a 1-dram shell vial, as depicted here. The plates or vials can be centrifuged, which is a critical step in optimizing the recovery of *Chlamydia*. Centrifugation should be performed at 35 to 37°C to maximize attachment and infection of the host cells by *Chlamydia*. After an incubation period ranging from 48 to 72 h, the plate or, in the case of the shell vial, the glass coverslip is stained to visualize infected cells. Culture is the recommended method to diagnose a *Chlamydia* infection for medical-legal cases.

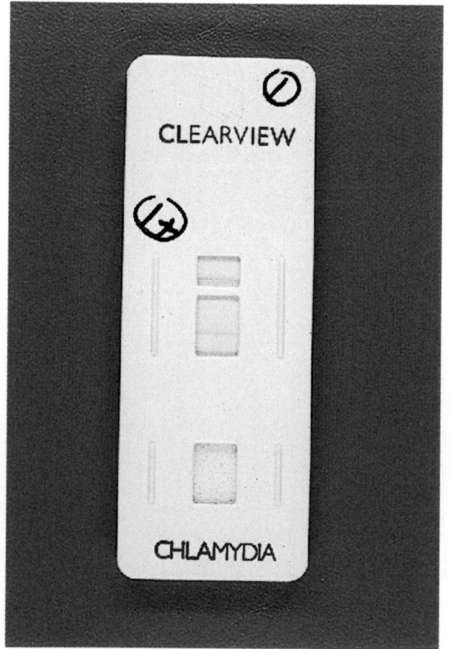

Figure 34-7 Rapid EIA for the direct detection of *Chlamydia trachomatis*. There are several commercially available antigen-based assays for the direct detection of *C. trachomatis* from genital specimens. None of these approach the sensitivity and specificity of NAATs. The main feature of the antigen assays is that they are rapid and are not technically demanding to perform. In the assay pictured, the Clearview Chlamydia (Alere, Waltham, MA), extracted specimens are placed on the filter in the bottom portion of the test device, which contains *Chlamydia* murine antibody that has been tagged with colored latex beads. If *Chlamydia* antigen is present in the sample, the antibody-antigen complex migrates up the filter. A band appearing in the middle portion of the device is a positive result due to the trapping of the complex by immobilized antibody. The top portion of the device is the control window, in which excess antibody is trapped, thus validating that the antibody migrated up the assay filter.

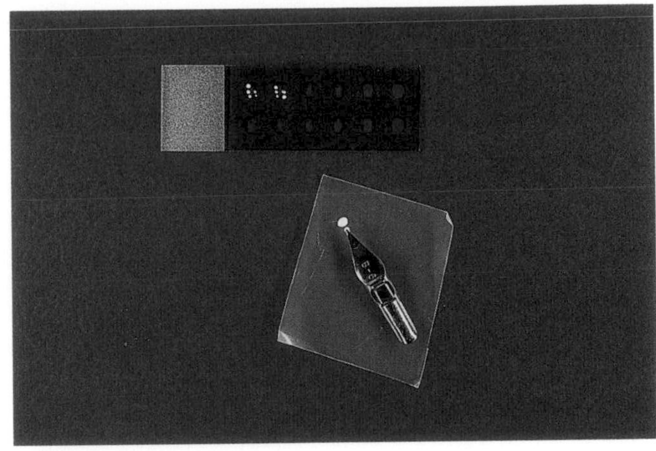

Figure 34-8 Preparation of a slide for the MIF assay. In the MIF assay, purified preparations of EBs are used as antigens to spot microscope slides. Pools of EBs that represent the major serotypes of *C. trachomatis*, *C. pneumoniae*, and *C. psittaci* can be used. A preparation of host cells used to raise the chlamydial antigens serves as a background or nonspecific control. Formalin-treated antigens are mixed with yolk sac and used to spot the slides. As shown, in a single well of a multiwell microscope slide, many antigen-containing dots are applied.

Figure 34-9 Positive MIF assay for *Chlamydia pneumoniae*. Shown here, a single antigen dot (see Fig. 34-8) of *C. pneumoniae* is positive when the EBs are distinct and fluorescent. In this assay, patient serum is serially diluted, applied to wells, incubated, and washed. A secondary antibody to human immunoglobulin tagged with fluorescein isothiocyanate is applied, and the sample is incubated and washed. The slide is then examined under ×400 magnification for the presence of fluorescent EBs. The serum titer to a given antigen is the reciprocal of the highest dilution of serum at which distinct fluorescent individual EBs are seen. Although this method is the gold standard of *Chlamydia* serological testing, it suffers from poor reproducibility due to the inherent variability in the antigen preparation and subjectivity in interpretation.

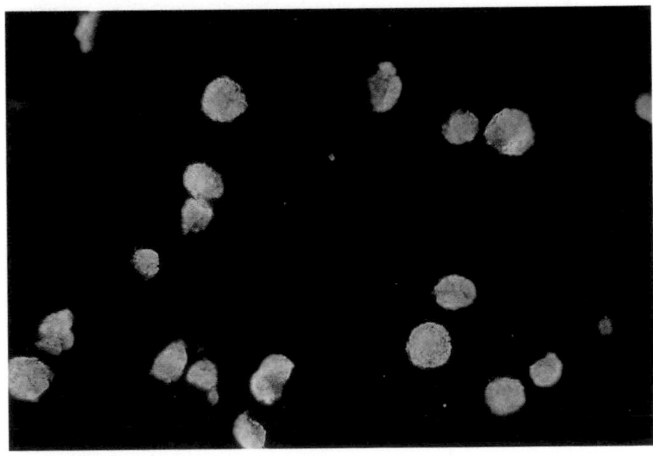

Figure 34-10 Positive inclusion indirect immunofluorescence assay for *Chlamydia trachomatis*. The inclusion indirect immunofluorescence assay is an alternative assay for the serological detection of *Chlamydia* antibodies. In this assay, infected host cells are grown on multiwell slides, fixed, and used to test sera. As described for the MIF (Fig. 34-8 and 34-9), serial dilutions of human sera are tested and the assay results are read microscopically. Here, unlike the MIF, in which the reader is searching for individual fluorescent EBs, fluorescent intracellular inclusions in the host cell are considered positive. In the example shown, the serum sample is positive for antibodies to *C. trachomatis*.

Mycoplasma and *Ureaplasma* 35

Mycoplasma and *Ureaplasma* are included within the class *Mollicutes*. More than 16 species are considered to be human pathogens; however, most of the infections involve *Mycoplasma pneumoniae*, *Mycoplasma hominis*, *Mycoplasma genitalium*, and *Ureaplasma urealyticum*. Mycoplasmas and ureaplasmas are most frequently found in the respiratory and urogenital mucosa but can disseminate, particularly in immunocompromised patients, and potentially may play a role in diseases such as arthritis. *M. genitalium* and *Mycoplasma penetrans* are frequently isolated from the genital tracts of patients with HIV type 1.

M. pneumoniae produces an "atypical pneumonia," also called walking pneumonia, that accounts for 10 to 20% of the reported pneumonias. These infections are frequently seen in young individuals, older persons, and those living in closed-in groups such as military personnel. Transmission is thought to be due to aerosol droplets, and most of the cases occur in the fall and winter. Most infections are asymptomatic, but in 5 to 10% of individuals, following an incubation period of 2 to 3 weeks, fever, headache, malaise, and anorexia occur. In these instances, a differential diagnosis from a *Chlamydia pneumoniae* infection is usually necessary. In rare occasions, extrapulmonary manifestations can occur. Isolation of the organism is considered significant since it does not occur as part of the normal flora.

M. hominis and *U. urealyticum* are associated with infections of the urogenital tract. However, both organisms can be isolated from a majority of asymptomatic, sexually active individuals, so their role in disease is still quite controversial. *M. hominis* has been found in patients with pelvic inflammatory disease and postabortal and postpartum fever. *U. urealyticum* appears to play a significant role in nongonococcal urethritis and female infertility. Both organisms can cause neonatal infections including sepsis, pneumonia, and meningitis. Transmission may be transplacental or can occur at the time of delivery. *M. genitalium* is associated with a significant number of cases of urethritis. Recent evidence suggests that this organism may be a more important genital pathogen than *U. urealyticum*.

Mycoplasma fermentans has been recovered from children and adults with respiratory infections. Isolation of *Mycoplasma amphoriforme* from individuals with antibody deficiencies and chronic pulmonary diseases has been described. The role of these two organisms in the etiology of these diseases is not yet well defined. There is now a significant body of evidence indicating that *M. genitalium* can be the etiological agent in cases of cervicitis and endometritis. However, its role in the induction of tubal infertility is still uncertain.

Mycoplasmas are the smallest known free-living organisms, with a genome size of less than 600 kb. They lack a cell wall and are surrounded only by a trilayered cell membrane. As a result, they are quite pleomorphic and may have a coccoid shape, measuring 0.2 to 0.3 μm in diameter, or they may have a rod structure that can be up to 2 μm in length. The lack of a cell wall makes mycoplasmas undetectable by Gram staining and insensitive to the activity of β-lactam antimicrobials.

Since mycoplasmas do not have a cell wall, they are very sensitive to environmental conditions. Thus, body fluids, tissue specimens, and swabs should optimally be inoculated at bedside; if that is not possible, they should be transported to the laboratory immediately in media such as 2-SP (containing sucrose, fetal calf serum, and phosphate buffer). Specimens that cannot be cultured within 24 h of collection should be frozen at −70°C.

These bacteria can grow in artificial media but require nucleic acid precursors and other components that can be supplied by serum. SP4 glucose broth and agar are probably the most appropriate media for culturing *M. pneumoniae* and *M. hominis*, although arginine must be added to isolate the latter organism. Shepard's 10B urea broth (pH 6.0) can be used to isolate *M. hominis* and *U. urealyticum* with the addition of A8 as the solid medium. Biphasic systems using a combination of a broth and agar are also commercially available. The broths should be incubated at 37°C under atmospheric conditions, and the agar plates should be incubated under 5 to 10% CO_2. Due to the fragility of this organism, broth cultures suspected of containing *U. urealyticum*, which are to be subcultured, should be observed twice daily for the first week to detect a change in color resulting from the hydrolysis of the urea.

Colonies of *M. hominis* measure 50 to 300 μm in diameter and exhibit a "fried egg" appearance resulting from the penetration of the growth in the center of the colony into the agar medium. *M. pneumoniae*, in contrast, produces spherical colonies. *M. hominis* grows rapidly and can form colonies in 1 to 2 days, while *M. pneumoniae* usually is a slow grower, taking 2 to 3 weeks before the colonies can be detected. Guinea pig red blood cells, which adhere to colonies of *M. pneumoniae* but not to those of *M. hominis*, can be useful in distinguishing between the two species. Overall, the recovery of *M. pneumoniae* in culture has very low sensitivity, and therefore a molecular test is recommended for the detection of this organism in clinical specimens. *U. urealyticum* colonies are smaller, ranging from 15 to 30 μm in diameter, which is the reason *U. urealyticum* is called the T (tiny)-strain mycoplasma. Cultures are usually positive within 24 to 48 h, and the characteristic colony morphology and production of urease are adequate criteria for identification. Colonies growing on agar containing urea and manganese chloride have a dark golden-brown color. Molecular techniques for the detection and identification of these organisms will probably replace culture in the future.

Several serological tests are available for the diagnosis of infections due to *M. pneumoniae*. Cold agglutinins have been used for this purpose for many years, but the test lacks sensitivity and specificity. Complement fixation is overall a better method but is technically very demanding. Enzyme immunoassays, indirect immunofluorescence, and indirect hemagglutination methods can also be used for the detection of antibodies to this organism. Serological tests have not been proven useful for detection of genital mycoplasma infections.

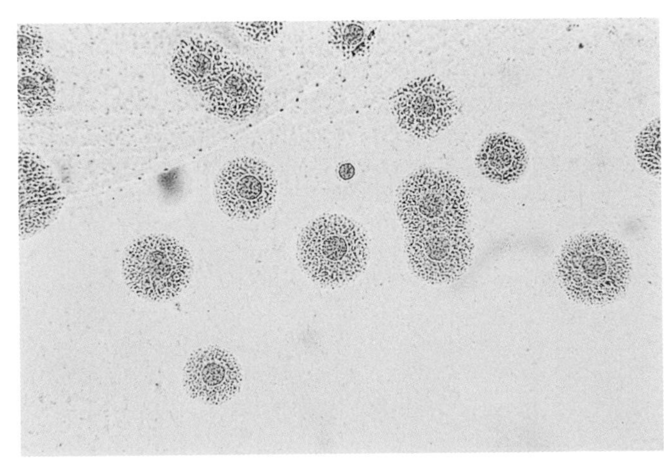

Figure 35-1 *Mycoplasma hominis* on A7 agar. Colonies of *M. hominis* have a typical "fried egg" appearance as a result of the organisms growing into the agar at the center of the colony and superficially on the periphery. The colonies appear in 1 to 5 days and are 50 to 300 μm in diameter. The typical colony morphology and the arginine positivity of *M. hominis* are usually adequate criteria for identification. Definitive identification can be performed using specific antisera to inhibit the growth of the organism.

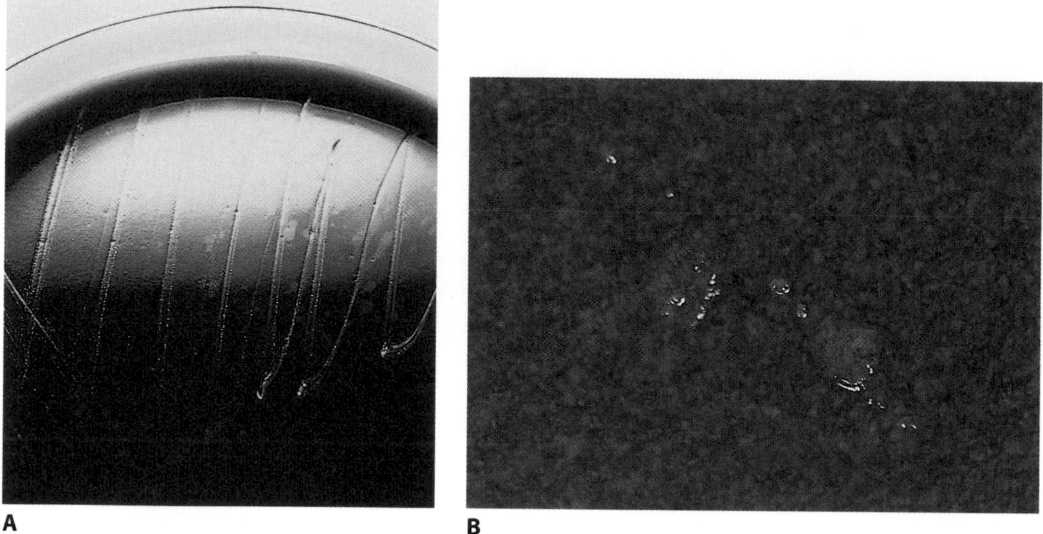

Figure 35-2 ***Mycoplasma hominis*** **on chocolate agar.** *M. hominis* is the only pathogenic mycoplasma that grows on bacteriological media such as chocolate or blood agar. Tiny translucent colonies can be observed after 3 to 4 days in culture (A). At higher magnification, the dewdrop appearance of the colony can be better observed (B). These colonies are often overlooked or the plates are discarded before they become visible.

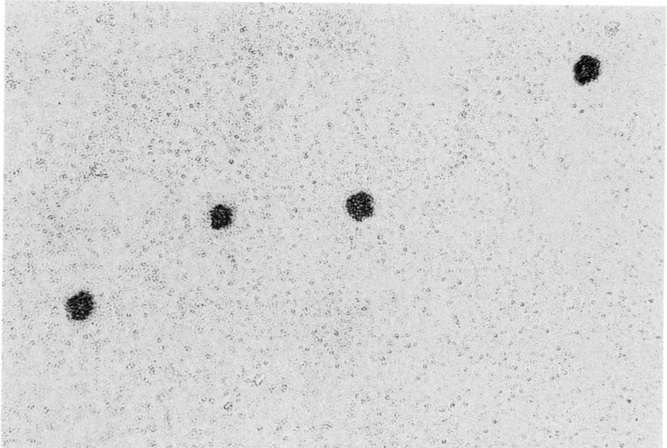

Figure 35-3 ***Ureaplasma urealyticum*** **on A7 agar.** *U. urealyticum*, originally called T (for "tiny") mycoplasma, produces very small colonies ranging in diameter from 15 to 30 μm. On A7 agar, which contains calcium chloride and urea, *U. urealyticum* forms a black precipitate of calcium ammonium chloride at the site of colony formation. Since the colonies are very small, they can be mistaken for several artifacts including air bubbles, cell debris, and other components of the medium. For that reason, it is important to confirm their identification using the urea test.

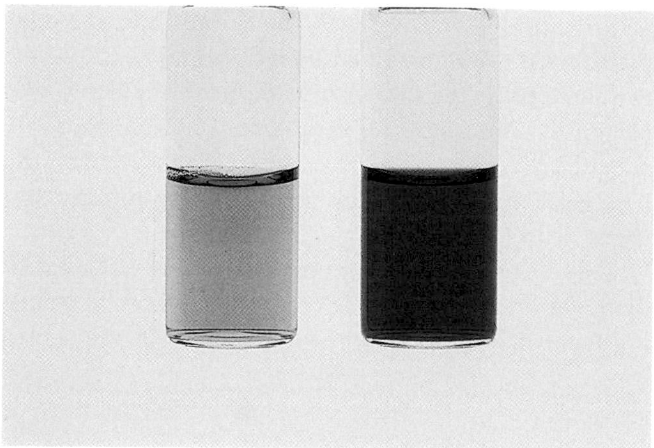

Figure 35-4 Urea test for the identification of ***Ureaplasma urealyticum.*** *U. urealyticum* rapidly hydrolyzes urea, turning the color of the medium from yellow (left tube) to red-purple (right tube) as a result of the change in the pH and the presence of phenol red in the medium as an indicator.

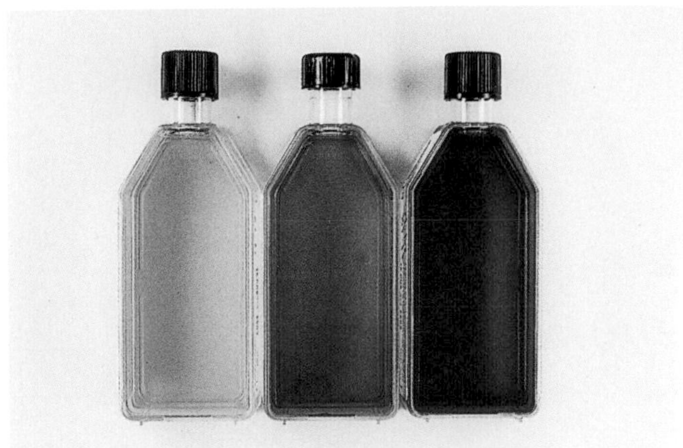

Figure 35-5 Mycotrim GU triphasic culture system. The commercial Mycotrim GU triphasic culture system (Irvine Scientific, Santa Ana, CA), designed for the detection of *M. hominis* and *U. urealyticum* in genitourinary specimens, consists of a diphasic medium containing agar and broth, with phenol red as an indicator. To minimize growth by other microorganisms, disks with nystatin and cefoperazone are added before inoculating the specimen. The flask is incubated at 34 to 37°C, and the agar is inoculated by allowing the broth to wash over it after 24 h of incubation. The flask should be checked every 24 h for a color change. Growth of *M. hominis* causes the medium to change from yellow (left flask) to orange-red (center flask), while growth of *U. urealyticum* results in a red color (right flask). When the color changes, the colonies on the agar phase can be observed under a microscope. A vial containing Dienes stain is provided to facilitate detection of the colonies. This stain should be used only when the flask is not going to be reincubated, since the organisms are killed. A similar system (Mycotrim RS; Irvine Scientific) is also available for the detection of *M. pneumoniae*.

Leptospira, *Borrelia*, and *Treponema* 36

LEPTOSPIRA

In the past, using serological methods, all pathogenic *Leptospira* serovars were included in the species *Leptospira interrogans*, while the nonpathogenic isolates were classified as *Leptospira biflexa*. More than 20 serovars were found to be pathogenic to humans, the most common being *Leptospira canicola* (dogs) and *Leptospira icterohaemorrhagiae* (rats). This classification has now been replaced with a genotypic classification, based on sequencing of the 16S rRNA, in which 20 genospecies include all serovars of *Leptospira*. Neither serogroup nor serovar classification predicts the species of *Leptospira*. As a result, both pathogenic and nonpathogenic serovars occur within the same species. Here we will use the serological terminology since there is still very limited epidemiological information based on the new genotypic classification.

Leptospira has a worldwide distribution; approximately 100 cases are reported yearly in the United States, particularly in Hawaii, with many cases probably going undiagnosed. *Leptospira* may be free living or live in association with animals, in particular dogs, rats, and other rodents. Humans are end hosts in the chain of transmission and become infected by direct or indirect exposure to the urine of animals. The most common source is contaminated water, and as a result, rice and dairy farmers, sewer workers, and swimmers are among the groups most commonly affected. Leptospires infect humans by entering through small breaks in the skin, mucosa, and conjunctiva.

Most infections with *L. interrogans* are asymptomatic, but in certain patients they cause a biphasic illness. During the first week, the leptospires disseminate via the blood. After a short quiescent period of 2 to 4 days, the immune phase begins; this phase may manifest with meningitis, leptospiruria, and jaundice. Clinical symptoms can vary from mild fever to a fatal disease, which occurs in 10% of patients as a result of hepatorenal failure: Weil's disease.

During the early stages of the disease, blood and cerebrospinal fluid (CSF) are the specimens of choice; later, urine is the preferred specimen. Acute- and convalescent-phase serum samples should always be collected to determine the presence of specific antibodies.

Members of the genus *Leptospira* are obligately aerobic, thin, tightly coiled rods, with one or both ends of the cell being hooked; the cells measure 0.1 μm in cross section and 6 to 12 μm in length. The name *L. interrogans* is derived from the shape of the organisms, which is in the form of a question mark with a single hook, while the name *L. biflexa* means "twice bent," for organisms having a hook at both ends. The spirals are right-handed and, in contrast to those of *Treponema* and *Borrelia*, are very close together, resulting in more than 18 coils per organism. Two subterminal periplasmic flagella make these organisms motile. By light microscopy, *Leptospira* is a faint-staining, gram-negative organism.

Although the sensitivity is low, direct wet mounts of urine or CSF can be positive by dark-field microscopy, phase-contrast microscopy, or direct fluorescent-antibody staining. Attention should be paid to artifacts, especially in urine, since they can give false-positive results.

Specimens including blood, CSF, and urine can be cultured by using serum-containing semisolid media such as Fletcher's, Stuart's, Ellinghausen's, or PLM-5. Addition of neomycin or 5-fluorouracil to the medium helps to reduce contaminating bacteria from the normal flora. Once growth is detected, either macroscopically or by dark-field microscopy, the culture can be transferred to a nonselective medium. Several tubes containing 5 ml of medium should initially be inoculated with 1 or 2 drops of blood or with 0.5 ml of CSF. Urine specimens need to be diluted before inoculation in order to minimize the chances of overgrowth by other organisms present in the urine. Tissues should be minced, and small fragments should be plated. Cultures are generally held at 28 to 30°C for up to 4 months. A drop of the culture should be microscopically examined weekly for the first 5 weeks and then every other week. Final identification can be performed using serological techniques and nucleic acid amplification tests. However, most cases of leptospirosis are diagnosed serologically using the microscopic agglutination test, in which a patient's serum is tested against suspensions of the *Leptospira* serovars. A rapid diagnosis can be made by detecting the presence of *Leptospira*-specific immunoglobulin M (IgM) in sera.

BORRELIA

Borrelia and *Treponema* (see below) are the two genera included in the family *Spirochaetaceae* that are human pathogens. All species of *Borrelia* are arthropod borne and, with the exception of *Borrelia recurrentis* and *Borrelia duttoni*, which infect only humans, are maintained by cycling from wild animals to the ticks that feed on them. Soft-shelled ticks of the genus *Ornithodoros* and hard-shelled ticks of the genus *Ixodes* are common vectors. *B. recurrentis*, on the other hand, is transmitted by the body louse *Pediculus humanus humanus*.

Borrelia spp. cause relapsing fever and Lyme disease. There are two forms of relapsing fever: the epidemic louse-borne disease caused by *B. recurrentis* and the endemic tick-borne form that can be caused by various organisms including *Borrelia hermsii*, *Borrelia turicatae*, and *Borrelia parkeri*. Louse-borne relapsing fever occurs under conditions of poor hygiene, crowding, and poverty, where organisms are maintained by passage between lice and humans. Tick-borne relapsing fever is transmitted via saliva during the attachment of ticks. Clinically, in both types of relapsing fever, after an incubation period of 2 to 15 days, there is a massive spirochetemia accompanied by high fever, muscle pain, headaches, and weakness. This episode usually ends suddenly after 3 to 7 days, when an immune response is mounted and the spirochetemia disappears. Several days or even weeks later, the disease often recurs with a less severe course. The relapses are caused by variation of the surface antigens of the organism, resulting in temporary avoidance of the immune system.

Borrelia burgdorferi sensu lato, the cause of Lyme disease, has been divided into three separate species that are pathogenic in humans: *B. burgdorferi* sensu stricto, found in the United States and Europe; and *Borrelia garinii* and *Borrelia afzelii*, found in Europe and Japan. In central to eastern Asia, *B. garinii* and *B. afzelli* are also the most common pathogens of Lyme borreliosis. Several other species of *B. burgdorferi* sensu lato have recently been described; some of them appear to be human pathogens, including *Borrelia valaisiana*, *Borrelia spielmanii*, and *Borrelia lusitaniae*. As in the case of syphilis, Lyme borreliosis has three clinical stages: early localized, early disseminated, and late-stage. It usually presents with fever, headaches, malaise, fatigue, and weight loss. Approximately 60% of patients develop erythema chronicum migrans, a skin lesion at the site of the *Ixodes* tick bite. The lesion begins as a macule, which expands to form an annular erythema with partial central clearing. Hematogenous dissemination to distant organs and tissues can occur days to weeks after the infection, and patients present with fever, fatigue, headache, myalgia, and arthralgia. Involvement of the heart, joints, and central nervous system may occur in the late stages of the disease. Arthritis, mainly involving the knees, is the most common long-term manifestation.

Members of the genus *Borrelia* are microaerophilic, gram-negative, helical bacteria that measure 0.2 to 0.5 μm by 5 to 30 μm. They have 3 to 10 spirals, and their motility is mediated by 7 to 20 endoflagella per terminus.

Direct staining of blood specimens with Giemsa or Wright's stain may be performed to detect *Borrelia*. The *Borrelia* organisms can usually be seen in the blood from patients with relapsing fever but not from those with Lyme disease. The Warthin-Starry silver stain or monoclonal antibodies can be used to stain tissues. Nucleic acid amplification techniques have high sensitivity when used with select specimens, including CSF, skin biopsies, and synovial fluid.

Although spirochetes causing relapsing fever can be cultured from human blood, the yield of positive cultures from blood samples from patients with Lyme disease is low; therefore, skin biopsy specimens, from the periphery of the erythema, are recommended. Cultures of joint fluid are recommended for patients with arthritis. The medium of choice is Barbour-Stoenner-Kelly broth, and the culture should be maintained in a microaerophilic environment at 30 to 33°C for 4 to 6 weeks. Periodic monitoring by dark-field microscopy and final identification can be performed using specific monoclonal antibodies or nucleic acid techniques.

Due to the low sensitivity of the direct assays, culture techniques, and molecular methods, serological tests using either enzyme immunoassays (EIAs) or indirect fluorescent-antibody tests are recommended for the diagnosis of Lyme disease. Positive and equivocal screening results should be confirmed by immunoblot analysis. An infection with *Treponema pallidum* could give a false-positive Lyme disease result. Therefore, a rapid plasma reagin (RPR) test should be performed. IgM antibody to *B. burgdorferi* can be detected 2 weeks after infection, and its level usually peaks by the second month; however, IgG may not be detectable for the first 3 to 6 months. IgM and IgG antibodies may persist for up to 20 years after infection. Antigenic variability and the stage of the disease may also affect the serological results.

TREPONEMA

Four species of *Treponema* are pathogenic for humans: *T. pallidum* subsp. *pallidum* (venereal syphilis), *T. pallidum* subsp. *endemicum* (endemic syphilis or bejel), *T. pallidum* subsp. *pertenue* (yaws), and *Treponema carateum* (pinta). The pathogenic treponemes are exclusively obligate human parasites, and there is no known animal reservoir. In addition, at least six nonpathogenic *Treponema* species are considered part of the normal flora.

Syphilis, the most common disease caused by treponemes, is usually transmitted by sexual contact by individuals who have an active primary or secondary lesion. In addition, congenital syphilis occurs as a result of transplacental transmission. It is estimated that the prevalence of syphilis worldwide is approximately 1%.

Three stages occur during the natural course of syphilis. The primary lesion develops in the first 3 months after exposure, as a result of the inflammatory response to the infection at the site of inoculation. The lesion starts as a papule and then becomes an ulcer, or chancre, that is firm, single or multiple, painless, and not tender, with a clean surface and a raised border, that can measure up to 1 to 2 cm in diameter and is accompanied by local lymphadenopathy. The chancre usually heals; however, as a result of the rapid dissemination of *T. pallidum* by the bloodstream, the secondary stage may appear 6 weeks to 6 months postinfection. The secondary stage can present with a rash on the mucosa and skin, typically including the palms and soles; fever; sore throat; headache; generalized lymphadenopathy; and sometimes involvement of the central nervous system. Alternatively, it may be asymptomatic or mild. During this stage, which lasts several weeks, patients are still highly contagious. In approximately 30% of cases the disease does not progress; in another 30% the infection becomes latent and does not produce clinical symptoms; but in the remaining 30 to 50% the tertiary stage develops 2 to 20 years later. During the tertiary stage, the heart and the central nervous system can be involved. Granulomatous lesions, called gummas, may appear, involving among other organs the skin, bones, and liver. In general, patients are not infectious during this stage.

Congenital syphilis results when treponemes cross the placenta and infect the fetus. When the mother becomes infected during pregnancy, acute infection of the fetus and stillbirth can occur. Babies born with congenital syphilis may have a multitude of malformations including interstitial keratitis, deafness, neurosyphilis, and bone and tooth deformities.

The other three diseases produced by human treponemes, bejel, yaws, and pinta, are nonvenereal infections. Bejel, or endemic syphilis, is found in the hot and arid regions of the world. The primary lesions are usually not detected. During the secondary stage, papules are formed that can progress to gummas involving the skin, bones, and oropharynx. Yaws is found in the tropical, humid areas of the world and resembles syphilis. The primary lesion, however, is elevated and granulomatous, and late, destructive lesions of the skin, bones, and lymph nodes occur. Pinta is found in the tropical areas of Central and South America and causes skin lesions, mainly papules that can result in scarring, accompanied by regional lymphadenopathy.

T. pallidum is 0.1 to 0.2 μm thick and 6 to 20 μm long and is spiral with 6 to 14 helices per cell. The ends of the organism are pointed and lack the hook shape of the nonpathogenic treponemes. Flagella at both ends give the organism its typical corkscrew motility.

Treponemes cannot readily be cultured, and so alternative methods are used for the diagnosis of syphilis. The gold standard is the rabbit infectivity test; however, this method is used only in research laboratories. During the primary and secondary stages and during early congenital syphilis, direct observation of motile treponemes from the base of the chancre or from the skin or mucosal lesion by dark-field microscopy or the direct fluorescent-antibody *T. pallidum* test is considered diagnostic. It is important, however, when using dark-field microscopy, particularly with oral lesions, to remember than nonpathogenic treponemes are part of the normal flora. Immunohistochemistry methods with specific antibodies are recommended for staining the organism in tissues.

For screening, a nontreponemal test is used for detection of serum antibodies. If the test shows a reaction, it is confirmed by performing a treponemal test. Serological tests may be negative until 1 to 4 weeks after the chancre has formed, but they have nearly 100% sensitivity during the secondary stages. However, during the late stage of the disease, the sensitivity of the nontreponemal tests is low.

The nontreponemal tests detect antibodies to lipid components released from the treponemes and from the host cells. The antigen used for these tests is an alcoholic solution containing cardiolipin, cholesterol, and lecithin. The RPR test and the Venereal Disease Research Laboratory (VDRL) test are the two most widely used nontreponemal tests. These tests are excellent screening methods, but they have to be confirmed by a treponemal test since they detect nonspecific antibodies.

Serological treponemal tests use treponemes grown in rabbit testicles to detect antibodies. These tests are used to confirm positive nontreponemal tests and are also helpful for detecting antibodies during the late stage of the disease. Furthermore, these tests remain positive in treated patients after the nontreponemal tests become negative. To perform these tests, the patient's serum is first absorbed with a non-*T. pallidum* treponeme, the Reiter treponeme, to remove antibodies to nonpathogenic treponemes. The fluorescent treponemal antibody absorption double-staining (FTA-ABS DS) test and the *T. pallidum* particle agglutination (TP-PA) test are the two most commonly used treponemal tests. The FTA-ABS DS test is an indirect fluorescent-antibody test that uses *T. pallidum*, fixed on a slide, as the antigen. After incubation with human serum, a tetramethylrhodamine isothiocyanate-labeled anti-human Ig is added and the specimen is observed under a fluorescence microscope. A fluorescein isothiocyanate-labeled anti-*T. pallidum* conjugate is also added to demonstrate the presence of the organisms on the slide. The TP-PA is a passive agglutination test that uses gelatin particles sensitized with *T. pallidum*. Specific antibodies react with the sensitized particles and form a smooth mat. EIAs are also commercially available for the serological diagnosis of syphilis.

In the "reverse sequence syphilis screening," the serum samples are first tested using a treponemal EIA. These EIAs use recombinant antigens (in particular the 15-, 17-, 44.5-, and 47-kDa proteins) that induce long-term antibody responses and are thought to be specific for pathogenic treponemes. Individuals with a negative treponemal enzyme-linked immunosorbent assay (ELISA) should be considered not infected with *T. pallidum*, unless an early primary infection is suspected. In persons with suspected early primary infection and a negative ELISA, a new sample should be tested in 2 to 4 weeks. Samples from patients with a positive ELISA should then be tested with the RPR. Those samples with a positive RPR should be titrated to determine the level of anticardiolipin antibodies, a result that subsequently can be used to assess the response to therapy. In these patients, treatment is indicated unless the patients were previously treated.

Patients with a positive treponemal ELISA and a negative RPR should be tested with another type of treponemal assay. If the treponemal test is nonreactive, the most likely explanation is that the treponemal screening ELISA was a false positive. A new specimen can be tested in 2 to 4 weeks to confirm the interpretation. If the second treponemal test is also positive, the patient most likely has been treated in the past for syphilis. However, treatment is indicated unless a history of syphilis exists. When the clinical assessment of a patient does not match with the laboratory results, a new sample should be tested in 2 to 4 weeks.

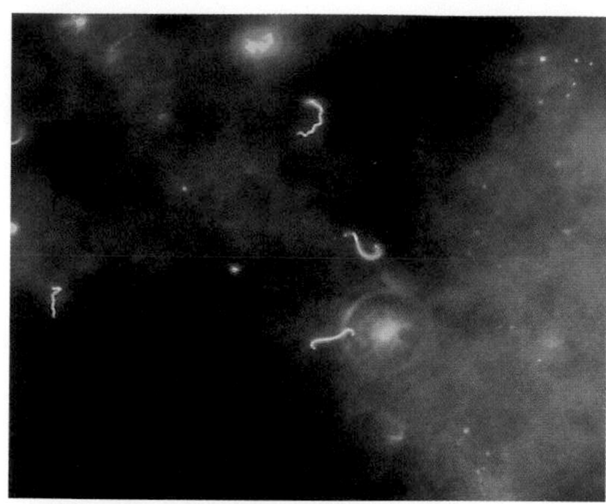

Figure 36-1 Dark-field micrograph of *Leptospira interrogans*. Members of this genus have tight coils and hooked ends. As the organisms die, they lose these coils and hooked ends. (Micrograph courtesy of Tamra Townsen, Orange County Health Department, Santa Ana, CA.)

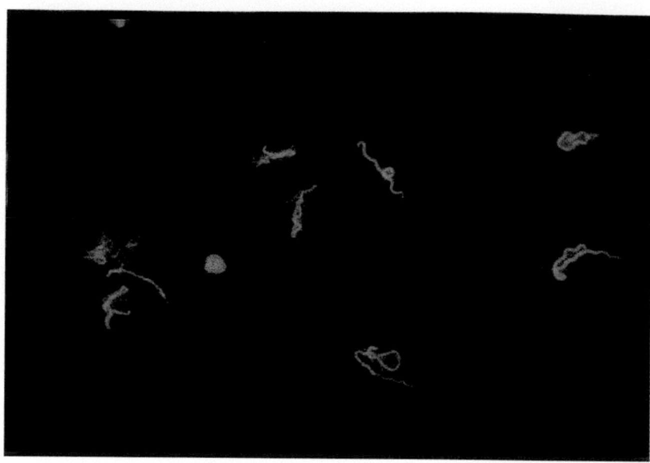

Figure 36-2 Fluorescent staining of *Leptospira interrogans*. As shown here, *L. interrogans* has tight coils. In one of these organisms, the hooked ends can be observed.

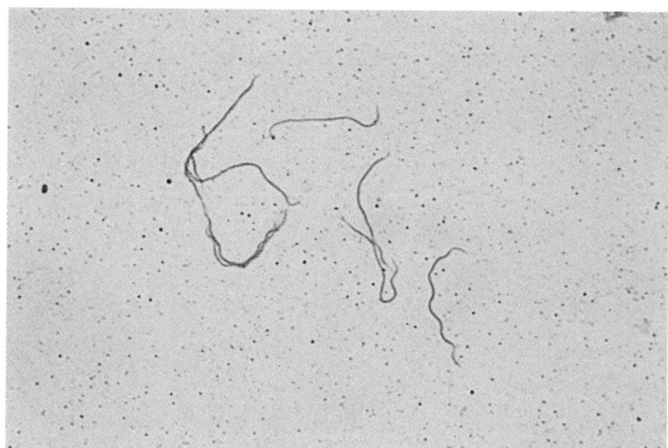

Figure 36-3 Gram stain of *Borrelia burgdorferi* counterstained with carbol fuchsin. *B. burgdorferi* is a coiled, gram-negative bacillus that measures 0.2 to 0.5 μm by 5 to 30 μm.

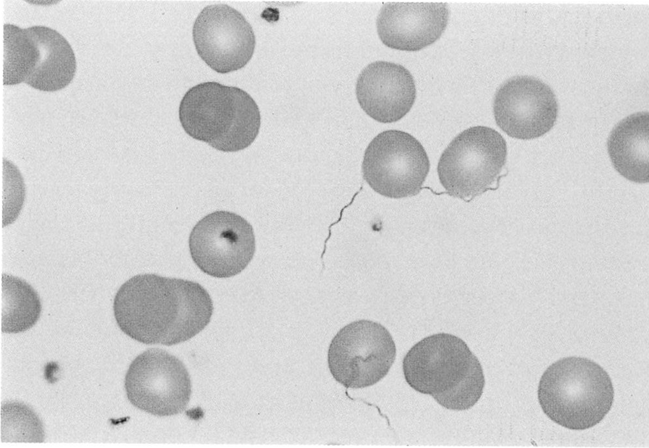

Figure 36-4 Wright-stained peripheral blood smear containing *Borrelia hermsii*. The preparation shown here was made by mixing a pure culture of *B. hermsii* and peripheral blood collected in a tube with heparin. Note the thin structure and loose coils of these organisms.

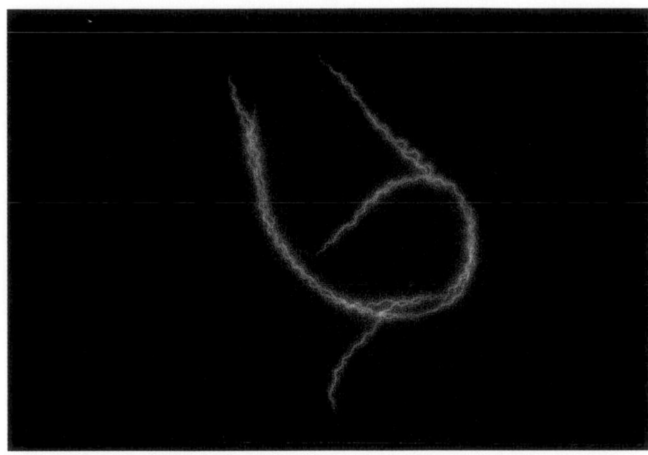

Figure 36-5 Peripheral blood stained with acridine orange for *Borrelia hermsii*. Acridine orange staining of blood specimens can greatly facilitate the detection of *Borrelia* organisms. The preparation shown here was made by mixing a pure culture of *B. hermsii* with heparinized peripheral blood.

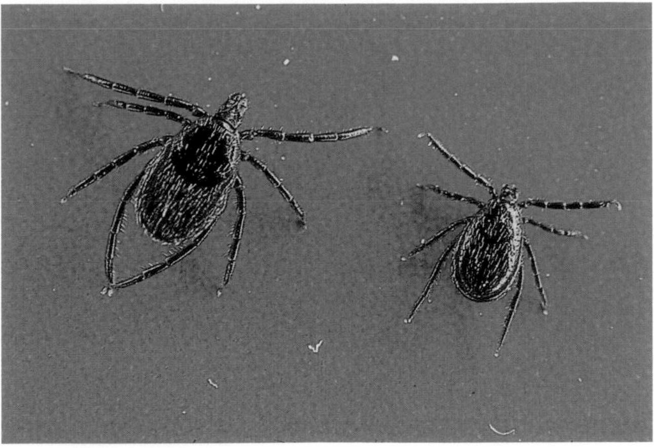

Figure 36-6 Female (left) and male (right) *Ixodes pacificus* ticks. *I. pacificus* is the arthropod vector of *B. burgdorferi* in the western United States. These hard ticks transmit the infection to humans after biting infected rodents. As shown here, the hard ticks are differentiated from the soft ticks by the presence of the scutum, a chitinous plate on the anterior portion of the dorsal surface of these parasites. (Specimens courtesy of Alan G. Barbour, University of California, Irvine.)

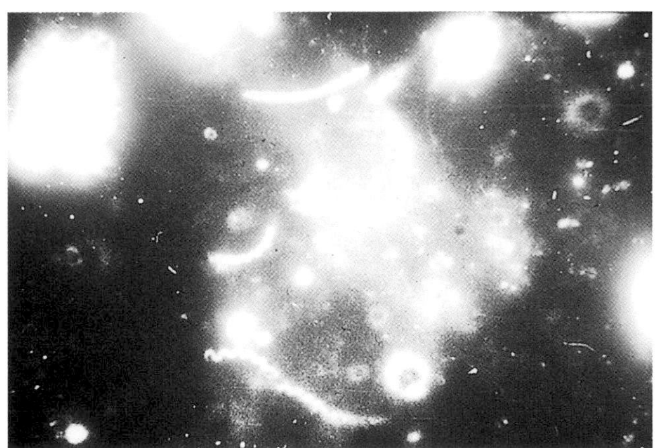

Figure 36-7 Dark-field micrograph of *Treponema pallidum* subsp. *pallidum*. Dark-field microscopic examination of a sample collected from a chancre reveals *T. pallidum*, which appears as an elongated helical corkscrew. Observations of fresh specimens should show the motility of *T. pallidum*. In this case, the motility has resulted in a blurry image. (Micrograph courtesy of J. Miller, University of California, Los Angeles.)

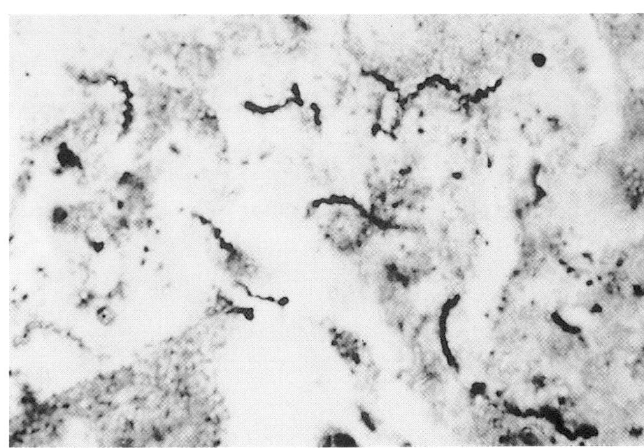

Figure 36-8 Silver stain preparation from the liver of a patient with congenital syphilis. This Warthin-Starry stain of the liver from a patient with congenital syphilis shows *T. pallidum* with its typical tight-spiral coils. (Micrograph courtesy of J. Miller, University of California, Los Angeles.)

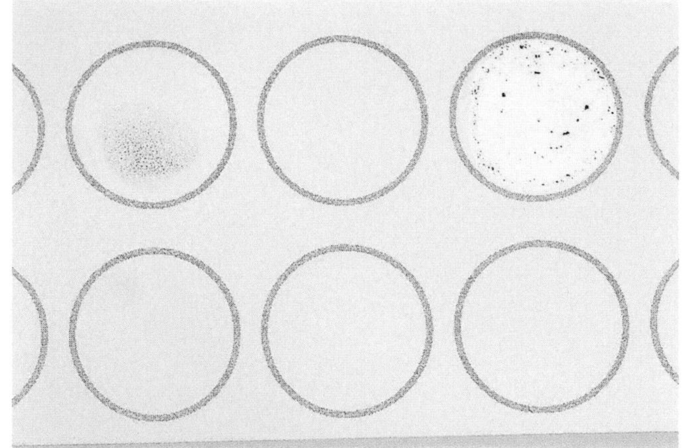

Figure 36-9 RPR card test. The RPR test is a nontreponemal test that uses the flocculation of lipoidal particles to indicate reactivity. Carbon particles, bound to the cardiolipin, make the reaction visible to the naked eye. Here the well at the top left shows a negative reaction and the well at the top right shows a positive reaction. The RPR test can be used to provide qualitative and quantitative results.

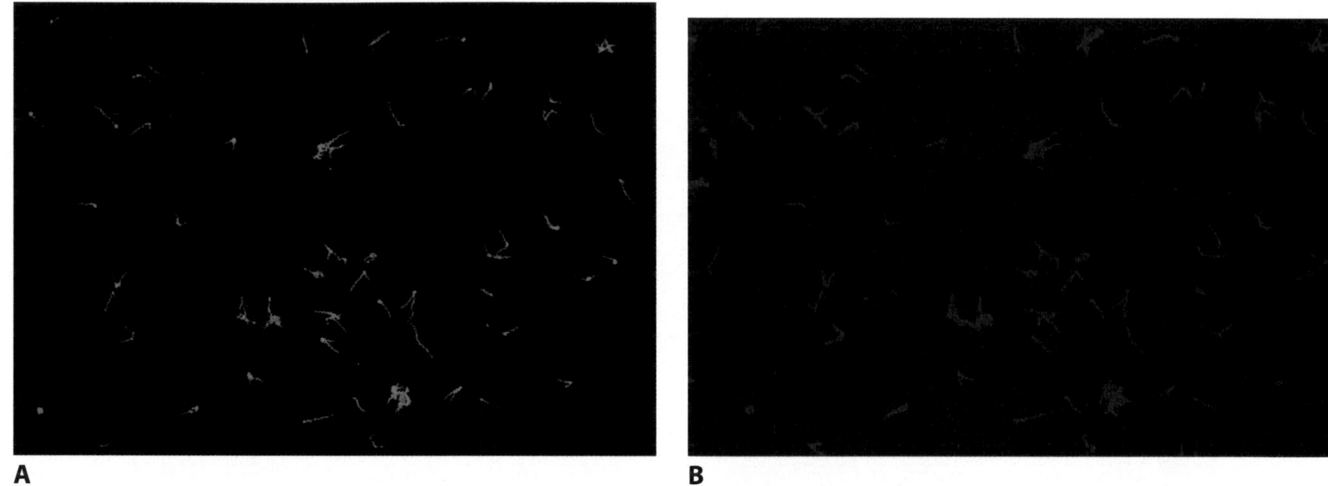

Figure 36-10 FTA-ABS DS test. *T. pallidum* subsp. *pallidum* Nichols is used as the antigen for the FTA-ABS DS test. After absorption of the patient's serum with the nonpathogenic *Treponema phagedenis* Reiter treponeme, the specimen is incubated with the antigen. (A) The fluorescein isothiocyanate-labeled anti-*T. pallidum* conjugate counterstain is used to locate the treponemes when there are no antibodies in the specimen. (B) Rhodamine-labeled anti-human Ig is then added, and in individuals with specific antibodies, the spirochetes are orange when observed by fluorescence microscopy.

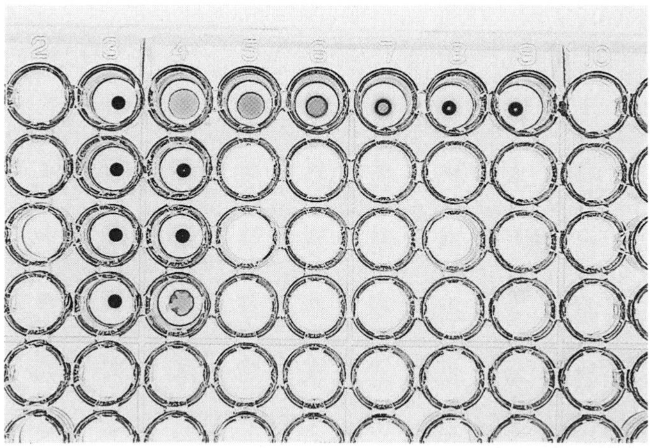

Figure 36-11 *Treponema pallidum* particle agglutination test. *T. pallidum* absorbed to gelatin particles is used as the antigen for the TP-PA test (Fujirebio Diagnostics, Inc., Malvern, PA). Here the top row shows the titration of the reactive control and the patient samples in the other wells. Unsensitized gelatin particles are included as a control for nonspecific reactivity (left column). The well with particles forming a large ring with a rough, multiform outer margin and peripheral agglutination surrounded by a small circle is considered 1+. A smooth mat of agglutinated gelatin particles covering the bottom of the well is considered 4+. This method is easy to perform and interpret in comparison with the FTA-ABS DS test and does not require expensive equipment. Overall, it is considered slightly less sensitive but a little bit more specific than the FTA-ABS DS test.

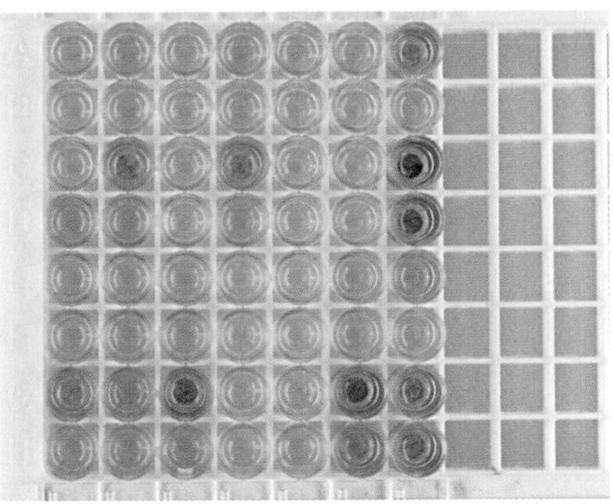

Figure 36-12 Trep-Sure EIA. The Trep-Sure EIA (Phoenix Bio-Tech, Oakville, Ontario, Canada) is a qualitative polyvalent sandwich assay that uses specific recombinant treponemal antigens immobilized on the microplate wells. Patient samples and controls are added and washed, and the antigen-antibody complexes are subsequently reacted with horseradish peroxidase-conjugated treponemal antigens. After a second wash, 3,3′,5,5′-tetramethylbenzidine, as a substrate for the peroxidase, is added. The resulting color is measured spectrophotometrically (450 nm) and the stop solution is added. Color intensity is proportional to the amount of antibody present in the patient's sample.

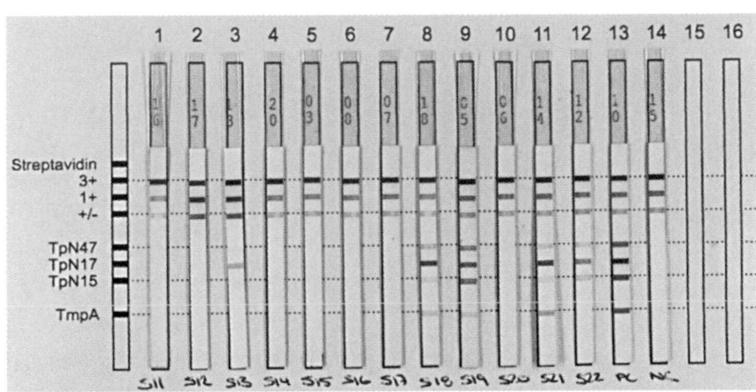

Figure 36-13 INNO-LIA Syphilis Score. The INNO-LIA (Innogenetics NV, Ghent, Belgium) is a line immunoassay that uses three recombinant antigens (TpN47, TpN17, and TpN15) and one synthetic peptide (TmpA) from *T. pallidum* (Nichols strain) to detect antitreponemal IgG antibodies in patients' sera. In addition to the syphilis antigens, four control lines are included for a semiquantitative assessment of the results and to verify the correct addition of the reagents and sample. This assay is being evaluated as a confirmatory test for the serological diagnosis of syphilis.

Rickettsia, Orientia, Ehrlichia, and *Coxiella* 37

RICKETTSIA AND *ORIENTIA* SPECIES

Rickettsia, *Orientia*, *Ehrlichia*, and *Coxiella* were initially classified as part of a single family, but recent genetic analysis has resulted in a reclassification. The family *Rickettsiaceae* now includes two genera, *Rickettsia* and *Orientia*. More than 20 species of *Rickettsia* have been described, while *Orientia tsutsugamushi* is the single species of the genus *Orientia*. These bacteria are small, measuring approximately 0.3 to 0.5 μm by 1 to 2 μm, and grow in the cytoplasm of eukaryotic cells; they were therefore originally considered to be viruses. Animals are their reservoir, and humans are only accidental hosts as a result of transmission by arthropod vectors.

Several species of *Rickettsia* can cause infections in humans. Table 37-1 lists some of the most important epidemiological characteristics of the organisms that cause human infections. Two main groups of human infections are recognized: spotted fever and typhus. In the United States, the most common pathogen is *Rickettsia rickettsii*, the agent of Rocky Mountain spotted fever (RMSF), which causes approximately 500 documented cases annually. The ticks *Dermacentor andersoni* and *Dermacentor variabilis* are the most common reservoirs and vectors for this disease. In the United States, most of these infections occur from April through October. Following approximately 1 week of incubation, a person bitten by a tick harboring *R. rickettsii* can develop fever, chills, headache, abdominal pain, vomiting, myalgias, and a rash. The rash usually starts in the extremities, involving the palms and soles, and spreads to the trunk. In certain cases, serious complications occur, including respiratory and renal failure, gastrointestinal symptoms, and encephalitis.

Rickettsia prowazekii causes epidemic typhus (louse-borne typhus) and is transmitted throughout the world by the human body louse, *Pediculus humanus humanus*. The spread of this infection occurs in situations where people live under crowded, unsanitary conditions such as during famines and wars. In the United States, this infection is more commonly found in the eastern states, where squirrels are infected. The initial symptoms are similar to those described for RMSF, but the rash occurs in only 30 to 40% of the patients. The mortality is as high as 60 to 70% in patients who develop myocarditis or central nervous system involvement. A recurrent form of the disease, called Brill-Zinsser disease, can occur years after the initial infection and usually has a mild clinical presentation.

Rickettsia typhi is the etiological agent of endemic or murine typhus, which has a worldwide distribution. Fewer than 50 cases are reported in the United States on an annual basis, but this disease is endemic in temperate and subtropical areas of the world. The main vector is the rat flea, *Xenopsylla cheopis*, and rodents are the primary reservoirs. After 1 to 2 weeks of incubation, the clinical presentation is similar to that described for *R. rickettsii*, although in most patients the rash is restricted to the chest and abdomen. Even in untreated patients the disease resolves within 3 to 4 weeks.

Table 37-1 Epidemiology of some of the most common *Rickettsia* and *Orientia* infections

Organism	Disease	Vector	Reservoir	Distribution
R. rickettsii	Rocky Mountain spotted fever	Ticks	Ticks, rodents	Western Hemisphere
R. africae	African tick bite fever	Ticks	Ticks	Africa, Caribbean
R. akari	Rickettsialpox	Mites	Mites, rodents	United States, Russia, Korea, Mexico, Turkey
R. conorii	Mediterranean spotted fever (boutonneuse fever)	Ticks	Ticks	Mediterranean countries, Asia, Africa
R. japonica	Japanese spotted fever	Ticks	Ticks	Japan, Korea
R. parkeri	Maculatum disease	Ticks	Ticks	North and South America
R. prowazekii	Epidemic typhus	Lice	Humans, rodents	Worldwide
R. typhi	Murine typhus	Fleas	Rodents	Worldwide
O. tsutsugamushi	Scrub typhus	Mites	Mites, rodents	Asia, Australia

Rickettsia parkeri causes a relatively mild disease with an eschar at the site of tick inoculation, myalgia, fever, headache, rash, and rarely regional lymphadenitis.

Scrub typhus is caused by *Orientia* (formerly *Rickettsia*) *tsutsugamushi*. Mites act as reservoirs and vectors of this infection. The disease occurs mainly in Asia and Australia, and cases in the United States are usually imported. Following 1 to 2 weeks of incubation, fever, headache, and myalgias appear and approximately 50% of patients develop a rash that starts on the trunk and spreads to the extremities. Involvement of the reticuloendothelial system, with cardiovascular and central nervous system complications, can occur.

For the diagnosis of rickettsial diseases, heparinized blood should be collected early in the course of the infection for isolation and serological testing. Samples for culture should be sent to the laboratory as soon as possible or stored at −70°C. A punch biopsy specimen from a skin lesion can also be used for immunohistochemistry, culture, or molecular analysis. Nucleic acid amplification techniques are the most sensitive method for detection, particularly from eschars. Rickettsiae can also be isolated in tissue culture or embryonated eggs. Tissue culture using cell lines such as Vero, L-929, or MRC5 are grown in shell vials, and the sample is inoculated by centrifugation. The monolayers are then stained after 48 to 72 h of incubation at 34°C in 5% CO_2. The organisms stain faintly with the Gram stain but can be better observed with Giemsa or Gimenez stains or with fluorescent antibodies. Monoclonal antibodies or nucleic acid amplification techniques are now used for the identification of clinical isolates.

The Weil-Felix test, which employs *Proteus* antigens, was used for many years as a serological test for the presumptive diagnosis of rickettsial diseases. However, currently the preferred method is an indirect fluorescent-antibody test. Commercially prepared antigens are now available for differentiating the spotted fever group from the typhus group. Latex agglutination, enzyme immunoassays, and Western blot analyses are also available for serological diagnosis. Optimally, acute- and convalescent-phase samples should be tested.

EHRLICHIA SPECIES

As a result of reclassification, human pathogens are now found in the genera *Ehrlichia* (*Ehrlichia ewingii* and *Ehrlichia chaffeensis*), *Anaplasma* (*Anaplasma phagocytophilum*), and *Neorickettsia* (*Neorickettsia sennetsu*) (Table 37-2). Like *Chlamydia*, these organisms produce intracellular inclusions. Elementary body-like organisms (200 to 400 nm in diameter) and reticulate body-like organisms (800 to 1,500 nm in diameter) grow to form morulae. Cell lysis eventually results, with the release of bacteria that infect adjacent cells.

Ehrlichia spp. are zoonotic agents that are transmitted to humans following a tick bite or consumption of infested fish. In the United States, human monocytic ehrlichiosis (HME), caused by *E. chaffeensis*, is distributed mainly in the southern regions corresponding to the location of the lone star tick (*Amblyomma americanum*), the primary vector for this organism. It now has also been reported in the mid-Atlantic region. HME may be the most serious tick-transmitted infection in the United States. *E. chaffeensis*, or a closely related organism, appears to be present in Europe, Africa, Asia, and Latin America. White-tailed deer and dogs are the main reservoirs. *E. ewingii* is the etiological agent of ewingii ehrlichiosis, largely affecting immunocompromised patients, and canine granulocytic ehrlichiosis. *A. phagocytophilum*, the etiological agent of human granulocytic anaplasmosis (HGA), is for the most part

Table 37-2 *Anaplasma, Ehrlichia,* and *Neorickettsia* species known to produce infections in humans

Organism	Disease	Vector	Reservoir	Distribution
A. phagocytophilum	Human granulocytic anaplasmosis	*Ixodes persulcatus* group	Deer, sheep, white-footed mice	America, Europe, Asia
E. chaffeensis	Human monocytic ehrlichiosis	*Amblyomma americanum, Dermacentor variabilis*	White-tailed deer, dogs	Worldwide
E. ewingii	Ewingii ehrlichiosis, canine granulocytic ehrlichiosis	*Amblyomma americanum, Dermacentor variabilis*	Canids, white-tailed deer	Worldwide
N. sennetsu	Sennetsu fever	Unknown; acquired by ingestion?	Fluke-infested fish	Asia

located in the northern midwestern and Atlantic regions of the United States. *Ixodes persulcatus* ticks are the vectors, and white-footed mice, deer, and sheep are the reservoirs. *N. sennetsu* causes Sennetsu fever, which occurs in Japan as a result of the ingestion of raw fish infested with flukes that contain *Neorickettsia*.

The clinical manifestations of HME and HGA parallel those observed in patients with RMSF. However, a rash occurs in fewer than 20% of the patients, while leukopenia and thrombocytopenia are frequently observed. Patients with Sennetsu fever, on the other hand, present with clinical manifestations similar to those of infectious mononucleosis.

Human ehrlichiosis can be diagnosed by collecting blood in EDTA or collecting cerebrospinal fluid and performing culture, histological analysis, nucleic acid amplification, or serological detection of specific antibodies. Several tissue culture cell lines, including DH82, THP-1, HEL-22, HL-60, and Vero cells, can be used for isolation. Culture requirements vary from a few days to a month, and the presence of the organisms is usually confirmed by a nucleic acid amplification technique. Giemsa or Wright stains of peripheral blood can detect intracellular organisms (morulae). Specific antibodies can also be used to stain the organisms. Morulae, however, are observed in only 10 to 20% of cases of HME and 50 to 80% of cases of HGA. Molecular tests, such as PCR, should be performed in specimens that contain infected leukocytes and not in plasma. An indirect fluorescent-antibody assay involving *Ehrlichia*/*Anaplasma*-infected cells on a glass slide or an immunoblot analysis can be used for serological testing. Testing of acute- and convalescent-phase sera can provide definitive diagnosis.

COXIELLA SPECIES

Infections by *Coxiella burnetii* can result in Q fever, which is usually an airborne infection in humans, although ticks occasionally serve as the vectors. *C. burnetii* infects macrophages and develops inside phagolysosomes. This organism has small-cell variants, 0.2 by 0.5 μm, that do not divide but are infectious and act like spores, and large-cell variants, 0.4 to 1.5 μm by 0.2 to 0.5 μm, that divide by binary fission. *C. burnetii* is widespread in nature and can survive for many years under harsh environmental conditions. Farm animals, in addition to dogs, cats, and rabbits, are the main reservoirs. Infections in humans are, for the most part, the result of aerosol transmission during delivery of an infected animal or the result of drinking raw cow's or goat's milk. Most of the infections in humans are asymptomatic, although in a few cases acute and chronic forms of the disease do produce manifestations. The acute infection usually appears, after a 3-week period of incubation, as fever, chills, headaches, and myalgias. An "atypical pneumonia" can develop, and some patients have hepatosplenomegaly. A liver biopsy on these patients will show a typical donut-shaped granuloma. Subacute endocarditis, in patients with prior heart damage, is the most common manifestation of chronic Q fever. Chronic infections occur mainly in immunocompromised patients. Also, a postinfectious chronic fatigue syndrome has recently been recognized. In pregnant females, *C. burnetii* can infect the placenta and the fetus, leading to abortion.

The laboratory diagnosis of Q fever is usually made serologically by testing acute- and convalescent-phase serum samples and using infected monolayers as the antigen. The indirect immunofluorescent-antibody assay is the test of choice for determination of both acute and chronic infections, but enzyme-linked immunosorbent assays also have good specificity and sensitivity. This organism undergoes phase variation; as a result, antibodies to phase I and II antigens can be detected. Phase I strains have intact lipopolysaccharide antigens, while phase II strains do not have complete lipopolysaccharide antigens. During the acute response the antibodies are directed mainly to phase II antigens, while in chronic infections the antibody response is mixed against phase I and II antigens. Seroconversion, or the presence of specific immunoglobulin M, is diagnostic for acute Q fever. Manipulation of infected animals and growth of this organism should be done only in Biosafety Level 3 facilities. Cultures can be performed using tissue culture in shell vials and infecting monolayers such as Vero and HEL cells. Embryonated egg yolk sacs and inoculation into laboratory animals such as mice and guinea pigs can also be used. Direct immunofluorescence can be used to directly detect *C. burnetii* in tissue samples from patients with endocarditis. Nucleic acid amplification techniques are now available to detect and identify this organism.

Figure 37-1 Microimmunofluorescence test for antibodies to *Rickettsia*. To perform the microimmunofluorescence assay, suspensions of the rickettsial antigens to be tested are fixed on a multiwell glass slide. The serum sample is placed on the slide and incubated, and a fluorescein-labeled anti-human immunoglobulin is then added. A positive reaction shows fluorescing microorganisms of the species with which the patient was infected. Here, the antigen spotted was *R. rickettsii*.

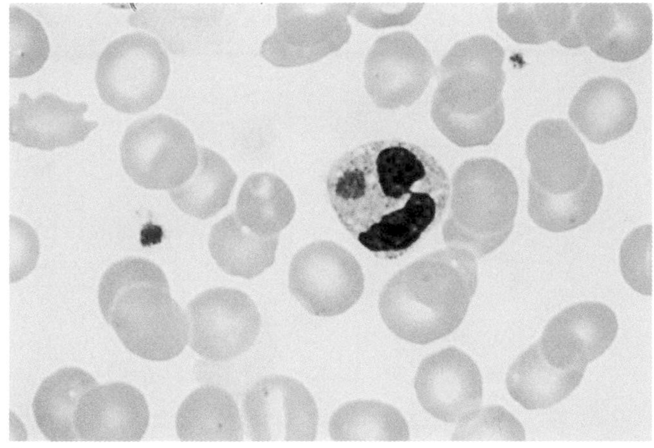

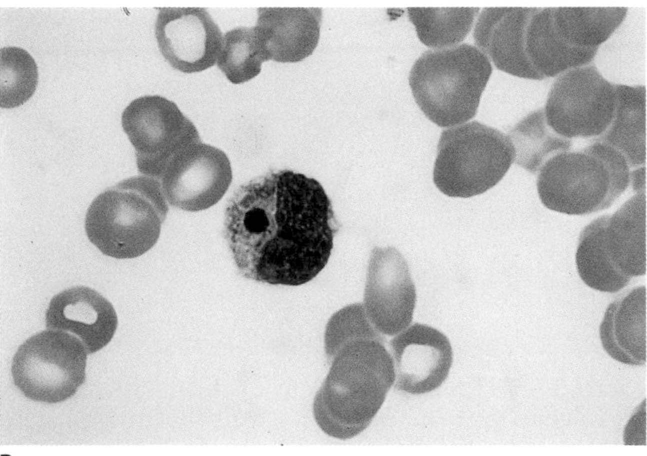

Figure 37-2 Wright-stained peripheral blood smear showing morulae of *Ehrlichia ewingii* (A) and buffy coat preparation demonstrating morulae of *Ehrlichia chaffeensis* (B). In peripheral blood of patients with ehrlichiosis, it is occasionally possible to detect the morulae produced by *E. ewingii* in granulocytes or those produced by *E. chaffeensis* in monocytes. As shown here, the morulae are small (2 to 3 mm in greatest diameter), basophilic, intracytoplasmic inclusions. These inclusions represent membrane-bound clusters of ehrlichiae replicating in the cytoplasm of the infected cell. (Blood smears courtesy of Christopher Paddock, Centers for Disease Control and Prevention, Atlanta, GA.)

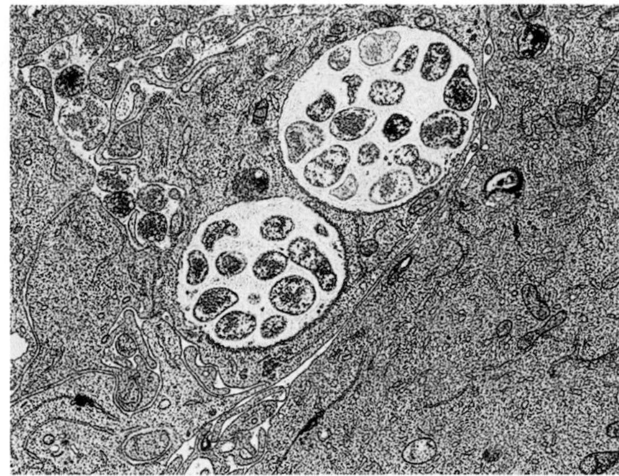

Figure 37-3 Electron micrograph of a monocyte infected with *Ehrlichia chaffeensis*. This electron micrograph shows two intracytoplasmic inclusions produced by *E. chaffeensis*. The morulae can eventually be extruded from the monocyte. (Electron micrograph courtesy of Ted Hackstadt, Rocky Mountain Laboratories, National Institute of Allergy and Infectious Diseases, Hamilton, MT.)

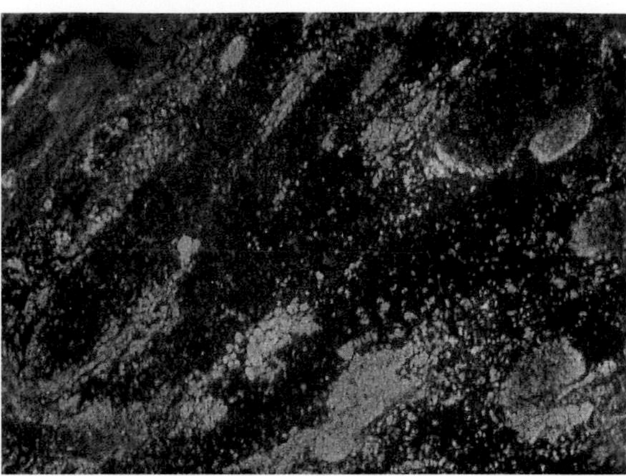

Figure 37-4 Shell vial culture of *Coxiella burnetii* stained with a fluorescence-labeled monoclonal antibody. A monolayer of HEL cells was inoculated with a positive sample and stained after 7 days with a specific fluorescence-labeled monoclonal antibody. The stain shows the organisms growing inside the phagolysosome. (Micrograph courtesy of Philippe Broughi, Unité des Rickettsies, CNRS UPRESA, Marseilles, France.)

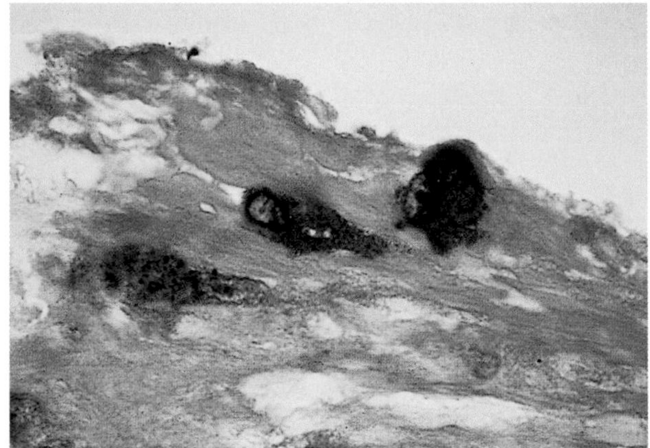

Figure 37-5 Heart section from a patient with endocarditis due to *Coxiella burnetii*. An alkaline phosphatase immunohistochemical stain of a human cardiac valve from a patient with *C. burnetii* endocarditis is shown. The organisms stain pink within the mononuclear cells. (Photograph courtesy of J. Stephen Dumler, The Johns Hopkins Medical Institutions, Baltimore, MD.)

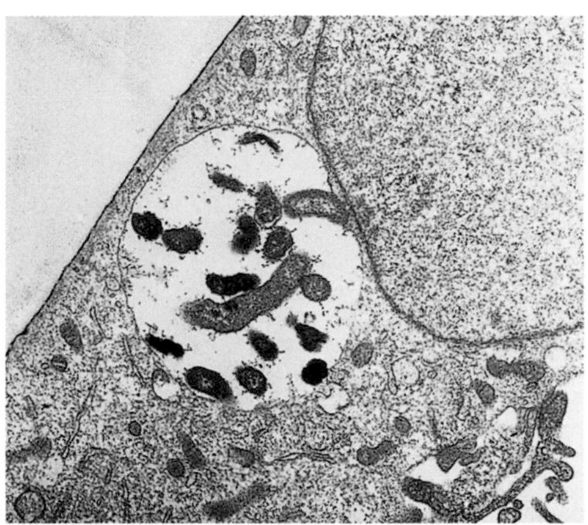

Figure 37-6 Electron micrograph of *Coxiella burnetii*. A cell infected with *C. burnetii* in culture is shown. Multiple organisms can be observed inside the cytoplasmic vacuole. (Electron micrograph courtesy of Ted Hackstadt, Rocky Mountain Laboratories, National Institute of Allergy and Infectious Diseases, Hamilton, MT.)

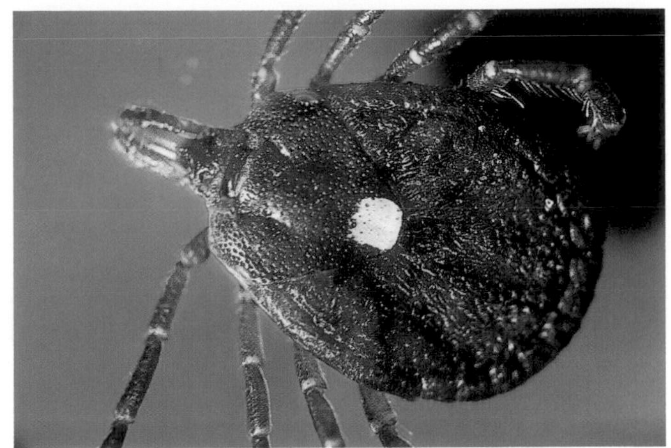

Figure 37-7 Female lone star tick: *Amblyomma americanum.* *A. americanum* is a hard-shell tick that transmits *R. rickettsii* (RMSF) and *E. chaffeensis* (HME) and is also a vector for *Borrelia lonestarii*. It is distributed throughout the United States, although it is most frequently found in Texas and Louisiana. As shown here, this tick can be identified by the white spot (lone star) on its back. (Specimen provided by Alan G. Barbour, University of California, Irvine.)

Antimicrobial Susceptibility Testing 38

Antimicrobial susceptibility testing (AST) is one of the most important functions of the clinical microbiology laboratory in that it provides information to the clinician to guide in selecting appropriate antimicrobial therapy. While there are several methods that one can use to perform AST, in general they are based on the same principles. Whether AST is performed using a totally manual or a fully automated system, or a combination of the two, methods must be reproducible and follow the basic principles outlined in published guidelines, whether they be from the Clinical and Laboratory Standards Institute, the U.S. Food and Drug Administration, or the European Committee on Antimicrobial Susceptibility Testing.

The majority of AST is performed to establish the MIC (minimal inhibitory concentration) of an antimicrobial. MIC values have been established for many drug-organism combinations. The MIC can be determined by broth macro- or microdilution or an agar assay. Here antimicrobials are diluted in broth or in agar and inoculated with a standard concentration of organism. The lowest antimicrobial concentration at which the growth of the organism is macroscopically inhibited is defined as the MIC. Disk diffusion, also referred to as the Kirby-Bauer method, named after the individuals who proposed this approach, relies on paper disks impregnated with a set concentration of antimicrobial. Disks are placed on a solid medium, e.g., Mueller-Hinton agar, that has been inoculated with a standardized lawn of bacteria. Upon incubation, the antimicrobial diffuses into the medium in a circular fashion. If the antimicrobial is able to inhibit the growth of the organism, a zone of inhibition is created around the disk and is measured in millimeters after a specified time of incubation. The Epsilometer test, or Etest, is also performed on solid media. Here a plastic strip that has been impregnated with a gradient of antimicrobial is placed on a standardized lawn of bacteria. If bacteria are inhibited by the antimicrobial, a zone of inhibition forms around the strip, resembling an ellipse. The concentration at which the interface of the zone of inhibition and growth crosses the strip is indicative of the MIC. In addition, several manufacturers have automated some or all the steps taken in these different AST methods.

Breakpoints are set for each antimicrobial as to the MIC (micrograms per milliliter) or zone diameter (millimeters) that corresponds to the likelihood that the antimicrobial will be effective in vivo, i.e., the organism is susceptible; or the antimicrobial has a high probability of clinical failure, i.e., the organism is resistant; or the antimicrobial is intermediate, which indicates that in some settings it may be adequate. This interpretation of susceptible, intermediate, or resistant is based on several factors, including the MIC distribution of known strains, clinical outcomes, pharmacodynamics, and pharmacokinetics.

The MIC and disk diffusion methods may fail to detect emergent resistant organisms. Phenotypic tests in which the basic susceptibility techniques have been modified have been used to predict whether an organism is capable of growing in the presence of a given antimicrobial or class of antimicrobials. An example of this is the D test to check for inducible clindamycin resistance, where, in the presence of erythromycin, organisms may be induced to express genes that confer resistance to clindamycin that would not have been detected using clindamycin alone. Phenotypic tests have also been employed for detecting carbapenemase (Hodge test) and extended-spectrum β-lactamase production.

Screening tests are commonly employed to identify patients colonized with a specific organism that is resistant to a particular class of antimicrobials. Screening is commonly performed using selective and differential media or nucleic acid amplification techniques. Examples of this are the screening of nares swabs for methicillin-resistant *Staphylococcus aureus* and rectal swabs for vancomycin-resistant *Enterococccus* spp. or fluoroquinolone- or carbapenem-resistant enterics.

Molecular testing has been limited mainly by the complexity of genes that code for resistance to certain antimicrobials. However, clustered mutations have made it possible to focus in on genes that have regions that are responsible for the majority of resistance expressed by a particular organism toward an antimicrobial or class of antimicrobials. Examples of this are the *mecA* gene in methicillin-resistant *Staphylococcus aureus* and the *rhoB* gene for rifampin resistance in *Mycobacterium tuberculosis*.

Less common tests that can also be useful in certain clinical situations include the determination of minimum bactericidal concentration. In a procedure similar to that for establishing a MIC, bacteria are added to known concentrations of an antimicrobial, and after overnight incubation broth cultures are subcultured to an agar medium free of antimicrobial. This allows one to determine the lowest concentration of antimicrobial that kills 99.9% of the original inoculum.

Testing for synergy between two antimicrobials can be accomplished using a macrodilution or microwell method, where various concentrations of each antimicrobial in combination and alone are tested against a standardized suspension of bacteria. Combinations of the two drugs for which the effect is greater than the sum of the effect of each drug alone are considered synergistic combinations. Testing for synergy using a single high concentration of an aminoglycoside, 500 μg/ml or higher, is commonly performed with *Enterococcus* spp. when this drug class is being considered as a treatment for endocarditis. Here susceptibility to the single high concentration of an aminoglycoside is predictive of effective treatment when used at therapeutic levels, i.e., low levels, with a cell wall-active antimicrobial.

In the serum bactericidal or Schlichter test, a patient's blood is drawn when the antimicrobial they have been receiving is at the lowest concentration, referred to as the trough, and also when the antimicrobial should be at the highest concentration, the peak. The patient's trough and peak serum samples are diluted in a nutrient broth to which a standardized solution of the bacteria that had been isolated from their blood, or other appropriate culture, is added. The broths are incubated overnight and then read for turbidity. The titer is established as the highest dilution of peak and trough sera that inhibits the growth of the organism.

Due to the slow growth rate of *Mycobacterium* spp., specialized susceptibility assays are required, with the majority of them focused on *Mycobacterium tuberculosis*. In addition to the agar proportion method, which is still referred to as the gold standard, some of the liquid-based systems, e.g., BACTEC MGIT (Mycobacteria Growth Indicator Tube) 960 (BD Diagnostic Systems, Franklin Lakes, NJ) and MB/BacT Alert 3D (bioMérieux, Inc., Durham, NC), have also been standardized to test first-line drugs for the treatment of *M. tuberculosis*. As mentioned above, molecular methods targeting the rifampin resistance-determining region of the *rpoB* gene and gene targets known to contribute to isoniazid resistance have been successfully used to rapidly identify strains that are resistant to first-line antimicrobials against *M. tuberculosis*. The Centers for Disease Control and Prevention has recommended that first-time sputum specimens from all patients suspected of having tuberculosis be tested by a molecular test in addition to traditional smears and culture. Many of these molecular tests also incorporate testing for rifampin and in some cases isoniazid resistance genes.

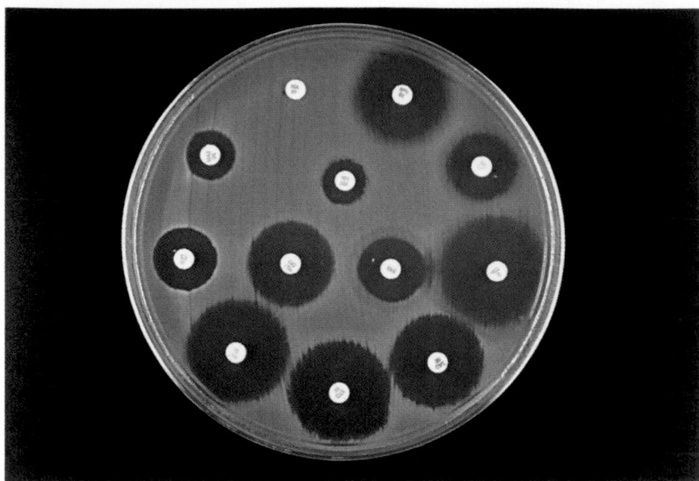

Figure 38-1 Disk diffusion (Kirby-Bauer) antimicrobial susceptibility test. In the disk diffusion method, a lawn of bacteria is spread onto a 150-mm Mueller-Hinton agar plate and paper disks impregnated with antimicrobial agents are placed onto the bacterial lawn. The plates are incubated at 35°C for 16 to 24 h, depending on the organism being tested; they are then examined, and the zones of bacterial growth inhibition are measured. This *Escherichia coli* isolate is resistant to ampicillin, as indicated by growth up to the disk and therefore no zone of inhibition, i.e., 6 mm, the diameter of the disk. For the remainder of the antimicrobial agents, the zone diameters of inhibition are measured in millimeters, and an interpretation of susceptible, intermediate, or resistant is made by comparing the zone with the established breakpoints for that particular antimicrobial-organism combination.

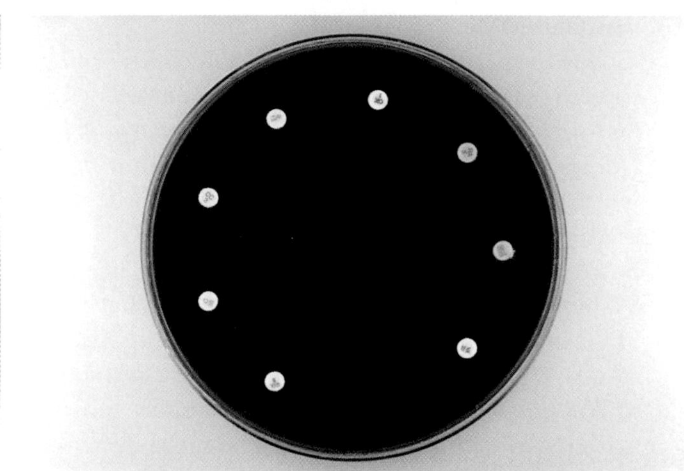

Figure 38-2 Disk diffusion (Kirby-Bauer) antimicrobial susceptibility test using Mueller-Hinton–blood agar. Rapidly growing organisms are usually tested on unsupplemented Mueller-Hinton agar, as shown in Fig. 38-1. However, more fastidious organisms, especially members of the genus *Streptococcus*, as shown in this picture, are tested on Mueller-Hinton supplemented with 5% sheep blood in order to improve growth. This organism is resistant to oxacillin, since this antimicrobial is unable to inhibit this organism, as shown by the bacterial lawn growing right to the edge of the antimicrobial-containing disk. For the other seven antimicrobials, the zone diameters will be measured and compared to breakpoints for this antimicrobial-organism combination to determine if the organism is susceptible, intermediate, or resistant.

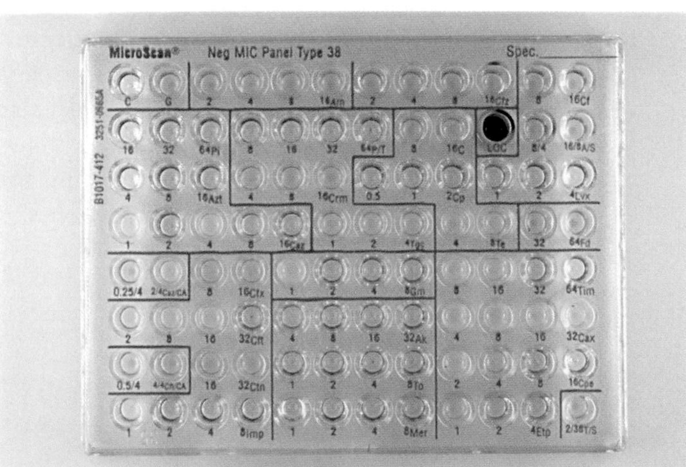

Figure 38-3 MIC testing by microdilution. The antimicrobial susceptibility assay shown here using *Pseudomonas aeruginosa* is performed in a microtiter plate. Serial dilutions of various antimicrobial agents are made in the microtiter plate. The plate is then inoculated with a standardized suspension of bacteria and incubated for 16 to 24 h at 35°C, and the individual wells are examined for growth. The MIC of a particular antimicrobial agent is the lowest concentration that inhibits visible growth. As with disk diffusion, MICs are compared to established standards to determine if the organism is susceptible, intermediate, or resistant to a particular antimicrobial agent. The dark well aids in orienting the plate to facilitate matching the wells with the correct antimicrobial and concentration.

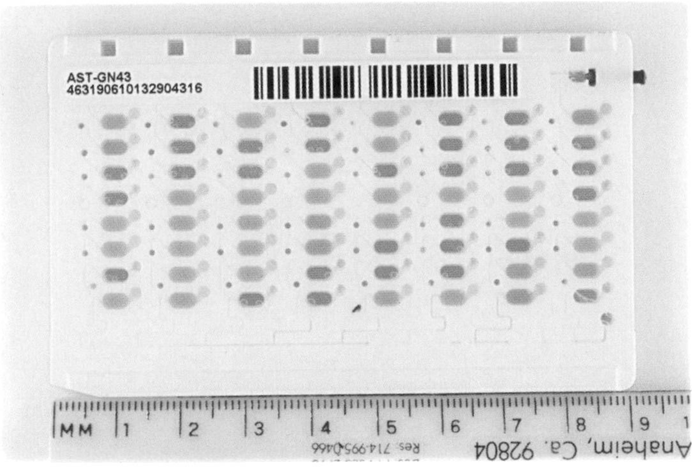

Figure 38-4 Automated antimicrobial susceptibility tests. Several systems are available for automated AST. Shown here is an antimicrobial susceptibility card used in the Vitek system (bioMérieux, Inc., Durham, NC). A standardized suspension of bacteria is used to inoculate a small card (as shown) that contains several antimicrobial agents at various concentrations. The card is then incubated in the Vitek reader/incubator and monitored by the instrument for bacterial growth. The instrument takes the readings, converts them into MICs, and provides an interpretation (susceptible, intermediate, or resistant).

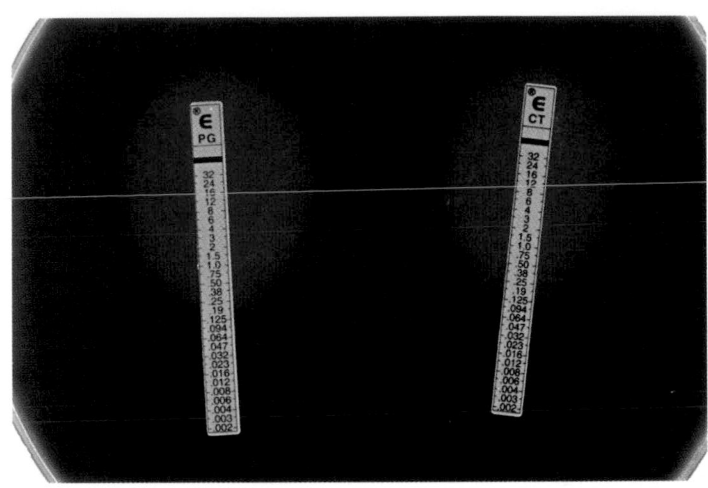

Figure 38-5 Etest. AST by the Etest is performed on solid media such as Mueller-Hinton agar. A standardized solution of bacteria is used to create a lawn of bacteria on the agar plate. A strip that contains a gradient of a particular antimicrobial is then laid over the bacterial inoculum. After incubation for 16 to 24 h at 35°C, the antimicrobial concentration at which the elliptical zone of bacterial inhibition intersects the antimicrobial strip is read as the MIC. The MIC is then compared to a standard chart for interpretation (susceptible, intermediate, or resistant). The organism pictured has a penicillin MIC (left strip) and a cefotaxime MIC (right strip) of 0.126 μg/ml.

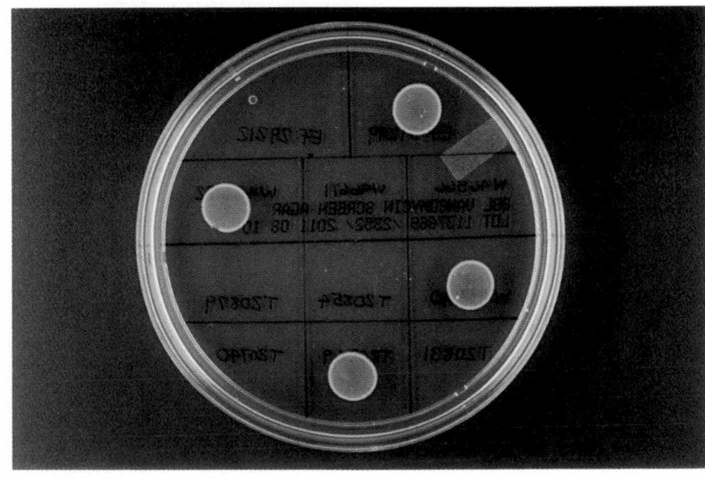

Figure 38-6 Screen plate to check for vancomycin-resistant *Enterococcus* spp. The plate shown here contains 6 μg/ml of vancomycin and is used to screen for isolates of *Enterococcus* spp. that are resistant to this antimicrobial (MIC, >6 μg/ml). Multiple isolates can be tested on the same plate by spotting standardized suspensions of isolates. On the plate shown here, there are four vancomycin-resistant *Enterococcus* isolates, as indicated by growth where the inoculum was placed; the other isolates inoculated are vancomycin-susceptible isolates.

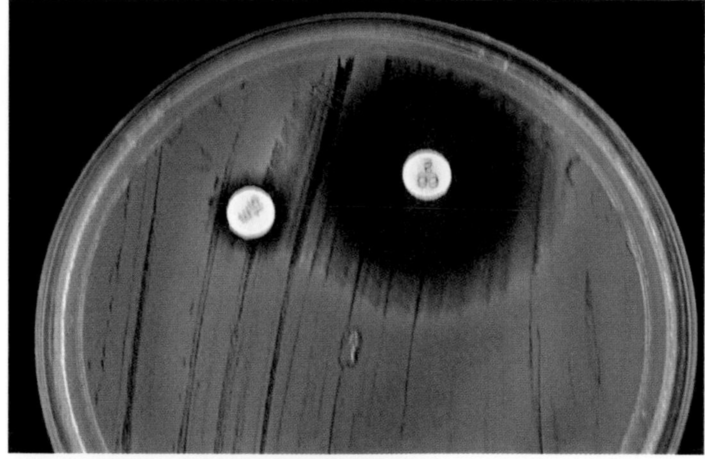

A

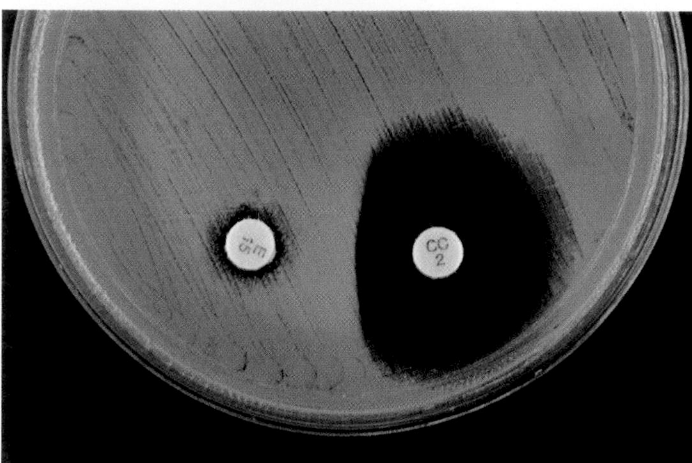

B

Figure 38-7 The D test, a phenotypic test to assess inducible clindamycin resistance. Phenotypic tests are often used to identify organisms that have the potential to express resistance in vivo, especially under antimicrobial pressure. While the definitive test would be DNA sequencing to identify genes or mutations that encode resistance mechanisms, at present this is not a practical approach. Standardized MIC or disk diffusion tests may fail to detect these isolates. Shown is the D test, in which erythromycin is used to test whether an isolate possesses the ability to express the *erm* gene, rendering it resistant to clindamycin. (A) The isolate is resistant to erythromycin but susceptible to clindamycin, indicating that erythromycin was not able to induce *erm* gene expression. This isolate is therefore most likely resistant to erythromycin due to an efflux mechanism commonly coded by the *msrA* gene. (B) The isolate is also resistant to erythromycin, but here the *erm* gene is expressed, which alters ribosome functioning and renders the isolate resistant to both erythromycin and clindamycin. This is indicated by a flattening of the zone of inhibition around clindamycin in the area juxtaposed to the erythromycin disk, making the zone of inhibition around clindamycin appear in the shape of the letter "D."

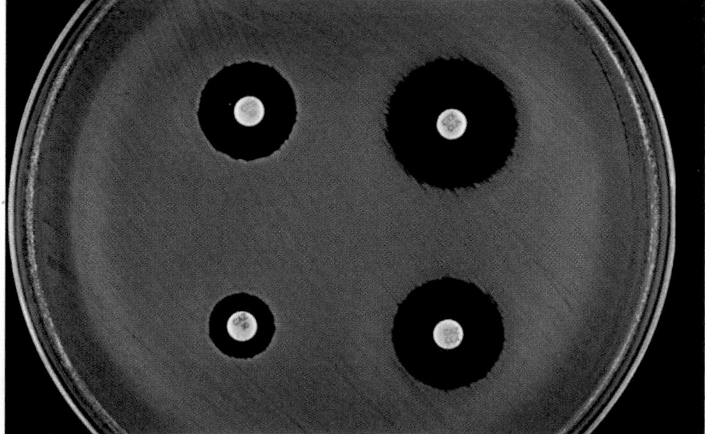

Figure 38-8 A phenotypic test for an extended-spectrum β-lactamase (ESBL). Traditional AST can miss the fact that an organism possesses the ability to express an ESBL. A phenotypic test for ESBL production by an organism can be performed using disks impregnated with ceftazidime and cefotaxime and disks containing both the cephalosporin and clavulanic acid, which can bind to and inactivate the ESBL enzyme. If the zone diameter increases by ≥5 mm in the presence of clavulanic acid in comparison to the cephalosporin disk without clavulanic acid, then it is assumed the organism expresses an ESBL. Shown is a *Klebsiella pneumoniae* isolate that is an ESBL producer, since both the disks containing cefotaxime + clavulanic acid (top right) and ceftazidime + clavulanic acid (bottom right) have zone diameters >5 mm larger than those of the cephalosporins cefotaxime (top left) and ceftazidime (bottom left) alone.

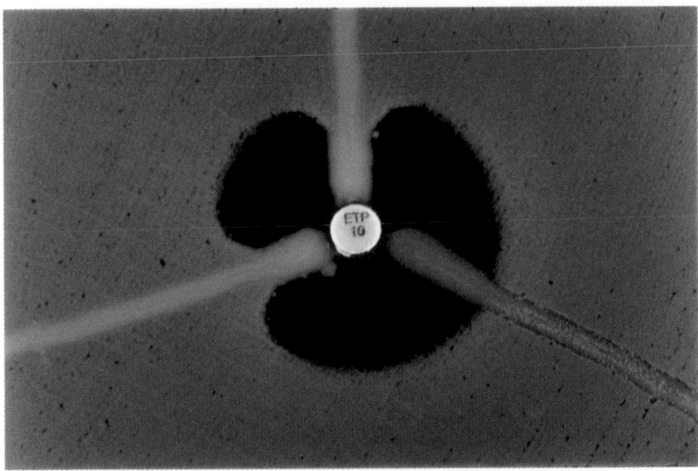

Figure 38-9 The Hodge test, a phenotypic test for a carbapenemase-producing organism. Carbapenemase production can be assessed by the Hodge test. In this test, a standardized suspension of *E. coli* that does not produce a carbapenemase and therefore is susceptible to the carbapenem class of antimicrobials is used to inoculate the surface of a Mueller-Hinton agar plate, forming a uniform lawn of bacteria. A carbapenem antimicrobial, as shown here, is placed on the lawn. The following organisms are then used to streak a line at a right angle to the antimicrobial-containing disk: a *K. pneumoniae* strain (KPC) known to produce a carbapenemase (top); an organism known not to produce carbapenemase (right); and the unknown test organism (left). The plate is incubated overnight and then read. The KPC organism at the top produces the carbapenemase that inactivates the carbapenem, allowing the *E. coli* indicator strain to grow into the zone of inhibition along the KPC inoculation line, as seen by an indentation of the zone. The negative control (right) does not alter the zone of inhibition and thus does not inactivate the antimicrobial. Finally, the test organism (left) is positive for the carbapenemase since the indicator *E. coli*, as with the known KPC-producing positive control, alters the zone of inhibition.

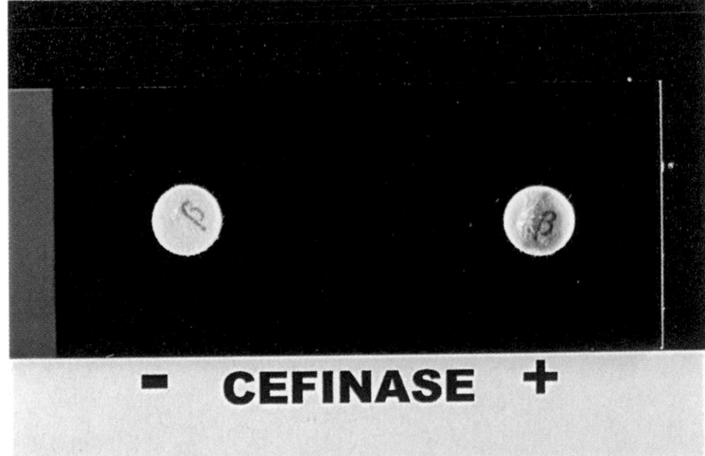

Figure 38-10 A phenotypic test for β-lactamase production. Testing for the enzyme β-lactamase can be performed using a disk impregnated with nitrocefin, a chromogenic cephalosporin. If an organism possesses the enzyme β-lactamase, which is able to hydrolyze the β-lactam ring of the penicillinase-labile penicillins, the chromogenic portion of this substrate is released, turning the disk from yellow to red, as shown in this figure.

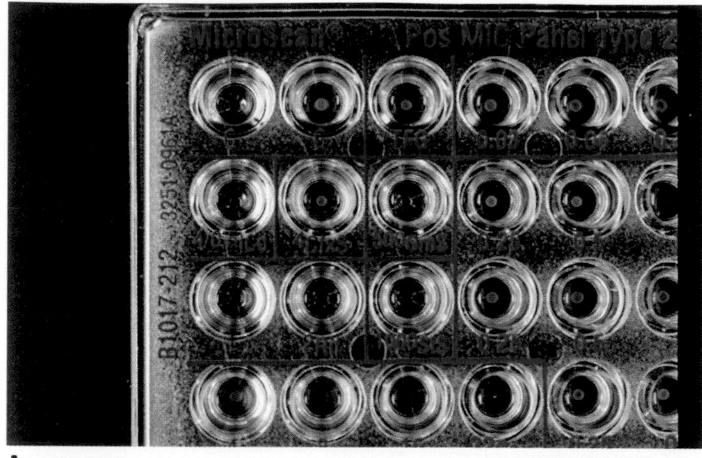

A

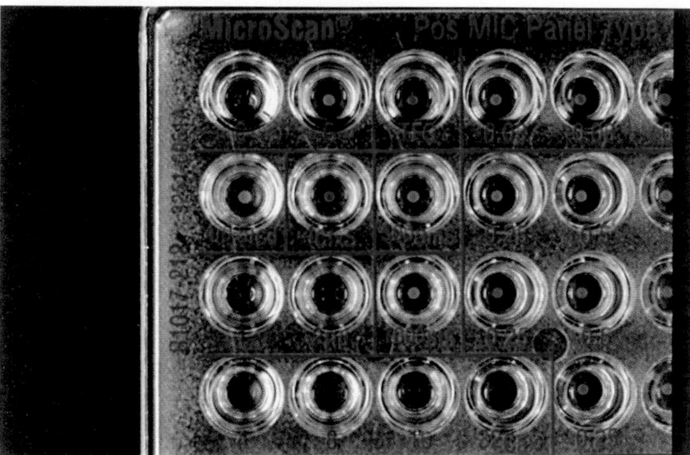

B

Figure 38-11 Synergy testing of *Enterococcus* species using high levels of aminoglycosides. Serious enterococcal infections may require treating a patient with an aminoglycoside and a cell wall-active antimicrobial. To predict whether the aminoglycoside would be synergistic with the cell wall-active antimicrobial, an in vitro synergy test can be performed. In this test, microtiter wells containing a single high concentration of gentamicin (GmS; 500 μg/ml) or streptomycin (StS; 1,000 μg/ml) are incorporated into a microtiter plate, as shown in Fig. 38-3. All wells of the microtiter plate are inoculated with a standardized suspension of the enterococcal isolate. After overnight incubation, the wells are read for visible signs of growth. The result of no growth in the GmS and StS wells for the isolate in panel A (row 2, well 3; row 3, well 3) predicts that the aminoglycosides will have a synergistic effect with a cell wall-active agent. In contrast, with the isolate in panel B, there is a button of growth in both aminoglycoside-containing wells (row 2, well 3; row 3, well 3), predicting a lack of synergy with cell wall-active antimicrobials.

Molecular Diagnosis of Bacterial Infections

39

The ability of the clinical microbiology laboratory to detect and identify bacterial pathogens in a timely fashion has been limited, for the most part, by the small number of organisms necessary to cause an infection. For example, less than 5 CFU (colony-forming units) of a bacterium are present per ml of blood in patients with septicemia. In addition, some pathogens grow slowly due to their unique metabolic requirements, which causes their identification to be delayed. An example of this is *Mycobacterium* sp., which can take up to 8 weeks to be detected on culture media.

Urine is cultured and evaluated today using methodology similar to what was employed in the 1950s. However, since that decade new technologies have been developed that have begun to revolutionize diagnostic bacteriology. It is not one branch of science or a unique technology that is making this change possible, but the convergence and integration of several of them. These technological advances are contributing to a major shift that is changing the way we practice diagnostic medical microbiology. From a fairly subjective art form, diagnostic bacteriology is evolving into an objective, chemically based science.

Some of the driving forces behind this change are our understanding of the biochemistry of microorganisms, our ability to rapidly amplify their nucleic acids, and the capacity to identify unique molecular signatures of each pathogen. In the late 19th century, Friedrich Miescher, a Swiss physician, first isolated and identified nucleic acids, and Albrecht Kossel, a German biochemist, found that nucleic acids are long-chain polymers of nucleotides made up of sugar (ribose in RNA and deoxyribose in DNA), phosphoric acid, and nitrogen-containing bases (adenine, cytosine, and guanine, plus thymine in DNA or uracil in RNA). In 1944, Oswald Avery, Colin MacLeod, and Maclyn McCarty discovered that DNA is the component that causes bacterial transformation. It had been shown that a killed form of the virulent *Streptococcus pneumoniae* type III-S strain, when inoculated into a test animal along with live organisms of the nonvirulent *S. pneumoniae* type II, resulted in a lethal infection due to the type III strain. Avery et al. extracted the virulent DNA and proved that it caused the infection. Until then, proteins had been thought to be the hereditary constituent of bacteria.

Less than 10 years after this discovery, James Watson and Francis Crick proposed a model for the structure of DNA. Based on X-ray diffraction data from Rosalind Franklin, showing that DNA has a helical structure with the phosphates on the outside, and Edwin Chargaff's findings about base pairs, Watson and Crick proposed a model with two chains of nucleotides, each in a helix going in an opposite direction and the matching bases interlocked in the middle of the double helix. Furthermore, Watson and Crick showed that each strand of the DNA was a duplicate of the other. They proposed that during cell division the DNA splits, with each strand acting as a template for a new strand, and by this means DNA can reproduce and maintain its structure. Soon after, Arthur Kornberg discovered DNA polymerase, an enzyme able to catalyze the template-directed synthesis of DNA. Julius Marmur, Paul Doty, and other investigators discovered DNA renaturation, which led to the study of nucleic acid homologies between organisms by using DNA:DNA and DNA:RNA hybridization.

From then on, our ability to characterize and manipulate nucleic acids quickly expanded. In the early

1970s, Daniel Nathans, Werner Arber, and Hamilton Smith discovered restriction endonucleases. These enzymes, found in bacteria, cut up foreign DNA at specific recognition nucleotide sequences, those acting as a defense mechanism against invading viruses. The availability of restriction enzymes allowed Stanley N. Cohen and Herbert W. Boyer to develop recombinant DNA technology, "cutting and pasting" pieces of DNA from one organism into the DNA of other organisms. In 1970, Howard Temin and David Baltimore independently described the activity of a new enzyme, reverse transcriptase. This enzyme transcribes single-stranded RNA (ssRNA) into single-stranded DNA (ssDNA). Due to its RNase activity, it also degrades the original RNA. Subsequently, a second DNA strand complementary to the reverse-transcribed ssDNA is then synthesized. The discovery of reverse transcriptase contradicted the accepted unidirectional dogma that DNA was transcribed into RNA which was then translated into proteins.

Additional methodologies were developed through the 1970s to further characterize RNA and DNA. New sequencing methods and studies included those of Walter Fiers to sequence RNA; the approach of Allan Maxam and Walter Gilbert, based on the chemical modification of DNA followed by cleavage at specific bases; and the chain-termination method of Frederick Sanger. The Maxam-Gilbert method was subsequently replaced by Sanger's technique when dideoxynucleotide triphosphates (ddNTPs) as DNA chain terminators became available. The development of fluorescent-labeled ddNTPs and primers by the laboratory of Leroy Hood greatly facilitated the implementation of automated high-throughput DNA sequencing using the Sanger method.

A new turning point occurred in the 1980s. It was in 1983 when, as the story goes, Kary Mullis, while driving with his girlfriend on the Pacific Coast Highway in California, came up with the idea of using a pair of primers to bracket a DNA sequence of interest that then could be amplified by using DNA polymerase. One limitation of the initial method was that the DNA polymerase was inactivated by the high temperature necessary to separate the two DNA strands, a necessary step to perform the polymerase chain reaction, or PCR. It was Mullis again who in 1986 came up with the idea of using *Thermophilus aquaticus* DNA polymerase, which is heat resistant and therefore can withstand the high temperatures necessary to denature double-stranded DNA (dsDNA).

Over the decades since then, new methods have been developed to amplify and characterize nucleic acids. These new approaches have simplified the application of these technologies, making them practical for use in the clinical laboratory. An important driving force behind many of these efforts was the appearance of the HIV-1 epidemic. A worldwide public and private effort was focused on identifying the cause of this disease and then in diagnosing and managing the infection. The application of molecular techniques played a critical role in these efforts.

Another molecular detection method that has moved from the research laboratory to the clinical laboratory is mass spectrometry. In the 19th century, physical and chemical characterization of the nature of matter laid the ground for the implementation of mass spectrometry. In 1918, Arthur J. Dempster established the basic theory and design of mass spectrometers, and Francis W. Aston built the first functional mass spectrometer in 1919. Working with isotopes of bromine, chlorine, and krypton, Aston was able to show that these naturally occurring elements are composed of various isotopes. Rapid advances have occurred since then, including the invention of the cyclotron by Ernest Lawrence; the concept of a time-of-flight mass spectrometer by William E. Stephens; the development of electrospray ionization by John B. Fenn and Malcolm Dole; and the ultra-fine metal plus liquid matrix method developed by Koichi Tanaka to ionize intact proteins. With all these advances, mass spectrometry, once used mainly in the research laboratory, is now becoming part of standard identification protocols in the clinical laboratory.

Implementation of all these new molecular methods, however, would not have been possible if not for advances in other fields, in particular computer and mechanical engineering sciences. The handling of massive amounts of sequencing data would not have been possible without the development and implementation of computational analysis. Charles Babbage, a mathematician and mechanical engineer, is credited with originating the concept of a programmable computer in the 1800s. Alan Turing in the early 1900s established the groundwork for computer science and artificial intelligence, and the "Turing machine" is considered the blueprint for the electronic digital computer. In 1941, Konrad Zuse constructed the first working, programmable, fully automatic computing machine. In the past 30 years the development of software and hardware that are both easy to use and relatively low-cost has made the use of computers accessible not only to the scientific community but also the public at large. Similarly, advances in mechanical engineering have resulted in the miniaturization of components and the application of robotics, thus facilitating the construction of instruments that can perform highly complex processing of clinical specimens at very high speed and at reasonable cost.

While it may take years, if not decades, to incorporate these new methodologies fully, they have the potential to significantly improve the management of patients with infectious diseases. Implementation of these methods will also require the reevaluation of how we diagnose and manage patients. From the point of view of specificity, techniques such as DNA sequencing probably provide as much information as we will ever need. The sensitivity of these methods, though, is going to require further work for at least some bacterial infections. For example, the very low number of organisms present in most cases of septicemia is still a challenge for our current molecular methods. The volume of the sample that can be processed and the presence of inhibitory substances can also contribute to the limited sensitivity of these assays. Similarly, in the case of *Mycobacterium tuberculosis,* culture continues to be the gold standard.

Interpretation of some of these results will also be a challenge. An increase in the analytical sensitivity of molecular methods cannot necessarily be directly applied to evaluate their clinical sensitivity. For example, some pathogens are present in low numbers as part of the normal flora. Quantitative molecular techniques may help to address this problem, but it will require extensive studies. In addition, the fact that these methods detect nucleic acids, and not necessarily viable organisms, necessitates further evaluation. This issue was extensively debated when molecular methods were implemented for the detection of *Chlamydia trachomatis* and *Neisseria gonorrhoeae.* By now, this concern has been incorporated in the management of patients. For example, it is not recommended to use nucleic acid amplification techniques as a test of cure to assess the efficacy of antibiotic therapy. In the future, simultaneous evaluation of host molecular markers in response to infection may also help address the limitations of these new diagnostic techniques.

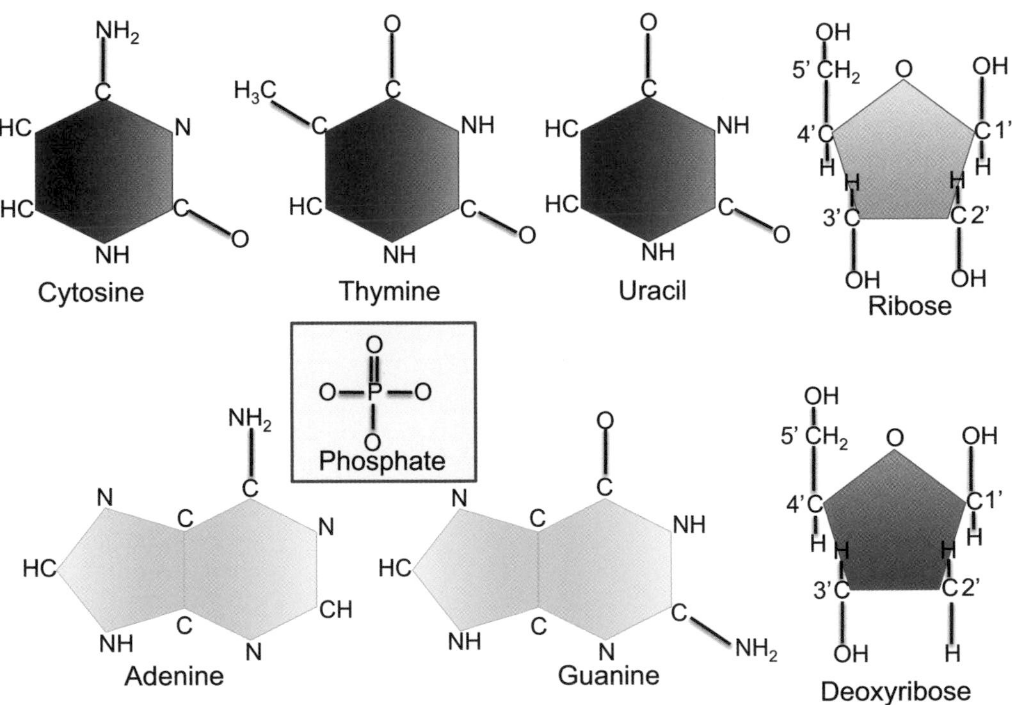

Figure 39-1 The building blocks of DNA and RNA. The building blocks of DNA and RNA are sugars, phosphate, and bases. The two main types of nucleic acids (DNA and RNA) differ in the type of sugar: the five-carbon sugar in DNA is deoxyribose whereas that in RNA is ribose. The four nitrogen-containing bases in DNA are adenine (A), guanine (G), cytosine (C), and thymine (T), while in RNA the thymine is replaced by uracil (U). Cytosine, thymine, and uracil are pyrimidines, while adenine and guanine are purines. Each numbered carbon on a sugar is followed by a prime symbol, and therefore they are called, for example: 3′ carbon.

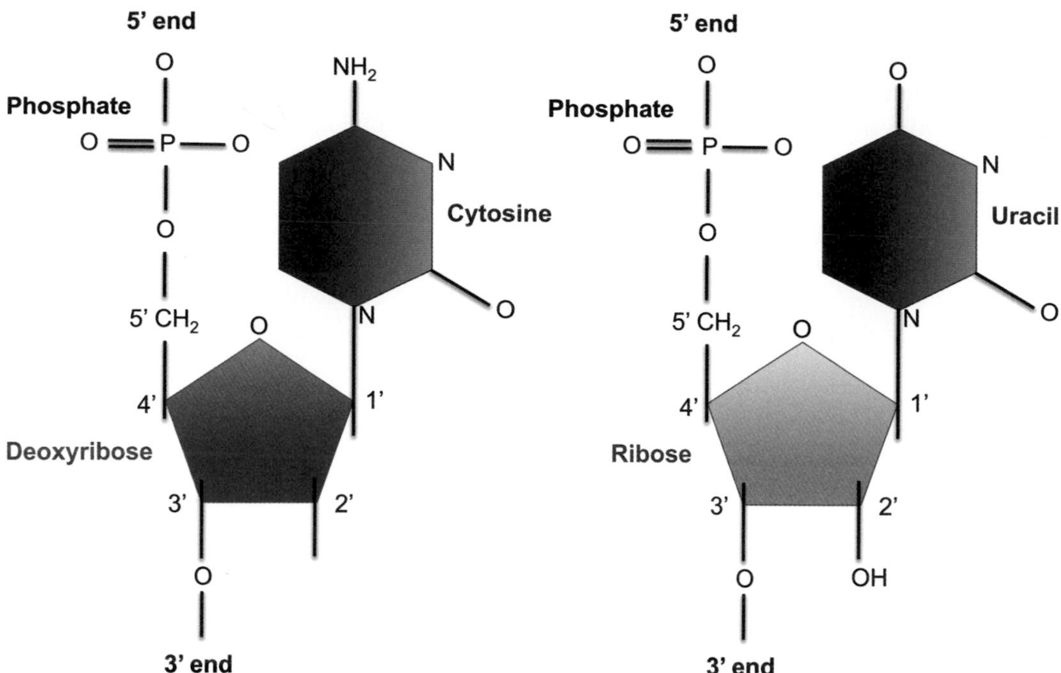

Figure 39-2 Nucleotides. DNA and RNA are polymers. The basic units of the polymer are nucleotides, which consist of a base, a sugar, and one or more phosphate groups. A nucleoside is only a base plus a sugar. Nucleotides are linked to each other by a phosphodiester linkage between carbon atoms of the sugar, known as the 5′ and 3′ atoms. As a result, the 5′ end of the polynucleotide chain has a free phosphate group while the 3′ end has a free hydroxyl group. The phosphates are joined to the C5 hydroxyl of the ribose, or the deoxyribose, while the bases are linked to the C1 of the sugar by an *N*-glycosidic bond. The nucleotides of DNA, since they contain the sugar deoxyribose, are called deoxyribonucleotides, while those of RNA, which contain ribose, are called ribonucleotides.

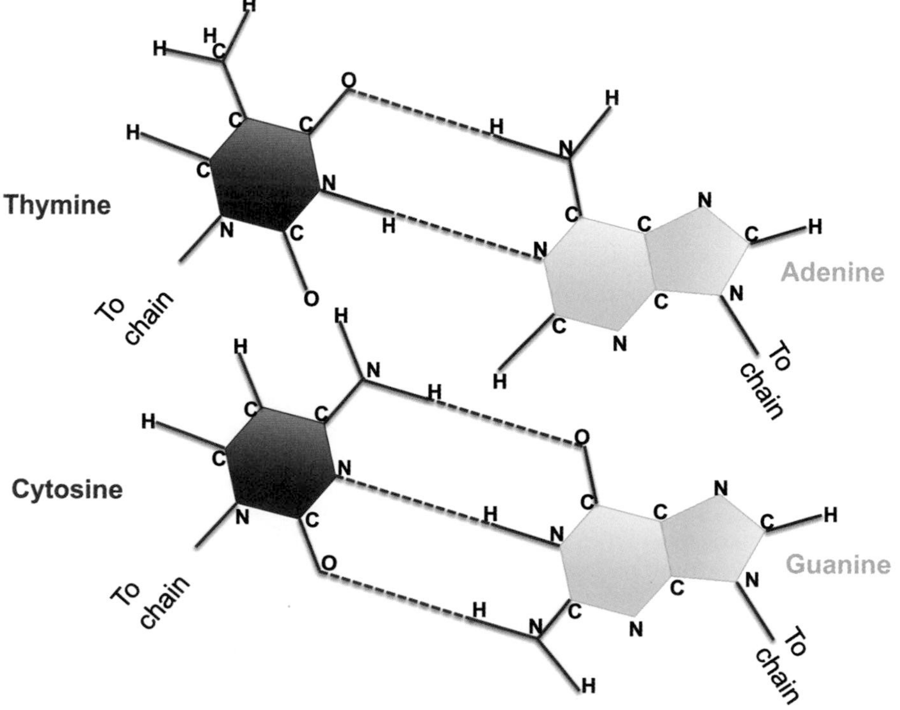

Figure 39-3 Hydrogen bonds. Pairs of bases, A-T and G-C, are linked by hydrogen bonds. There are two hydrogen bonds between A and T and three hydrogen bonds between G and C. Therefore, the G-C bond is more difficult (requires more energy) to break than the A-T bond. In this type of bond the hydrogen is located between two electron-attracting atoms, such as nitrogen and oxygen. When dsDNA is denatured, for example by heat or an alkaline pH, the hydrogen bonds between the bases break. Molecules that form hydrogen bonds to each other can form hydrogen bonds to water molecules.

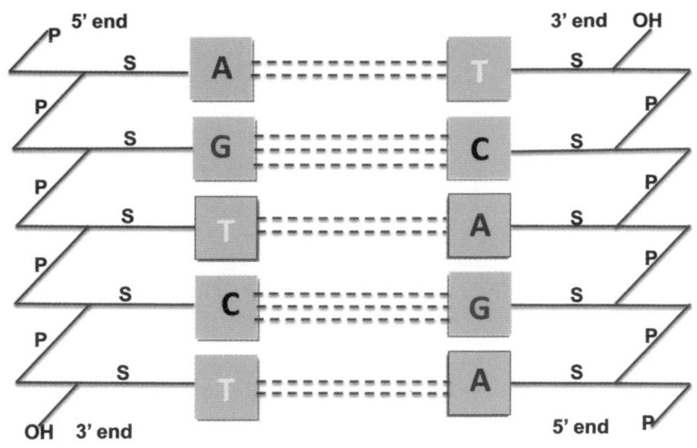

Figure 39-4 Double-stranded DNA. dsDNA is composed of two long polynucleotide chains that are complementary to each other; that is, their base sequence matches with each other: A-T and G-C. The structure of a dsDNA molecule resembles a ladder. The sugar (S) and phosphate (P), known as the "backbone" of the molecule, form the rails of the ladder while the bases correspond to the steps. The two chains have different polarity and run antiparallel to each other. As a result, the two ends of a dsDNA will have a deoxyribose at the 3′ end and a phosphate at the 5′ end. The linear sequence in a polynucleotide chain is always read starting from the 5′ end.

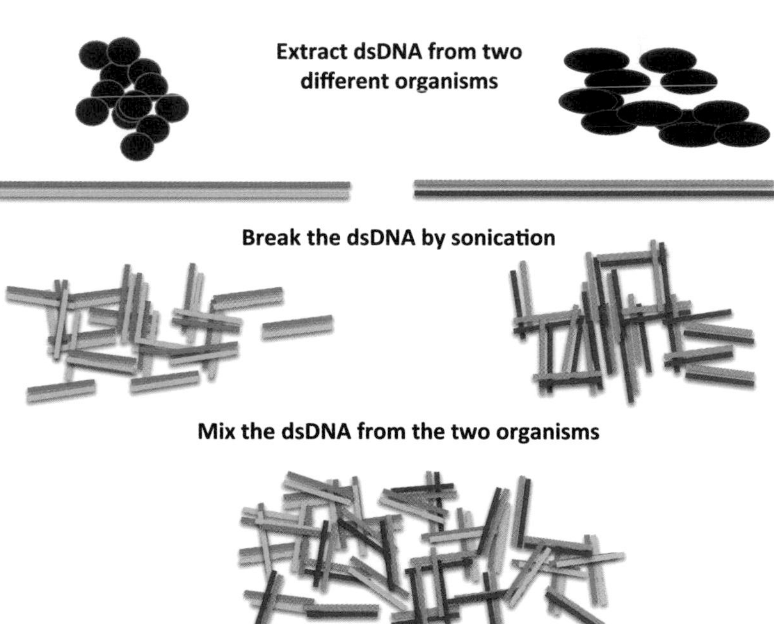

Figure 39-5 DNA:DNA and DNA:RNA hybridization. When a dsDNA molecule is denatured with heat, the two ssDNA molecules are not necessarily irreversibly separated. If a heated DNA solution is allowed to cool down slowly, an ssDNA may be able to reassociate with its complementary strand and reform the original dsDNA molecule. Similarly, if a complementary RNA sequence is added, a hybrid DNA:RNA molecule will be formed. Among the factors that affect the degree of specificity of the reassociation reaction, temperature, salt concentration, and the pH are very important. The "stringency" of the hybridization reaction can be restricted with those parameters, and therefore the degree of mismatched bases along the strands can be controlled. In this figure, the dsDNA from two unrelated organisms was first extracted, then sheared by sonication to make fragments 500 to 1,000 bp in length, and finally heated. The amount of heat required to dissociate the fragments of dsDNA is mainly dependent on the number of G-C bases present in each dsDNA fragment. The higher the number of G-C pairs, the higher the temperature. The melting temperature (*Tm*) of the dsDNA can be used to determine its base composition and is frequently utilized to verify the specificity of the amplified product of a nucleic acid amplification reaction. In this illustration it is assumed that there is no sequence homology between the DNA of the two organisms, so that upon reassociation the two genomes are independently reassociated.

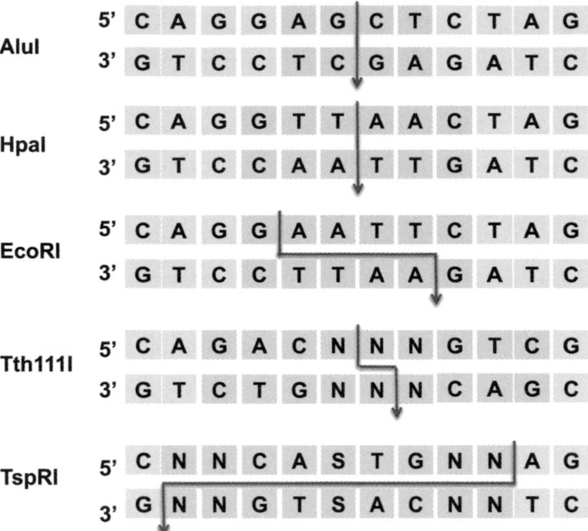

Figure 39-6 Restriction endonucleases. Restriction endonucleases are enzymes from bacteria that cleave the phosphodiester bond of DNA at specific sequences known as restriction sites. These sites are usually 4 to 8 base pairs (bp) in length and frequently have a palindromic structure, meaning that the sequence on one strand is identical to that of the complementary strand when read in the same orientation (e.g., 5′ to 3′). Assuming a random DNA sequence, there is an inverse relationship between the length of the recognition DNA sequence as cut by the enzyme and its frequency of occurrence. These enzymes are usually named after the bacterial species from which they were isolated. For example, as shown in this figure, EcoRI was isolated from *Escherichia coli* while HpaI was extracted from *Haemophilus parainfluenzae*. Restriction enzymes usually cut the DNA within the recognition sequence, although some of them cut at a nearby position. Enzymes that cut the same DNA sequence are called isoschizomers. Some of these enzymes, although they recognize the same sequence, may be affected differently by methylation. These enzymes make it possible to determine whether a segment of DNA is or is not methylated by comparing the fragments produced by cleaving the DNA with a methylation-sensitive and a methylation-insensitive isoschizomer. Abbreviations: S, C or G; N, A or T or C or G.

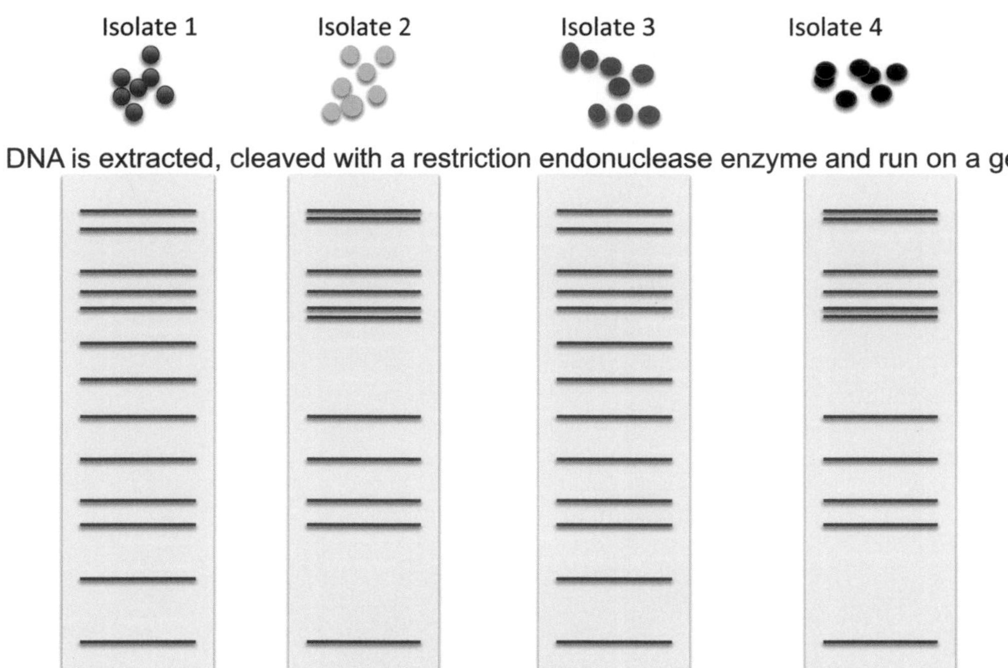

Figure 39-7 Restriction fragment length polymorphism (RFLP). In RFLP, DNA is digested with restriction endonucleases and the cleaved products are separated by gel electrophoresis. When DNA is cleaved with a restriction enzyme, several fragments are generated. The number and size of the fragments are a result of the distance between restriction sites in the DNA. Closely spaced restriction sites result in short-length DNA fragments, while those located at a greater distance yield long DNA fragments. Assuming that the bases in a particular DNA fragment are randomly distributed, we expect that a restriction enzyme that recognizes 4-bp sequences will generate more fragments than one that recognizes 8-bp sequences. The DNA fragments generated by the restriction endonucleases can be separated by electrophoresis in agarose or polyacrylamide gels. Because of the ionized phosphate groups at a mild alkaline pH, the DNA is negatively charged and migrates towards the anode. Small DNA fragments migrate faster than large segments. After electrophoresis, the DNA can be visualized in the gel by using fluorescent dyes. The DNA bands can be stained with ethidium bromide, and the cleavage pattern of different bacterial isolates can be compared. RFLP was one of the first techniques extensively used for genetic fingerprinting of pathogenic isolates. Based on the results shown in this figure, we can say that isolate 1 is closely related to isolate 3 and isolate 2 is related to 4.

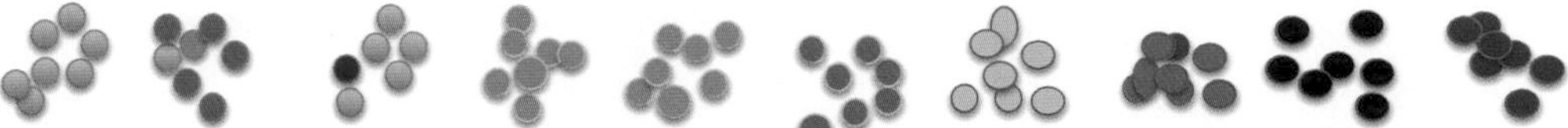

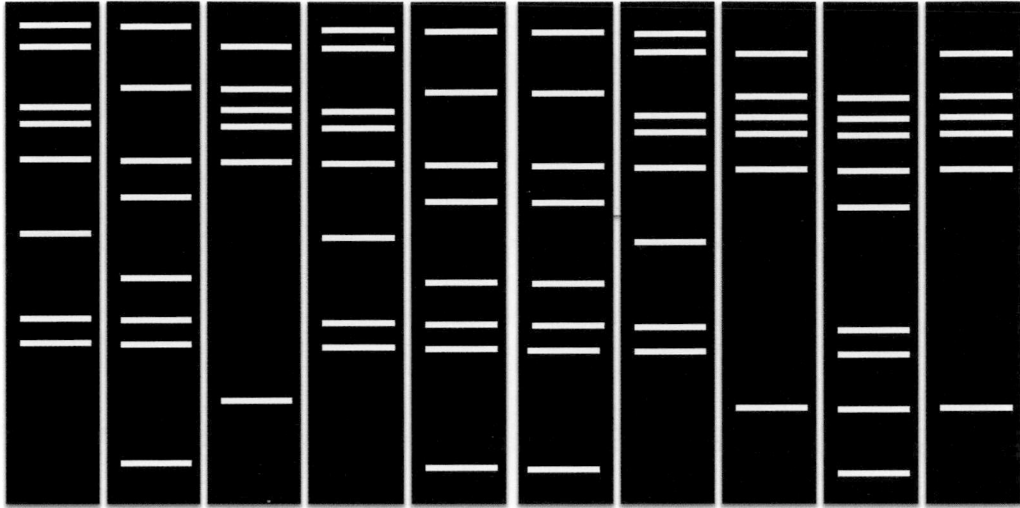

Figure 39-8 Pulsed-field gel electrophoresis (PFGE). PFGE is used for genotyping prokaryotes, and it was the gold standard for epidemiological studies until DNA sequencing became readily available. Large DNA fragments, 20 kb to >1 Mb, are separated by gel electrophoresis utilizing pulsed electrical fields. These large fragments are usually generated by digesting the DNA with "rare-cutting" restriction endonucleases, in general enzymes that recognize eight or more nucleotide bases. This technique is used because DNA fragments larger than 30 to 50 kb run at the same rate in standard gel electrophoresis. In contrast to the standard gel electrophoresis method, in which the voltage is constantly running in one direction, for PFGE the voltage is periodically switched among three directions. One direction is the central axis of the gel, and the other two run at a 60° angle on either side. This periodic change in field direction allows various lengths of DNA to change at different rates. Larger fragments of DNA will realign more slowly than smaller pieces when the field direction is changed. The separated fragments can be visualized, for example by using ethidium bromide. This figure shows that control 1 is related to isolates 3 and 6 while control 2 is related to isolates 2 and 7.

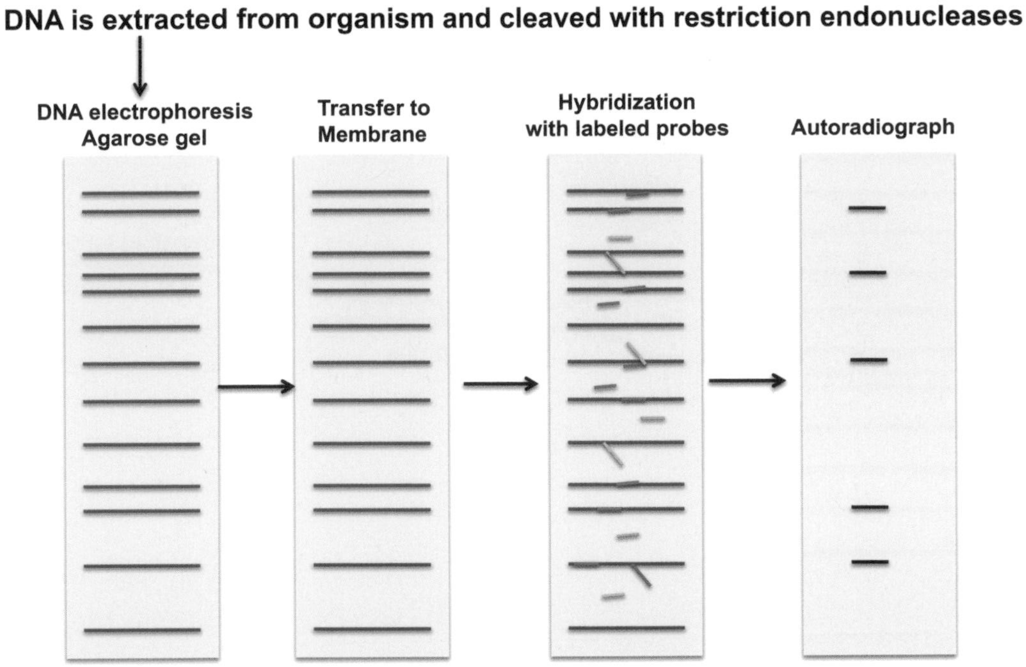

Figure 39-9 Southern blot. For Southern blots, since gels are fragile, after electrophoresis of the restriction endonuclease-digested fragments, the DNA is transferred (blotted) to a positively charged membrane, usually nitrocellulose or nylon, where the DNA binds. To make the transfer, the DNA is treated with alkali, which results in the formation of ssDNA. To identify specific fragments on the membrane, the Southern blot uses labeled ssDNA probes unique to the regions of interest. The probe hybridizes to the complementary sequence blotted on the membrane. Factors that significantly affect the specificity of the binding include the salt concentration of the buffer and the temperature. This technique can be used to test for mutations, deletions, and the presence of specific gene sequences, among others.

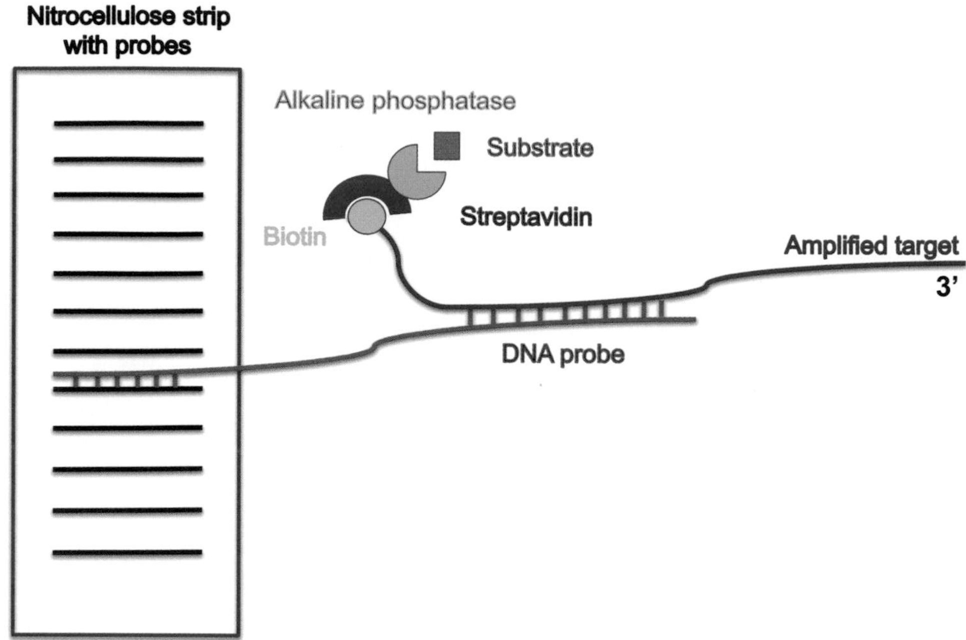

Figure 39-10 Line probe assays. In line probe assays (Immunogenetics, Ghent, Belgium), oligonucleotides specific for the target of interest are attached to nitrocellulose strips. The biotin-labeled amplified target nucleic acid to be identified is hybridized to the immobilized probes on the nitrocellulose membrane. Following hybridization, streptavidin-labeled probes with alkaline phosphatase are added and incubated to bind to the hybrids. Addition of a chromogen results in the production of a color precipitate. DNA probes that hybridize to rRNA are frequently utilized to detect bacteria. The number of copies of rRNA present per bacterial cell is at least 10,000, and therefore it is a good target for detection. This assay has been used for the identification of *Mycobacterium tuberculosis*, for analysis of drug resistance in *M. tuberculosis* and *Helicobacter pylori*, and for the genotyping of several viruses.

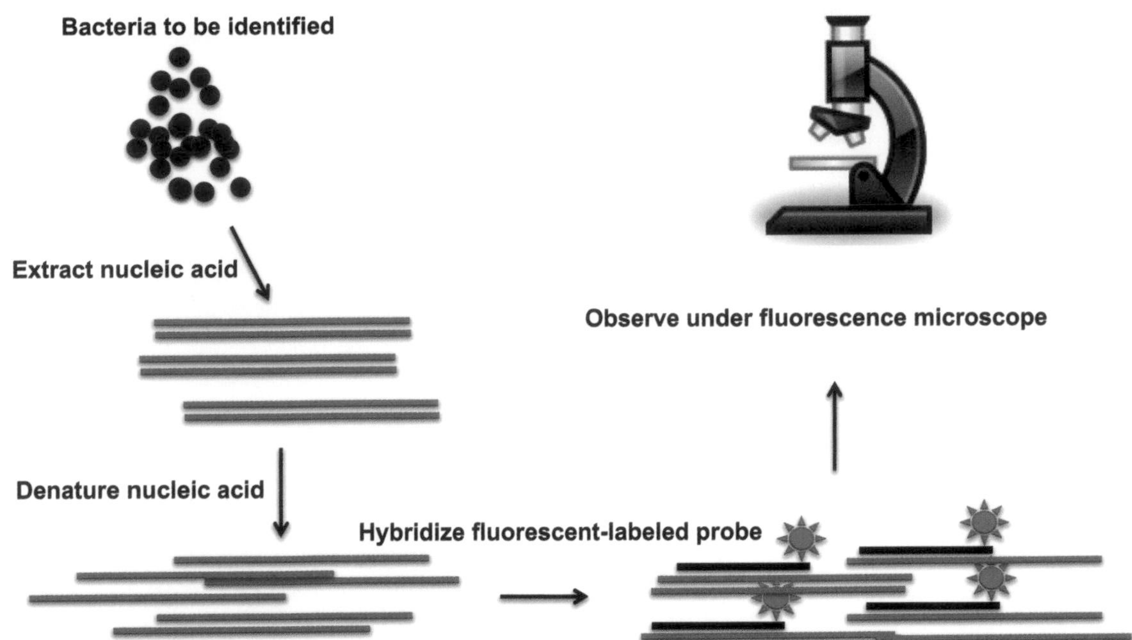

Figure 39-11 Fluorescent in situ hybridization (FISH). FISH is a method in which a fluorescent-labeled probe is hybridized to the target nucleic acid. The probes either can be directly labeled (direct technique) or have a hapten, such as biotin or digoxigenin, that can be detected by a fluorescently labeled conjugate (indirect technique). The direct technique is shown here. This assay is used in cases of sepsis to discriminate between *Staphylococcus aureus* and coagulase-negative staphylococci and also to differentiate *Candida albicans* from other *Candida* species.

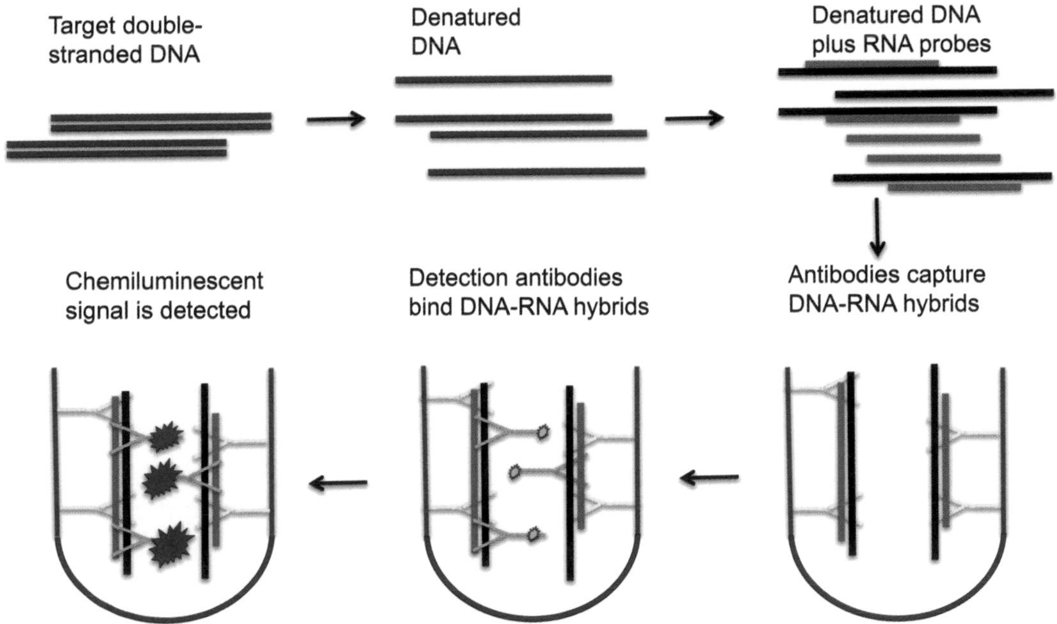

Figure 39-12 Hybrid capture assay. In the hybrid capture assay (Qiagen, Germantown, MD), the target DNA is denatured and then hybridized to a complementary RNA probe. Antibodies bound to a solid phase, specific for the DNA-RNA hybrid, capture this complex. Alkaline phosphatase-conjugated anti–RNA-DNA hybrid antibodies are subsequently added. The bound antibody conjugate is detected by using a chemiluminescent substrate, and the light is measured in a luminometer. Hybrid capture assays are available for the detection of *Neisseria gonorrhoeae*, *Chlamydia trachomatis*, and several viruses.

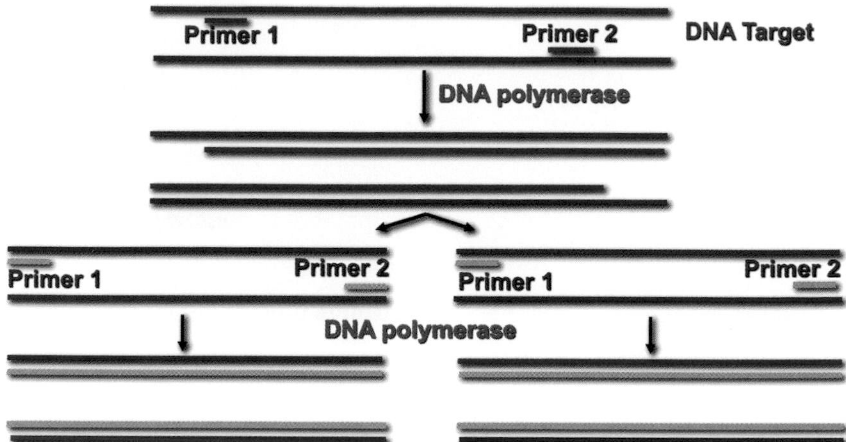

Figure 39-13 PCR (polymerase chain reaction). In PCR amplification, in addition to the target dsDNA, two oligonucleotides (primers), a heat-stable DNA polymerase, and the four deoxyribonucleotide triphosphates (dNTPs) are added in a buffer solution. The two primers are complementary to opposite strands of the target and are usually at a distance of 100 to 500 bp from each other. The reaction starts by increasing the temperature to approximately 95°C to denature the target dsDNA. This is followed by cooling to approximately 60 to 65°C to allow the primers to anneal to the target DNA. The DNA polymerase then initiates the extension of the primers, producing new dsDNA copies. Under ideal conditions, the number of target sequences doubles at each cycle. In a 100% efficient reaction, after 20 cycles a 10^6-fold amplification occurs and after 30 cycles a 10^9-fold amplification is obtained. The amplified DNA can be detected by using various methods including fluorescent dyes, such as ethidium bromide after running a gel, or by using labeled oligonucleotides complementary to the amplified target. Internal controls can be included in the reaction to make sure that no inhibitory substances such as hemoglobin interfered with the amplification. Numerous commercial kits are available for the detection of pathogens using PCR.

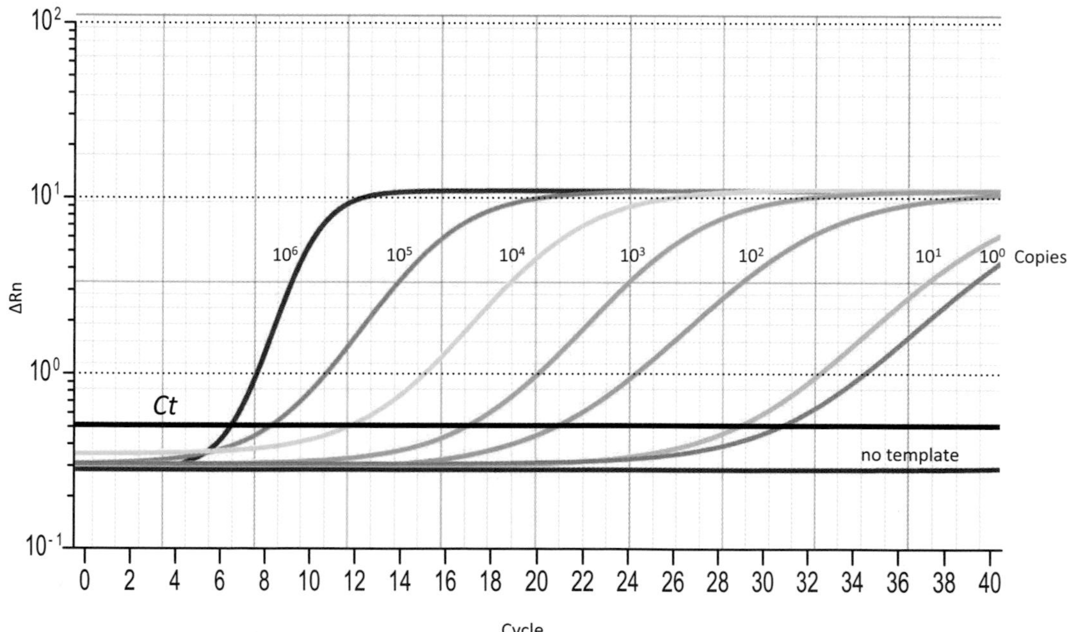

Figure 39-14 Real-time PCR. In this type of PCR, the amplification of the target and the detection of the amplified product occur simultaneously. Using different dyes, fluorescence emission is generated proportional to the amount of the amplified product. This figure shows the normalized fluorescence signal from the reporter dye depending on the initial input of target sequences. The cycle threshold (*Ct*) is the cycle number at which fluorescence passes the fixed threshold. The number of copies in the sample is calculated by determining the *Ct* and using a standard curve to determine the starting number of nucleic acid copies. Several commercially available kits are available for the detection of a wide variety of bacterial pathogens, including *Mycobacterium tuberculosis*, *Clostridium difficile*, *Chlamydia trachomatis*, *Neisseria gonorrhoeae*, *Staphylococcus aureus*, and *Streptococcus agalactiae*.

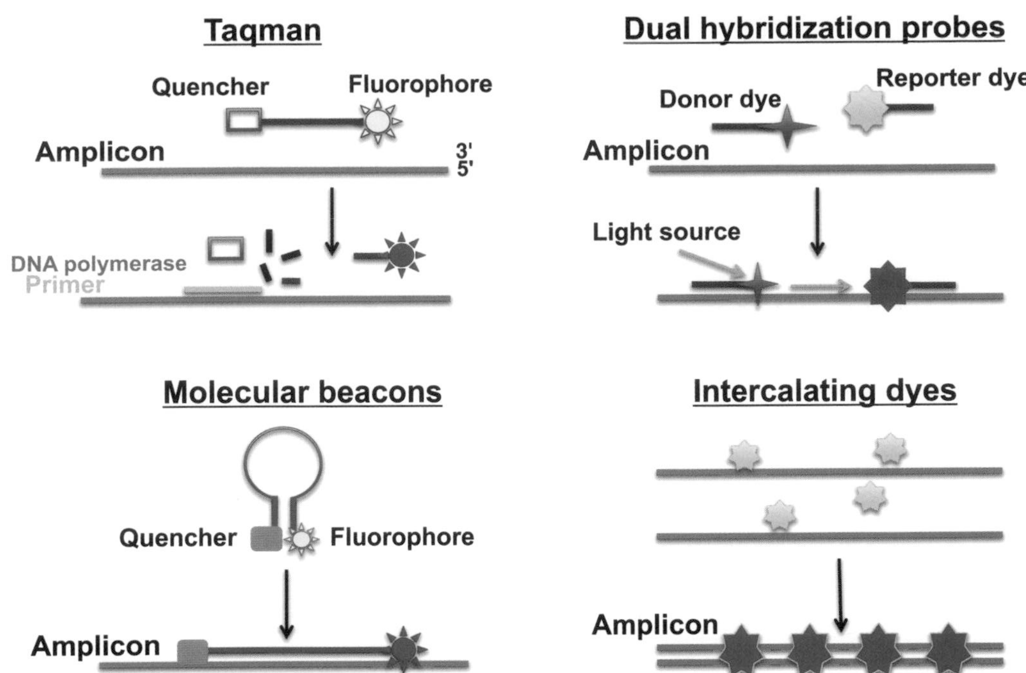

Figure 39-15 Molecular probes. Different approaches can be used to detect the product of an amplification reaction in real time. Dyes such as SYBR Green I intercalate into dsDNA and can therefore be used to determine the amount of dsDNA product during nucleic amplification reactions. The FRET probes are labeled with a fluorescent dye and a quencher. The distance in the probe between the dye and the quencher is such that the fluorescence of the dye is absorbed by the quencher. In the case of the TaqMan method, the probe hybridizes to the target DNA, and when the exonuclease activity of the *Taq* DNA polymerase digests the probe, the fluorescent dye is released. Alternatively, as also shown in this figure, dual hybridization probes have the dye and the quencher in different oligonucleotides which come into proximity only after they both anneal to the amplified target DNA.

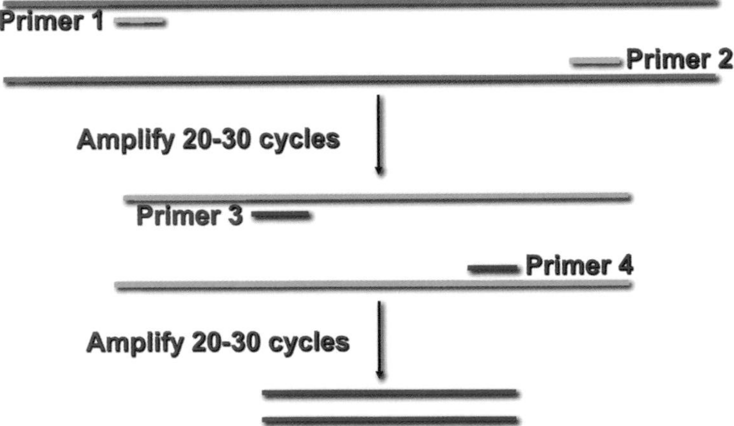

Figure 39-16 Nested PCR. The nested PCR uses two sets of primers. Following amplification with the first set of primers, a second set of oligonucleotides, complementary to the sequence that was amplified during the first round, is added and the amplification continues. The main purpose of the nested PCR is to increase the sensitivity of the assay. Problems of contamination due to carryover are difficult to avoid with this method unless it is a completely closed system.

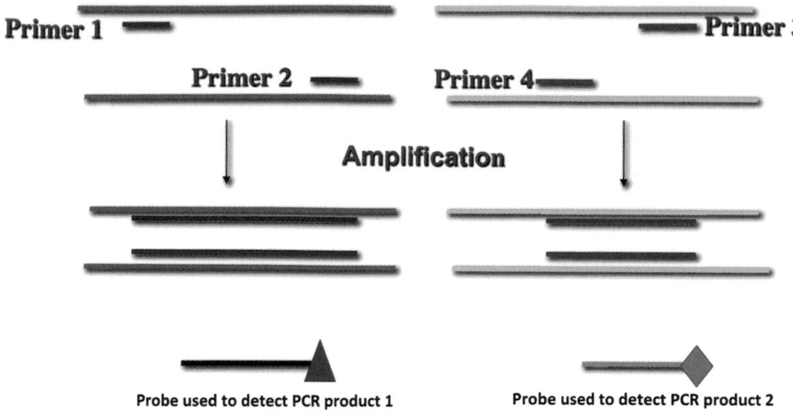

Figure 39-17 Multiplex PCR. The purpose of the multiplex PCR is to amplify different targets in the same reaction. Primers have to be selected that have similar annealing temperatures and are not complementary to each other. Following amplification, the products of each set of primers can be detected by using probes specific for each amplified product. Several companies have kits for the detection of multiple bacterial and viral pathogens, including Prodesse (Gen-Probe, San Diego, CA), Luminex Corp. (Austin, TX), and BioFire (Salt Lake City, UT).

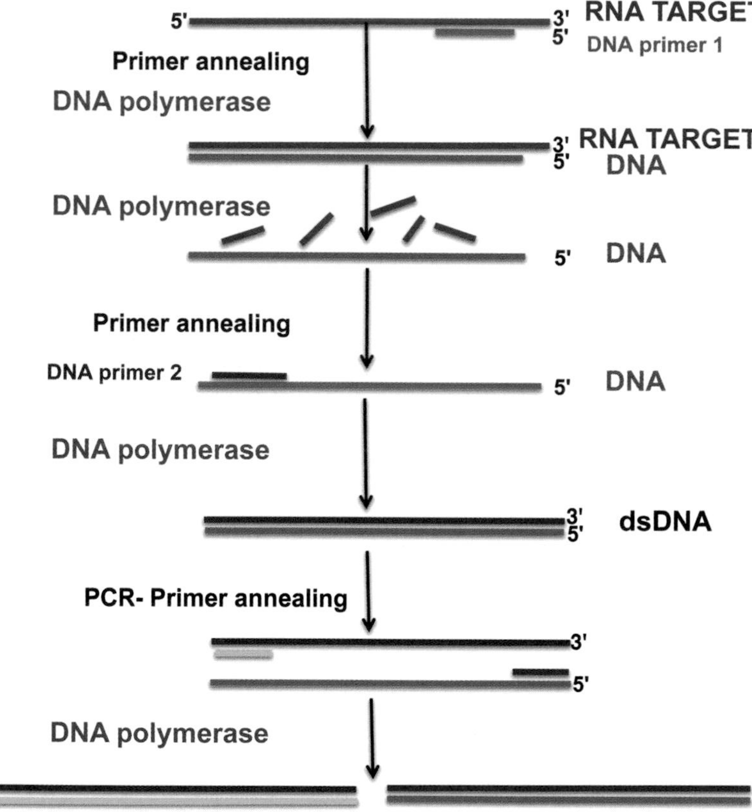

Figure 39-18 Reverse transcriptase PCR. Most of the work originally performed with PCR involved the amplification of DNA. To amplify RNA, a reverse transcription step was incorporated to produce complementary DNA (cDNA) to the target RNA. The use of a thermostable DNA polymerase that, under the appropriate conditions, has both reverse transcriptase and DNA polymerase activity permits the complete reaction to occur using a single enzyme.

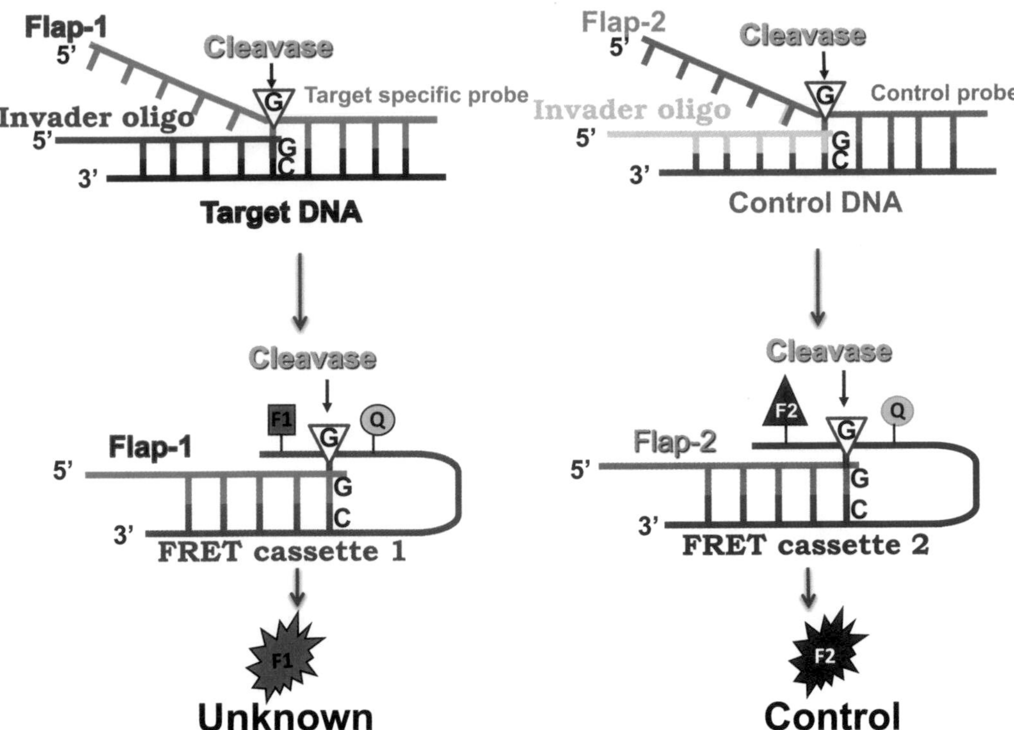

Figure 39-19 Hologic-Cervista molecular assay. The Cervista (Hologic, Bedford, MA) method uses the Invader chemistry, a signal amplification method, for the detection of specific nucleic acid sequences. Two isothermal reactions, a primary reaction directed to the target DNA and a secondary reaction that generates a fluorescent signal, occur simultaneously. In the primary reaction the probe and the Invader oligonucleotide bind to the DNA target. When this oligonucleotide overlaps by at least 1 bp with the target DNA, an invasive structure forms that serves as the substrate for the Cleavase enzyme. The cleaved flap then binds to the hairpin fluorescence resonance energy transfer (FRET) oligonucleotide, forming another invasive structure that the Cleavase also cuts. This separates the fluorophore from the quencher, producing the fluorescence signal. The probes are added in large molar excess, and they cycle rapidly, resulting in a 10^6- to 10^7-fold signal amplification per hour. When human specimens are tested, a positive internal control, the human histone 2 gene, is also present and is detected with different primary and secondary probes. This internal control helps to confirm that negative results are not due to insufficient sample or inhibitory substances, and to ensure that the testing procedure was performed correctly.

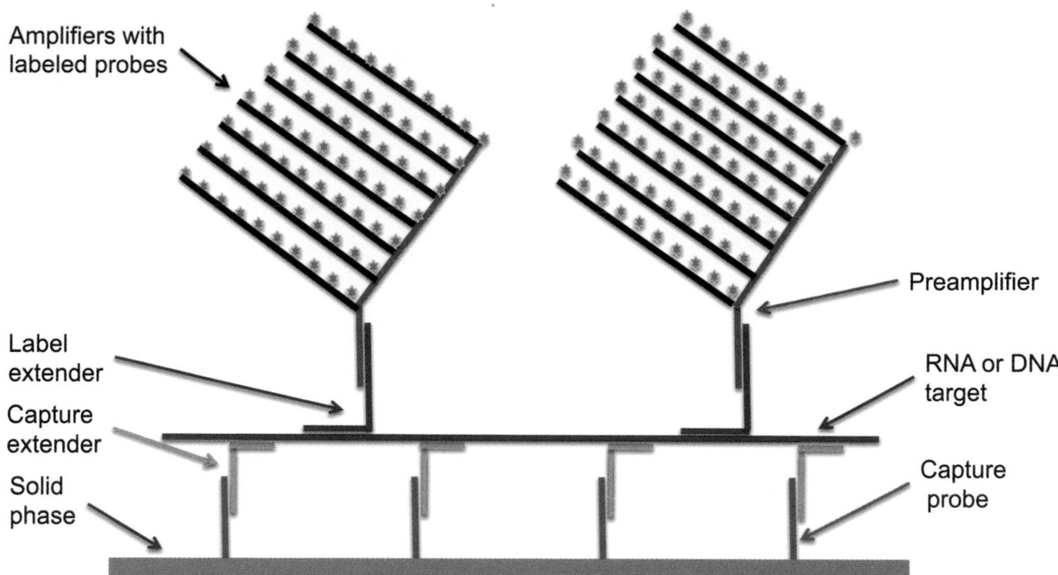

Figure 39-20 Branched DNA. Branched DNA (Siemens Healthcare Diagnostics, Deerfield, IL) is a signal amplification sandwich hybridization system that incorporates the addition of multiple synthetic oligonucleotide probes. As shown in the figure, capture probes attached to a solid phase, such as a microtiter plate, bind to capture extenders that are also complementary to the DNA or RNA target of interest. Label extender probes, also complementary to the DNA or RNA target, are then added. Preamplifier molecules subsequently bind to the label extender probes and to amplifiers. Alkaline phosphatase-labeled probes hybridize to the amplifiers. When dioxetane is added, the light emission produced is measured by a luminometer. The amount of signal is proportional to the quantity of the target in the sample, and the number of target copies is calculated by using an external standard curve. So far this method has been used for the identification and quantitation of viruses.

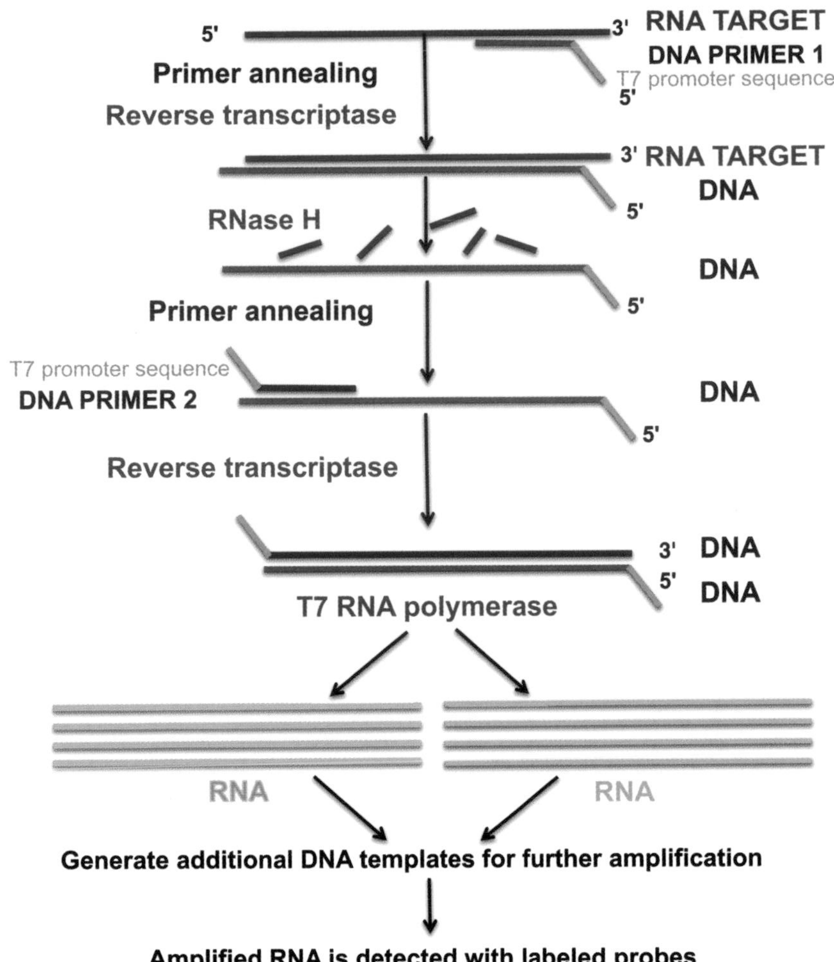

Figure 39-21 Transcription-based amplification. Transcription-based amplification (Gen-Probe Inc., San Diego, CA) and nucleic acid sequence-based amplification are isothermal methods that amplify RNA targets using retroviral replication as the model. A DNA primer, containing sequences complementary to the target RNA and the T7 RNA polymerase promoter, is hybridized to the target RNA. The reverse transcriptase synthesizes complementary DNA (cDNA). The RNase H enzyme then degrades the target RNA of the RNA-DNA hybrid. A second primer binds to the cDNA, and the DNA polymerase activity of the reverse transcriptase extends the primer, resulting in the formation of a dsDNA containing the T_7 RNA polymerase promoter at both ends. Using the cDNA as template, the T_7 RNA polymerase synthesizes multiple copies of ssRNA that reenter the cycle. The RNA products of the reaction can be detected and quantitated by using oligonucleotide probes. Alternatively, the amplification products can be measured using real-time methods. These assays are commercially available for *Mycobacterium tuberculosis*, *Mycoplasma genitalium*, *Chlamydia trachomatis*, *Neisseria gonorrhoeae*, and other bacterial and viral pathogens.

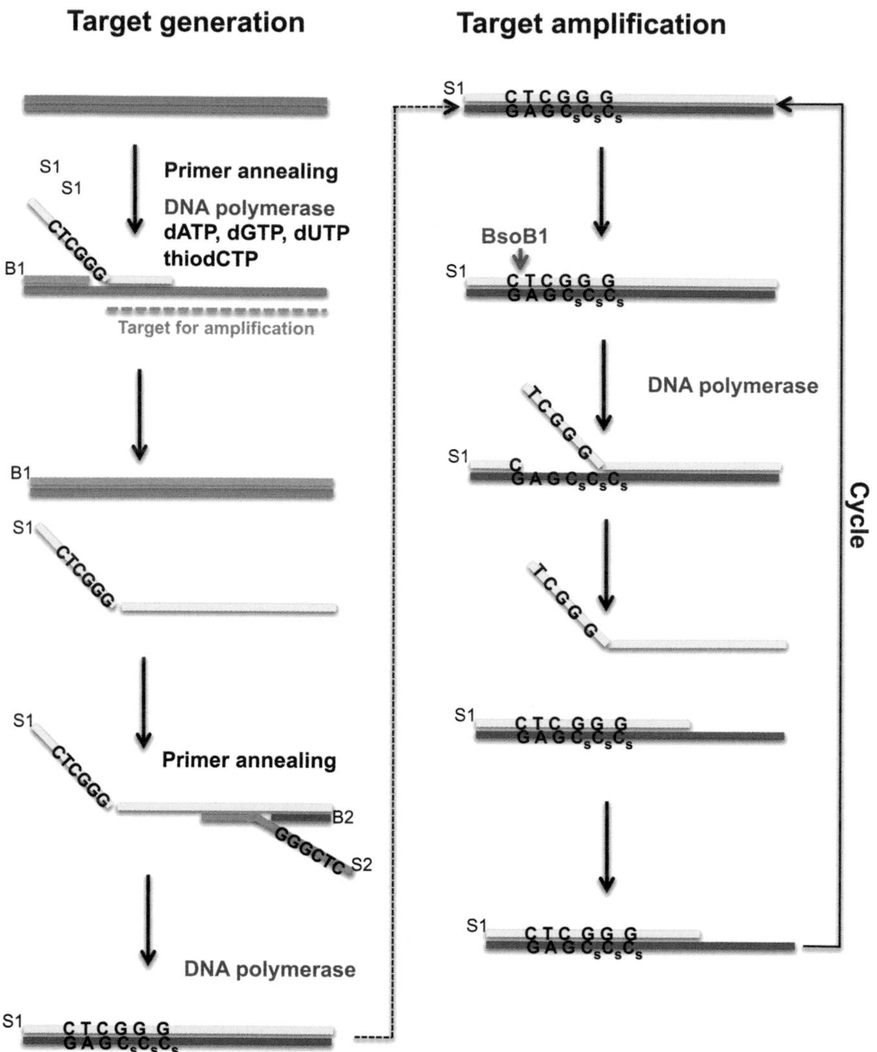

Figure 39-22 Strand displacement amplification. Strand displacement amplification (BD Diagnostic Systems, Franklin Lakes, NJ) is an isothermal method that can be used to amplify DNA or RNA. As shown in this figure, dsDNA is denatured and hybridized to two different oligonucleotides, called bumper and amplification primers. The amplification primer includes the single-stranded restriction endonuclease enzyme sequence of BsoBI at the 5′ end. The bumper primer anneals to the target DNA upstream from the segment to be amplified. Three standard deoxynucleotide triphosphates, dATP, dGTP, and dUTP, in addition to a thiolated dCTP (C_s), are added. Simultaneous extension of both primers results in the displacement of the amplification primer, which can then hybridize with the opposite strand. The BsoBI enzyme binds to the amplified products and, due to the C_s, only nicks the strand rather than cleaving it. The DNA polymerase binds to the nicked site and synthesizes a new strand while simultaneously displacing the downstream strand, thus generating dsDNA with the same structural characteristics which reenters the cycle. Labeled probes can be used to detect the amplified products by using a real-time method. The figure only shows amplification for one strand, but both strands of the dsDNA are amplified simultaneously. Commercially available kits are available for the detection of *Chlamydia trachomatis* and *Neisseria gonorrhoeae* using this approach.

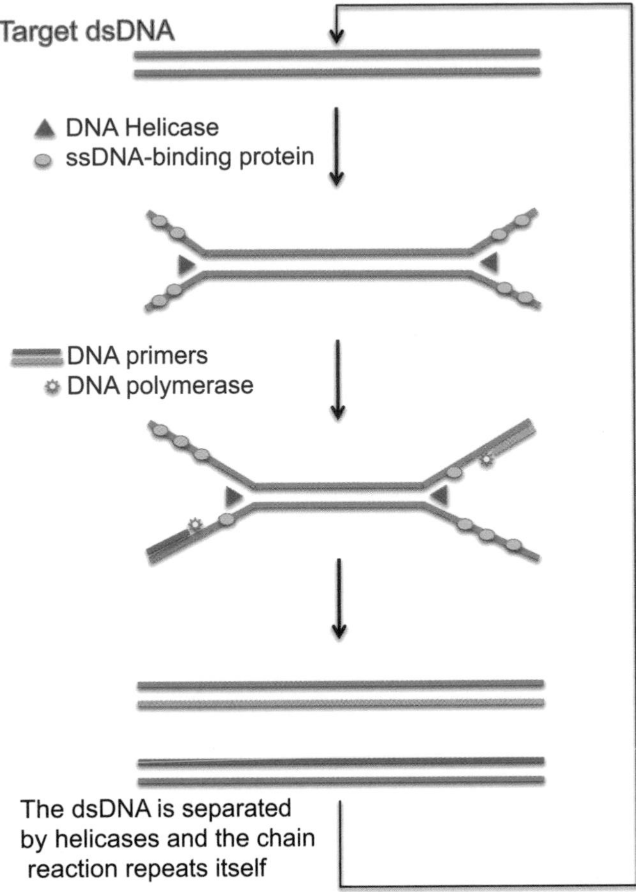

Figure 39-23 Helicase-dependent amplification. In this isothermal amplification method (BioHelix, Beverly, MA), the dsDNA is separated by two enzymes, helicase and the ssDNA-coated ssDNA binding protein, resulting in two ssDNA templates. These two enzymes, therefore, replace the increase in temperature that is used in a standard PCR to separate the two DNA strands. Specific primers are added and a DNA polymerase extends the strands. The newly synthesized products continue to cycle and can be detected with a variety of probes. Assays to detect *Chlamydia trachomatis*, *Neisseria gonorrhoeae*, *Helicobacter pylori*, and other pathogens are under development. (Adapted from Vincent et al., *EMBO Rep.* 5:793–800, 2004.)

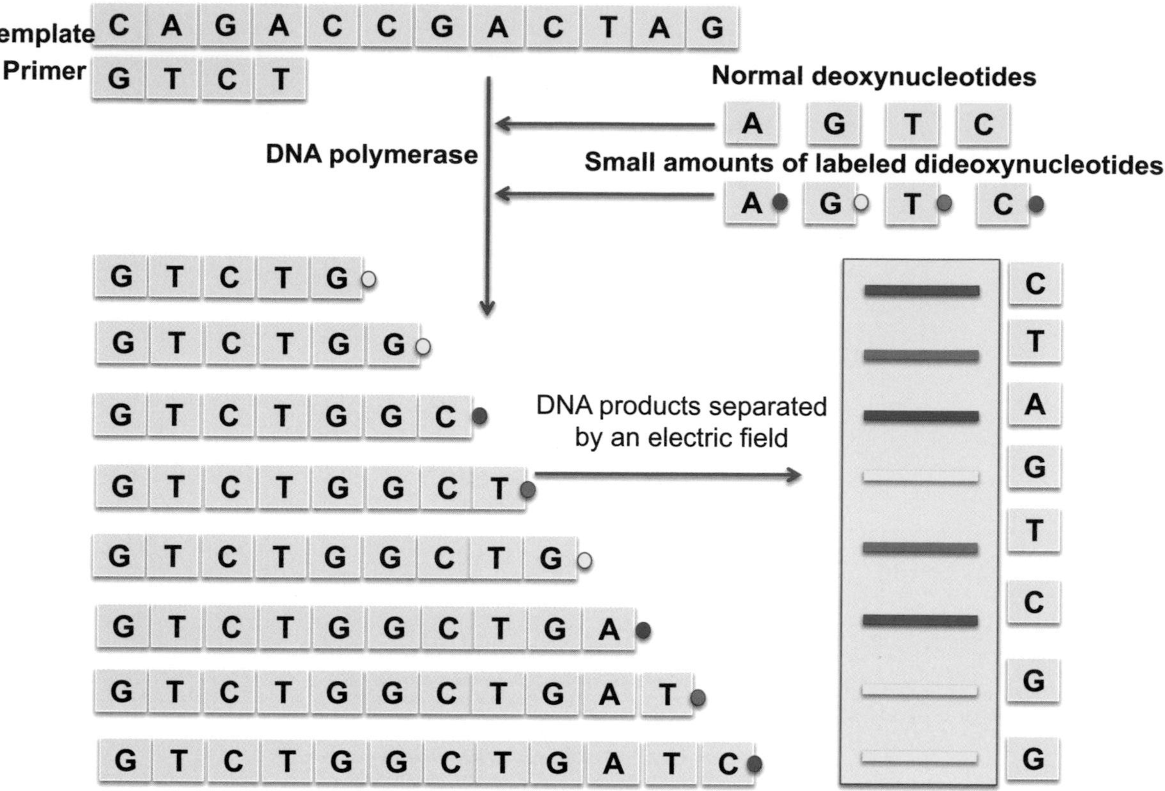

Figure 39-24 DNA sequencing (Sanger method). To perform DNA sequencing using the Sanger method, PCR is performed. In addition to the four regular deoxynucleotides, small amounts of four fluorescent-labeled 2′,3′-dideoxynucleotides are included in the reaction. Incorporation of a 2′,3′-dideoxynucleotide by the DNA polymerase results in termination of the elongation reaction. Therefore, the last base incorporated into that DNA strand will correspond to the labeled 2′,3′-dideoxynucleotide. The DNA fragments are size analyzed by gel or capillary electrophoresis. A laser beam can be used to read the four different fluorescent labels corresponding to the four different bases.

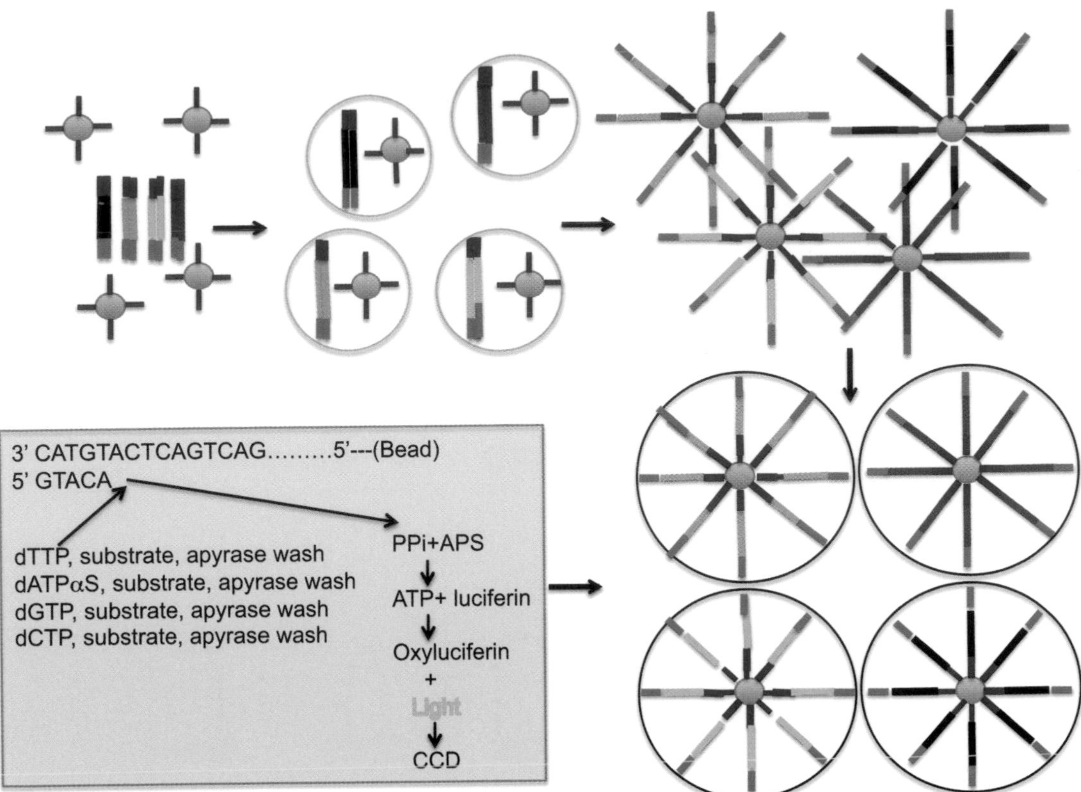

Figure 39-25 Pyrosequencing. In the pyrosequencing method (Roche 454; Roche, Basel, Switzerland), an adaptor-flanked shotgun library of the DNA to be sequenced is constructed in vitro. The adaptor sequences are all the same and can be used to perform a multitemplate PCR with a single primer pair. The other primer has a 5′-biotin tag that binds to micrometer-scale (28 μm) streptavidin-coated beads. After binding to the beads, a PCR is performed in water-in-oil emulsions at a very low concentration of the template so that, in the majority of the bead compartments, there is only one template molecule. The products of the PCR are then captured by primers on the surface of the beads. The water-in-oil emulsion is subsequently broken, and the beads are treated with denaturant to remove untethered strands, enriched for amplicon-bearing beads, and transferred to arrays of picoliter wells so that only one bead can fit inside a well. The sequencing primers are hybridized to the universal adaptor immediately adjacent to the start of the segment to be sequenced. Each microwell has channels that allow the addition of the enzymes required for sequencing and reaction detection, including the *Bacillus stearothermophilus* polymerase, single-stranded binding protein, ATP sulfurylase, luciferase, and the substrates luciferin and adenosine 5′-phosphosulfate. For sequencing, one side of the array functions as a flow cell for introducing and removing reagents and the other side has a charge-coupled device (CCD) for signal detection. At each cycle, a single unlabeled nucleotide is introduced in each well (dATPαS, which is not a substrate for luciferase, is added instead of dATP). On the templates where the complementary nucleotide is present, this results in the incorporation of the incoming nucleotide, and pyrophosphate is released. For each nucleotide incorporated, a pyrophosphate is generated that is detected by the CCD. On the other hand, if the complementary nucleotide is not present, no light is produced. The well is then washed with apyrase to remove unincorporated nucleotide, and then the next nucleotide is flowed. A limitation of this approach is the presence of segments with the same base, such as TT or CCCCC. Although the intensity of the luminescence should be proportional to the number of nucleotides incorporated, this is not easy to quantitate. An advantage of the system is that it can sequence 400×10^6 to 600×10^6 bp per run at lengths of 400 to 500 bp. (Adapted from Shendure and Ji, *Nat. Biotechnol.* **26:**1135–1145, 2008.)

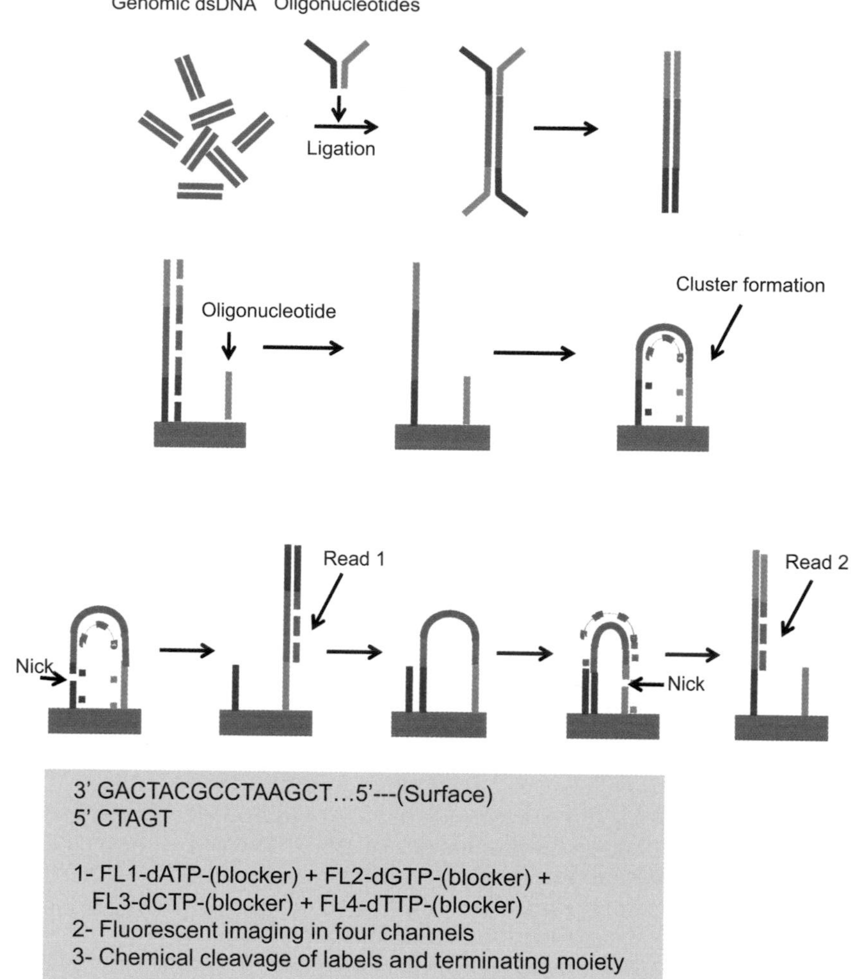

Figure 39-26 Cluster DNA sequencing using reversible dye terminators. In cluster DNA sequencing (Illumina Genome Analyzer; Illumina Inc., San Diego, CA), the dsDNA from the genome to be sequenced is sheared and ligated to a pair of oligonucleotides. The DNA is then amplified using two oligonucleotide primers, yielding double-stranded blunt-ended fragments with a different adapter on either end. To generate clonal single molecule arrays, the dsDNA is denatured and the single strands are annealed to oligonucleotides attached to the surface of a flow cell. A new strand is copied from the original ssDNA, using as a primer the surface-bound oligonucleotide. The original ssDNA is removed by denaturation, and the adapter sequence at the 3′ end of each copied strand is annealed to a new complementary oligonucleotide that is attached to the surface of the flow cell, generating a bridge-like structure. A dsDNA is subsequently synthesized, and multiple cycles of annealing, extension, and denaturation result in the synthesis of DNA clusters. Bridge amplification, therefore, yields multiple clusters attached to a surface, with each cluster representing a single template. To sequence each cluster, the DNA is linearized using a cleavage site within one adapter oligonucleotide. These templates are now sequenced by utilizing reversible dye terminator nucleotides. Each nucleotide is labeled with a different color of fluorophore, and every time one of these nucleotides is incorporated the extension reaction is terminated. The fluorophore is linked to the pyrimidine or purine bases through a cleavable disulfide linker. The steric hindrance of the cleavable fluorophore is what confers terminating properties to the free 3′-OH-modified nucleotides. In each cluster, the nucleotide that has been incorporated is detected before the terminator group is removed and the next labeled reversible dye terminator nucleotide is added. Imaging, using four channels to detect the incorporation of each of the four nucleotides in each cluster, determines the sequence of the DNA. (Adapted from Bentley et al., *Nature* **456:**53–59, 2008; Turcatti et al., *Nucleic Acids Res.* **36:**e25, 2008; and Shendure and Ji, *Nat. Biotechnol.* **26:**1135–1145, 2008).

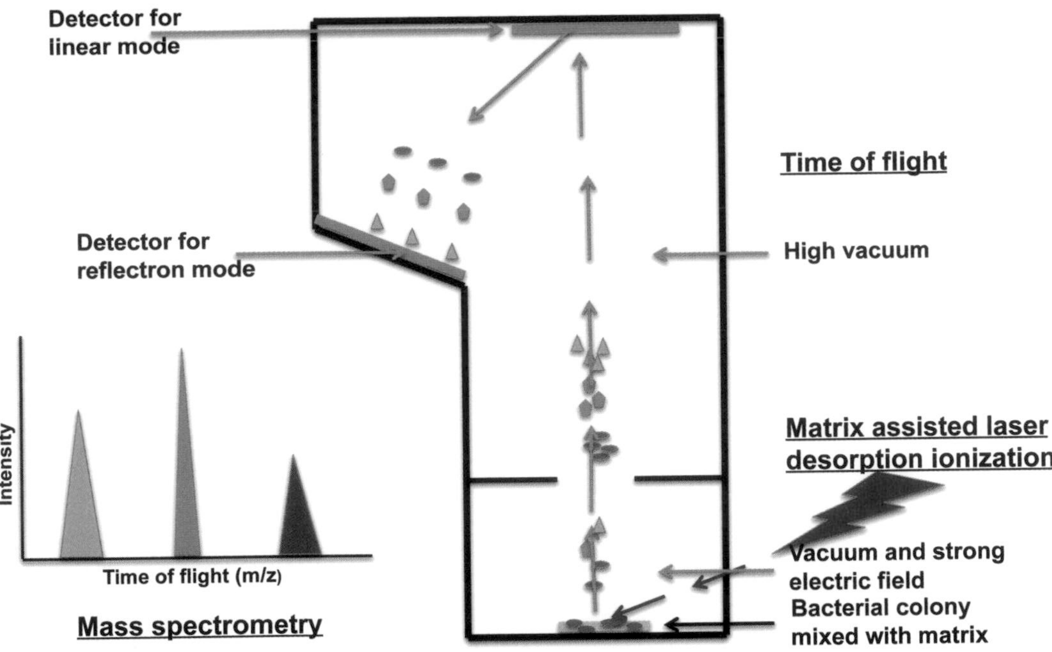

Figure 39-27 Matrix-assisted laser desorption/ionization time-of-flight mass spectrometry (MALDI-TOF). Mass spectrometry is an analytical method that allows fast and precise determination of the mass of molecules, including proteins and nucleic acids, in a range from 100 Da to 100 kDa. In the case of MALDI-TOF, molecules such as proteins are embedded in a matrix consisting of low-molecular-weight organic acids, frequently α-cyano-4-hydroxy-cinnamic acid. As a result of exposure to laser pulses, energy is transferred from the matrix to the analyte molecule. The analyte is desorbed (removed) into the gas phase, and the ionized molecules are accelerated in the flight tube by electric potentials based on their mass/charge ratio (*m*/*z*). The ionized molecules collide with a detector, generating a profile that is then compared with a collection of patterns of well-characterized controls. The method used for the identification of bacteria requires approximately 10^4 to 10^5 CFU from a well-isolated colony. In some systems the bacteria are directly transferred to the mass spectrometry plate. Alternatively, the bacteria, or other pathogens such as fungi, are first fixed with ethanol, and the proteins are extracted with formic acid and acetonitrile before they are mixed with the matrix solution. Most of the bacterial components detected by MALDI-TOF are intracellular proteins in the 4- to 15-kDa range, including ribosomal and mitochondrial proteins, cold- and heat-shock proteins, DNA binding proteins, and RNA chaperone proteins. Mass spectrometry is also being used to detect and identify amplified nucleic acids and to do sequencing.

Stains, Media, and Reagents 40

Bacteria are identified in the clinical laboratory by a variety of methods including microscopy, growth characteristics, reactions to organic and inorganic compounds, and molecular techniques. The purpose of this chapter is to present images of the more common stains, media, and tests used in the diagnostic medical microbiology laboratory. The Gram stain is the most widely used method to visualize bacteria. Shown here are examples of the various sizes, shapes, and arrangements of both aerobic and anaerobic bacteria found in clinical specimens. Also included are some of the most common culture media used in the laboratory for demonstrating growth, isolation, colonial morphology, hemolysis, pigment production, and other distinguishing bacterial characteristics. The following images illustrate some of the key tests that have been shown over the years to be most helpful for the identification of clinical isolates.

STAINS

Gram Stain

The Gram stain is one of the most important procedures in bacteriology. It is used to classify bacteria on the basis of their size, shape, arrangement, and Gram reaction. It was originally described in 1884 by Christian Gram; the modification currently in use was developed by Hucker in 1921. The reagents and stains used in Hucker's modification include crystal violet, Gram's iodine, acetone alcohol, and safranin. The figures in this section demonstrate a variety of morphotypes as well as Gram reactions.

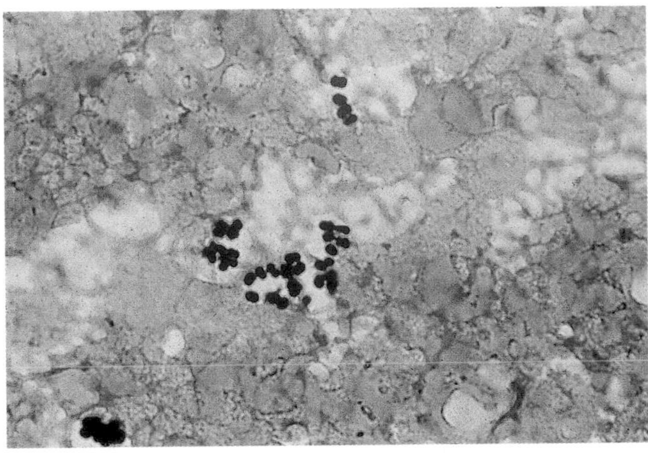

Figure 40-1 Gram-positive cocci in pairs and clusters.

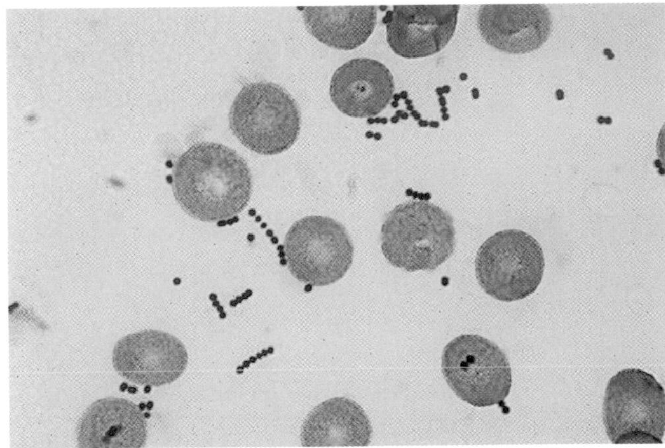

Figure 40-2 Gram-positive cocci in pairs and short chains.

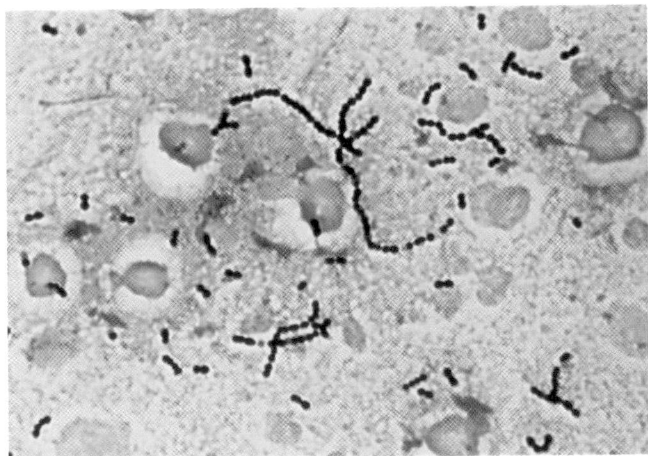

Figure 40-3 Gram-positive cocci in pairs and chains.

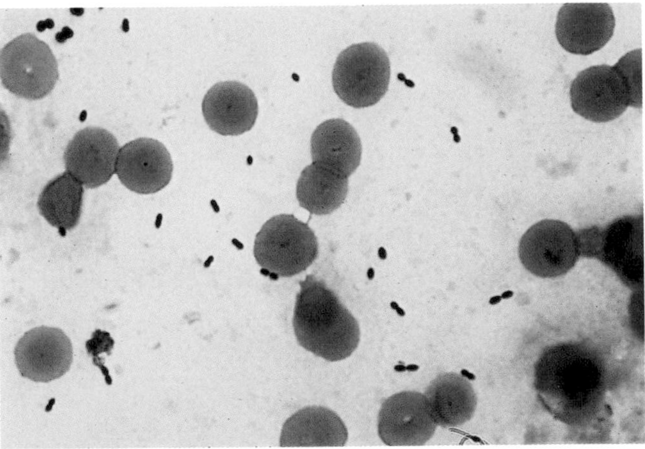

Figure 40-4 Lancet-shaped, gram-positive diplococci.

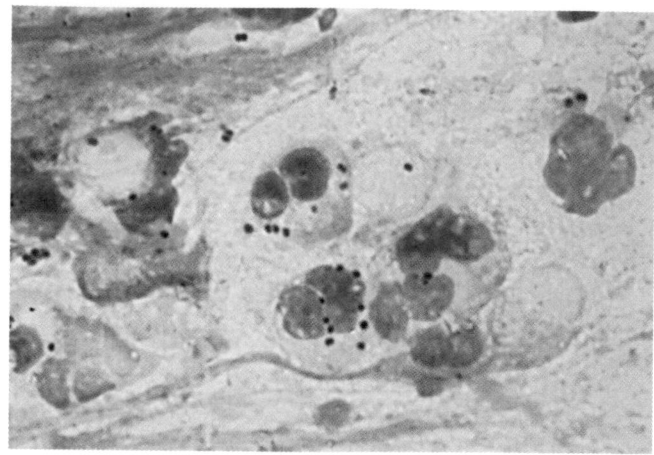

Figure 40-5 Intracellular, gram-negative diplococci.

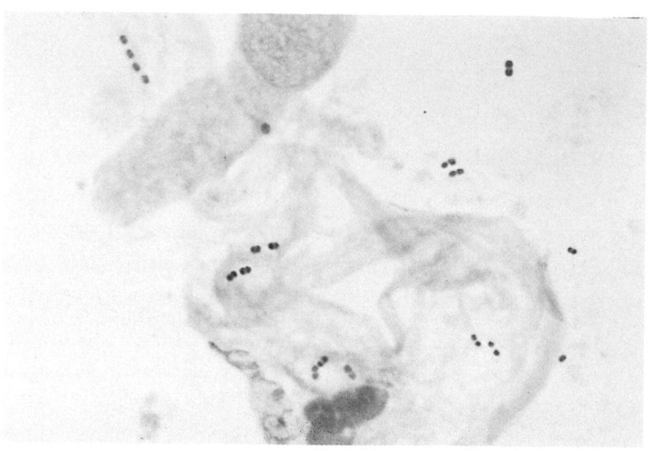

Figure 40-6 Small, gram-negative coccobacilli.

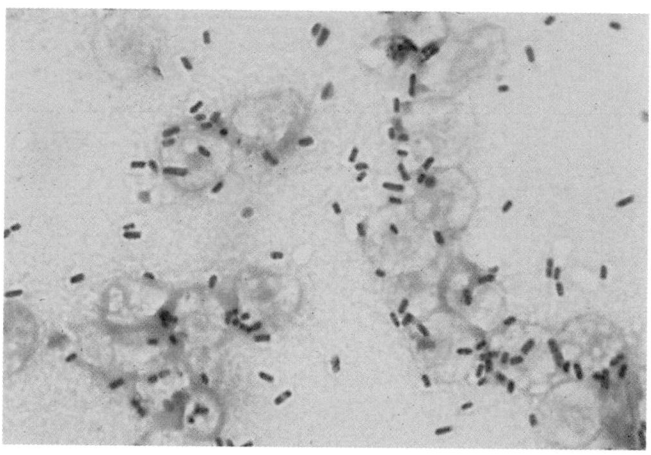

Figure 40-7 Short, gram-negative bacilli with bipolar staining.

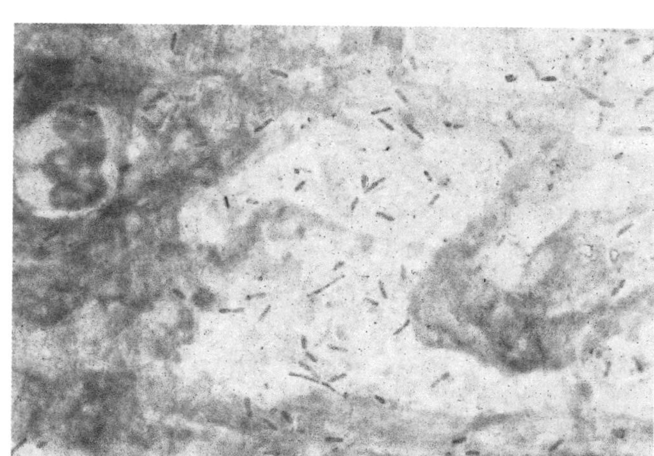

Figure 40-8 Long, slender, gram-negative bacilli.

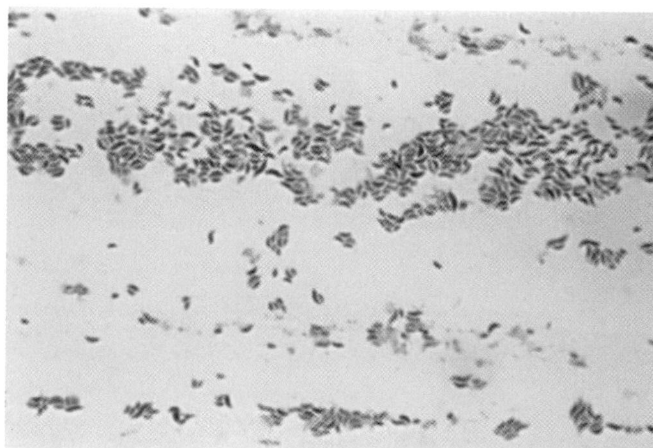

Figure 40-9 Curved, pleomorphic, gram-negative bacilli resembling *Campylobacter* spp.

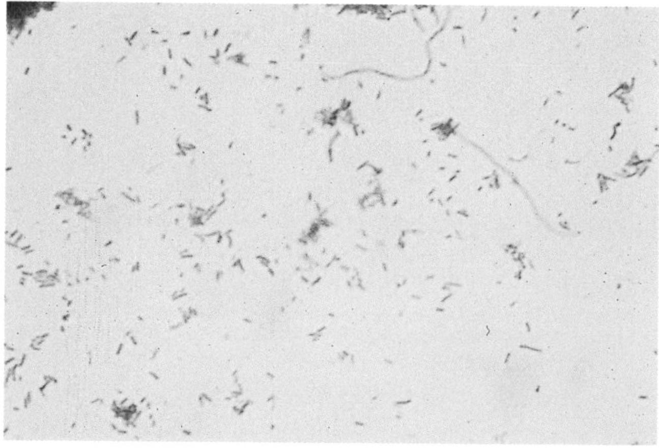

Figure 40-10 Long, slender, gram-negative bacilli resembling anaerobes.

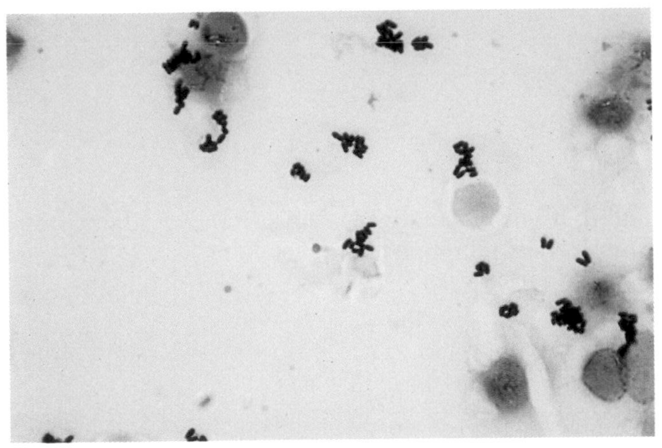

Figure 40-11 Short, gram-positive bacilli in palisade formation.

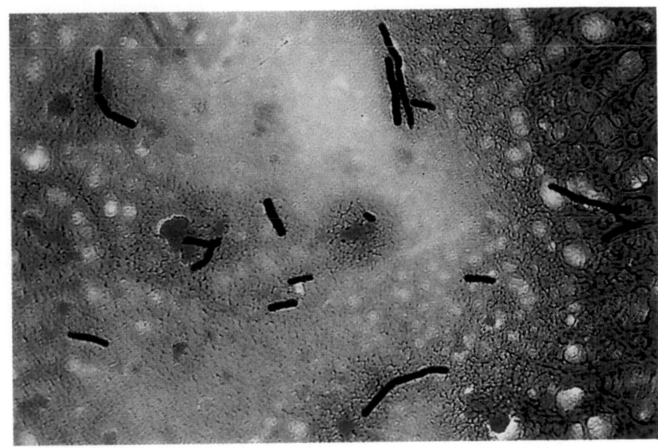

Figure 40-12 Long, gram-positive bacilli.

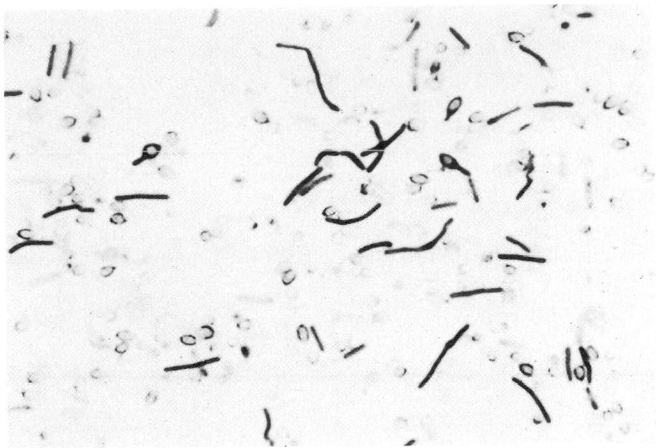

Figure 40-13 Large, gram-positive bacilli with terminal spores.

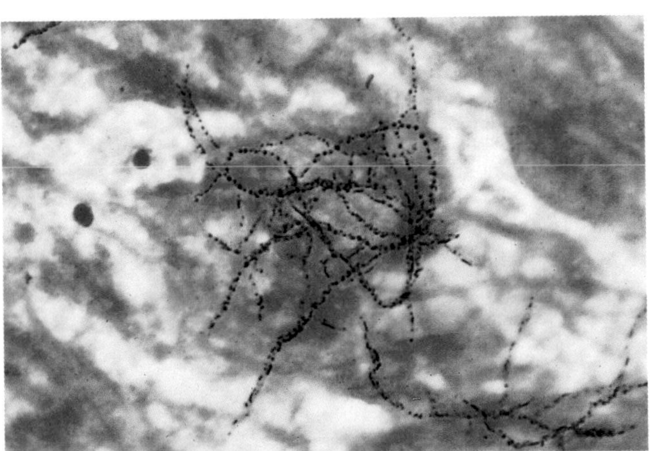

Figure 40-14 Branching, gram-positive bacilli.

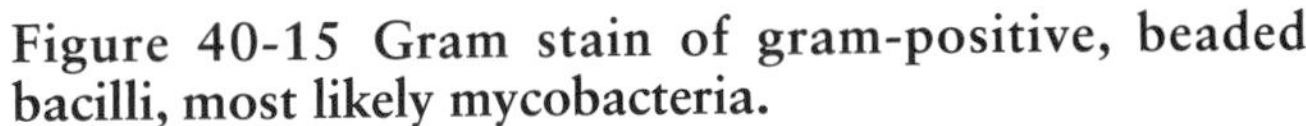

Figure 40-15 Gram stain of gram-positive, beaded bacilli, most likely mycobacteria.

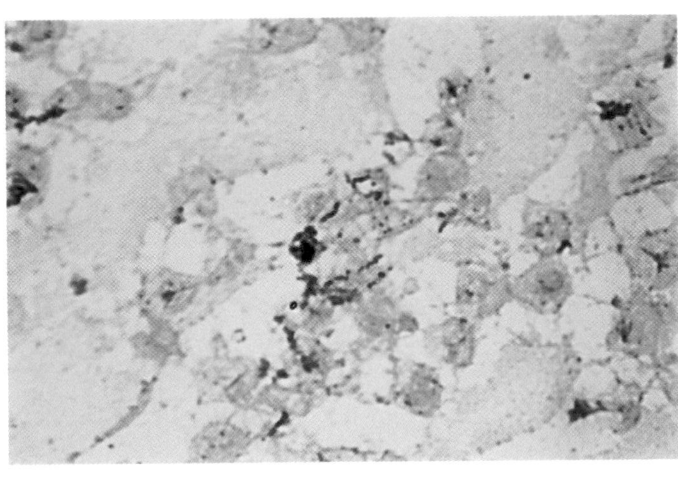

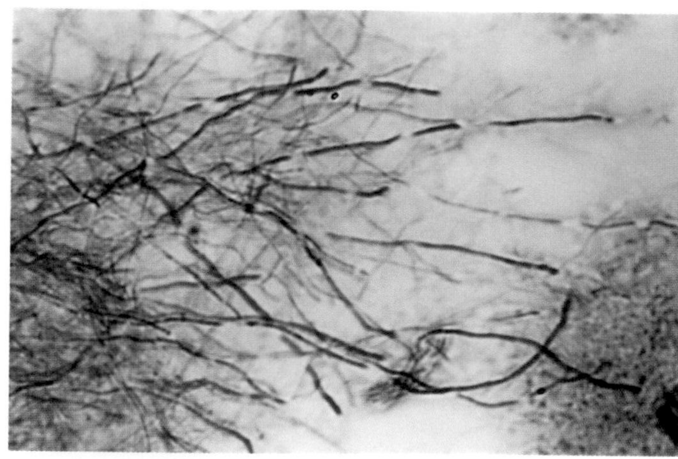

Figure 40-16 Partially acid-fast stain of filamentous branches resembling *Nocardia* spp.

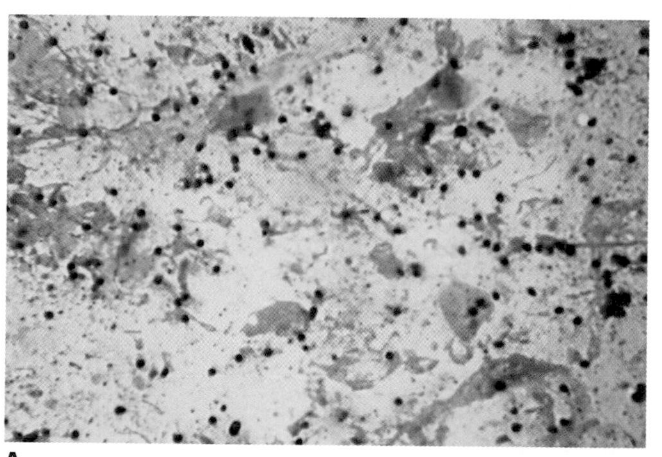

A

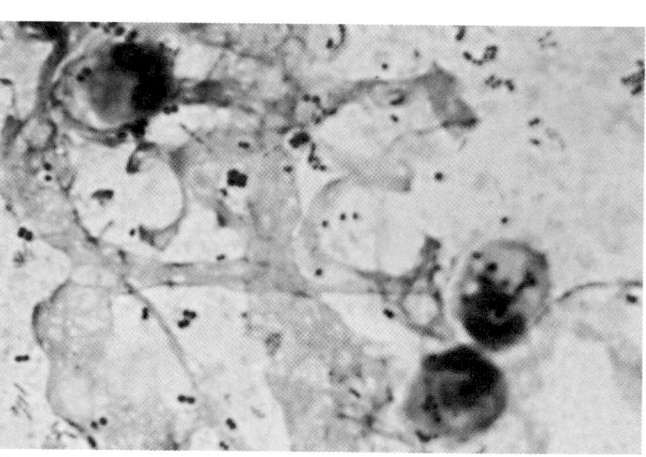

B

Figure 40-17 Gram stain of a good-quality sputum specimen. The presence of many polymorphonuclear leukocytes (PMNs) is suggestive of a good-quality specimen that is acceptable for further workup. Here there appear to be several polymorphonuclear leukocytes when observed under ×10 magnification (A). This is confirmed by examining the PMNs under ×100 magnification (B).

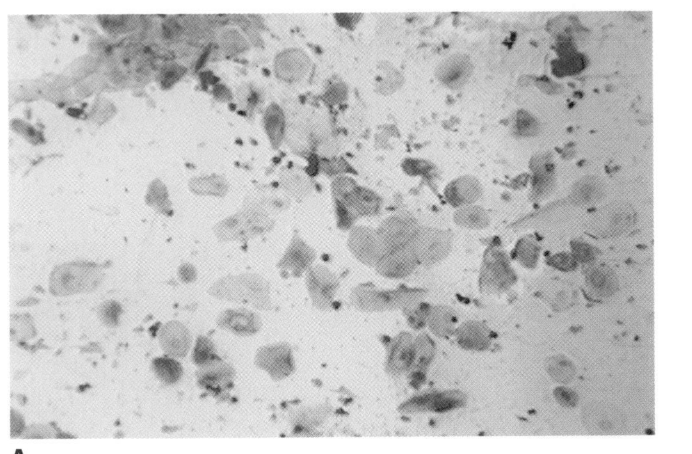

A

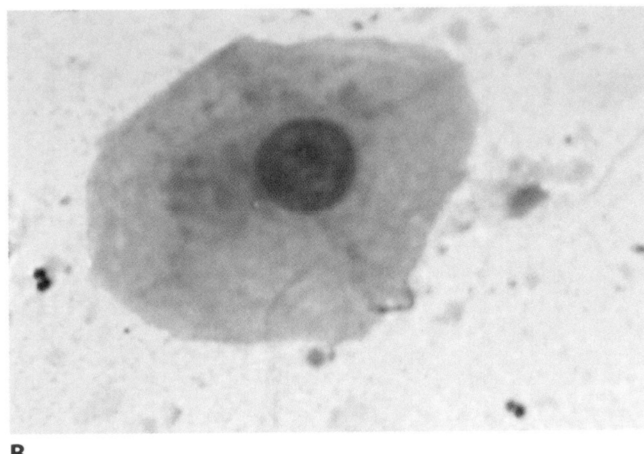

B

Figure 40-18 Gram stain of a poor-quality sputum specimen. The presence of many squamous epithelial cells suggests that the specimen may have been contaminated with normal oral pharyngeal flora, and a repeat specimen should be requested if possible. Shown here are squamous epithelial cells observed under lower-power magnification (×10) (A) and under oil immersion (×100) (B), indicating that the specimen was contaminated with oral pharyngeal flora.

Figure 40-19 Poorly stained Gram stain. The organisms, cellular material, and background appear purple, suggesting that the slide has not been properly decolorized.

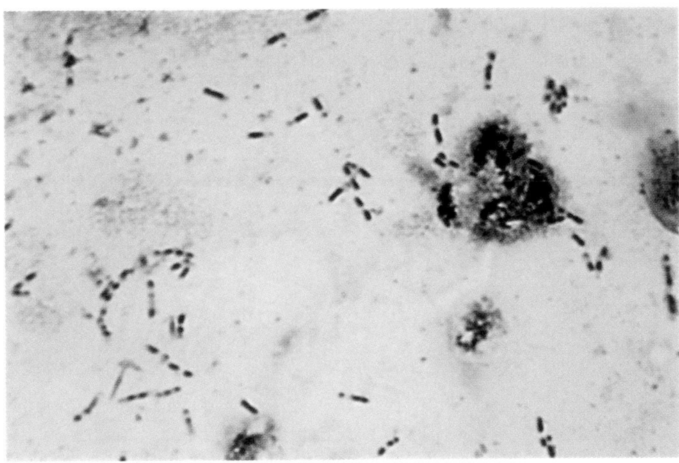

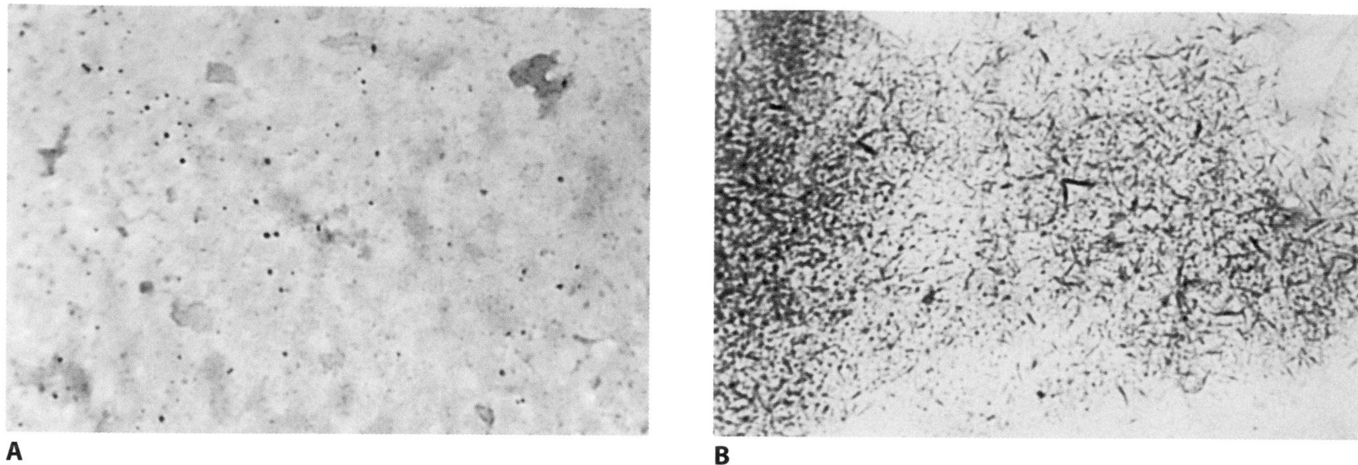

Figure 40-20 Gram stains containing artifacts, crystals, and precipitated stain. (A) Shown here are purple-staining coccoid structures of uneven sizes, which may be confused with gram-positive cocci. However, no organisms grew aerobically and anaerobically; therefore, these were determined to be artifacts. (B) These rod-like structures, which can be confused with gram-positive bacilli, are deposits from the crystal violet stain. Precipitated stain appears in the background.

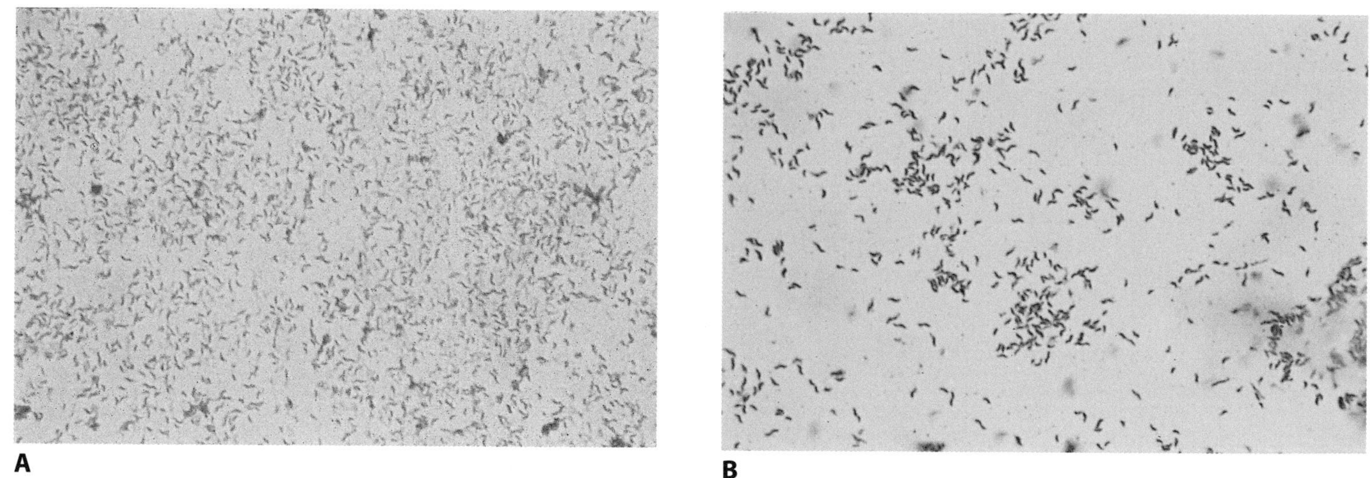

Figure 40-21 Gram stain with carbol fuchsin counterstain. Carbol fuchsin can be used to counterstain faintly staining, gram-negative organisms. In this modification, the decolorizer is a 1:3 mixture of reagent-grade acetone and 95% ethanol and the counterstain is carbol fuchsin or 0.8% basic fuchsin. Gram-negative organisms such as *Bacteroides*, *Fusobacterium*, *Legionella*, *Campylobacter*, and *Brucella* spp. stain a darker pink when carbol fuchsin is used as the counterstain. In these examples, *Campylobacter* is stained with the routine Gram stain (A) and the carbol fuchsin modification (B).

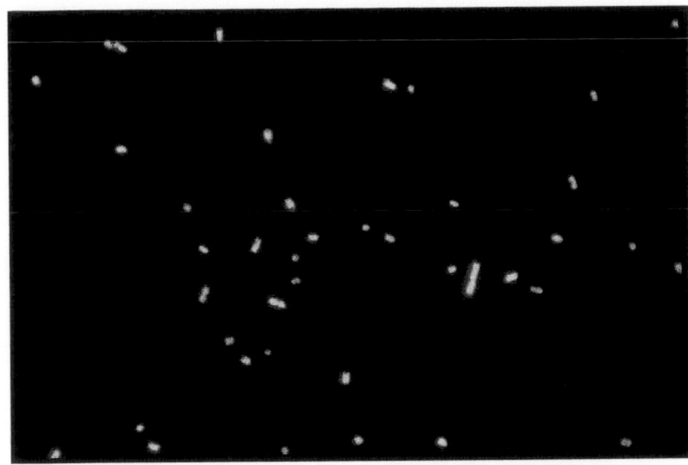

Figure 40-22 Acridine orange stain. Acridine orange is a fluorochrome dye that can bind nucleic acid. When stained with this dye in a buffered low-pH solution, bacteria and fungi appear orange, whereas host nucleic acid is green to yellow. The stain cannot be used to discriminate viable from dead microorganisms. The smear shown here represents a broth culture that grew gram-negative bacilli. This stain has been reported to be more sensitive than the Gram stain for detecting small numbers of bacteria and is used by some laboratories for blood culture broths, body fluids, and other specimens where small numbers of bacteria may be expected.

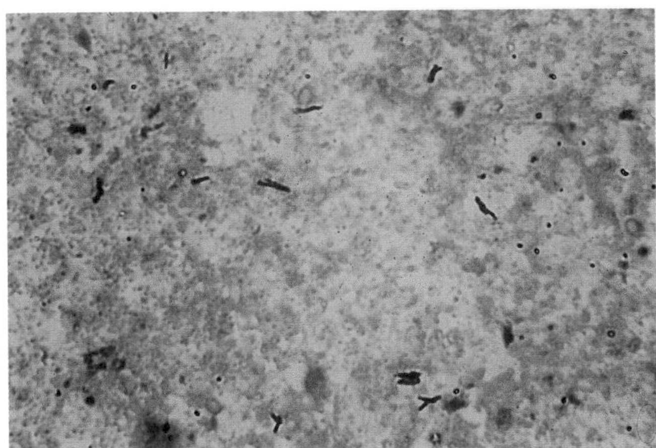

Figure 40-23 Acid-fast stain: Kinyoun stain of a sputum specimen. Pictured are *Mycobacterium tuberculosis* cells, which appear as red against a blue background. Mycobacteria have a high lipid content in their cell walls, which allows the binding of a fuchsin dye to mycolic acid so that it is not decolorized by acid alcohol. Two types of carbol fuchsin, a mixture of fuchsin and carbolic acid (phenol), stains are used: the Ziehl-Neelsen method requires heating during staining with carbol fuchsin, whereas the Kinyoun procedure is done at room temperature. Following staining, the preparation is decolorized using a solution containing ethanol and HCl followed by counterstaining with methylene blue. Acid-fast smears are useful not only for making the primary diagnosis but also for monitoring response to antimycobacterial drug therapy. In general, cultures become negative before the smears because the organisms are no longer capable of replicating. Thus, quantitation of the organisms on the smear and the correlation with growth may provide an indication of the effectiveness of the therapy.

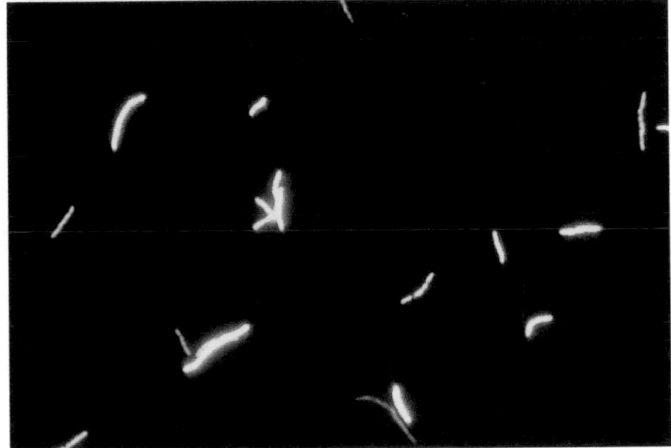

Figure 40-24 Acid-fast stain: auramine fluorochrome. Auramine O, with or without rhodamine, can also be used to stain mycobacteria. In this case, fluorochromes dissolved in ethanol and phenol are used to stain the preparation. The specimen is then decolorized with ethanol-HCl, and potassium permanganate is used as the counterstain. As shown here, mycobacteria appear yellow (golden when rhodamine is used) on a black background when observed under a fluorescence microscope. The advantage of the fluorochrome-stained smears is that mycobacteria can be seen with a 25× objective, significantly reducing the time required to scan a preparation. However, it is important to emphasize that this type of staining is the direct result of a physicochemical binding of the dye to the lipid-rich cell of the organisms, and not an antigen-antibody reaction. Therefore, the staining is not specific.

PRIMARY PLATING MEDIA

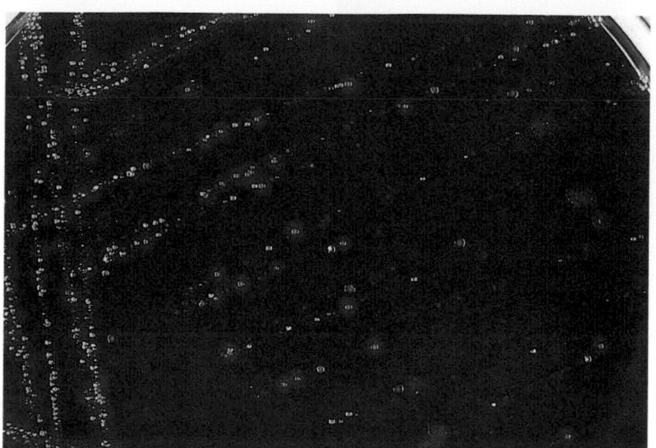

Figure 40-25 Blood agar. Blood agar is a common medium used for the primary plating of clinical material as well as for the propagation of many laboratory bacterial strains. In general, blood agar is nonselective but is differential, in particular for species for which hemolysis is a key characteristic. Shown here is 5% sheep blood agar with a Trypticase soy broth base. There are several variations to this formulation, including the type of red cells used, the percentage of cells, and the broth base used to prepare the medium. Throughout this book, when blood agar is shown, sheep blood is used unless otherwise noted. In this figure, the beta-hemolytic organism shown is *Streptococcus pyogenes*.

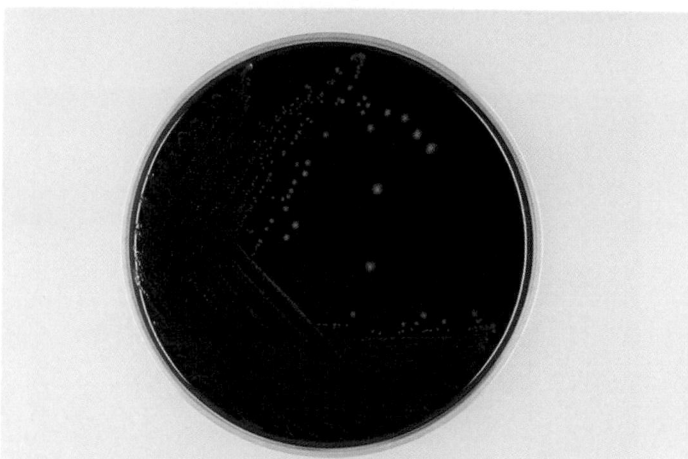

Figure 40-26 Brucella agar with hemin and vitamin K. Brucella agar with hemin and vitamin K is a nonselective, enriched medium used for the isolation of anaerobic bacteria, especially gram-negative organisms. The medium contains casein peptones, dextrose, and yeast extract. Hemin and vitamin K are added enrichments. The addition of defibrinated blood allows for the determination of hemolytic reactions, which may have a greenish color because of the high carbohydrate concentration. Shown here are gray colonies of *Bacteroides*. *Clostridium perfringens* produces double zones of beta-hemolysis when grown on brucella medium, as shown in Fig. 29-15.

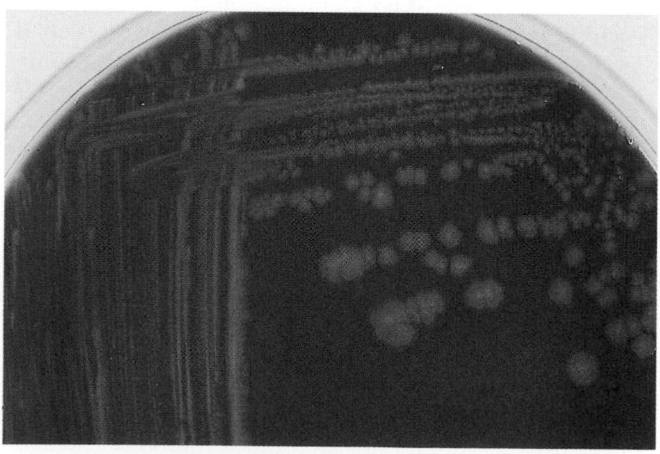

Figure 40-27 Chocolate agar. Chocolate agar is a highly enriched medium commonly used for growth of a variety of bacteria including fastidious microorganisms. While there are several variations of the formulation, in general it is composed of a GC agar base to which hemoglobin is added, which serves as a source of hemin (X factor) and gives the medium a brown or chocolate appearance. Other enrichments are also used, such as yeast extract or IsoVitaleX, which provides a source of NAD (V factor). Examples of organisms able to grow on chocolate agar but not on blood agar include some members of the genera *Neisseria* and *Haemophilus*.

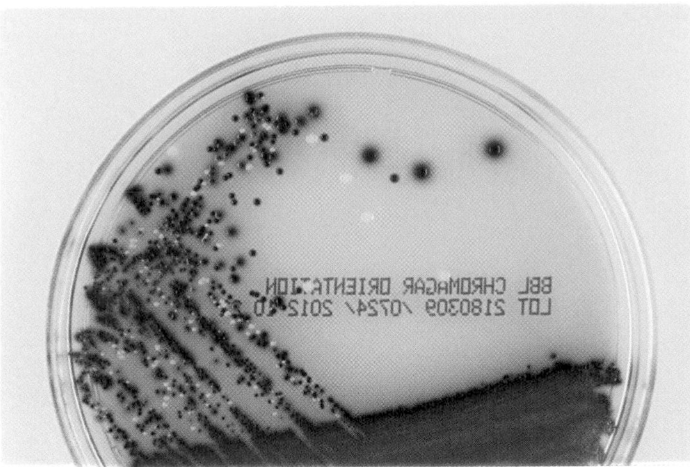

Figure 40-28 CHROMagar. CHROMagar is a chromogenic medium for the isolation and identification of a variety of microorganisms. The medium has also been referred to as Rambach agar, named after Alain Rambach, the developer. First-generation media were monochromogenic, developed specifically for the detection of *Escherichia coli* and *Salmonella* spp. Second-generation agars are multicolor and are widely used for the isolation and identification of several organisms. Shown here, BBL CHROMagar Orientation medium (BD Diagnostic Systems, Franklin Lakes, NJ) is used to identify potential pathogens of urinary tract infections. The medium has been seeded with *E. coli* (pink colonies), *Enterococcus* sp. (blue/turquoise colonies), and coagulase-negative staphylococci (golden opaque/white colonies).

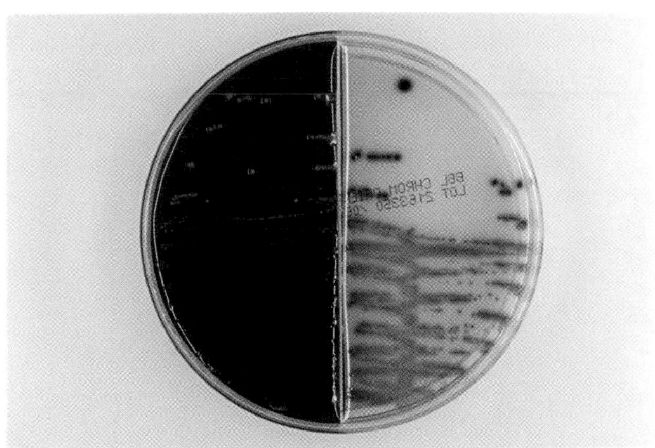

A

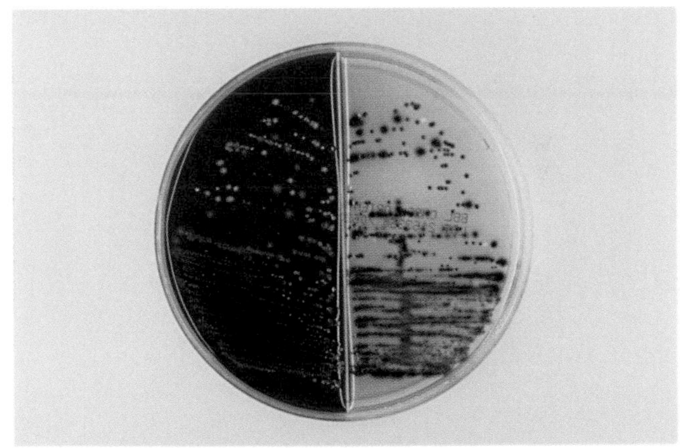

B

Figure 40-29 BBL CHROMagar and BBL Trypticase Soy Agar with 5% Sheep Blood (TSA-II)-I Plate. The BBL CHROMagar and BBL Trypticase Soy Agar with 5% Sheep Blood (TSA-II)-I Plate (BD Diagnostic Systems, Franklin Lakes, NJ) is used primarily to isolate and identify microorganisms from urine specimens. (A) It is difficult to determine whether the organism on the sheep blood agar is gram positive or gram negative; however, based on the color reaction on the CHROMagar medium, the organism is likely *E. coli* (right). (B) A mixed culture is shown on the blood agar; however, the color reactions on the CHROMagar medium suggest the presence of *E. coli, Enterococcus,* and coagulase-negative staphylococci (right) as described in Fig. 40-28.

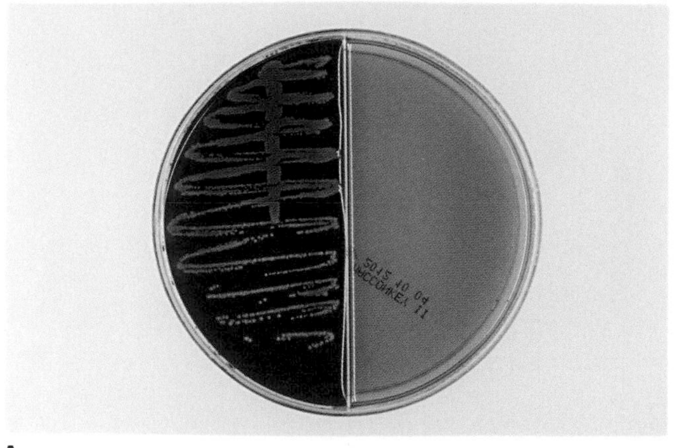

A

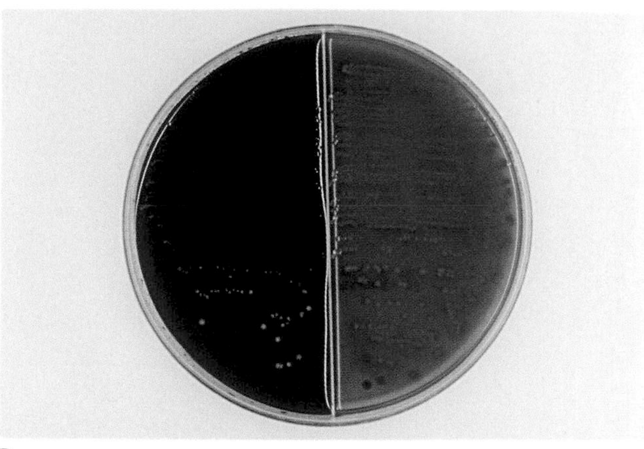

B

Figure 40-30 Columbia CNA/MacConkey agar biplate. CNA (colistin-nalidixic acid blood agar) is selective for the growth of gram-positive cocci. The colistin and nalidixic acid in the medium inhibit the growth of gram-negative bacilli. (A) A gram-positive organism is growing on the left half of the plate containing CNA, and there is no growth on the MacConkey agar side. (B) *Enterococcus* was identified on CNA and *E. coli* on MacConkey agar.

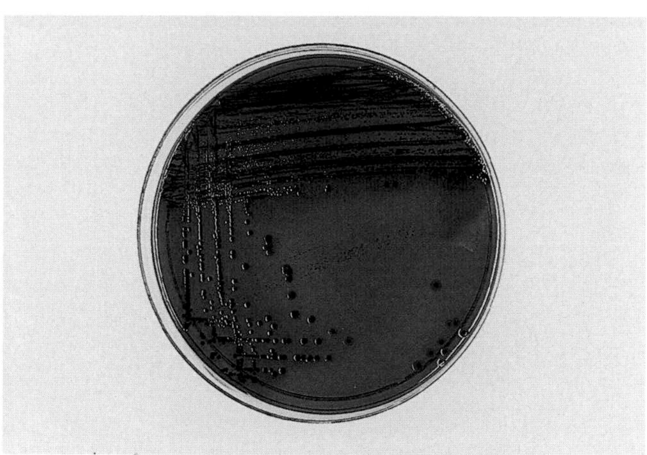

Figure 40-31 Eosin methylene blue agar. Eosin methylene blue agar, like MacConkey agar, is moderately inhibitory and was developed to inhibit the growth of gram-positive organisms and to detect lactose fermentation. Eosin Y and methylene blue are the inhibitors used in this medium. Due to the precipitation of dye, rapid lactose fermenters such as *E. coli* form colonies with a metallic sheen, as shown here; other strong acid producers can give the same appearance.

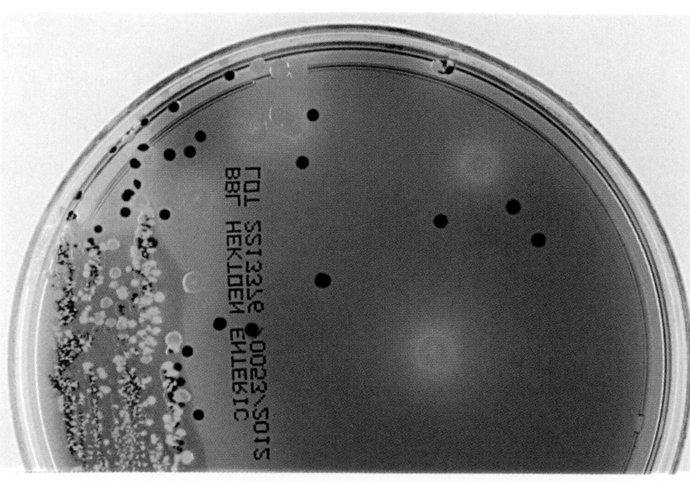

Figure 40-32 Hektoen enteric (HE) agar. HE agar is a selective and differential medium used for the isolation of *Salmonella* spp. and *Shigella* spp. from fecal specimens. The medium contains lactose, sucrose, and salicin. *Salmonella* spp. and *Shigella* spp. do not generally ferment these carbohydrates. Also, differentiation of species occurs with the addition of sodium thiosulfate and ferric ammonium citrate, which allow detection of hydrogen sulfide production. Organisms producing H_2S appear with a black precipitate on the colony. Examples of reactions on HE agar are *E. coli* organisms, which appear as yellow or salmon colored; *Shigella* spp., which are green or transparent; and *Salmonella* spp., which are green or transparent with black centers. Shown here are lactose-positive colonies (yellowish color) and H_2S-producing colonies (black).

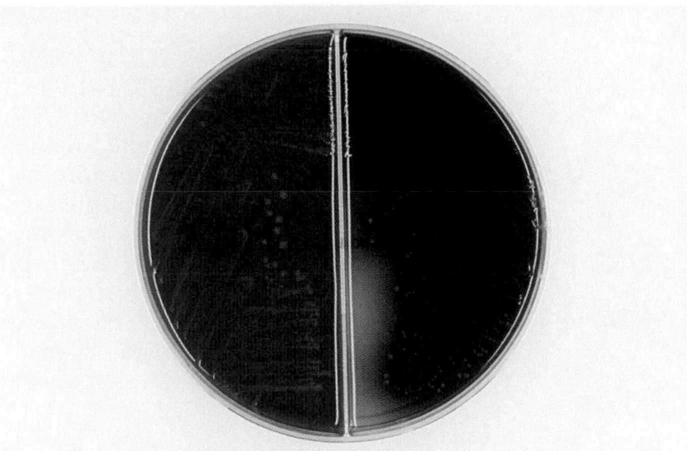

Figure 40-33 Kanamycin-vancomycin-brucella-laked blood agar/bacteroides bile esculin agar. Kanamycin-vancomycin-brucella-laked blood agar is an enriched, selective, and differential medium used for the isolation of anaerobic bacteria, especially *Bacteroides* spp.; pigmented, anaerobic, gram-positive bacilli; and *Prevotella* spp. The sheep blood in the medium is laked, and vitamin K_1 is added to facilitate the recovery of *Prevotella melaninogenica*. The base is CDC anaerobe blood agar, and the selective agents are kanamycin and vancomycin. Kanamycin inhibits the growth of gram-negative, facultative anaerobic bacilli, and vancomycin inhibits the growth of gram-positive organisms. Bacteroides bile esculin agar is also an enriched medium for the isolation of the *Bacteroides fragilis* group. It contains gentamicin, which inhibits most facultative anaerobes. The bile in the medium inhibits anaerobic, gram-negative bacilli, with the exception of the *B. fragilis* group and other bile-resistant, gram-negative bacilli. Most members of the *Bacteroides* group hydrolyze esculin, and therefore the esculin in the medium produces a brown/black color around the colonies, as shown on the right side of the biplate, which confirms the identification of the organism grown on the left side of the biplate.

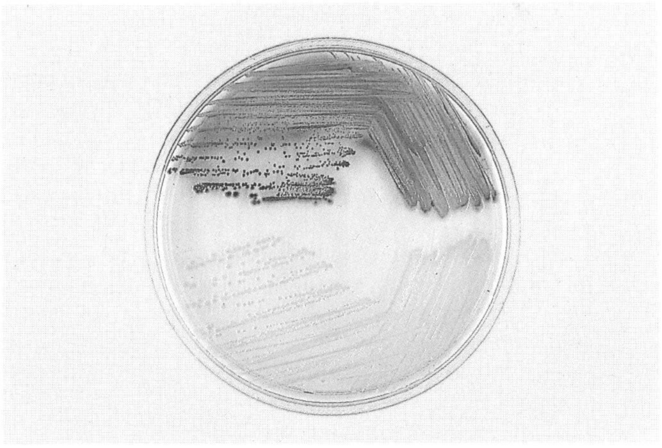

Figure 40-34 MacConkey agar. MacConkey agar contains a peptone base with lactose and is used to distinguish rapid lactose fermenters from delayed lactose fermenters or nonfermenters. Crystal violet and bile salts in the medium inhibit gram-positive organisms. Neutral red is the pH indicator. Colonies vary in color from pink to colorless and from dry with a donut shape to mucoid. Rapid lactose fermenters appear as pink colonies on MacConkey agar after overnight incubation, and their size and color intensity vary with different species. In this example, colonies of *E. coli* appear dark pink, 2 to 3 mm in diameter, surrounded by precipitated bile. Colonies of nonfermenters are colorless or the color of the medium.

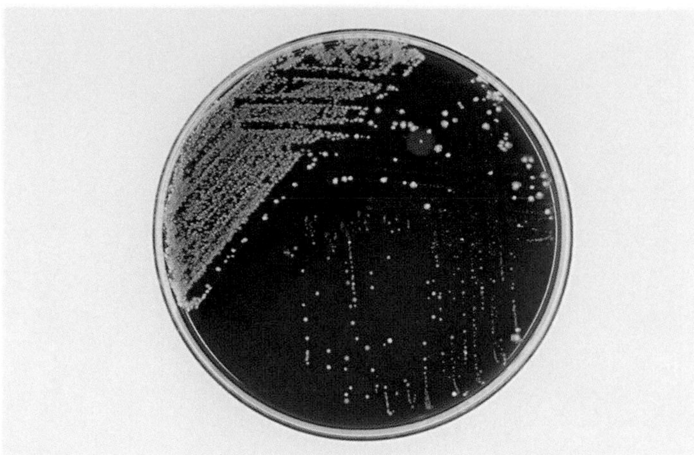

Figure 40-35 Phenylethyl alcohol agar. Phenylethyl alcohol agar with 5% sheep blood is a selective medium for the isolation of gram-positive organisms, particularly gram-positive cocci, from specimens of mixed gram-positive and gram-negative flora. It also inhibits gram-negative bacteria, particularly *Proteus* spp. The medium should not be used for determination of hemolytic reactions since atypical reactions may be observed. Shown here are organisms isolated directly from a fecal culture. As expected, the gram-negative organisms have been inhibited.

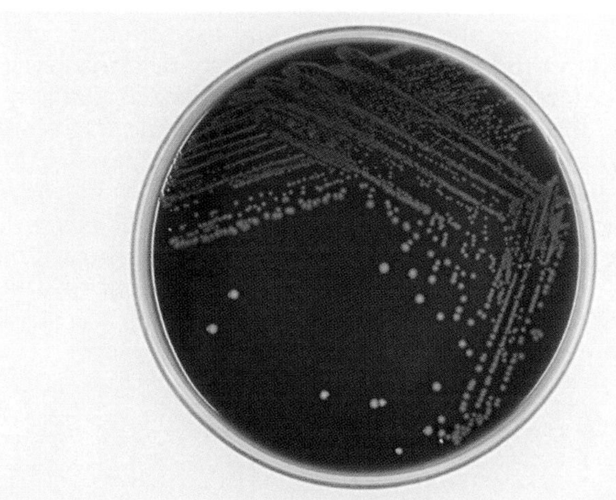

Figure 40-36 Modified Thayer-Martin agar. Modified Thayer-Martin (MTM II; BD Diagnostic Systems, Franklin Lakes, NJ) agar is based on Chocolate II Agar, which contains an improved GC agar base, bovine hemoglobin, and BBL IsoVitaleX enrichment (BD Diagnostic Systems). Hemoglobin provides X factor (hemin) for *Haemophilus* species. IsoVitaleX enrichment is a defined supplement that provides V factor (NAD) for *Haemophilus* species and vitamins, amino acids, coenzymes, dextrose, ferric ion, and other factors that improve the growth of pathogenic *Neisseria* spp. This selective medium also contains the antimicrobial agents vancomycin, colistin, nystatin (V-C-N inhibitor), and trimethoprim to suppress the normal flora. Vancomycin inhibits gram-positive organisms, while colistin inhibits gram-negative organisms, including *Pseudomonas* species, but not *Proteus* species. Trimethoprim is added to inhibit *Proteus* species, and nystatin inhibits fungi. Shown here are colonies of *Neisseria gonorrhoeae*.

BIOCHEMICAL TESTS

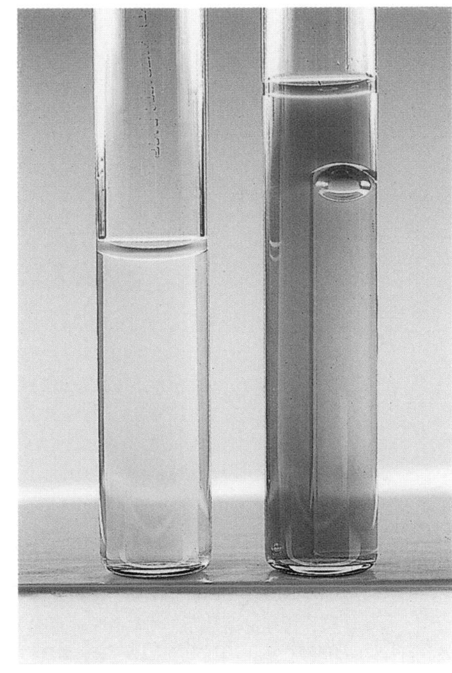

Figure 40-37 Andrade's broth. Andrade's broth supplemented with carbohydrates is used to determine fermentation by bacteria, particularly members of the *Enterobacteriaceae*. The medium contains a sugar-free peptone broth to which a specific carbohydrate is added. A decolorized acid fuchsin is used as the pH indicator. When the organism metabolizes the carbohydrate, the pH of the medium decreases as a result of the acid production and changes the color of the indicator from colorless to pink or red, depending on the amount of acid generated. As shown here, a Durham tube may be inserted to detect the formation of gas (right). As a control, a tube without the added carbohydrate should be inoculated and processed in parallel (left).

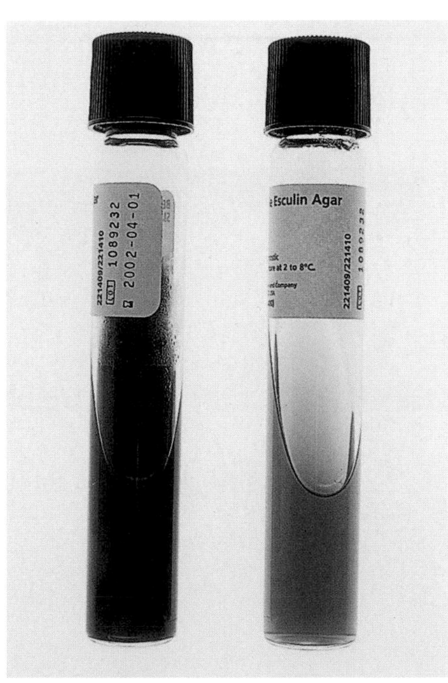

Figure 40-38 Bile esculin agar. Bile esculin agar is both a differential and selective medium. This agar is commonly used in plates or, as shown here, slants. It is used for the differentiation of *Enterococcus* spp. and the *Streptococcus bovis* group (group D) from other streptococci. The medium consists of 40% bile (oxgall), which inhibits streptococci other than enterococci or group D streptococci. Enterococci and group D streptococci are able to hydrolyze esculin, resulting in the formation of esculetin and dextrose. The former complexes with ferric citrate in the medium, resulting in a dark brown to black precipitate. Shown here are *Enterococcus faecalis* (left), which is bile esculin positive, and *Streptococcus pyogenes* (right), which is bile esculin negative.

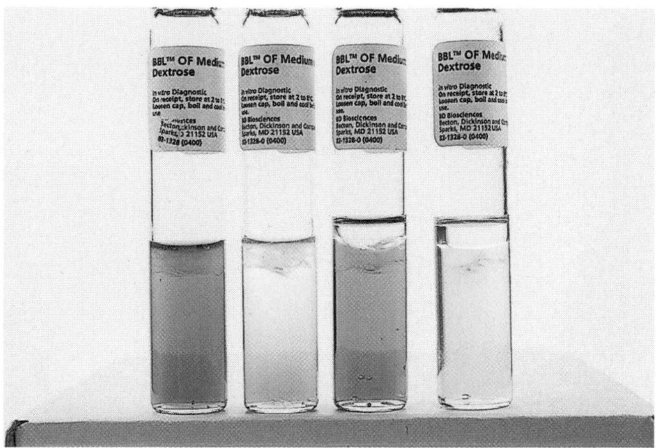

Figure 40-39 Carbohydrate oxidative-fermentative (OF) medium. Bacteria can degrade glucose by the anaerobic pathway (also called the glycolytic or fermentative pathway), producing strong acids that can easily be detected with regular media, or by the aerobic (oxidative) pathway, producing weak acids that can be detected using the Hugh and Leifson (OF) medium. This medium has three unique characteristics: (i) a low (0.2%) concentration of peptone, thus preventing the formation of alkaline products that may neutralize small quantities of acids; (ii) a high (1.0%) concentration of carbohydrates, which allows large amounts of acid to be formed; and (iii) a low (0.3%) concentration of agar, which results in a semisolid medium that permits acids formed on the surface to permeate throughout the medium. Two tubes are used for the test. One is covered with melted paraffin to block out oxygen (mineral oil is frequently used but does not block oxygen very efficiently). Both tubes are inoculated with the unknown organism by using a straight needle and are incubated at 35°C for several days. A yellow color in both tubes indicates that the organism is fermentative, since it can produce acid without oxygen. A yellow color only in the uncovered tube means that the organism is oxidative, since it requires oxygen to metabolize the carbohydrates. If both tubes remain green, this indicates that the organism is asaccharolytic.

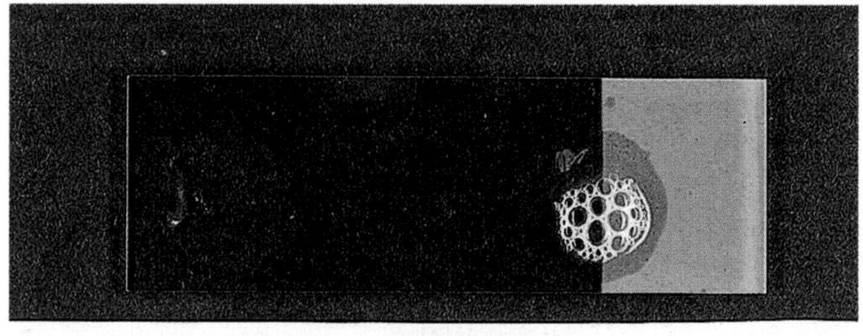

Figure 40-40 Catalase test. The rapid catalase test uses a solution of 3% hydrogen peroxide to determine whether a microorganism contains the enzyme catalase. Microorganisms are added to a drop of hydrogen peroxide. If catalase is present, bubbles appear as a result of the release of O_2 from the breakdown of the hydrogen peroxide by the enzyme.

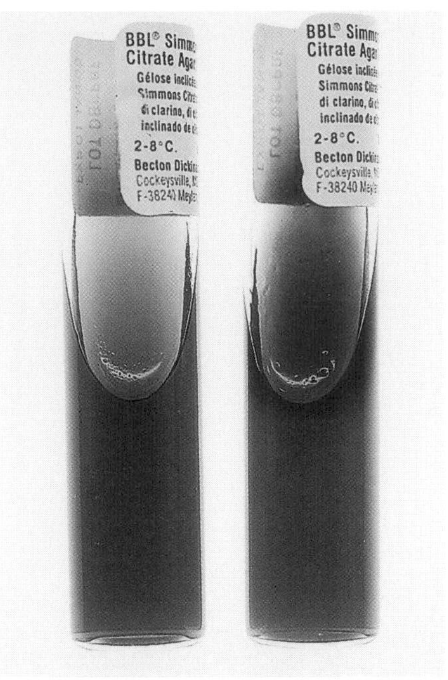

Figure 40-41 Citrate utilization. Some microorganisms have the ability to utilize sodium citrate as the sole carbon source. Therefore, the medium used to detect citrate utilization cannot contain proteins or carbohydrates as the source of carbon. The medium includes sodium citrate as the sole source of carbon and ammonium phosphate as the only source of nitrogen. By utilizing the nitrogen from the ammonium phosphate, bacteria that can use the citrate will excrete ammonia, leading to the alkalinization of the medium. Bromthymol blue is used as the indicator. This characteristic helps in the identification of several members of the *Enterobacteriaceae*. The negative slant appears on the left, and the positive slant is shown on the right.

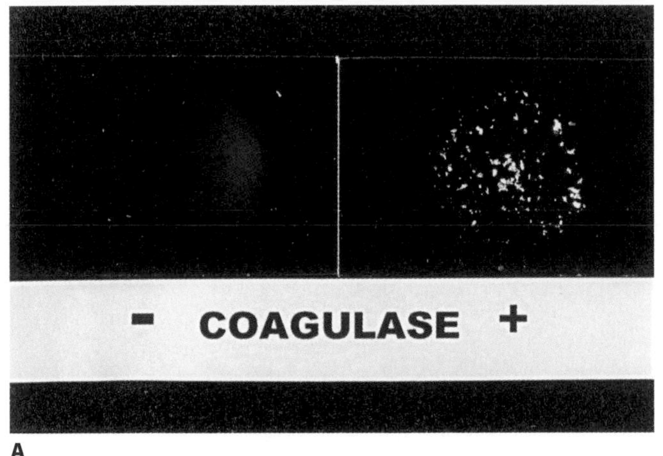

A

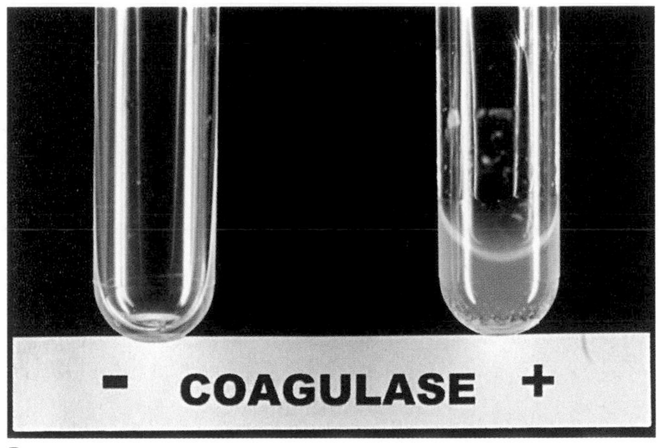

B

Figure 40-42 Coagulase slide and tube test. The coagulase test is widely used for differentiating *Staphylococcus aureus* from most other *Staphylococcus* spp. Most *S. aureus* strains produce two forms of coagulase, free and bound. Bound coagulase, or clumping factor, is bound to the bacterial cell wall and reacts directly with fibrinogen. The fibrinogen precipitates on the staphylococcal cell, causing the organisms to clump when the bacterial suspension is mixed with plasma. The slide coagulase test is positive in the presence of bound coagulase, whereas the tube coagulase test measures free coagulase. In most cases, the presence of bound coagulase correlates well with free coagulase. However, some *S. aureus* strains produce only free coagulase. Also, *Staphylococcus lugdunensis* and *Staphylococcus schleiferi* have only bound coagulase and therefore are slide coagulase positive but tube coagulase negative. (A) In the slide coagulase test, clumping of cells suspended in rabbit plasma is observed on the right side of the slide (positive test), whereas there is no clumping on the left side (negative test). (B) In the tube coagulase test, a clot is observed in the right tube, indicating a positive test, and the left tube remains liquid (negative test). The tube should be read after a 4-h incubation to look for clot formation and reincubated for up to 24 h if negative. It is important to note that once a clot is formed, if it is not observed early (4 h) it can dissolve, causing a false-negative result.

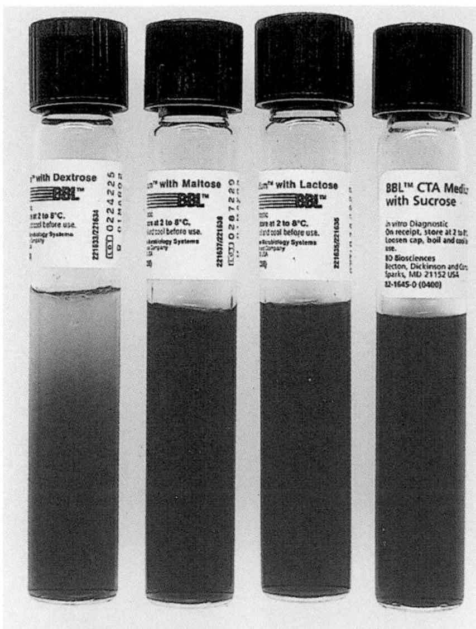

Figure 40-43 Cystine Trypticase agar (CTA) carbohydrates. The fermentation of carbohydrates by bacteria can be detected using CTA containing maltose, sucrose, lactose, and glucose, and phenol red as the pH indicator. A positive reaction is indicated by a yellow color, which occurs when the pH drops below 6.8 as a result of the fermentation of the carbohydrate. Shown is an isolate of *Neisseria gonorrhoeae* that exhibits a typical pattern of positive glucose but negative maltose, lactose, and sucrose fermentation (left to right).

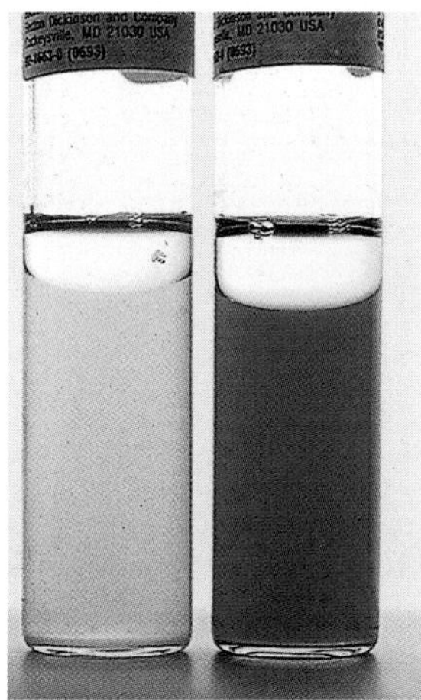

Figure 40-44 Decarboxylase/dihydrolase test. The decarboxylase/dihydrolase test is based on the principle that certain organisms have the ability to remove a carboxy or hydroxyl group (hydrolyze) from an amino acid to form an amine, resulting in an alkaline pH. The test medium contains both glucose and one of the three amino acids lysine, ornithine, or arginine. Under anaerobic conditions, certain organisms can ferment glucose, resulting in a decrease in pH detected by a change in color to yellow. The low pH activates the decarboxylase that converts the lysine to cadaverine and converts the ornithine to putrescine. Arginine is first converted to citrulline by a dihydrolase. Citrulline is then converted to ornithine, which is decarboxylated to putrescine. The formation of alkaline amines increases the pH, and the medium returns to a purple/reddish purple color. An alkaline reaction in the medium containing the amino acid is interpreted as a positive test (right tube), whereas an acidic reaction is considered negative (left tube).

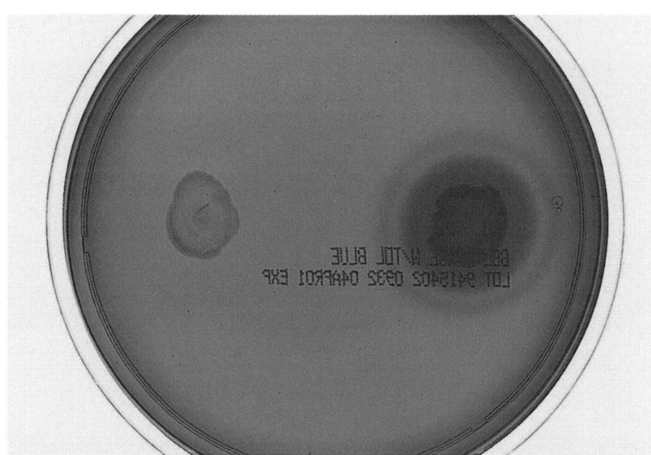

Figure 40-45 DNase test. The DNase test can be used to differentiate between certain groups of microorganisms. In this test, the presence of DNase is assessed by its ability to digest DNA, producing oligonucleotides. A common method of testing for DNase is to inoculate the isolate of interest onto an agar plate that incorporates DNA and the metachromatic dye toluidine blue. If DNase is not present, the area surrounding the bacterial growth remains unchanged. However, when the DNA is hydrolyzed by DNase, the resulting oligonucleotides form a complex with the toluidine blue, resulting in metachromatic (pink) staining. In the example shown, *Moraxella catarrhalis* is DNase positive (pink halo, right), whereas the other organism shown is negative for DNase since there is no change in the original blue color of the medium (left).

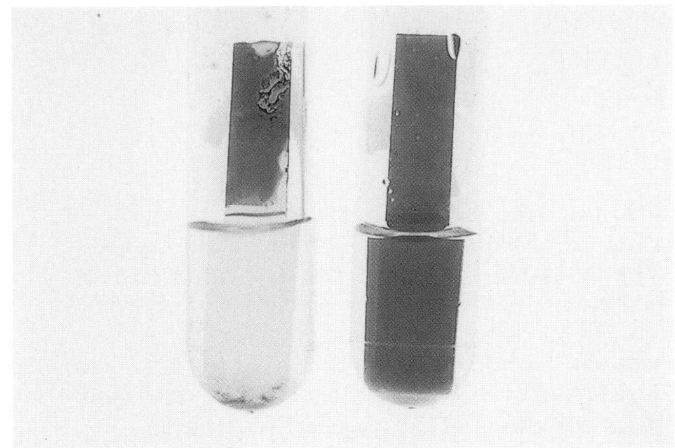

Figure 40-46 Gelatin hydrolysis test. Gelatin is incorporated into various media to detect the presence of the proteolytic enzyme gelatinase, which hydrolyzes gelatin into its constituent amino acids with the subsequent loss of its gelling characteristic. The use of exposed, undeveloped X-ray film is one method to test for the presence of the enzyme. When hydrolysis occurs, the film loses its gelatin coating, resulting in a clear, bluish photographic film (left tube).

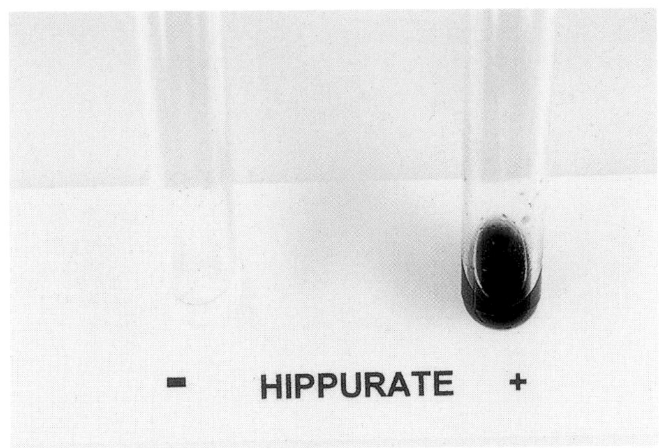

Figure 40-47 Hippurate hydrolysis test. The hippurate hydrolysis test detects hippuricase; this reaction can be used to differentiate between groups of streptococci as well as *Gardnerella vaginalis* and *Campylobacter jejuni*. Hippuric acid is hydrolyzed by hippuricase to form glycine and sodium benzoate. In the hippurate test shown, a heavy suspension of organisms is made in a 1% aqueous hippurate solution and incubated for 2 h at 37°C. Subsequently, ninhydrin is added, which complexes with glycine and produces a purple color (right).

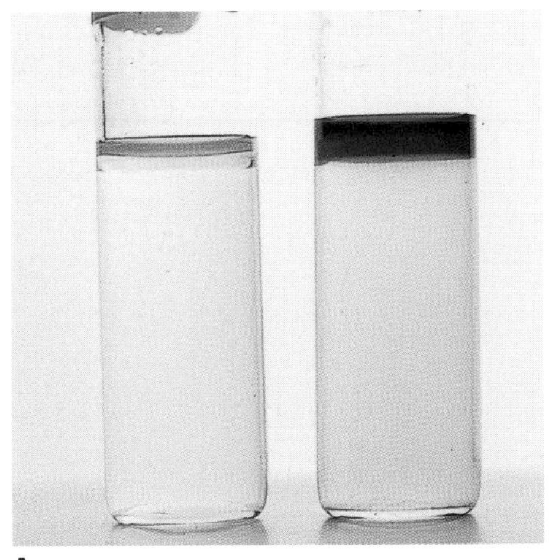

A

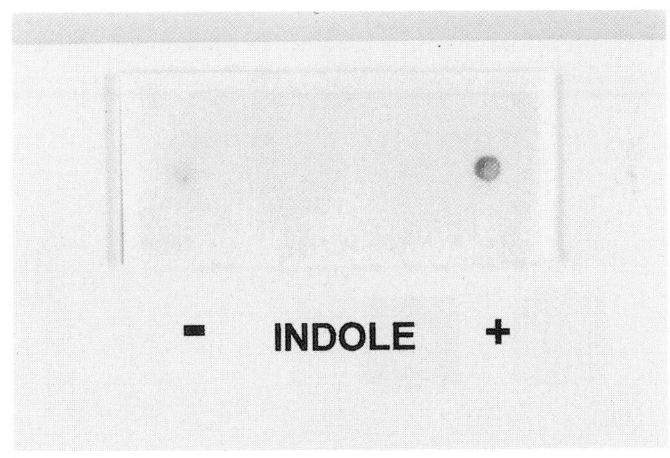

B

Figure 40-48 Indole test. Some organisms contain the enzyme tryptophanase, which converts tryptophan to indole. (A) Indole is detected by the addition of *p*-dimethylaminobenzaldehyde (Ehrlich's or Kovac's reagent) to a broth solution (tube test). If a ring of red appears at the interface between the top of the broth and the reagent, the test is positive (right). (B) Alternatively, using filter paper impregnated with *p*-dimethylcinnemaldehyde, a positive reaction results in the formation of a green color (spot test).

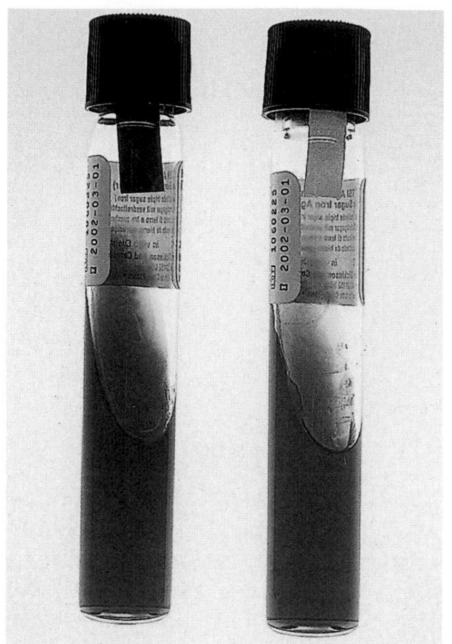

Figure 40-49 Lead acetate test. Certain organisms are capable of enzymatically liberating sulfur from sulfur-containing amino acids or other compounds. The hydrogen sulfide gas released can then react with ferric ions or lead acetate to yield a black precipitate, i.e., ferrous sulfide or lead acetate. The sensitivity of each indicator varies. Lead acetate is the most sensitive method and should be used for organisms that produce trace amounts of H_2S. A positive lead acetate test is indicated by brownish-black coloration of the paper strip (left tube).

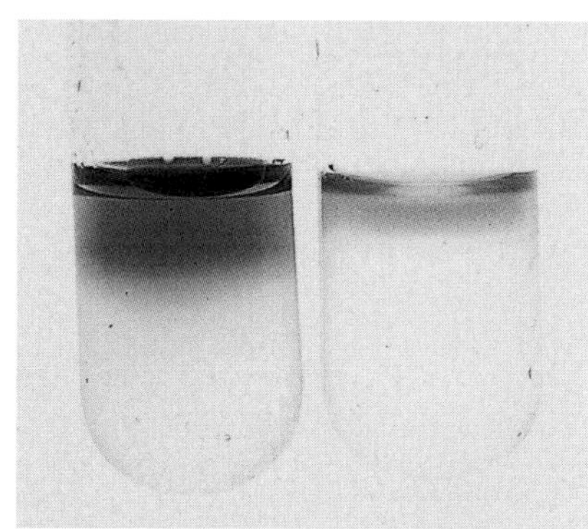

Figure 40-50 Methyl red test. When glucose is metabolized through the mixed acid fermentation pathway, strong acids such as lactic acid, acetic acid, and formic acid are produced, resulting in a decrease of pH below 4.5. At this pH, the broth turns red (left tube) upon addition of methyl red.

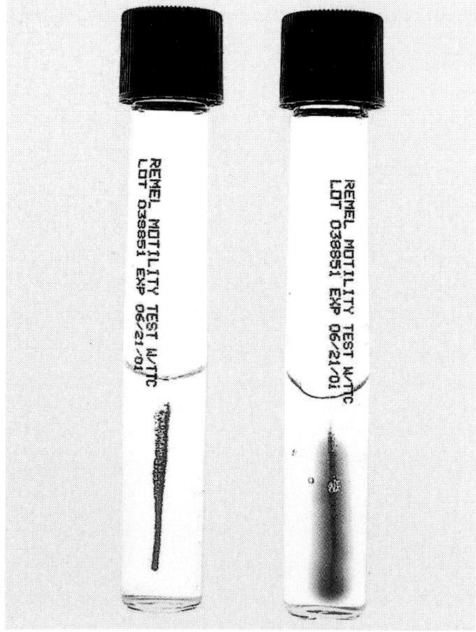

Figure 40-51 Motility test. Organisms can be differentiated based on motility. An agar deep, containing tryptose and the dye triphenyltetrazolium chloride, is inoculated with a microorganism and incubated at 35°C overnight. Motile bacteria are able to migrate from the original inoculation site or stab line. This migration is visualized with the aid of triphenyltetrazolium chloride, which is incorporated into the bacterial cells and is reduced to form an insoluble red pigment (formazan). In the example shown here, the nonmotile organism is on the left and the motile organism is on the right.

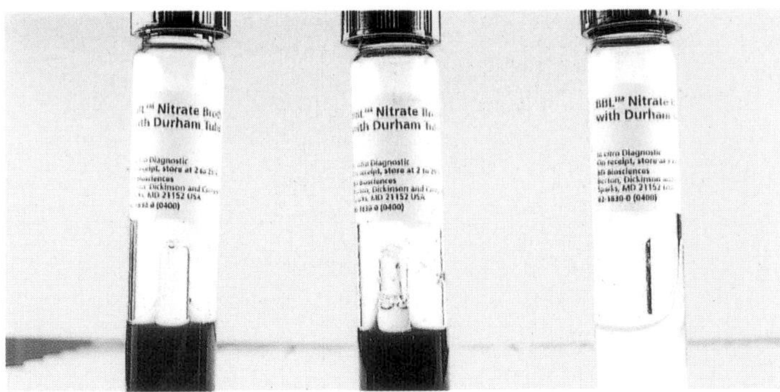

Figure 40-52 Nitrate test. Certain bacteria reduce nitrates to nitrites. Adding α-naphthylamine and sulfanilic acid results in the formation of *p*-sulfobenzene-azo-α-naphthylamine, a red diazonium dye which indicates that nitrite has been reduced to nitrate (left tube). A negative result indicates that either no nitrites are present or that nitrates have been reduced to other compounds such as ammonia, molecular nitrogen, nitric oxide, or nitrous oxide (right tube). To determine if a colorless broth is truly negative or if the nitrates have been reduced to products other than nitrites, zinc dust is added. Zinc reduces nitrate to nitrite and produces a red color. Thus, if the broth turns red when zinc is added, the test is interpreted as negative (middle tube). If the broth remains colorless, the nitrates have been reduced to other products (right tube).

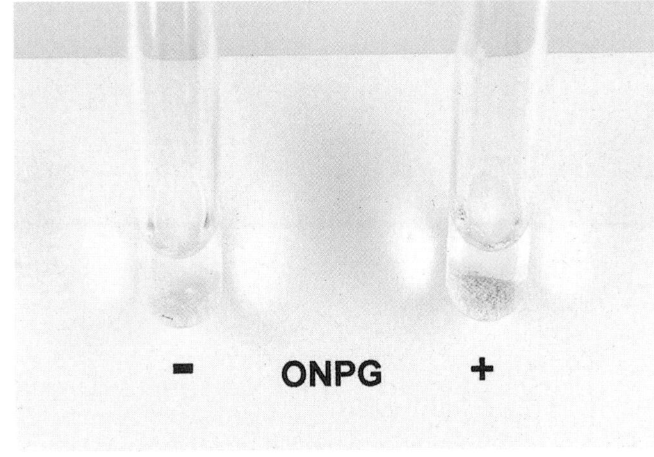

Figure 40-53 *o*-Nitrophenyl-β-D-galactopyranoside (ONPG) test. Late lactose fermenters are very difficult to distinguish from lactose nonfermenters because both appear as colorless colonies on MacConkey agar. The ONPG test is used to detect the enzyme β-galactosidase, present in late lactose fermenters. Organisms that produce this enzyme hydrolyze the substrate ONPG, and orthonitrophenol is formed (right tube). Orthonitrophenol is yellow in its free form and colorless when bound to D-galactopyranoside. It should be noted that the ONPG test detects β-galactosidase activity only and hence cannot be equated with determination for lactose fermentation, which is also dependent on the enzyme permease.

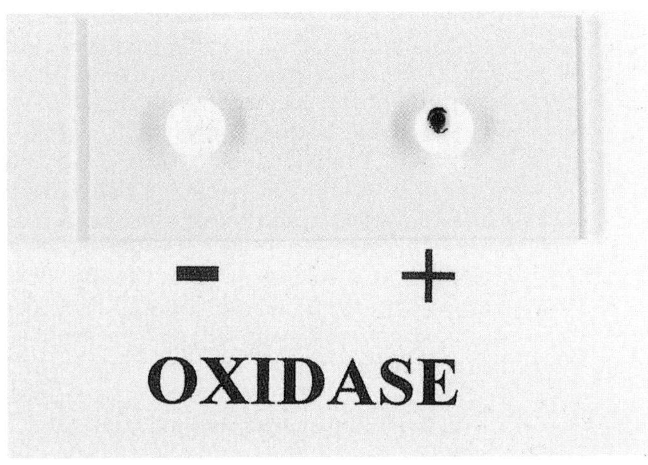

Figure 40-54 Oxidase test. Certain bacteria possess either cytochrome oxidase or indophenol oxidase, which catalyzes the transport of electrons (hydrogen) from donor compounds (NADH) to electron acceptors (usually oxygen) with the formation of water. In the presence of atmospheric oxygen and cytochrome oxidase, a colorless dye such as 1% tetramethyl-*p*-phenylenediamine dihydrochloride (Kovac's reagent) is oxidized and forms indophenol blue. This test can easily be performed directly by applying Kovac's reagent onto the colonies or indirectly by rubbing the colonies onto filter paper moistened with the reagent. If colonies rubbed onto filter paper moistened with the reagent turn dark blue or purple within 10 to 30 s, the test is positive, as shown on the right.

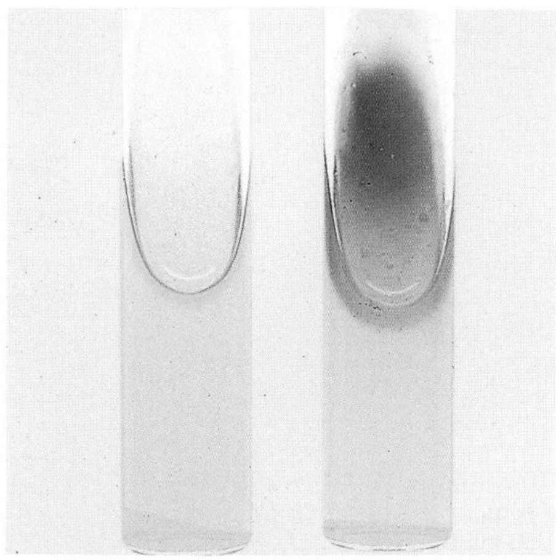

Figure 40-55 Phenylalanine deaminase (PAD) test. Amino acids can be oxidatively deaminated to form a keto acid. In the presence of PAD, the amino acid L-phenylalanine is converted to phenylpyruvic acid, a keto acid. On addition of 10% ferric chloride, a green compound is formed (right). *Proteus* spp., *Providencia* spp., and *Morganella* spp. are PAD positive.

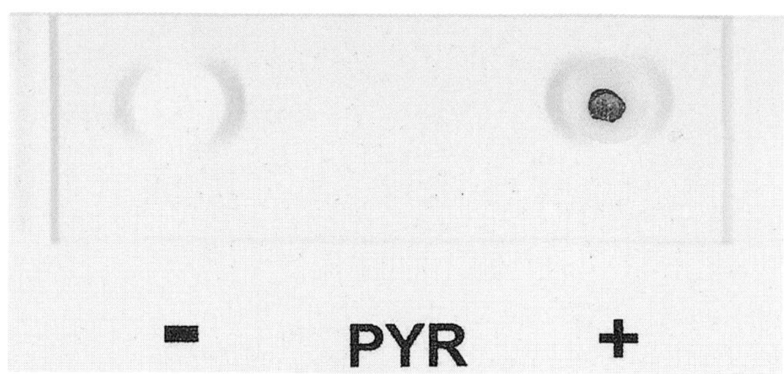

Figure 40-56 L-Pyrrolidonyl-β-naphthylamide (PYR) test. The PYR test is commonly used to identify *Streptococcus pyogenes* and *Enterococcus* spp., which are PYR positive. In this test, the enzyme L-pyrrolidonyl arylamidase hydrolyzes the substrate PYR, resulting in the formation of a free β-naphthylamine. Subsequently, this by-product is detected with *N*,*N*-methyl-aminocinnamaldehyde, resulting in a bright red color. The figure shows negative (*Streptococcus agalactiae*) and positive (*S. pyogenes*) reactions.

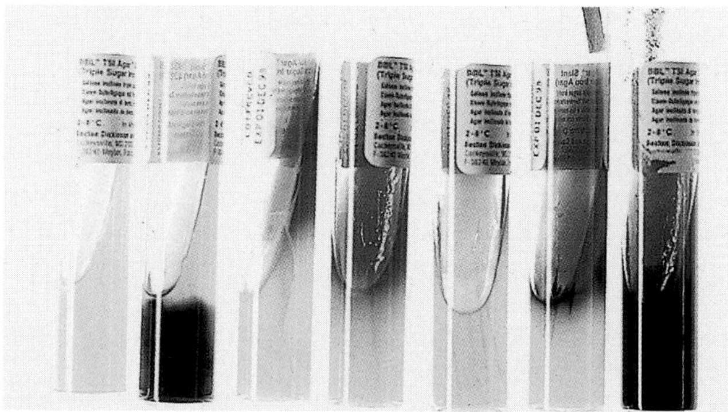

Figure 40-57 Triple sugar iron (TSI) agar. TSI agar slants contain three carbohydrates, glucose, lactose, and sucrose, at a ratio of 10:10:1. For the detection of H_2S, sodium thiosulfate is present in the medium as the source of sulfur atoms. Two iron salts, ferrous sulfate and ferric ammonium citrate, react with the H_2S to form a black precipitate of ferrous sulfide. In the TSI tube, half of the length of the agar is at a slant and thus is aerobic due to the exposure to oxygen, while the butt is protected from air and as a result is considered anaerobic. Production of the gases CO_2 and H_2 is also detected by observing cracks or bubbles in the agar. The tubes should be inoculated with a single, well-isolated colony by using a long, straight wire. No change in the medium (alkaline/alkaline [Alk/Alk]) indicates that the organism cannot ferment any of the sugars present, thereby excluding the *Enterobacteriaceae*. If glucose alone is fermented, the bottom (butt) portion of the slant will be yellow due to the acid production by the fermentation of glucose under anaerobic conditions; however, the top (slant) portion will be alkaline (pink) due to the oxidative degradation of the peptones under aerobic conditions (Alk/Acid). Fermentation of glucose and lactose or of sucrose results in both an acidic slant and an acidic butt (Acid/Acid). As shown in this figure, members of the *Enterobacteriaceae* demonstrate a variety of reactions (see also Table 10-3). Because they all ferment glucose, the butt will always be acidic (yellow). The second tube from the right shows a characteristic reaction for *Salmonella enterica* serovar Typhi because of the slight H_2S production. An alternative to the TSI system is Kligler iron agar, which does not contain sucrose. The advantage of the sucrose in TSI is that *Salmonella* spp. and *Shigella* spp. do not metabolize either lactose or sucrose. Thus, any acid-acid reaction on a TSI will exclude *Salmonella* spp. and *Shigella* spp. *Yersinia enterocolitica* ferments sucrose but not lactose, giving an Acid/Acid in TSI and Alk/Acid in Kligler iron agar.

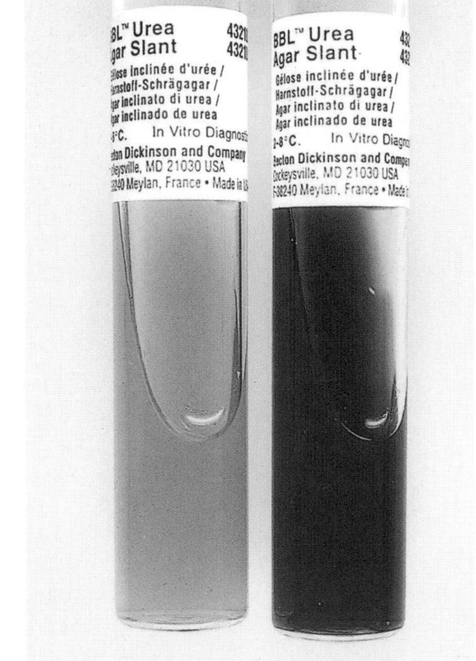

Figure 40-58 Urease test. Organisms that possess the enzyme urease hydrolyze urea, resulting in the production of ammonia and CO_2, forming ammonium carbonate, an alkaline end product (pH 8.1). In the presence of a phenol red indicator, the color changes from a tan to cerise color (bright pink, right tube).

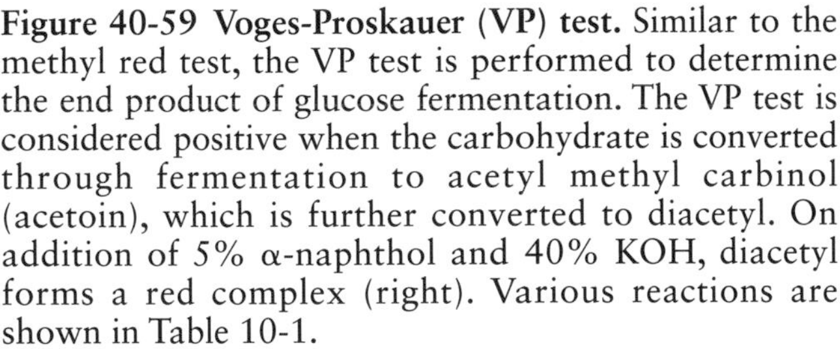

Figure 40-59 Voges-Proskauer (VP) test. Similar to the methyl red test, the VP test is performed to determine the end product of glucose fermentation. The VP test is considered positive when the carbohydrate is converted through fermentation to acetyl methyl carbinol (acetoin), which is further converted to diacetyl. On addition of 5% α-naphthol and 40% KOH, diacetyl forms a red complex (right). Various reactions are shown in Table 10-1.

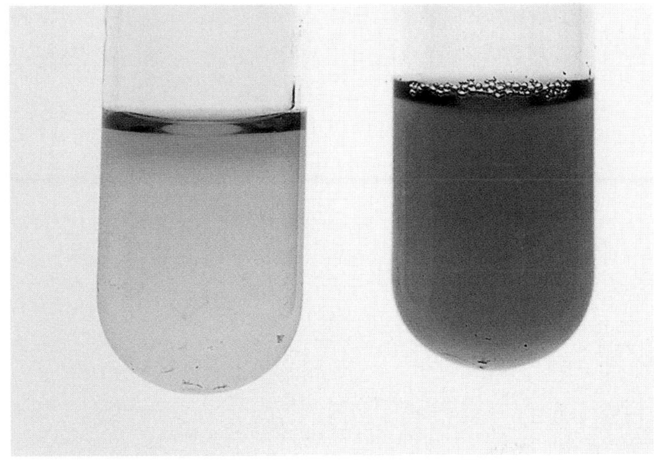

Index

Note: Page numbers followed by "f" indicate a figure; page numbers followed by "t" indicate a table.

D

E

F

G

I

N